Complex Anorectal Disorders

Steven D. Wexner, MD, FACS, FRACS, FRCS(Ed)
Andrew P. Zbar, MD, FRCS, FRACS
Mario Pescatori, MD, FRCS, EBSQ

Complex Anorectal Disorders

Investigation and Management

With 162 Illustrations

With a Foreword by Robin Phillips

Springer

Steven D. Wexner
MD, FACS, FRACS, FRCS(Ed)
Chairman and Residency
Hospital Program Director
Department of Colorectal Surgery
Cleveland Clinic Florida
Weston, FL
USA

Andrew P. Zbar
MD, FRCS, FRACS
Department of Clinical Medicine
and Research
University of the West Indies
Queen Elizabeth Hospital
Cave Hill Campus
Barbados

Mario Pescatori
MD, FRCS, EBSQ
Coloproctology Unit
Villa Flaminia Hospital
Rome, Italy
Honorary President
Italian Society of
Colo-Rectal Surgery (SICCR)

British Library Cataloguing in Publication Data
Complex anorectal disorders: investigation and management
1. Anorectal function tests 2. Defecation disorders—Treatment
I. Wexner, Steven D. II. Zbar, Andrew P., 1955– III. Pescatori, Mario
616.3′42

ISBN 978-1-84996-896-6 e-ISBN 978-1-84628-057-3
Springer Science+Business Media
springeronline.com

Printed in the United States of America. (BS/EB)

Printed on acid-free paper

This book is dedicated to my wife, Nicolette,
for all of her love, support, and wisdom.

SDW

As always, to my parents for their constant
inspiration to strive for intellectual betterment.

APZ

To my father, Alan Parks, and Vic Fazio,
who taught me honesty, surgery, and science.

MP

Foreword

A large cross-section of the world's great and good in colorectal surgery have been enticed, inveigled, I suspect at times brow-beaten, to produce this *tour de force*. The editors, themselves famous for their own extensive contributions in this area, must be congratulated for their fine achievements.

Every card-carrying specialist needs a reference book of this sort. My own are well worn by many years' reference, for when confronted by big problems, big issues, senior clinicians must be able to lay their hands on a well-thumbed old favourite: not a small, "where are we now" sort of book, or an exam crammer, but on one that is large, sedate and of "traditional build."

Rather than being a supergiant covering all of colorectal surgery, this book has focused on the broad structural investigation of the anorectum and on the focused management of largely "functional" problems. And it has done so in style. For this is a core area of specialist practice; your more general colleagues may think twice before referring you new cases of cancer and inflammatory bowel disease (both also central areas in colorectal surgery), but they will not hesitate in referring the patients whose investigation and management are described here. And they will expect you to know how to deal with them.

These are some of the most challenging patients to manage. Rightly have the editors covered the physiological areas, rightly the psychological issues, rightly the medicolegal aspects: here is the making of a specialist—the sword and the shield.

Robin Phillips
St Mark's Hospital
Harrow, Middlesex

Preface

The recent profusion of colorectal and anal surgical techniques and investigative procedures has made it comparatively difficult for both the general surgeon with a colorectal interest and the specialist coloproctologist to keep up with the body of new literature and the regular appearance of new surgical procedures. The introduction of capital-intensive imaging modalities discussed in this book (including endoanal ultrasonography, 3-dimensional reconstructed axial anal sonography, thin-slice high spatial-resolution magnetic resonance imaging and endoanal MR imaging), has rendered the management and research of some complex anorectal disorders within the perview of a few specialized colorectal centers. Balanced against this, the standardization of rectal cancer resection has shown that workshop practices can readily be translated into noncolorectal environments and has highlighted the improvement in cancer-specific outcomes for specialists trained specifically in these techniques. We felt that this book was timely to condense these complex disorders into a workable format for the colorectal clinician.

This book is divided into two main sections. Section 1 discusses the investigative aspects of specialist proctological practice with heavy emphasis on the complex physiology of the region in health and disease. The abundance of literature here makes the subject somewhat difficult to comprehend for the busy colorectal surgeon and the aim is to précis relevant physiology which defines anorectal pathology and which may be clinically useful in referrals to a tertiary practice. Here, there is detailed discussion of conventional (and vectorvolume) anorectal manometry, the nuances of rectoanal inhibition (and its clinical significance), the research role of ambulatory anorectal manometry, mucosal electrosensitivity, and the new field of impedance planimetry. The complex subject of rectal biomechanics is deliberately highlighted in an effort to show the pitfalls (and meaning) of simple rectal compliance measurement. The selected use of colonic (and rectal) transit assessment in the patient presenting with intractable constipation and evacuatory difficulty is discussed along with the ever diminishing place (in view of endoanal sonography), of electromyography and other neurophysiologic testing.

Here too, there is discussion of the expanded role of endoanal sonography and its extensions, (namely 3-dimensional reconstructed axial endosonography and dynamic transperineal sonography), along with an outline of defecography as it is clinically used in two different European centers. The importance in functional disorders of dynamic sequence MR imaging and its endoanal counterpart is included for the assessment of patients with pelvic floor disorders along with the place of surface pelvic phased-array MR imaging which has become the "gold standard" for selected use in recurrent and specific perirectal sepsis and for the preoperative determination of rectal cancer stage. In the latter circumstance, accurate staging before surgery defines those patients who will benefit from definitive downstaging neoadjuvant chemoradiation and those likely to benefit in terms of reduced locoregional recurrence and enhanced cancer-specific survival from pre- and postoperative adjuvant radiotherapy.

This section continues with an extensive discussion of internal anal sphincter neurotransmission and pharmacology; a burgeoning field for the topical therapy of passive fecal incontinence and chronic anal fissure. Finally there is consideration of the specialized histopathology of the anus and anal canal and the newer area of cytology and "high-resolution anoscopy" of the region; an important field with limited longitudinal data for human papillomavirus (HPV) -associated preinvasive anal intraepithelial neoplasia. This latter disease is becoming increasingly recognized in the HIV-positive population and in other immunosuppressed patients.

Section 2 assesses the specific management decisions of importance in particular proctological practice, as recommended from many renowned units throughout the world dedicated to complex anorectal disorders. It begins with an overview of the surgical approach towards patients presenting with intractable constipation, examining the importance of paradoxical puborectalis contraction and its management, colectomy, biofeedback therapies and the coloproctological approach to symptomatic rectocele. Fecal incontinence is broadly reviewed along with its prevention, surgical management, biofeedback strategies, quality of life considerations and the place of new operative procedures including dynamic electrically-stimulated graciloplasty, artificial anal sphincter replacement (either as a primary procedure or in total anorectal reconstruction) and the exciting developments in sacral neuromodulation.

The gynecological perspective of patients with complex postoperative evacuatory dysfunction, rectocele and enterocele and mixed fecal and urinary incontinence, is covered as well as the technical clinical problems encountered after failed sphincteroplasty, graciloplasty, artificial bowel sphincter deployment and following construction of a neorectal reservoir. When patients present with functional problems following these surgeries, management is particularly difficult and renowned units present their experience in this book of these discrete specialized problems. There is discussion of the functional problems encountered in patients with particular neurological disorders as well as consideration of the specific psychological problems in patients with defecation difficulty along with the psychologist's approach and integration within the dedicated colorectal unit. Finally, our authors outline the "nuts and bolts" of setting up an anorectal laboratory and the medicolegal issues entailed in the assessment and management of these complex patients; many of whom present after failed surgeries and treatments. It is hoped that this textbook will serve as a useful resource reference for the busy coloproctologist faced with a range of complicated and challenging patients who present with complex proctological disorders.

The production of our textbook could not have been possible without the unwavering assistance of Elektra McDermott whose constant cajoling of authors to complete their chapters on time was the difference between whether the product would be finished or simply just remain on the drawing board. Both Melissa Morton and Eva Senior of the medical editorial staff of Springer in London were also essential for the project to come to fruition and their tireless efforts, organization and energy made the task an editor's joy.

Steven D. Wexner, MD
Andrew P. Zbar, MD
Mario Pescatori, MD

Contents

Contributors

Homayoon Akbari, MD, PhD
Department of Colorectal Surgery, St Luke's/Roosevelt Hospital Center, New York, NY, USA

Donato F. Altomare, MD
Department of Emergency and Organ Transplantation, General Surgery and Liver Transplantation Unit, University of Bari, Italy

Ponnandai J. Arumugam, MS, FRCS
Department of Colorectal Surgery, Royal Cornwall Hospital, Truro, UK

Cornelius G.M.I. Baeten, MD, PhD
Department of General Surgery, Academic Hospital Maastricht, The Netherlands

Nancy Baxter, MD
University of Minnesota, Minneapolis, MN, USA

David E. Beck, MD
Department of Colon and Rectal Surgery, Ochsner Clinic Foundation, New Orleans, LA, USA

Marc Beer-Gabel, MD
Gastroenterology Institute, Kaplan Medical Center, Rehovot, Israel

Mitchell Bernstein, MD, FACS
Center for Pelvic Floor Disorders, St Luke's/Roosevelt Hospital Center, New York, NY, USA

John Beynon, BSc, MS, FRCS
Department of Colorectal Surgery, Singleton Hospital, Swansea, UK

Gina Brown, MBBS, MD, MRCP, FRCR
Department of Radiology, Royal Marsden Hospital, Sutton, UK

Linda Brubaker, MD
Departments of Obstetrics and Gynecology and Urology, Female Pelvic Medicine and Reconstructive Surgery, Loyola University Medical Center, Maywood, IL, USA

G. Willy Davila, MD
Department of Gynecology, Section of Urogynecology and Reconstructive Pelvic Surgery, Cleveland Clinic Florida, Weston, FL, USA

Graeme S. Duthie, MD, FRCS
Academic Department of Colorectal Surgery, University of Hull, Castle Hill Hospital, Cottingham, UK

Richelle J.F. Felt-Bersma, MD, PhD
Department of Gastroenterology, Erasmus University Medical Center, Rotterdam, The Netherlands

Claus Fenger, MD, DrMSci
Department of Pathology, Odense University Hospital, Denmark

Andrea Ferrara, MD, FACS, FASCRS
Colon and Rectal Disease Center, Orlando, FL, USA

Tanja Fischer, MD
Department of Diagnostic Radiology, Ludwig-Maximilians-Universität, Munich, Germany

Andrea Frudinger, MD
Department of Obstetrics and Gynecology, Medical University Graz, Austria

Joseph T. Gallagher, MD, FASCRS
Colon and Rectal Disease Center, Orlando, FL, USA

Ezio Ganio, MD
Colorectal Eporediensis Center, Ivrea, Italy

Julio Garcia-Aguilar, MD, PhD
Section of Colon and Rectal Surgery, Department of Surgery, University of California, San Francisco, CA, USA

Angela B. Gardiner, MPhil
Academic Department of Colorectal Surgery, University of Hull, Castle Hill Hospital, Cottingham, UK

Jeanette Gaw, MD
Department of Surgery, Yale University School of Medicine, New Haven, CT, USA

Marc A. Gladman, MBBS, MRCOG, MRCS
Academic Department of Surgery and Gastrointestinal Physiology Unit, Barts & The London, Queen Mary School of Medicine and Dentistry, The Royal London Hospital, London, UK

Hans Gregersen, MD, DrMSci, MPM
Center of Excellence in Visceral Biomechanics and Pain, Aalborg Hospital and Center for Sensory-Motor Interaction, Aalborg University, Denmark

Altomarino Gugliclmi, MD
Department of Emergency and Organ Transplantation, General Surgery and Liver Transplantation Unit, University of Bari, Italy

Tracy L. Hull, MD, FACS
Department of Colorectal Surgery, Cleveland Clinic Foundation, Cleveland, OH, USA

J. Marcio N. Jorge, MD
Department of Coloproctology, Anorectal Physiology Laboratory, University of São Paulo, Brazil

Sergio W. Larach, MD, FACS, FASCRS
Colon and Rectal Disease Center, Orlando, FL, USA

Andreas Lienemann, MD
Department of Diagnostic Radiology, Ludwig-Maximilians-Universität, Munich, Germany

Walter E. Longo, MD, MBA, FACS, FASCRS
Department of Surgery, Section of Gastrointestinal Surgery, Yale University School of Medicine, New Haven, CT, USA

Annika López, MD, PhD
Department of Obstetrics and Gynecology, Karolinska Institutet, Danderyd Hospital, Stockholm, Sweden

David Z. Lubowski, MB BCh, FRACS
Department of Colorectal Surgery, St. George Hospital, Sydney, Australia

Carlos M. Lumi, MD, MAAC, MASCRS
Department of Proctology, Hospital Enrrique Erill, Buenos Aires, Argentina

Robert D. Madoff, MD
Division of Colon and Rectal Surgery, University of Minnesota, Minneapolis, MN, USA

Michelle M. Marshall, MB BS, BSc, MRCP
Department of Intestinal Imaging, St. Mark's Hospital, Harrow, UK

Anders F. Mellgren, MD, PhD
Division of Colon and Rectal Surgery, Department of Surgery, University of Minnesota, Minneapolis, MN, USA

Neil J. McC Mortensen, MD, FRCS
Department of Colorectal Surgery, John Radcliffe Hospital, Oxford, UK

Minda Neimark, MD
Department of Gynecology, Cleveland Clinic Florida, Weston, FL, USA

Juan J. Nogueras, MD
Department of Colorectal Surgery, Cleveland Clinic Florida, Weston, FL, USA

Lucia Oliveira, MD
Department of Anorectal Physiology, Policlínica Geral do Rio de Janeiro, Brazil

Bharat Patel, MB BCh, FRCR
Department of Radiology, Singleton Hospital, Swansea, UK

John H. Pemberton, MD
Division of Colon and Rectal Surgery, Mayo Graduate School of Medicine, Mayo Clinic and Mayo Foundation, Rochester, MN, USA

Mario Pescatori, MD, FRCS, EBSQ
Coloproctology Unit, Villa Flaminia Hospital, Rome, Italy

Johann Pfeifer, MD
Department of General Surgery, University Clinic Medical School Graz, Karl-Franzens University School of Medicine, Graz, Austria

Jennifer T. Pollak, MD
Department of Gynecology, Section of Urogynecology and Reconstructive Pelvic Surgery, Cleveland Clinic Florida, Weston, FL, USA

Thanesan Ramalingam, BSc, FRCS
University Department of Pharmacology, University of Oxford, UK

Kim F. Rhoads, MD
Department of Surgery, University of California, San Francisco, San Francisco, CA, USA

Marcella Rinaldi, MD
Department of Emergency and Organ Transplantation, General Surgery and Liver Transplantation Unit, University of Bari, Italy

Patricia L. Roberts, MD
Department of Colon and Rectal Surgery, Lahey Clinic, Burlington, MA, USA

Mart J. Rongen, MD
Department of General Surgery, Academic Hospital Maastricht, The Netherlands

Guillermo O. Rosato, MD, MAAC, FASCRS
Department of Proctology, Hospital Enrrique Erill, Buenos Aires, Argentina

Annalisa Russo, PhD
Coloproctology Unit, Villa Flaminia Hospital, Rome, Italy

Theodore J. Saclarides, MD
Section of Colon and Rectal Surgery, Rush Medical College, Chicago, IL, USA

Dana R. Sands, MD
Anorectal Physiology Laboratory, Department of Colorectal Surgery, Cleveland Clinic Florida, Weston, FL, USA

T. Cristina Sardinha, MD
Department of Colorectal Surgery, Cleveland Clinic Florida, Weston, FL, USA

John H. Scholefield, MB ChB, ChM, FRCS
Department of Surgery, Division of GI Surgery, University Hospital, Nottingham, UK

S. Mark Scott, PhD
Academic Department of Surgery and Gastrointestinal Physiology Unit, Barts & The London, Queen Mary School of Medicine and Dentistry, The Royal London Hospital, London, UK

Andrew A. Shelton, MD
Department of Colorectal Surgery, Stanford University School of Medicine, Stanford University Medical Center, Stanford, CA, USA

Philip J. Shorvon, MB BS, MA, MRCP, FRCR
Department of Radiology, Central Middlesex Hospital, London, UK

Jaap Stoker, MD, PhD
Department of Radiology, Academic Medical Center, University of Amsterdam, The Netherlands

Michelle J. Thornton, FRACS, LLB
Department of Colorectal Surgery, St. George Hospital, Sydney, NSW, Australia

Dawn E. Vickers, RN
Department of Gastroenterology, Cleveland Clinic Florida, Weston, FL, USA

Steven D. Wexner, MD, FACS, FRACS, FRCSED
Department of Colorectal Surgery, Cleveland Clinic Florida, Weston, FL, USA

Norman S. Williams, MS, FRCS
Academic Department of Surgery and Gastrointestinal Physiology Unit, Barts & The London, Queen Mary School of Medicine and Dentistry, The Royal London Hospital, London, UK

Andrew P. Zbar, MD, FRCS, FRACS
Department of Clinical Medicine and Research, University of the West Indies, Queen Elizabeth Hospital, Cave Hill Campus, Barbados

Jan Zetterström, MD, PhD
Department of Obstetrics and Gynecology, Karolinska Institutet, Danderyd Hospital, Stockholm, Sweden

Section I
Anorectal Testing

Chapter 1
Anorectal Anatomy: The Contribution of New Technology

Andrew P. Zbar

Introduction

Recent imaging utilizing direct coronal and sagittal images, as well as reconstructed axial anatomical images, has largely clarified the disposition of the sphincters in humans and the relevant gender differences (1,2). Despite these studies, there is no uniform consensus regarding their anatomic nomenclature (3). Recent attempts to incorporate matched images obtained by three-dimensional (3D) reconstructions of the anal canal with attendant level-orientated physiologic readings, where morphologically demonstrable and separable recognizable muscle groups have been equated with resting and squeeze contributions to recorded pressures (4), have provided results that are somewhat contradictory to manometric reports, particularly in what is represented by the anal high-pressure zone (5). In this chapter, an outline of basic anorectal embryology is provided, along with an anatomical description of the internal anal sphincter (IAS), external anal sphincter (EAS)–puborectalis complex, the longitudinal muscle, and the rectogenital septum of relevance to the colorectal surgeon based on anatomical dissections and recent imaging. The specific pharmacology of the IAS as it pertains to proctologic practice may be found in Chapter 4.

Anorectal Embryology for the Adult Coloproctologist

A working knowledge by the adult coloproctologist of current concepts in anorectal embryology permits an understanding of congenital anorectal anomalies and their surgical aftermath. For the adult surgeon, description, diagnosis, and management of neonates and young children with congenital anorectal anomalies appears confusing. Little is known about the genetic and teratogenic influences on hindgut development, and this is compounded by an incomplete knowledge concerning normal anorectal growth and its interrelationship with the developing pelvic musculature and inner-

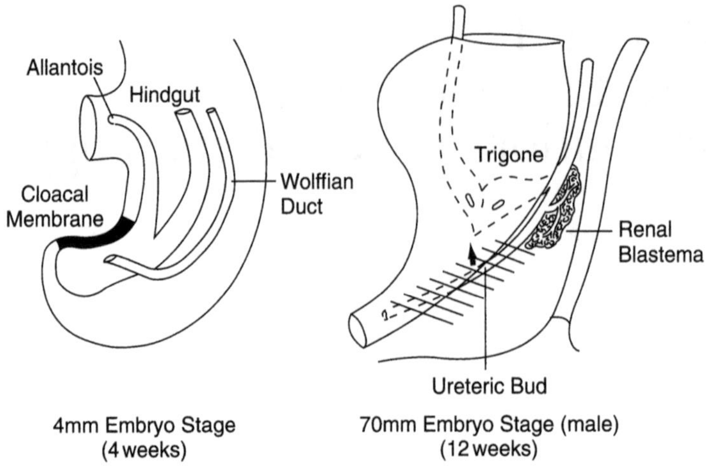

FIGURE 1.1. Traditional concepts in cloacal development. (Left) At the 4-week stage, a common cloaca incorporates the allantois, hindgut, and Wolffian ducts. The cloacal membrane joins the ectodermal edge and separation of the urorectal septum proceeds in the craniocaudal and lateral directions. (Right) By the 12th week, the bladder and rectum are separated by the urorectal septum. The distal Wolffian duct atrophies and the ureteric bud fuses with its contralateral partner to form the trigone (male). In the female, the Mullerian ducts intervene and fuse in a craniocaudal direction. The formed sinovaginal bulb represents the distal vaginal vault. In the male, these ducts atrophy and persist as the utriculus masculinus.

vation. Recent advances in whole embryo scanning electron microscopy and immunostaining have permitted 3D reconstruction of hindgut structures in well-established animal models, allowing their re-characterization and providing avenues for working classifications of the main types of anomalies (6).

Classical descriptions of the developing rectum have been based upon early independent work by Tourneux (7) and Retterer (8) towards the end of the last century that postulated the formation of a primitive cloaca subdivided by a urorectal septum into an anterior urogenital sinus and a posterior anorectal tract (Figure 1.1). Caudal continuity with a proctodeal anlage was separable from the ectoderm by a cloacal membrane whose abnormal development was believed to result from either craniocaudad arrest (resulting in some variant of anal/anorectal agenesis or an imperforate anal membrane) or a disturbance in lateral fusion (producing an H-type complex rectourinary fistula between the blind-ending rectal pouch and some portion of the urinary tract). Although the cloacal concept is useful in practical definition of low anomalies in the female (9), this simplistic view has been challenged by detailed studies largely performed in pig embryos with a high hereditary expressivity of anorectal malformations resembling those observed in humans (10). This misunderstanding about the nature of the cloacal membrane and the urorectal septum has been compounded by the traditional concept originally proposed by Bill and Johnson that the rectum and anal anlage tends to migrate backwards relatively late in the course of embryonic growth (11). This view purported to explain the observed anal ectopia in both sexes, as manifested by the covered anus, perineal anus, and anocutaneous fistula in the male and the anovestibular fistula in the female. These anomalies present in association with a normally disposed sphincter complex and are dealt with satisfactorily via a perineal approach with excellent long-term functional outcomes. This traditional view of anorectal embryology provided a basic division of anomalies into high, intermediate, and low dependent upon their relationship to the levator plate and into those either communicating or not communicating with the genitourinary tract.

What has become evident from the work of van der Putte (10) and Kluth and Lambrecht (6) is that there is no embryological evidence of such a dorsal shift in the anal anlage, but rather a ventral outgrowth of the cloacal membrane (with a failure of normal posterior membrane development), as well as an impairment in the movement of the membrane from a vertical to a horizontal orientation (Figure 1.2). This "new" description has resulted

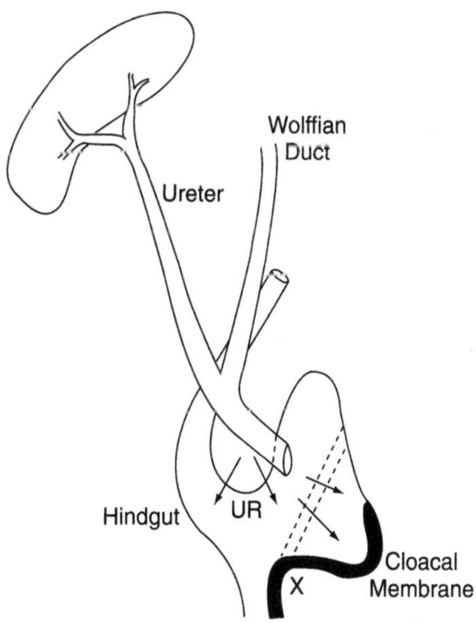

FIGURE 1.2. Newer concepts in disposition of the cloacal membrane. The cloacal membrane re-orientates to a horizontal disposition with ventral outgrowth (movement by arrows of the dotted line). This pushes the anal anlage posteriorly at its fixed point (marked as X), provided that the dorsal cloaca develops normally. The urorectal septum (UR) moves downward to separate the hindgut from the urogenital sinus.

from the work of these groups using whole embryo scanning electron microscopy at different stages of gestation for on-line 3D assessment. Both studies failed to show either lateral septation of the cloacal elements or dorsal anal migration, as previously described (12,13). This work has been assisted by the presence of characterized animal models of anorectal malformations, most notably the Danforth SD-mouse mutant, which carries a gene affecting tail, rectal and urogenital development, and which phenotypically demonstrates a range of anorectal anomalies that bear a striking resemblance to those observed in pigs and humans (14–16). This model has been re-examined recently using the new whole-embryo techniques (17).

In summary, improved genetic understanding of anorectal deformities will occur through mutational analyses of candidate loci in patients with recognizable syndrome complexes or co-existent dysganglionoses. New whole-embryo immunostaining and scanning has provided a different view of cloacal membrane development as the primary abnormality in many cases and has highlighted the inadequacy of conventional concepts of hindgut embryology as they pertain to observable categories of human anorectal malformations. Consequently, no simple classification system for anorectal anomalies based upon embryological considerations currently exists (18).

The Internal Anal Sphincter

Historically, there have been many conflicting anatomical reports of the IAS and its relationship to the EAS. Prior to 1950, it was believed that the IAS was the main contributing influence to resting continence, although subsequently it had been suggested that preservation of the EAS was critical in the maintenance of overall continence (19,20). Resting pressure analyses in human subjects during general and spinal anesthesia independently conducted by Duthie, Ihre, and von Euler had shown that the IAS is the main contributor to resting anorectal pressure (21–23). Only recently has it has become evident that IAS division or damage by itself may be associated with troublesome soiling (24), and this finding may be allied to those studies that have shown that resting anal function, anorectal sampling (the ability to differentiate between flatus and fluid), and the presence of the IAS-driven rectoanal inhibitory reflex (RAIR) are all impaired following low anterior resection and coloanal anastomosis where there is extensive endoanal manipulation (25). The restoration of both the anorectal sampling mechanism and the return of the RAIR both correlate with clinical improvement in functional outcome and less nocturnal incontinence and urgency after this type of restorative rectal resection (26). In this regard, incontinence has been shown to occur (although not be strictly predictable) after isolated IAS injury (27), with inherent differences in basal IAS manometry and sphincter graphics in those patients prospectively followed through their internal anal sphincterotomy for topically resistant anal fissure where differences were represented in those who remained continent and those who became incontinent based entirely on their IAS manometric pattern (5,28). Moreover, the inherent parameters of the RAIR (an IAS function) appear to be different in those patients with different anorectal disorders (29–31) whereby a more rapid recovery is demonstrable in those cases where there is already fecal incontinence and EAS atrophy, implying that IAS function itself may differentially contribute towards continence defense where continence is already compromised.

Recently, endoanal ultrasound (US) [as well as magnetic resonance imaging (MRI)] has clarified the expected age and gender variations of the IAS, as well as the IAS/EAS, disposition in what may be regarded as the constitutive overlap of these sphincter components (32). This effect has proved of clinical relevance where it has been shown in some patients that there is such poor constitutive overlap, particularly in chronic anal fissure. In these cases, injudicious internal anal sphincterotomy may render the distal anal canal relatively unsupported, leading to predictable postoperative leakage (33).

Although there are no longitudinal studies, there is ample evidence to show morphological increases in the IAS thickness with age, probably associated with degeneration in the muscle component and its replacement with fibrous tissue (34). This effect has been equated with the development of passive leakage consequent upon isolated IAS degeneration (35). Although the exact morphological interrelationship between the IAS and the other sphincter musculature in health and disease remains to be determined, direct comparisons between endoluminal US and MRI cannot strictly be made because both modalities variably identify the intersphincteric space and US appears less capable of defining the outer extremity of the EAS muscle. An overall greater IAS dimension determined by US may be indicative of the relationship of the IAS to variable components of the longitudinal muscle (vide infra, 36).

Overall, the physiological and clinical significance of IAS integrity is increasingly being recognized, where all attempts are made to preserve the muscle by avoidance of excessive anal distraction, particularly in patients where continence is already compromised (37,38). This view recently has carried over to deliberate IAS preservation in anorectal surgery where normally the IAS is deliberately destroyed, most notably in high transsphincteric fistula-in-ano, where resting pressures and continence appear to be maintained when cutting setons are rerouted through the intersphincteric space for attendant EAS division with concomitant IAS repair (39).

The External Anal Sphincter

Recent endoluminal imaging has clarified the widely held view that the EAS is represented by a three-tiered structure (1,40,41). This view owes much to the original anatomical descriptions of the subcutaneous, superficial, and deep components of the EAS as espoused by Riolan and Santorini

(42,43) and by von Holl (44), Milligan and Morgan (45), and Gorsch (46). These new imaging modalities have permitted the abandonment of confusing systems of bi-tiered anatomical configurations as reported by Courtney (47), Fowler (48), and Wilson (49), as well as more recent often-quoted expositions (50). This also has cast doubt on the more controversial models of interconnecting muscle loops as proffered by Shafik (51). Some of the confusions of the component muscle parts of the EAS have arisen as a result of descriptions of encasing fascia that extended laterally and that are inserted into the perianal skin, a point of some importance in defining and classifying the spread and presentations of perirectal infections (52). However, this area still requires considerable work because both endoanal and transvaginal imaging have failed to delineate adequately the anatomical composition of the perineal body (53), a difficulty that may account for variation in the reported incidence of anterior postobstetric anal EAS defects following vaginal delivery (54). The "misimpression" provided by conventional unreconstructed endoanal ultrasonography of a shorter anterior EAS in women has resulted in a more complex and sophisticated view of a greater relative physiological contribution by the posterior puborectalis muscle. Given that there is a clear plane of cleavage between these two muscle entities (namely the puborectalis and the deep component of the EAS; 55), this area needs to be revisited in the dissecting room (56,57).

The Longitudinal Muscle and Distal Anal Supporting Structures

There is remarkably little data concerning the disposition of the anal longitudinal muscle. It is evident during intersphincteric rectal dissection and has been demonstrated by routine endoanal ultrasonography (58) and endoanal MRI (59). This muscle is in direct contiguity with the outer muscle coat of the rectum and has been variously reported as supplemented by striated musculature derived from the levator ani (45,60), the puboanalis (61), and the pubococcygeus (62), as well as by the levator muscle fascia (47,63). The complexity of the intersphincteric musculofibrous contribution and the way it splits to attach to the perianal skin has formed the basis of Shafik's classification of attendant perianal spaces and has given rise to his complex classification of perirectal sepsis (64).

The medial and lateral extensions of these bands and contributions abound in a series of historical eponyms that are used in various texts. Communications between the submucosal and intersphincteric planes have been described (65,66), being labeled by Milligan and Morgan as the anal intermuscular septum, limiting the spread of rectal infection to the inferior termination of the IAS, as well as surrounding the lowermost border of the subcutaneous portion of the EAS muscle (45). These fascial bands were considered of some clinical importance both in the understanding of the spread of perirectal infection and in their classification, being labeled by Parks as the mucosal suspensory ligament that medially confined the ductal system of the anal glands (and crypts) and that inferolaterally separated the perianal from the ischiorectal space (67–70). Extensions of this musculofascial band have been described as running submucosally for variable distances, independently being labeled as the musculis canalis ani (71), Treitz's muscle (72), the sustentator tunicae mucosae (73), and the musculus submucosæ ani (74,75). Lateral extensions of the longitudinal muscle have been described by Courtney (47) as encircling the urethra and contributing to the rectourethralis muscle as the most medial fibers of the levator ani complex (76–78). This muscle is a principal landmark in the anterior aspect of the rectal dissection during perineal proctectomy by angulating the rectum, where division of the right and left columns of the rectourethralis muscle permits the rectum to fall backwards, protecting the prostate (or vagina) from inadvertent injury. The most caudal extensions of these fibers extend to the skin in a variably reported way, enclosing the perianal space and separating it from the ischiorectal fossa, with formation of the corrugator cutis ani muscle bands extending into the perianal skin. This latter muscular component originally described by Ellis (79) has been attributed as part of the *panniculus carnosus*, and its existence in many cases has been questioned (48).

The Rectovaginal Septum

There has been a long-standing debate concerning the existence and integrity of the rectovaginal septum. Several early anatomical studies, which were entirely histologic in nature (where there were no correlative anatomical dissections), were unable to define its presence (80,81). These frequently quoted studies have been contradicted by the fetal and adult cadaveric work of Uhlenluth et al. (82,83) and Nichols and Milley (84,85), who were able to identify a definitive anatomic and histologic fascial structure between the rectum and the vagina in all dissections. More recently, Fritsch and colleagues, revisiting this area using transparent plastinated fetal and adult pelvic specimens with sectional radiographic [computed tomography (CT) and MR] correlations, also were unable to demonstrate visceral fasciae surrounding the pelvic organs (86–89), suggesting that the disposition of pelvic connective tissue and the designation of potential pelvic spaces bound by visceral and parietal pelvic fascia are actually less complicated than previously reported in classical textbooks of anatomy and embryology (90–93). Very recent comparative fetal and adult dissections by Fritsch and her team specifically addressing the rectovaginal septum have confirmed its presence in plastinated specimens, showing it to be completely developed in the newborn (94–98).

These early studies recently have been confirmed by the cadaveric work of DeLancey, who showed the fibers of the rectovaginal septum running vertically and blending with the muscular wall of the vagina. He has suggested a multifaceted posterior vaginal support reliant upon the endopelvic fascia, levator ani muscle, and perineal membrane. Distally, the perineal membrane fibers are effectively horizontal and become parasagittal in the mid vagina, connecting the vaginal channel to the pelvic diaphragm. It has been suggested that these structures may become important in vaginal support in the pelvis if the main levator muscle is damaged or denervated (99,100).

Anatomically, it is believed that the rectovaginal septum represents the female analogue of the male rectovesical fascia first described by Denonvilliers in 1836 (101–105). The surgical importance of this fascia was first recognized by Young during radical perineal prostatectomy for cancer as a surgical landmark for urologists (106). Its anatomy was confirmed independently at the turn of the century by Cuneo and Veau (107) and Smith (108) and has been re-highlighted extensively in the dissection of the extraperitoneal rectum for rectal cancer. Recently our group has used macroscopic dissections on embalmed human pelves and plastination histology in both fetal and newborn pelvic specimens, showing that the rectogenital septum is formed by a local condensation of mesenchymal connective tissue during the early fetal period and that the longitudinal muscle bundles can be traced back to the longitudinal layer of the rectal wall. Immunohistochemical staining methods using mono- and polyclonal antibodies for tissue analysis and neuronal labeling (most notably PGP 9.5, S-100, Substance P, and Choline acetyl transferase) has revealed that autonomic nerve fibers and ganglia appear to innervate these muscle cells, suggesting that parasympathetic co-innervation of both the rectal muscle layers and the adjacent longitudinal muscle fibers of the septum is relevant in the function between the two structures and that the rectogenital septum has intrinsic sensory innervation that might be important in rectal filling and asymmetric rectal distension (109).

In recent years, Richardson has called attention to the presence of "breaks" within this septum that are anatomically evident using a transvaginal approach to rectocele repair, highlighting the importance of what he has described as "defect-specific" rectocele repairs (110,111). In this sense, although short-term follow-up data is coming out in the literature of such repair types for symptomatic rectocele, it really represents a gynecological "rediscovery" of the importance of defect-specific repair, which has been the cornerstone of the endorectal route (as advocated by the coloproctological fraternity) for many years. In Richardson's cadaveric and clinical operative work, he has described a taxonomy of fascial breaks, with the most common type appearing as a transverse posterior separation above the attachment of the perineal body, resulting in a low rectocele. The most recent work assessing the ultrastructural anatomy of the rectogenital septum, as described above, shows that this septum is formed within a local condensation of collagenous fibers from the beginning of the fetal period as early as the 9th week. In plastination studies, it has been found that the tissue components of the rectogenital septum in both sexes are not derivatives of any fascial structures demonstrable at any developmental stage that have undergone fusion either from the lateral pelvic wall or from the peritoneal pouch. Instead, it is suggested that they result more from an anatomic separation between the rectum and the bladder and prostate in men and the rectum and the vagina in women, where longitudinal muscle bundles can be found both within the rectogenital septum extending to and intermingling with the anal sphincter musculature and terminating in the perineal body in both sexes. This is of clinical and operative significance because this component of the levator ani complex (namely the rectourethralis muscle) is an important landmark in the anterior perineal dissection of the rectum during abdominoperineal resection, where it tethers and angulates the rectum against the membranous urethra (*vide supra*, 78).

Conclusions

An improved understanding of rectal and anal canal anatomy has resulted from advances in coronal and sagittal modality imaging *in vivo*, as well as from ultrastructural whole-image work and fetal and adult plastination (112). This improvement in anatomical definition has re-highlighted the clinical importance of the IAS as a central component in the maintenance of continence and has shown the significance of the rectogenital septum repair in low and mid rectocele (113).

References

1. deSouza NM, Puni R, Zbar A, Gilderdale DJ, Coutts GA, and Krausz T. MR imaging of the anal sphincter in multiparous females using an endoanal coil: correlation with *in vitro* anatomy and appearances in fecal incontinence. AJR Am J Roentgenol. 1996;167:1465–71.
2. Gold DM, Bartram CI, Halligan S, Humphries KN, Kamm MA, and Kmiot WA. Three-dimensional endoanal sonography in assessing anal canal injury. Br J Surg. 1999;86:365–70.
3. Zbar AP and Kmiot WA. Anorectal investigation. In: Phillips RKS, editor. A companion to specialist surgical practice—Colorectal surgery. 1st ed. London: W.B. Saunders Company Ltd; 1998. p. 1–32.
4. Williams AB, Cheetham MJ, Bartram CI, Halligan S, Kamm MA, Nicholls RJ, and Kmiot WA. Gender differences in the longitudinal pressure profile of the anal canal related to anatomical structure as demonstrated by three-dimensional anal endosonography. Br J Surg. 2000;87:1674–9.
5. Zbar AP, Beer-Gabel M, Chiappa AC, and Aslam M. Fecal incontinence after minor anorectal surgery. Dis Colon Rectum. 2001;44:1610–23.
6. Kluth D and Lambrecht W. Current concepts in the embryology of anorectal malformations. Semin Pediatr Surg. 1997;6(4):180–6.

7. Tourneux F. Sur le premiers developments du cloaque du tubercle genitale et de l'anus chez l'embryon moutons avec quelques remarques concernant le development des glandes prostatiques. J Anat Physiol. 1888;24:503–17.
8. Retterer E. Sur l'origin et de l'evolution de la region ano-genitale des mammifieres. J Anat Physiol. 1890;26:126–210.
9. Stephens FD. Embryology of the cloaca and embryogenesis of anorectal malformations. In: Stephens FD and Durham-Smith E, editors. Anorectal malformations in children: Update. New York: Alan R Liss Inc.; 1988. p. 177–209.
10. Van der Putte SCJ. Normal and abnormal development of the anorectum. J Pediatr Surg. 1986;21(5):434–40.
11. Bill AH and Johnson RJ. Failure of migration of the rectal opening as the cause for most cases of imperforate anus. Surg Gynecol Obstet. 1958;106:643–51.
12. Ikebukuro K-I and Ohkawa H. 3-dimensional analysis of anorectal embryology. A new technique for microscopic study using computer graphics. Pediatr Surg Int. 1994;9:2–7.
13. Kluth D, Hiller M, and Lambrecht W. The principles of normal and abnormal hindgut development. J Pediatr Surg. 1995;30:1143–7.
14. Danforth CH. Developmental anomalies in a special strain of mice. Am J Anat. 1930;45:275–87.
15. Dunn LC, Gluecksohn-Schoenheimer S, and Bryson V. A new mutation in the mouse affecting spinal column and urogenital system. J Hered. 1940;31:343–8.
16. Gluecksohn-Schoenheimer S. The morphological manifestation of a dominant mutation in mice affecting tail and urogenital systems. Genetics. 1943;28:341–8.
17. Kluth D, Lambrecht W, Reich P, et al. SD-mice—an animal model for complex anorectal malformations. Eur J Pediatr Surg. 1991;1:183–8.
18. Hassink EA, Riev PN, and Severijnen RS. Are adults content or continent after repair for high anal atresia? Ann Surg. 1993;218:196–2000.
19. Gaston E. Physiological basis for preservation of fecal continence after resection of the rectum. JAMA. 1952;146:1486–9.
20. Hollinshead H. Anatomy for surgeons, Vol 2. Thorax, abdomen and Pelvis. 2nd ed. New York: Harper & Row; 1971. p. 708–9.
21. Duthie HL and Watts J. Contribution of the external anal sphincter to the pressure zone in the anal canal. Gut. 1965;6:64–8.
22. Ihre T. Studies on anal function in continent and incontinent patients. Scand J Gastroenterol. 1974;9 Suppl 25:1–64.
23. Frenckner B, von Euler B. Influence of pudendal block on the function of the anal sphincters. Gut. 1975;16:482–9.
24. Lund JN and Scholefield JH. Aetiology and treatment of anal fissure. Br J Surg. 1996;83:1335–44.
25. Lewis WG, Williamson ME, Miller AS, Sagar PM, Holdsworth PJ, and Johnston D. Preservation of complete sphincteric proprioception in restorative proctocolectomy: the inhibitory reflex and fine control of continence need not be impaired. Gut. 1995;36:902–6.
26. Tuckson W, Lavery I, Fazio VW, Oakley J, Church J, and Milsom J. Manometric and functional comparison of ileal pouch anal anastomosis with and without anal manipulation. Am J Surg. 1991;161:90–6.
27. Abbasakoor MG, Nelson M, Beynon J, Patel B, and Carr ND. Anal endosonography in patients with anorectal symptoms after haemorrhoidectomy. Br J Surg. 1998;85:1522–4.

28. Zbar AP, Aslam M, and Allgar V. Faecal incontinence after internal sphincterotomy for anal fissure. Tech Coloproctol. 2000;4:25–8.
29. Zbar AP, Aslam M, Gold DM, Gatzen C,Gosling A, and Kmiot WA. Parameters of the rectoanal inhibitory reflex in patients with idiopathic fecal incontinence and chronic constipation. Dis Colon Rectum. 1998;41:200–8.
30. Kaur G, Gardiner A, and Duthie GS. Rectoanal reflex parameters in incontinence and constipation. Dis Colon Rectum. 2002;45:928–33.
31. Zbar AP and Jonnalagadda R. Parameters of the rectoanal inhibitory reflex in different anorectal disorders. Dis Colon Rectum. 2003;46:557–8.
32. Sultan AH, Kamm MA, Hudsson CN, Nicholls JR, and Bartram CI. Endosonography of the anal sphincters: normal anatomy and comparison with manometry. Clin Radiol. 1994;49:368–74.
33. Zbar AP, Kmiot WA, Aslam M, Williams A, Hider A, Audisio RA, Chiappa AC, and deSouza NM. Use of vector volume manometry and endoanal magnetic resonance imaging in the adult female for assessment of anal sphincter dysfunction. Dis Colon Rectum. 1999;42:1411–8.
34. Burnett SJD and Bartram CI. Endosonographic variations in the normal internal anal sphincter. Int J Colorectal Dis. 1991;6:2–4.
35. Vaizey CJ, Kamm MA, and Bartram CI. Primary degeneration of the internal anal sphincter as a cause of passive faecal incontinence. Lancet. 1997; 349:612–5.
36. Schafer A, Enck P, Furst G, Kahn T, Frieling T, and Lubke HJ. Anatomy of the anal sphincters: comparison of anal endosonography to magnetic resonance imaging. Dis Colon Rectum. 1994;37:777–81.
37. Sangwan YP and Coller JA. Internal anal sphincter: advances and insights. Dis Colon Rectum. 1998;41:1297–1311.
38. Zbar AP, Jayne DG, Mathur D, Ambrose NS, and Guillou PJ. The importance of the internal anal sphincter (IAS) in maintaining continence: anatomical, physiological and pharmacological considerations. Colorectal Dis. 2000; 2:193–202.
39. Zbar AP, Salazar R, Ramesh J, and Pescatori M. Conventional cutting versus internal anal sphincter-preserving seton for high trans-sphincteric fistula: a prospective randomized manometric and clincal trial. Tech Coloproctol. In press 2003.
40. Zbar AP. Magnetic resonance imaging and the coloproctologist. Tech Coloproctol. 2001;5:1–7.
41. Kmiot WA, Zbar AP, and deSouza NM. MRI in anorectal disease. In: Nicholls RJ and Dozois RR, editors. Surgery of the colon and rectum. New York: Churchill Livingstone. p. 68–98.
42. Riolan J. Anatomia 162 (1577–1657). As quoted in Dalley AF. The riddle of the sphincters: the morphophysiology of the anorectal mechanisms reviewed. Am Surgeon. 1987;53:298–306.
43. Santorini GD. Septum decum tabulae edit et explicit. Parone: Mich. Gerardi. 1715;tabula 15.
44. von Holl M. Handbuch der anatomie des menchen von Bardeleben. 1897;7 book 2, section 7.
45. Milligan ETC and Morgan CN. Surgical anatomy of the anal canal with special reference to ano-rectal fistulae. Lancet. 1934;2:150–6, 1213–7.

46. Gorsch RV. Proctologic anatomy. 2nd ed. Baltimore (MD): Williams & Wilkins; 1955.
47. Courtney H. Anatomy of the pelvic diaphragm and anorectal musculature as related to sphincter preservation in anorectal surgery. Am J Surg. 1950;79:155–73.
48. Fowler R. Landmarks and legends of the anal canal. Aust N Z J Surg. 1957;27:1–8.
49. Wilson PM. Anchoring mechanisms of the anorectal region. S Afr Med J. 1967;41:1127–32, 1138–43.
50. Oh C and Kark AE. Anatomy of the external anal sphincter. Br J Surg. 1972;59:717–23.
51. Shafik A. A new concept of the anatomy of the anal sphincter mechanism and the physiology of defecation. I. The external anal sphincter: a triple loop system. Invest Urol. 1975;13: 412–9.
52. Milligan ETC. The surgical anatomy and disorders of the perianal space. Proc R Soc Med. 1942;36:366–78.
53. Frudinger A, Bartram CI, and Kamm MA. Transvaginal versus anal endosonography for detecting damage to the anal sphincter. AJR Am J Roentgenol. 1997;168:1435–8.
54. Bollard RC, Gardiner A, Phillips K, and Duthie GS. Natural gaps in the female anal sphincter and the risk of postdelivery sphincter injury. Br J Surg. 1999;86 Suppl 1:50–1(A).
55. Fucini C, Elbetti C, and Messerini L. Anatomical pnae of seperation between the external anal sphincter and puborectalis muscle: clinical implications. Dis Colon Rectum. 1999;42:374–9.
56. Bogduk N. Issues in anatomy: the external anal sphincter revisited. Aust N Z J Surg. 1996;66:626–9.
57. Zbar AP and Beer-Gabel M. Gender differences in the longitudinal pressure profile of the anal canal related to anatomical structure as demonstrated on three-dimensional anal endosonography. Br J Surg. 2001;88:1016.
58. Bartram CI and Frudinger A. Handbook of endoanal endosonography. Petersfield, UK: Wrightson Biomedical Publishing; 1997.
59. Zbar AP and deSouza NM. The anal sphincter. In: deSouza, editor. Endocavitary MRI of the pelvis. The Netherlands: Harwood Academic Publishers; 2001. p. 91–109.
60. Cruvelhier H. Traite d'anatomie descriptive. Paris: Labe; 1852.
61. Lawson JON. Pelvic anatomy. I. Pelvic floor muscles. Ann R Coll Surg Engl. 1974;54:244–52.
62. Shafik A. A new concept of the anatomy of the anal sphincter mechanism and the physiology of defecation. III. The longitudinal anal muscle: anatomy and role in sphincter mechanism. Invest Urol. 1976;13:271–7.
63. Ayoub SF. The anterior fibres of the levator ani muscle in man. J Anat. 1979;128:571–80.
64. Shafik A. A new concept of the anatomy of the anal sphincter mechanism and the physiology of defecation. IV. Anatomy of the perianal spaces. Invest Urol. 1976;13:424–8.
65. Rudinger N. Topographisch chirurgische Anatomie des Menschen. Stuttgart: JG Cotta;1878. p. 111–2.
66. Roux C. Contribution to the knowledge of the anal muscles in man. Arch Mikr Anat. 1881;19:721–3.

67. Parks AG. A note on the anatomy of the anal canal. Proc R Soc Med. 1954;47:997–8.
68. Wilde FR. The anal intermuscular septum. Br J Surg. 1949;36:279–85.
69. Lunniss PJ and Phillips RKS. Anatomy and function of the anal longitudinal muscle. Br J Surg. 1992;79:882–4.
70. Gerdes B, Kohler HH, Stinner B, Barth PJ, Celik I, and Rothmund M. The longitudinal muscle of the anal canal. Chirug. 1997;68:1281–5.
71. Hansen HH. Die Betendung des Musculus canalis ani für die Kontinenz und anorectale Erkrangungen. Langenbecks Arch Chir. 1976;341:23–7.
72. Treitz W. Uber Einen neuen Muskel am Doudenum des Menschen, uber elastische Sehnen, und einige andere anatomische Verhaltuisse. Viertal-Jahrschrift für die praktische Heilkunde. 1853;37:113–44.
73. Levy E. Anorectal musculature. Am J Surg. 1936;34:141–98.
74. Fine J and Wickhma Lawes CH. On the muscle fibres of the anal submucosa, with special reference to the pectin band. Br J Surg. 1940;27:723–7.
75. Haas PA and Fox TA. The importance of the perianal connective tissue in the surgical anatomy and function of the anus. Dis Colon Rectum. 1977;20:303–13.
76. Morgan CN and Thompson HR. Surgical anatomy of the anal canal with special reference to the surgical importance of the internal sphincter and conjoint longitudinal muscle. Ann R Coll Surg Engl. 1956;19:88–114.
77. Goligher JC. Surgery of the anus, rectum and colon. 4th ed. London: Baillière Tindall; 1980. p. 7–20.
78. Brooks JD, Eggener SE, and Chao W-M. Anatomy of the rectourethralis muscle. Eur Urol. 2002;41:94–100.
79. Ellis GV. Demonstrations of anatomy. 8th ed. London: Smith Elder; 1878. p. 420.
80. Goff BH. Histological study of the perivaginal fascia in nullipara. Surg Gynecol Obstet. 1931;52:32–42.
81. Ricci JV and Thom CH. The myth of a surgically useful fascia in vaginal plastic reconstructions. Q Rev Surg Obstet Gynecol. 1954;11:253–61.
82. Uhlenluth E, Wolfe WM, Smith EM, and Middleton EB. The rectovaginal septum. Surg Gynecol Obstet. 1948;86:148–63.
83. Uhlenluth E and Nolley GW. Vaginal fascia,a myth? Obstet Gynecol. 1957;10:349–58.
84. Milley PS and Nichols DH. A correlative investigation of the human rectovaginal septum. Anat Rec. 1969;163(3):443–51.
85. Nichols DH and Milley PS. Surgical significance of the rectovaginal septum. Am J Obstet Gynecol. 1970;15:215–20.
86. Fritsch H. The connective tissue sheath of uterus and vagina in the human female fetus. Ann Anat. 1992;174:261–4.
87. Fritsch H. Topography and subdivision of the pelvic connective tissue in human fetuses and in the adult. Surg Radiol Anat. 1994;16:259–65.
88. Fritsch H and Hotzinger H. Tomographical anatomy of the pelvis, visceral pelvic connective tissue and its compartments. Clin Anat. 1995;8:17–24.
89. Fröhlich B, Hötzinger H, and Fritsch H. Tomographical anatomy of the pelvis, pelvic floor, and related structures. Clin Anat. 1997;10:223–30.
90. Kocks J. Normale und Pathologische Lage und Gestalt des Uterus Sowie Deren Mechanik, Bonn: Cohen; 1880. p. 1–60.
91. Thompson P. On the arrangement of the fasciae of the pelvis and their relationship to the levator ani. J Anat Physiol. 1901;35:127–41.

92. Pernkopf E. Topografische Anatomie. Bd 2, 1. und 2. Hälfte. Berlin: Urban and Schwarzenberg; 1941. p. 191–7, 513–23.
93. Courtney H. Anatomy of the pelvic diaphragm and anorectal musculature as related to sphincter preservation in anorectal surgery. Am J Surg. 1959; 79:155–73.
94. Fritsch H, Bruch H-P, and Kühnel W. Development and topography of the perirectal spaces. Proceedings of the First European Congress of Clinical Anatomy; September 1991; Bruxelles.
95. Fritsch H, Fröhlich B. Development of the levator ani muscle in human fetuses. Early Hum Dev. 1994;37:15–25.
96. Fritsch H. Klinische anatomie des kontinenzorgans. Zentralb Chir. 1996; 121:613–6.
97. Fritsch H, Kühnel W, and Stelzner F. Entwicklung und klinische anatomie der adventita recti; Bedeutung für die Radikaloperation eines Mastadrmkrebses. Langenbecks Arch Chir. 1996;381:237–43.
98. Ludwikowski B, Hayward IO, and Fritsch H. Rectovaginal fascia: An important structure in pelvic visceral surgery? About its development, structure, and function. J Pediatr Surg. 2002;37:634–8.
99. DeLancey JO. Standing anatomy of the pelvic floor. J Pelv Surg. 1996;2:260–3.
100. DeLancey JOL. Structural anatomy of the posterior pelvic compartment as it relates to rectocele. Am J Obstet Gynecol. 1999;180:815–23.
101. Denonvilliers C.P-D. Anatomie du perinée. Bull Soc Anat, Paris. 1836;11:105–6.
102. Denonvilliers C. Propositions et observations d'anatomie, de physiologie et de pathologie. Theses 285, Paris; 1837. As cited in Wesson MB, 1922.
103. Wesson MB. The development and surgical importance of the rectourethralis muscle and Denonvilliers' fascia. J Urol. 1922;8:339–59.
104. Dietrich H. Giovanni Domenico Santorini (1681–1737) Charles-Pierre Denonvilliers (1808–1872). First description of urosurgically relevant structures in the small pelvis. Eur Urol. 1997;32(1):124–7.
105. Van Ophoven A and Roth S. The anatomy and embryological origins of the fascia of Denonvilliers: a medico-historical debate. J Urol. 1997;157:3–9.
106. Young HH. The early diagnosis and radical cure of carcinoma of the prostate. Being a study of 40 cases and a presentation of a radical operation which was carried out in 4 cases. Johns Hopkins Hosp Bull. 1905;16:315.
107. Cuneo B and Veau V. De la signification morphologique des aponeuroses perivesicales. J Anat Physiol. 1899;35:235.
108. Smith GE. Studies in the anatomy of the pelvis, with special reference to the fasciae and visceral supports. Part 1. J Anat Physiol. 1908;42:198, 252.
109. Aigner F, Zbar AP, Ludwikowski B, Kreczy A, Kovacs P, and Fritsch H. The rectogenital septum: morphology, function and clinical relevance. Dis Colon Rectum. In press 2003.
110. Richardson AC. The rectovaginal septum revisited: its relationship to rectocele and its importance in rectocele repair. Clin Obstet Gynecol. 1993;36:976–83.
111. Richardson AC. The anatomic defects in rectocele and enterocele. J Pelv Surg. 1995;1:214–21.
112. von Hagens G, Tiedemann K, and Kriz W. The current potential of plastination. Anat Embryol (Berl). 1987;175:411–21.
113. Zbar AP, Lienemann A, Fritsch H, Beer-Gabel M, and Pescatori M. Rectocele: pathogenesis and surgical management. Int J Colorectal Dis. 2003;18:369–84.

Chapter 2
Anorectal Physiology

Chapter 2.1
History, Clinical Examination, and Basic Physiology

J. Marcio N. Jorge

Introduction

Several studies have documented a relatively limited usefulness of the history and physical examination for the diagnosis of the causes of functional anorectal disorders, including both constipation and fecal incontinence (1–4). While anorectal physiologic testing is important in diagnosis, management, and objective follow-up, it can be uncomfortable for the patient, time consuming, and costly, as well as requiring well-trained professional staff experienced in its use in order to avoid over-interpretation of the results obtained. In this regard, an accurate and detailed history and physical examination is crucial in directing the investigation algorithm in order to avoid unnecessary, and even conflicting, testing.

In 1988, a survey of methods utilized for anorectal physiology was conducted amongst members of the Coloproctology Section of the Royal Society of Medicine (UK) and the American Society of Colon and Rectal Surgeons (ASCRS) (5). Although 90% of the respondents relied mainly on three traditional methods (namely history, digital examination, and sigmoidoscopy), the majority of respondents polled confirmed that specialized tests such as colonic transit studies, defecography, and anorectal manometry also were considered of some clinical utility. This process of opinion formation is dynamic, and testing methods will continue to fluctuate in their popularity and use. Although new surveys may reveal different directions of investigative efforts in the assessment of the physiology of the colon, rectum, and anus, there is little doubt that patient history and physical examination are considered crucial in the assessment of functional disorders. However, in the assessment of such a complex subject as anorectal physiology, more objective methods are required, not only for research purposes, but also in the clinical decision-making process.

The first and one of the most commonly used methods for assessing anorectal physiology is anorectal manometry. This chapter will outline the historical and clinical features of relevance in the approach to the patient with functional disorders and discuss conventional techniques of anorectal manometry.

Patient History

Anorectal physiological evaluation may be indicated for a myriad of disorders, most notably before any anorectal or colorectal procedure in which the status of anal continence may be jeopardized. However, primary functional disorders clinically manifest as constipation, fecal incontinence, or a combination of the two. The clinical history is addressed in this chapter under these two main symptom groups.

Constipation

The definition of constipation can vary tremendously among patients. In the past, several definitions have been used, including (6):

1. *Undefined self-reported symptom.* Constipation is a frequent complaint when the patient feels the situation to be unsatisfactory; the prevalence using this definition may reach 34% of the surveyed population.
2. *Stool frequency.* Constipation has been defined on the basis of infrequent bowel movements, typically less than three per week, which is the 98th percentile for self-reported stool frequency among adults in the United States, England, France, and Italy; the overall prevalence is about 2% of surveyed populations using these definitions.
3. *Whole gut transit time.* An upper limit for normal defined as the 95th percentile for healthy controls of approximately 68 hours (6).

Generally, the Rome criteria have been accepted as the more comprehensive definition for constipation (6). These criteria are based on the presence of at least two of the following four symptoms without the use of laxatives for at least 12 months; namely, straining for 25% or greater of bowel movements, a feeling of incomplete evacuation for 25% or greater of bowel movements, hard or pellet-like stools for 25% or greater of bowel movements, and bowel movements less than three times per week. In addition, if fewer than two stools per week on a regular basis are reported (even in the absence of any other symptom), the criteria for the definition of constipation are fulfilled.

The onset of constipation is also an important question. Most patients who have constipation due to congenital disorders such as Hirschsprung's disease or meningocele have this symptom from birth. When constipation occurs later in life, the symptom may be of chronic or recent onset. Constipation of recent onset, specifically if less than two years in duration, frequently is related to secondary causes and the exclusion by the clinician of organic colonic or extracolonic disorders, including malignancy, is mandatory (7). Questioning should emphasize which symptom the patient rates as most distressing. It is important to distinguish if the main complaint is infrequent bowel movements per se, or straining, hard stools, unsatisfied/unsatisfactory defecation, or symptoms that occur between infrequent bowel movements suggesting irritable bowel syndrome, such as bloating or abdominal pain.

A constipation scoring system has been proposed by Agachan et al. (8) in order to achieve uniformity in the assessment of the severity of this symptom. This scoring system was based upon eight parameters, including frequency of bowel movements, difficult or painful evacuatory effort, completeness of evacuation, abdominal pain, time (minutes) per attempt for evacuation, type of assistance (laxatives, digitation, or enema), number of unsuccessful attempts for evacuation per 24 hours, and duration (years) of constipation. Based on the questionnaire, scores ranged from 0 to 30, with 0 indicating normal and 30 indicating severe constipation. According to the authors' experience with 232 patients, the proposed scoring system correlated well with objective physiologic findings. This type of objective scoring recently has been supplemented by Knowles et al. (9), who have validated a symptom scoring system in pathophysiologic subgroups of patients, correlating this with the Cleveland Clinic Constipation Score (8) and with colonic transit studies, standard anorectal physiologic testing, and evacuation proctography. What is clear is that these forms of objective scoring instruments are valuable in coloproctological practice since the definition of chronic constipation based on infrequency of bowel movements alone or its correlation with slow transit are too insensitive and nonspecific for particular forms of disordered defecation (10).

Incontinence

As fecal incontinence is an under-reported and often silent condition, the clinical history is crucial and requires careful attention by the interviewer (11). The history should assess the age at onset and the progression of symptoms. It also should include a detailed search for a possible etiology, including extrasphincteric causes such as diabetes, neurologic disease, and the extraneous use of medications. Additionally, sphincteric causes such as obstetric birthing injury, prior anorectal surgery, or pelvic/perineal accidental trauma also should be considered. The coexistence of urinary incontinence—also known as double incontinence—and a history of constipation strongly suggest injury to the pudendal nerves.

A relationship between sphincter trauma and the onset of symptoms must be established; however, there is not always a clear correlation. For instance, lesions from obstetric trauma may remain dormant for many years until they manifest as symptoms of incontinence triggered by the effects of age or associated diseases such as irritable bowel syndrome. In patients who suffer primarily from diarrhea and who are incontinent, assessment should focus on the evaluation of their diarrhea—dietary factors and drug intake. A detailed questionnaire should assess the frequency and type of incontinence and its effects on the patient's quality of life. In order to assess the severity of incontinence, data from these factors are compiled to generate an incontinence score (Table 2.1-1) (12). This score ranges from 0, indicating perfect continence, to 20, indicating total incontinence. An incontinence scoring system is helpful to convert subjective to objective results, thereby permitting objective comparison of levels of incontinence among groups of patients, evaluation of treatment results, and comparison of data between centers. Although this particular incontinence scoring system addresses some aspects related to quality of life, a more in-depth evaluation on this matter is desirable. In practice, it is not uncommon to encounter patients with "minor" incontinence (loss of control for gas and occasional liquid stool soiling), who experience a considerable psychosocial impact as a direct consequence of their incontinence. Likewise, some patients with "major" incontinence, such as involuntary loss of solid stool, may have a less-than-expected alteration in their lifestyle. Therefore, the patient's perspective is crucial in the evaluation of anal incontinence, as well as in the results of treatment.

The Fecal Incontinence Quality of Life (FIQL) scale has gained widespread acceptance as a specific instrument to quantify the impact of fecal incontinence on the patient's quality of life (13). The FIQL is composed of 29 questions grouped into four scales: lifestyle, coping/behavior, depression/self-perception, and embarrassment. Although a more in-depth psychological evaluation may be required in some patients, the contents of these four scales address important quality-of-life issues for patients with fecal incontinence that may affect self-image and social functioning. Along with these validated and well-accepted scales, several other important scales appear in the literature and may be used for incontinence reporting, as well as for research tools (14–16).

TABLE 2.1-1. Incontinence scoring system.*

Type of incontinence	Frequency**				
	Never	Rarely	Sometimes	Usually	Always
Solid	0	1	2	3	4
Liquid	0	1	2	3	4
Gas	0	1	2	3	4
Use of pad	0	1	2	3	4
Lifestyle alteration	0	1	2	3	4

* The incontinence score is determined by adding points from the above grid, which takes into consideration the type and the frequency of incontinence and the extent to which it alters the patient's life.

** 0 perfect; 20 complete incontinence; never = 0 (never); rarely = <1 per month; sometimes = <1 per week and ≤1 per month; usually = <1 per day and ≤1 per week; always = ≤1 per day.
From Jorge and Wexner (12).

Physical Examination

Aspects of difficult defecation and fecal incontinence may overlap during physical examination as a conundrum. Patients with constipation may have signs of anal incontinence during physical examination due to progressive chronic neural injury or as part of an associated neuromuscular lesion secondary to childbirth. Occasionally, incontinence is suspected only during physical examination or during formal physiological testing. This circumstance may occur due to the patient's embarrassment and unwillingness to seek medical therapy or as a subclinical finding. In any event, physical examination of a patient with a functional anorectal disorder must be thorough in order to rule out a systemic etiology. Evidence of systemic illness, including neurologic or muscular deterioration and endocrine or metabolic disorders, should be sought. Furthermore, an abdominal examination may detect evidence of neoplasic or inflammatory bowel diseases.

Both the lateral decubitus and prone positions are used for routine anorectal examination. Although the prone position is purported to provide better exposure, the left lateral decubitus is a good alternative and better accepted by patients, particularly the elderly or those otherwise incapacitated. The evaluation of dynamics (squeeze and simulated defecation) is crucial during inspection and palpation. Occasionally, the examination requires extensive observation with the patient in a squatting position in order to uncover an occult rectal prolapse (17).

The anorectal examination should begin by inspection of the patient's undergarment and perineal skin for evidence of fecal soiling. Causes of perineal soiling (pseudoincontinence) include hemorrhoidal prolapse, pruritus ani, perianal fistula, rectal mucosal prolapse, and anorectal venereal diseases, each of which should be excluded. Descent of the perineum can easily be recognized during physical examination where, with the buttocks separated, descent and elevation of the perineum can be seen during simulated defecation and squeeze. During simulated defecation, the anal verge should be observed for any patulous opening or frank rectal prolapse. Cutaneous sensation around the anus may be absent in patients with neurogenic disorders and may indicate the level and side of the lesion. An intact bilateral anal reflex (as tested by a light pinprick or scratch) demonstrates that innervation of the external sphincter mechanism is present.

The next step is gentle palpation with a well-lubricated gloved index finger to evaluate resting tone. Fecal impaction, especially in the elderly, may be the sole cause of fecal incontinence. The lower rounded edge of the internal anal sphincter can be felt on physical examination, approximately one to two centimeters distal to the dentate line. The groove between the internal and external anal sphincter (the intersphincteric sulcus) can be visualized or easily palpated (Figure 2.1.1A). The entire circumference of the anorectum

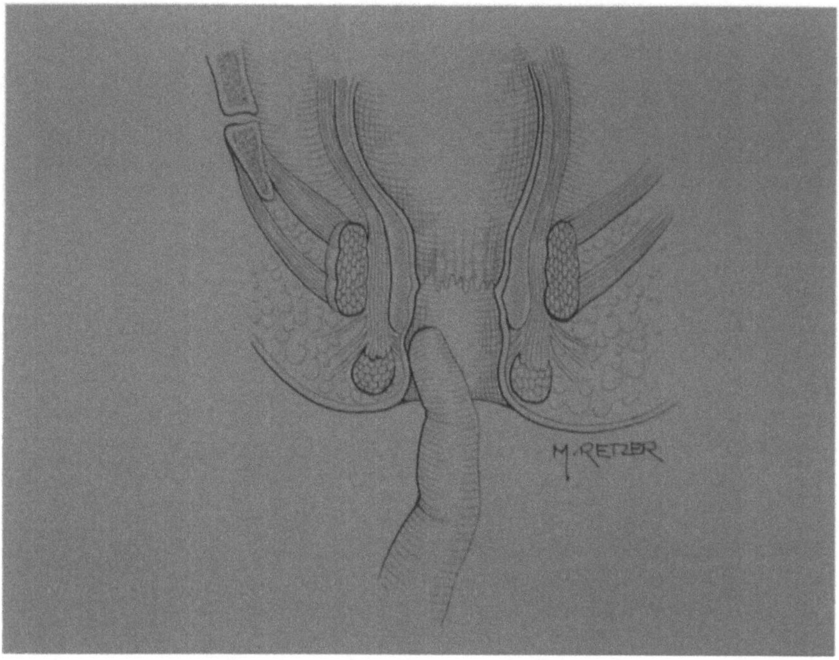

A

FIGURE 2.1.1. Anatomical landmarks during rectal examination—(A) intersphincteric groove; (B) Anorectal ring; (C) Puborectalis sling.

should be palpated by gentle circumanal rotation of the examining finger to assess the integrity of the anorectal ring, a term coined by Milligan and Morgan (18). This is a strong muscular ring that represents the upper end of the anal sphincter (more precisely the puborectalis) and the upper border of the internal anal sphincter around the anorectal junction (Figure 2.1.1B). Despite the lack of embryologic significance, it is an easily recognized boundary of the anal canal appreciated on physical examination. Furthermore, the anorectal ring is clinically relevant, as division of this structure during surgery for abscess or fistula invariably results in fecal incontinence.

During inspection and palpation, the presence of any sphincter defect should be noted, as well as the integrity of the perineal body or rectovaginal septum. Endoanal ultrasound is an excellent method of identifying and documenting internal and external sphincter defects (see Chapter 3.2). During dynamic palpation, the examiner should note both the increase in anal canal tone and the mobility of the posterior loop of the puborectal muscle during squeeze (Figure 2.1.1C).

In patients with spinal lesions, return of the anal resting tone after digital examination is characteristically very slow. However, the incidence of these

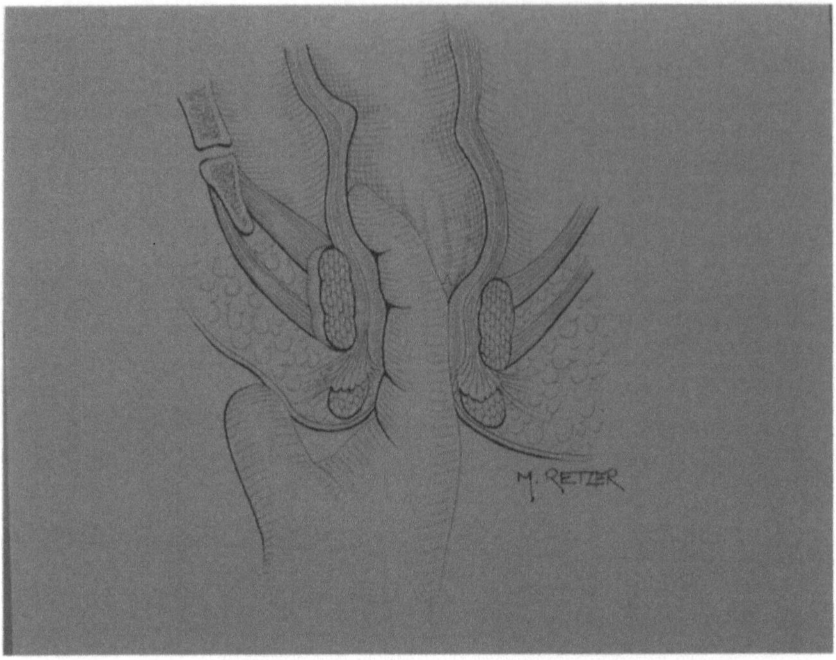

B

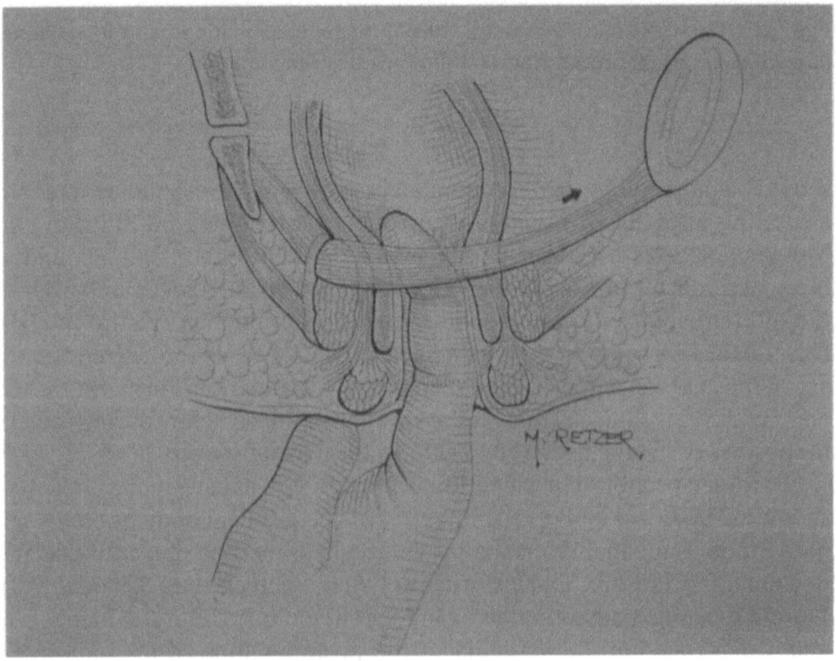

C

FIGURE 2.1.1. *Continued*

abnormalities and their exact etiologic significance remain uncertain. In cervical transection. for example, the anus remains closed and a balloon can be retained in the rectum, whereas in low flaccid lesions of the medulla, the anus is patulous and unable to prevent extrusion of the balloon (19). To assess the presence of anismus, the patient is asked to strain while the examiner's finger is kept in the rectum. Patients with anismus will squeeze, and some will have intermittent contractions. However, prior to diagnosing paradoxical contraction, this procedure should be repeated several times to ensure that the Valsalva's maneuver could not be accomplished due to true paradoxical contraction and not as a result of the patient's misunderstanding or embarrassment (20).

The presence of a rectocele can be assessed during physical examination by curving the examining finger and pressing it against the anterior rectal wall until it appears in the vagina, on the other side of the perineal body (Figure 2.1.2) (21). Bulging of the rectum because of an internal prolapse may be confused with rectocele, whereas internal (mucosal) prolapse can be palpated by the examining finger as a descending mass during straining on digital examination. At times, however, the differential diagnosis can be made only by defecography, which also can assist in determining the size of the rectocele. Moreover, by providing data on rectal emptying, defecography will allow differentiation of any secondary findings from a concomitant clinically relevant rectocele (see Chapter 3.1). An overt rectal prolapse or procidentia can be diagnosed by examining the patient while straining on a commode.

A combined vaginal and digital rectal examination can be very helpful in some patients, where, with the patient in a standing position, the examiner's index finger is inserted into the rectum and the thumb is inserted into the vagina. During this examination, the patient should be asked to strain (Figure 2.1.3). A peritoneal sac containing omentum or a loop of bowel dissecting the rectovaginal septum can be palpable between the thumb and the index finger, indicating the presence of a peritoneocele or enterocele (22,23). This examination can be an effective method of distinguishing between enterocele, prolapse of the vaginal vault (following hysterectomy), rectocele, or a combination of these weakened conditions (24–26). Again, defecography is a crucial method of confirming these findings and evaluating their role in the dynamics of defecation. The puborectalis muscle should be palpated and compressed between the forefinger and external thumb. Acute localized pain triggered by pulling or compressing the border of the muscle is a feature of levator spasm syndrome.

Finally, endoscopy is indicated. The patient should be prepared with a cleansing enema where possible. Both anoscopy and proctosigmoidoscopy are useful to exclude anatomic causes of soiling such as prolapsing hemorrhoids or rectoanal intussusception. In addition, solitary rectal ulcer, melanosis coli, inflammatory bowel disease, and rectal/anal tumors can be diagnosed. Rigid proctosigmoidoscopy is a more accurate method

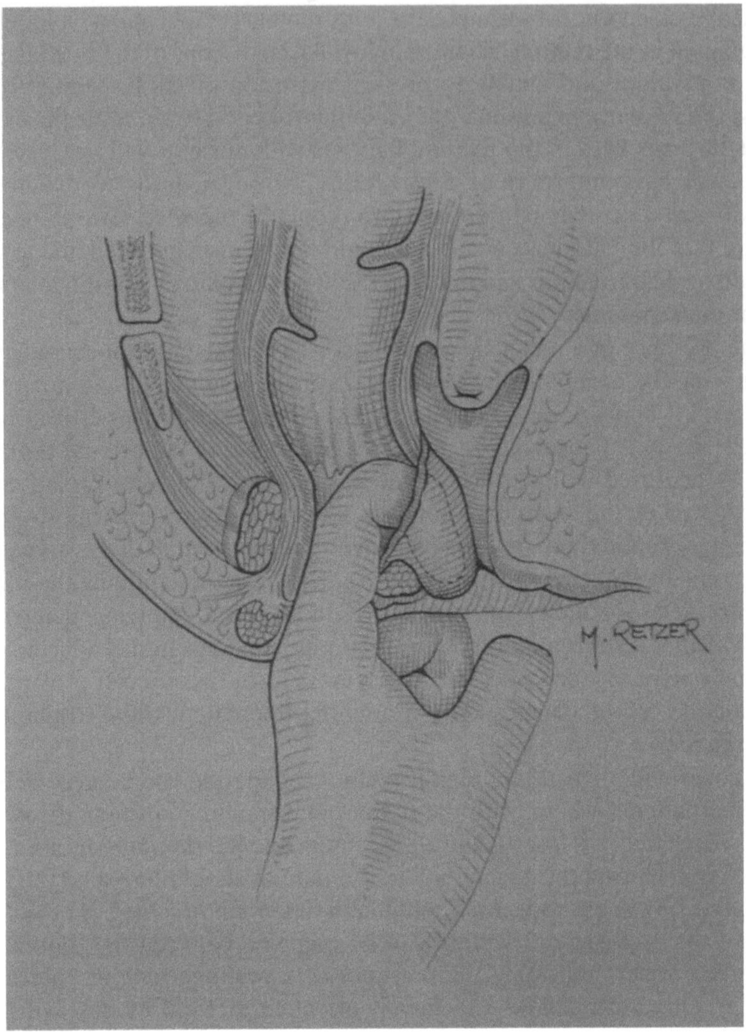

FIGURE 2.1.2. Anterior rectocele noted in the vagina during rectal examination.

of measuring distance from the anal verge; however, the average reached length is approximately 20 centimeters. Flexible sigmoidoscopy has a three to six times higher yield and is more comfortable for the patient. Ancillary colonoscopy may be indicated depending on the specific patient's complaints, family history, and the findings on anorectal examination.

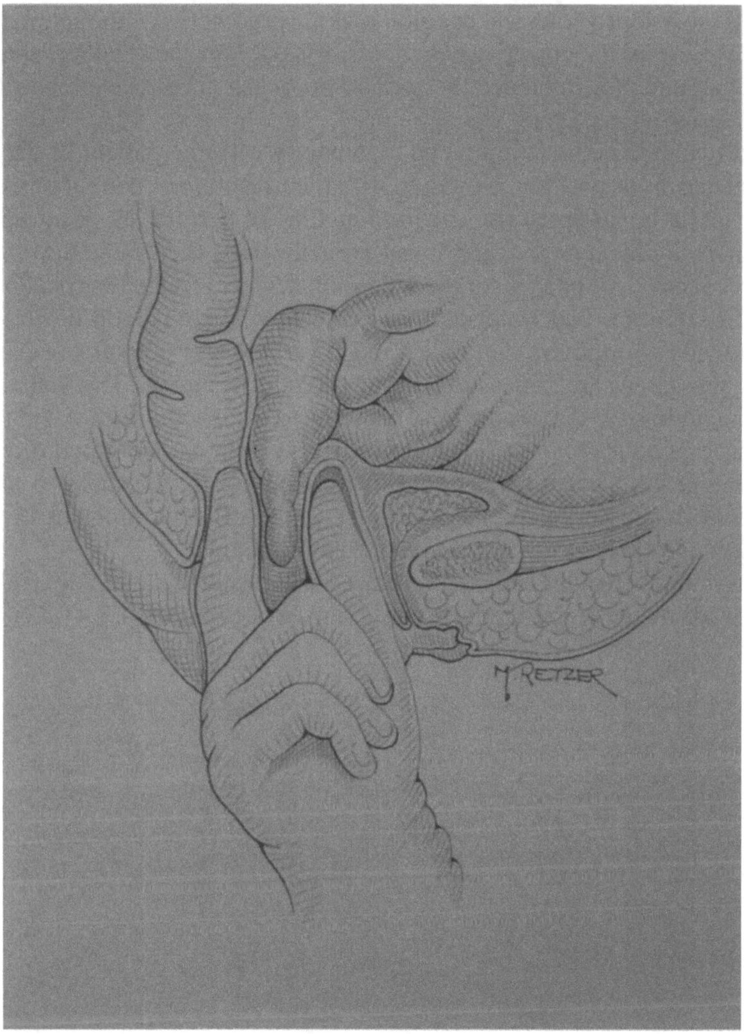

FIGURE 2.1.3. Palpation of a prolapsed bowel-filled sac dissecting the rectovaginal septum (enterocele).

Anorectal Manometry

Anorectal manometry is an objective method of studying the physiologic apparatus of defecation provided by the anorectal sphincter where it appears to be essential if a more accurate and detailed assessment is desired. Furthermore, the sensitivity, specificity, and predictive values of digital examination in estimating normal resting and squeeze pressures have been proven less than optimal (27,28). Despite this, there is still considerable controversy as to whether routine preoperative manometry affects the coloproctological decision-making process (29) although it quite clearly provides the objective data necessary to follow the results of sphincter repair and may influence the surgical approach in rectocele repair (30) and fissure surgery (31).

Most centers perform anorectal manometry with the patient in the left lateral decubitus position. However, with the exception of patient position, there is still no accepted standardized method of performing or interpreting anorectal manometry (32). Local normal values need to be developed and recognized for each institution. Sensing devices include microballoons, microtransducers, and water-perfused catheters. Microballoon devices do not provide information that reflect radial variations in pressure; instead, a single pressure value is measured based on collective forces. This technique has the additional disadvantage of the effect the balloon itself has on the averaged pressure reading. Microtransducers can be incorporated directly into the probe to eliminate the need for perfusion systems and to allow ambulatory measurement (see Chapter 2.6). Although still costly and fragile, microtransducers may have a promising future.

Plastic multichannel catheters perfused with water by a microperfusion system are the most commonly used sensing devices (Figure 2.1.4) (33). The

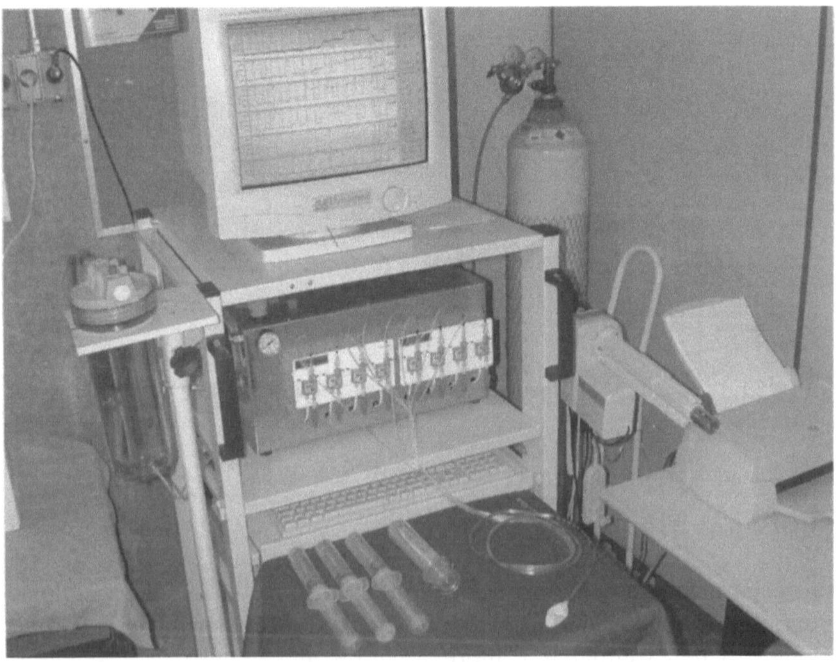

FIGURE 2.1.4. Manometry apparatus—multichannel water-perfused catheter, perfusion system, polygraph, and computer hardware.

principle of this technique is to measure the resistance in terms of pressure that the sphincters offer to a constant flow of water through the port. A constant perfusion rate (usually 0.3 mL per channel per minute) is required to measure adequately the outflow from the tube (34,35). High flow rates can result in considerable fluid accumulation in the rectum and can adversely effect the reproducibility, whereas low rates may not promptly reflect changes in pressures. In order to minimize anatomic distortion, catheters must be flexible and no more than four to eight millimeters in maximal diameter.

The most important advantage of perfused catheters is that multiple channels (commonly 4 to 8 in number) can be set on a single catheter. Depending on the purpose of the study, catheters may have their channel ports displayed in either a radial (for station measurement) or a stepwise oblique (for averaged anal canal pressure profile) fashion. The technique of manometric measurement also varies between anorectal laboratories. The catheter can be left at one position (stationary technique), can be manually moved at continuous intervals (manual or station pull-through technique), or can be continuously withdrawn (continuous manual or automated pull-through). Theoretically, the manual pull-through technique provides a more accurate pressure at a single point because a stabilization period is obtained before each interval recording. The pull-through techniques provide a longitudinal profile, which is important because of the considerable variation in pressures along the axis of the anal canal. Although a constantly moving catheter may produce some artifact due to sphincter stimulation, it can be minimized if the steady withdrawal of a well-lubricated catheter is done by a mechanical device (automated pull-through). The automated pull-through of an eight-channel catheter can provide more-detailed recording of the radial and longitudinal pressure profiles where the greater the number of ports, the less the inter-port interpolation (36). The vector diagrams of these profiles can be plotted together, thus generating a three-dimensional representation of the entire pressure profile of the anal canal. Although the true value of this sphincter graphic remains controversial, the calculation of the sphincter asymmetry index seems to be useful in detecting occult sphincter defects (37) (see Chapter 2.3).

Conventional anorectal manometry enables measurement of both resting and squeeze pressures, as well as the high-pressure zone or functional anal canal length, each of which will be discussed in this chapter. Adjunct studies using an intrarectal balloon include assessment of the rectoanal inhibitory reflex (see Chapter 2.2), rectal sensory threshold (see Chapter 2.8), rectal capacity, and rectal compliance (see Chapter 2.4), all of which are discussed in other chapters of this book.

Resting Tone

In healthy adults, the mean anal canal resting tone is generally in the range of 50 to 70 mmHg and tends to be lower in women and in the elderly population (38). In the composition of the resting tone, the internal anal sphincter is responsible for 50 to 85%, the external anal sphincter accounts for 25 to 30%, and the remaining 15% is attributed to expansion of the anal cushions (39–41). As a smooth muscle in a state of continuous maximal contraction, the internal anal sphincter, due to both intrinsic myogenic and extrinsic autonomic neurogenic properties, represents a natural barrier to the involuntary loss of stool. Although the internal anal sphincter relaxes in response to rectal distension, it gradually reacquires tone as the rectum accommodates to the distension. Profound impairment of internal anal sphincter function has been noted in 25% of patients with idiopathic fecal incontinence; spontaneous relaxation of the internal anal sphincter without compensatory increase in external anal sphincter activity may be an important factor leading to fecal incontinence (42). Moreover, it has been shown that in patients where there is already reported fecal incontinence and attendant external anal sphincter atrophy that the inherent parameters of the rectoanal inhibitory reflex (an internal anal sphincter function) are altered (43). In particular, the rapidity of recovery of the rectoanal inhibitory reflex on rectal distension may function as an innate mechanism of continence preservation in those patients where continence is already compromised (44,45).

High-Pressure Zone (Functional Anal Canal Length)

A gradual increase in pressure is noted from proximal to distal in the anal canal; the highest resting pressures are usually recorded one to two centimeters cephalad to the anal verge (Figure 2.1.5). This high-pressure zone (or functional anal canal length) corresponds anatomically to the condensation of the smooth muscle fibers of the internal anal sphincter and is shorter in women (2.0–3.0 cm) when compared with men (2.5–3.5 cm) (35). Interestingly, although parity may contribute to this difference, nulliparous women still have a significantly shorter functional anal canal than do men (37).

The anal canal is relatively asymmetric in its radial profile (46,47). The normal values for the radial asymmetry index are less than or equal to 10%; however, these values are subject to the technique and equipment used (37,48). This functional asymmetry is found for both resting and squeeze pressure profiles and follows the inherent anatomic asymmetry in the arrangement of the sphincter muscles. In the upper third of the anal canal, higher pressures are found posteriorly due to the activity of the puborectalis, along with the deep portion of the internal anal sphincter; however, in the lower third of the anal canal, pressures are higher anteriorly due to the

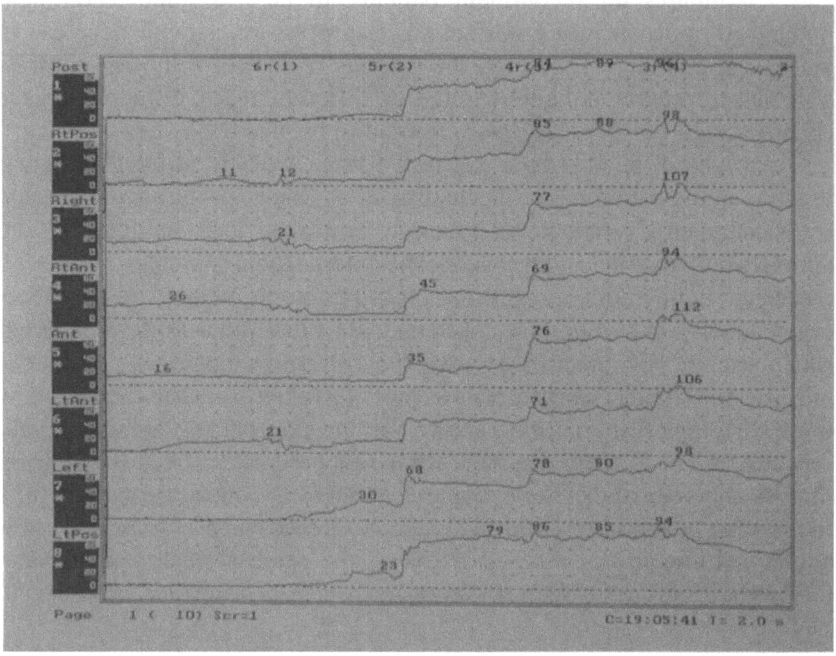

FIGURE 2.1.5. Resting tone profile in eight quadrants at 45-degree intervals from six to one centimeter above the anal verge. Note the increase in pressures as the catheter is pulled distally in the anal canal (high-pressure zone).

posteriorly directed superficial loop of the external anal sphincter. These differential pressure gradients have been implicated in the maintenance of the normal continence mechanism (49).

Squeeze Pressures and Skeletal Muscle Responses

During maximal voluntary contraction or squeeze effort, intra-anal pressures usually escalate to two or three times the baseline resting tone (100 to 180 mmHg) (Figure 2.1.6). However, due to muscular fatigue, maximal voluntary contraction of the external anal sphincter can be sustained for only 40 to 60 seconds. The squeeze pressures are largely related to the contraction of the external anal sphincter, although the levator ani muscles also contribute. More recently, the fatigue rate index has been proposed by Marcello et al. (50) as a new manometric parameter to evaluate the voluntary component of the anal sphincter function. This parameter is a calculated measure (minutes) of the time necessary for the sphincter to be completely fatigued to a pressure equivalent to the resting tone. According to their results, the mean fatigue rate index was 3.3 minutes for volunteers, 2.8 minutes for constipated patients, 2.3 minutes for patients with seepage, and 1.5 minutes for incontinent patients. In fact, in some incontinent patients, despite an initial normal squeeze pressure, a rapid decrease in values can be noted. Therefore, the inability to sustain voluntary contraction may represent either an initial or different mechanism of damage (Figure 2.1.7). Further studies are needed to resolve this issue.

Garavoglia et al. (51) have suggested three types of striated muscular function in the maintenance mechanism of continence: lateral compression (pubococcygeus), sphincteric function (external anal sphincter), and anorectal angulation (puborectalis). The external anal sphincter, along with the pelvic floor muscles, has three types of activity, namely, resting tone, reflex activity, and voluntary contractions. Unlike other skeletal muscles, which usually are inactive at rest, the sphincters maintain continuous unconscious resting electrical tone as part of a reflex arc at the cauda equina level. Histological studies have shown that the external anal sphincter, puborectalis, and levator ani muscles each have a predominance of type I fibers that are characteristic of skeletal muscles with tonic contractile activity (52). In response to conditions of threatened continence (such as increased intra-abdominal pressure or rectal distension), the external anal sphincter and the puborectalis reflexively or voluntarily contract further in order to

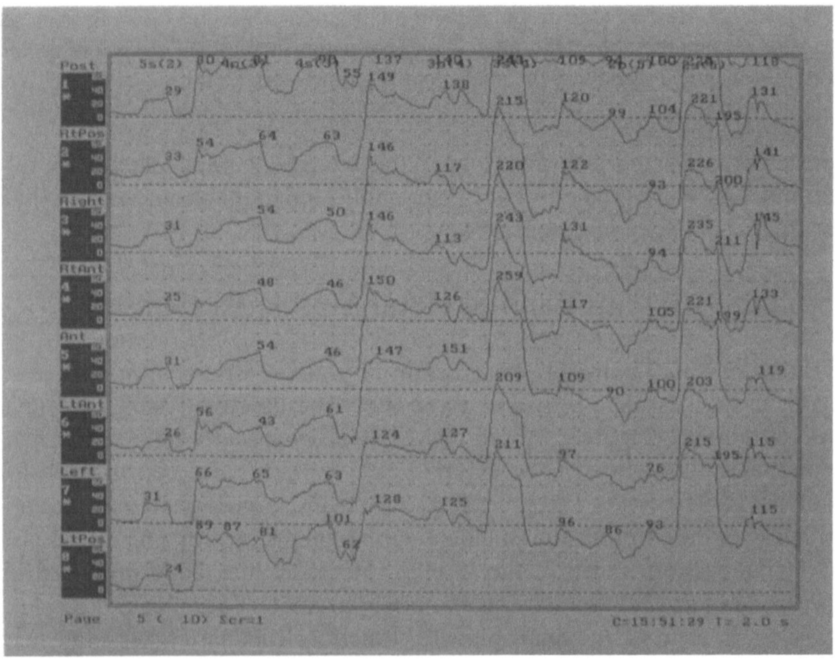

FIGURE 2.1.6. Voluntary contraction pressure profile in eight quadrants at 45-degree intervals. During normal squeeze effort, intra-anal pressures can reach two to three times the baseline resting tone, reflecting the activity of the external anal and levator ani muscles.

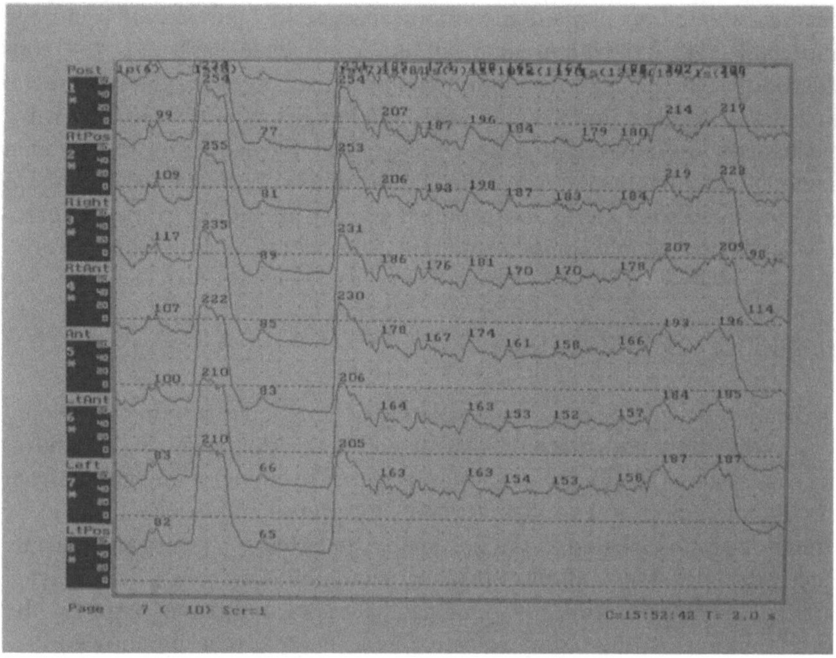

FIGURE 2.1.7. Tracing shows the maximum voluntary contraction during a 40-second period for the calculation of the fatigue index rate.

prevent fecal leakage (53). The automatic continence mechanism is then formed by the resting tone governed by the internal anal sphincter and magnified by reflex external anal sphincter contraction. This extra pressure gradient is essential to minimize voluntary attention to the sphincters.

Although manometry assesses important aspects of anorectal physiology, the mechanism of defecation and continence includes other elements such as stool consistency, the anorectal angle, anal sensation, pelvic floor muscle integrity and function, and central neurologic pathways. Therefore, a comprehensive evaluation of anorectal function will require a combination of tests. Some of these aspects related to basic anorectal physiology and its impact on understanding and diagnosing continence disorders are discussed below.

The Puborectalis Muscle and the Anorectal Angle

The anorectal angle is reportedly the result of the anatomic configuration of the U-shaped sling of puborectalis muscle around the anorectal junction. Whereas the anal sphincters are responsible for closure of the anal canal to retain gas and liquid stool, the puborectalis muscle and the anorectal angle are designed to maintain gross fecal continence. Different theories have been postulated to explain the importance of the puborectalis and the anorectal angle in the maintenance of fecal continence. Parks et al. (54) considered that increasing intra-abdominal pressure forces the anterior rectal wall down into the upper anal canal, occluding it by a type of flap valve mechanism, thereby creating an effective seal. Subsequently, it has been demonstrated that the flap valve mechanism does not occur, but rather there is a continued sphincteric occlusion, an activity attributed to the puborectalis and external anal sphincter musculature operating in tandem (55,56).

Sequence of Defecation

Defecation is a complex and incompletely understood phenomenon related to several integrated mechanisms, all under the influence of the central nervous system (57,58). Defecation is triggered by filling of the rectum from the sigmoid colon. Rectal distension is interpreted at a conscious level by stretch receptors located in the pelvic floor muscles as a desire to defecate. Rectal distension also initiates the rectoanal inhibitory reflex. The internal anal sphincter relaxation, by opening the upper anal canal, exposes the rectal contents to the highly sensitive anal mucosa, thereby allowing differentiation between flatus and stool. This "sampling" mechanism (59) determines the urgency of defecation whereas the simultaneous reflex contraction of the external anal sphincter maintains continence. If defecation is to be deferred, conscious contraction of the external anal sphincter, assisted by the mechanism of rectal compliance, yields time for recuperation of the internal anal sphincter function.

If the call to stool is answered, either the sitting or squatting position is assumed and the anorectal angle is "opened." Increases in both the intrarectal and intra-abdominal pressures result in reflex relaxation of the internal and external anal sphincter and puborectalis; at this point, defecation may occur without straining. Nevertheless, some degree of straining usually is necessary to initiate rectal evacuation. Straining will ensure further relaxation of the sphincteric and puborectalis musculature and the anorectal angle becomes even more obtuse. Consequently, pelvic floor descent and funneling occurs and the rectal contents are expelled by direct transmission of the increased abdominal pressure through the relaxed pelvic floor. Stool consistency will determine either mass peristaltic emptying of the left colon or the intermittent passage of stools. Transient external anal sphincter and puborectalis contraction after completion of rectal evacuation, the "closing reflex," restores the internal anal sphincter tonus and closes the anal canal.

References

1. Wexner SD, and Jorge JMN. Colorectal physiological tests: use or abuse of technology? Eur J Surg. 1994;160:167–74.

2. Keating JP, Stewart PJ, Eyers AA, Warner D, and Bokey EL. Are special investigations of value in the management of patients with fecal incontinence? Dis Colon Rectum. 1997;40:896–901.
3. Halverson AL, and Orkin BA. Which physiologic tests are useful in patients with constipation? Dis Colon Rectum. 1998;41:735–739.
4. Vaizey CJ, and Kamm MA. Prospective assessment of the clinical value of anorectal investigations. Digestion. 2000;61:201–14.
5. Karulf RE, Coller JA, Bartolo DCC, Bowden DO, Roberts PL, Murray JJ, Schoetz DJ Jr, and Veidenheimer MC. Anorectal physiology testing: a survey of availability and use. Dis Colon Rectum. 1991;34:464–8.
6. Whitehead WE, Chaussade S, Corazziari E, and Kumar D. Report of an international workshop on management of constipation. Gastroenterol Int. 1991; 4;99–112.
7. Kruis W, Thieme C, Weinzierl M, Schussles P, Holl J, and Paulus W. A diagnostic score for irritable bowel syndrome. Its value in the exclusion of organic disease. Gastroenterology. 1984;87:1–7.
8. Agachan F, Chen T, Pfeifer J, Reissman P, and Wexner SD. A constipation scoring system to simplify evaluation and management of constipated patients. Dis Colon Rectum. 1996;39:681–5.
9. Knowles CH, Eccersley AJ, Scott SM, Walker SM, Reeves B, and Lunniss PJ. Linear discriminant analysis of symptoms in patients with chronic constipation. Validation of a new scoring system (KESS). Dis Colon Rectum. 2000; 43:1419–26.
10. Koch A, Voderholzer WA, Klauser AG, and Müller-Lissner S. Symptoms in chronic constipation. Dis Colon Rectum. 1997;40:902–6.
11. Leigh RJ, and Turnberg LA. Faecal incontinence: the invoiced symptom. Lancet. 1982;1:1349–51.
12. Jorge JMN, and Wexner SD. Etiology and management of fecal incontinence. Dis Colon Rectum. 1993;36:77–97.
13. Rockwood TH, Church JM, Fleshman JW, Kane RL, Mavrantonis C, Thorson AG, Wexner SD, Bliss D, and Lowry AC. Fecal incontinence quality of life scale: quality of life instrument for patients with fecal incontinence. Dis Colon Rectum. 2000;43:9–17.
14. Pescatori M, Anastasio G, Bottini C, and Mentasti A. New grading and scoring for anal incontinence. Evaluation of 335 patients. Dis Colon Rectum. 1992; 35:482–7.
15. Vaizey CJ, Carapeti E, Cahill JA, and Kamm MA. Prospective comparison of faecal incontinence grading systems. Gut. 1999;44:77–80.
16. Reilly WT, Talley NJ, Pemberton JH, and Zinsmeister AR. Validation of a questionnaire to assess fecal incontinence and associated risk factors. Fecal Incontinence Questionnaire. Dis Colon Rectum. 2000;43:146–54.
17. Pescatori M, and Quandamcarlo C. A new grading of rectal internal mucosal prolapse and its correlation with diagnosis and treatment. Int J Colorectal Dis. 1999;14:245–9.
18. Milligan ETC, and Morgan CN. Surgical anatomy of the anal canal: with special reference to anorectal fistulae. Lancet. 1934;2:1150–6.
19. Connell AM, Frankel H, and Guttman L. The motility of the pelvic colon following complete lesions of the spinal cord. Paraplegia. 1963;104: 98–115.

20. Miller R, Duthie GS, Bartolo DC, Roe AM, Locke-Edmunds J, and Mortensen NJ. Anismus in patients with normal and slow transit constipation. Br J Surg. 1991;78:690–2.
21. Heslop JH. Piles, and rectoceles. Aust N Z J Surg. 1987;57:935–8.
22. Bremmer S. Peritoneocele. A radiologic study with defaeco-peritoneography. Acta Radiologica. 1998;413 Suppl:1–33.
23. Holley RI. Enterocele: a review. Obstet Gynecol Surv. 1994;49:284–93.
24. Nichols DH, and Randall CL. Vaginal surgery. 3rd ed. Baltimore (MD): Williams & Wilkins; 1989. p. 313–327.
25. Imparato E, Aspesi G, Rovetta E, and Presti M. Surgical management and prevention of vaginal vault prolapse. Surg Gynecol Obstet. 1992;175:233–7.
26. Kenton K, Shott S, and Brubaker L. The anatomic and functional variability of rectocele in women. Int Urogynecol J Pelvic Floor Dysfunct. 1999;10:96–9.
27. Felt-Bersma RJF, Klinkenberg-Knol LB, and Meuwissen SGM. Investigation of anorectal function. Br J Surg. 1988;75:53–5.
28. Eckardt VF, and Elmer T. Reliability of anal pressure measurements. Dis Colon Rectum. 1991;34:72–7.
29. Carty NJ, Moran B, and Johnson CD. Anorectal physiology measurements are of no value in clinical practice. True or false? Ann R Coll Surg Engl. 1994;76:276–80.
30. Ayabaca SM, Zbar AP, and Pescatori M. Anal continence after rectocele repair. Int J Colorect Dis. 2002;45:63–9.
31. Pescatori M, Maria G, and Anastasio G. "Spasm related" internal sphincterotomy in the treatment of anal fissure. A randomized prospective study. Coloproctology. 1991;1:20–2.
32. Zbar AP, and Kmiot WA. Anorectal Investigation. In: Phillips RKS, editor. A companion to specialist surgical practice; colorectal surgery. 1st ed. London: WB Saunders; 1997. p. 1–33.
33. Smith LE. Practical guide to anorectal testing. 2nd ed. New York: Igaku-Shoin; 1995.
34. Coller JA. Clinical application of anorectal manometry. Gastroenterol Clin North Am. 1987;16:17–33.
35. Jorge JMN, and Wexner SD. Anorectal manometry: techniques and clinical applications. South Med J. 1993;86:924–31.
36. Zbar AP, Aslam M, Hider A, Toomey P, and Kmiot WA. Comparison of vector volume manometry with conventional manometry in anorectal dysfunction. Tech Coloproctol. 1998;2:84–90.
37. Jorge JMN, and Habr-Gama A. The value of sphincteric asymmetry index analysis in anal incontinence. Int J Colorectal Dis. 2000;15:303–10.
38. Frenckner B, and Euler CHRV. Influence of pudendal block on the function of the anal sphincters. Gut. 1975;16:482–9.
39. Lestar B, Penninckx F, and Kerremans R. The composition of anal basal pressure. An in vivo and in vitro study in man. Int J Colorect Dis. 1989;4:118–22.
40. Gibbons CP, Trowbridge EA, Bannister JJ, and Read NW. Role of anal cushions in maintaining continence. Lancet. 1986;1:886–7.
41. Zbar AP, Jayne DG, Mathur D, Ambrose NS, and Guillou PJ. The importance of the internal anal sphincter (IAS) in maintaining continence: anatomical, physiological and pharmacological considerations. Colorectal Dis. 2000; 2:193–202.

42. Sun WM, Read NW, and Donnelly TC. Impaired internal anal sphincter in a subgroup of patients with idiopathic fecal incontinence. Gastroenterology. 1989;97:130–5.
43. Kaur G, Gardiner A, and Duthie GS. Rectoanal reflex parameters in incontinence and constipation. Dis Colon Rectum. 2002;45:928–33.
44. Zbar AP, Aslam M, Gold DM, Gatzen G, Gosling A, and Kmiot WA. Parameters of the rectoanal inhibitory reflex in patients with idiopathic fecal incontinence and chronic constipation. Dis Colon Rectum. 1998;41:200–8.
45. Zbar AP, and Ramesh J. Parameters of the rectoanal inhibitory reflex in different anorectal disorders. Dis Colon Rectum. 2003;46:557–8.
46. Collins CD, Brown BH, Whittaker GE, and Duthie HL. New method of measuring forces in the anal canal. Gut. 1969;10:160–3.
47. Taylor BM, Beart RW, and Phillips SF. Longitudinal and radial variations of pressure in the human anal sphincter. Gastroenterology. 1984;86:693–7.
48. Braun JC, Treutner KH, Dreuw B, Klimaszewski M, and Schlumpelick V. Vectormanometry for differential diagnosis of fecal incontinence. Dis Colon Rectum. 1994;37:989–96.
49. Goes RN, Simons AJ, Masri L, and Beart RW Jr. Gradient of pressure and time between proximal anal canal and high-pressure zone during internal anal sphincter relaxation: its role in the fecal continence mechanism. Dis Colon Rectum. 1995;38:1043–6.
50. Marcello PW, Barrett RC, Coller JA, Schoetz DJ Jr, Roberts PL, Murray JJ, and Rusin LC. Fatigue rate index as a new measurement of external sphincter function. Dis Colon Rectum. 1998;41:336–43.
51. Garavoglia M, Borghi F, and Levi AC. Arrangement of the anal striated musculature. Dis Colon Rectum. 1993;36:10–5.
52. Swash M. Histopathology of pelvic floor muscles in pelvic floor disorders. In: Henry MM and Swash M, editors. Coloproctology and the pelvic floor. Oxford: Butterworth-Heinemann Ltd.; 1992. p. 173–83.
53. Farouk R, Duthie GS, and Bartolo DCG. Functional anorectal disorders and physiological evaluation. In: Beck DE and Wexner SD, editors. Fundamentals of anorectal surgery. New York: McGraw-Hill; 1992. p. 68–88.
54. Parks AG, Porter NH, and Hardcastle J. The syndrome of the descending perineum. Proc R Soc Med. 1966;59:477–82.
55. Bartolo DCC, Roe AM, Locke-Edmunds JC, Virjee J, and Mortensen NJM. Flap-valve theory of anorectal continence. Br J Surg. 1986;73:1012–4.
56. Bannister JJ, Gibbons C, and Read NW. Preservation of faecal continence during rises in intra-abdominal pressure: is there a role for the flap valve? Gut. 1987;28:1242–5.
57. Kumar D, and Wingate DL. Colorectal motility. In: Henry MM and Swash M, editors. Coloproctology and the pelvic floor. Oxford: Butterworth-Heinemann Ltd.; 1992. p. 72–85.
58. Wexner SD, and Bartolo DCC. Constipation. Etiology, evaluation and management. London: Butterworth-Heinemann Ltd.; 1995.
59. Miller R, Bartolo DCC, Cervero F, Mortensen NJM. Anorectal sampling: a comparison of normal and incontinent patients. Br J Surg. 1988;75:44–7.

Editorial Commentary

Dr. J. Marcio N. Jorge has given a detailed but easy to understand description of basic anorectal physiology including clinical examination and manometry. He has shown the clinical practical aspects of the necessary facets for evaluation of these patients with both faecal incontinence and chronic constipation. This chapter highlights the fact that, when appropriate, applied anorectal physiology can yield significant quanta of useful information for the evaluation and management of patients with fecal incontinence and constipation but these tests are not always necessary in every individual presenting with these complaints.

SW

Chapter 2.2
Rectoanal Inhibition

Patricia L. Roberts

Introduction

The rectoanal inhibitory reflex is defined as transient relaxation of the internal anal sphincter in response to rectal distention. It was first described by Gowers in 1877 (1) and confirmed by Denny-Brown and Robertson (2) in 1935. A consensus statement of definitions for anorectal physiology has defined the rectoanal inhibitory reflex as "the transient decrease in resting anal pressure by ≥25% of basal pressure in response to rapid inflation of a rectal balloon with subsequent return to baseline." (3) While the exact role of the rectoanal inhibitory reflex is unknown, it has been postulated to serve as a "sampling reflex" and is felt to be a factor in the maintenance of continence (4,5). Thus, the upper anal canal is able to discriminate between flatus and fecal material.

Physiology

This reflex is believed to be mediated through the intramural neuronal plexus (6). It is present following spinal cord injury and cauda equina syndrome, and it can remain intact after full rectal mobilization or presacral blockade. It is absent in Hirschsprung's disease and absent initially after low anterior resection and ileoanal pouch procedure. Regeneration of the reflex may occur after hand-sewn coloanal anastomosis and after low stapled anastomosis (7–10), in some cases clinically correlating with less-reported nocturnal fecal urgency. A false-negative reflex may be obtained if the resting pressure is extremely low and if the patient has a hyposensitive rectum, as frequently is seen in patients with megarectum. Failure to elicit such a reflex in some patients with full-thickness rectal prolapse may mitigate against a perineal approach to repair. In such patients, large inflation volumes may be necessary to elicit a recognizable reflex.

The role of nitric oxide, an endogenous bioactive substance and important inhibitory neurotransmitter in the gastrointestinal tract, in the mediation of the rectoanal inhibitory reflex also has been examined (11). Nitric oxide is a mediator of internal anal sphincter relaxation in response to nonadrenergic, noncholinergic nerve stimulation (12) (see Chapter 4).

Methods

There are a variety of methods for the performance of anal manometry and eliciting the rectoanal inhibitory reflex, although none has been standardized. Various catheter and balloon systems have been used, including semiconductor strain-gauge catheters, air-filled or water-filled balloons, and water-perfused catheters. The following describes the method of eliciting the rectoanal inhibitory reflex in our unit.

In our laboratory, anal manometry is performed with an eight-channel water-perfused catheter with an external diameter of 5.5 millimeters (Mui Scientific, Mississauga, Ontario, Canada). A computerized system with menu-driven software developed by Dr. John Coller is used. Analysis of data, graphic presentation, and generation of reports is facilitated by interfacing the pressure recorder with a computer. The protocol for eliciting the reflex has been described previously and is detailed here in brief (13,14). A Coller type B catheter, which is a spiral catheter (Figure 2.2.1) is used for eliciting the rectoanal inhibitory reflex. A 100-second run is performed, and at 50 seconds, the balloon is inflated with 60 cubic centimeters of air that allows it to attain a preset trigger pressure signaling the onset of balloon distention to the computer. Pressure events during the first 20 seconds after balloon distention indicate the reflex response (Figure 2.2.2). Rectoanal inhibitory and excitatory responses are considered present when pressure increases or decreases within two standard deviations below or above the resting pressure. The degree of relaxation varies in the proximal, middle, and distal sphincter, with the greatest degree of relaxation in the proximal internal anal sphincter. Latency of the rectoanal inhibitory (RAIR) or rectoanal excitatory (RAER) reflex is measured in seconds from the start of balloon inflation to the onset of the RAIR or RAER as defined by the computer setting.

Although some laboratories have reported the rectoanal inhibitory reflex as a discrete variable, that is, being either "present" or "absent," other units, such as ours, have looked at the significance of various parameters of the rectoanal inhibitory reflex, including the latency, the duration of the reflex, and the amplitude of the reflex in the proximal and distal portion of the sphincter (15,16).

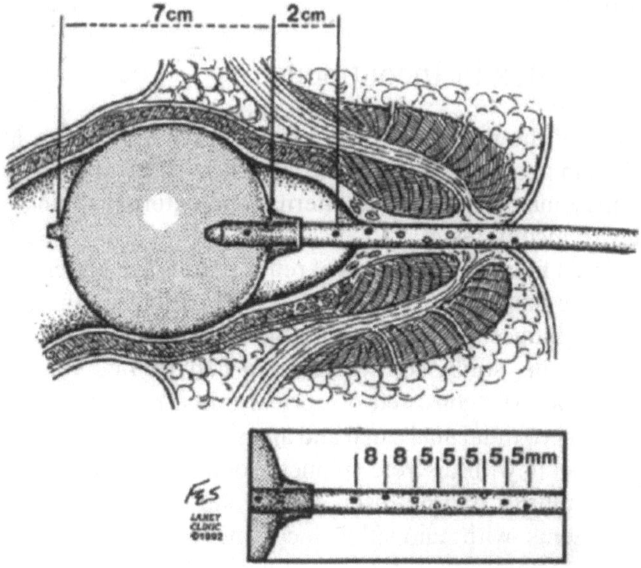

FIGURE 2.2.1. The Coller type B catheter, a balloon, and side-perfused multiple port catheter is used to elicit the rectoanal inhibitory reflex. The spacing of the ports is depicted in the inset. One port measures the intraluminal pressure of the rectum, one measures pressures in the balloon, and the others take measurements along the anal canal. (Reprinted with permission of the Lahey Clinic)

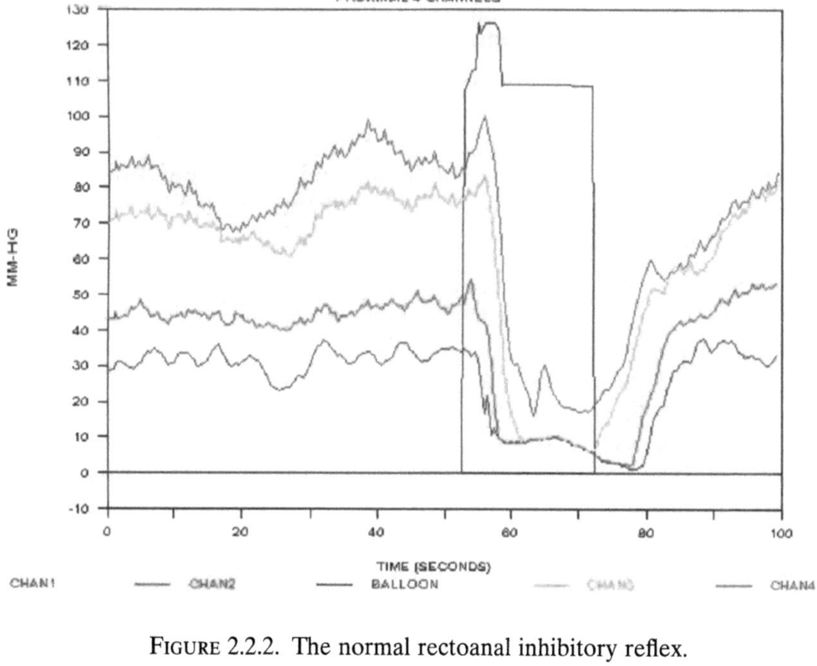

FIGURE 2.2.2. The normal rectoanal inhibitory reflex.

Rectoanal Reflex in Incontinence

Abnormalities of the rectoanal inhibitory and excitatory reflex have been well described in patients with fecal incontinence. These abnormalities may reflect the anatomic defects of the internal and external sphincter muscle associated with incontinence.

We have noted five different types of reflex patterns in patients with fecal incontinence. We have previously compared 43 patients with idiopathic or traumatic incontinence with 29 control subjects who had no anorectal complaints (17). In this study, control subjects had normal reflex patterns. Normal reflex patterns consisted of normal initial excitation followed by inhibition in the proximal anal canal and an excitatory response in the distal anal canal. Patients with discrete sphincter defects such as those patients with obstetric injuries had no distal excitation, but had normal proximal inhibition. Patients with idiopathic incontinence had normal proximal response, but an inhibitory instead of an excitatory response in the distal anal canal. An additional group had a normal reflex pattern while the remaining two groups, including one group with iatrogenic trauma, had no excitatory response in the proximal or distal anal canal, but had a normal inhibitory reflex. One group with idiopathic incontinence had excitatory response in the entire anal canal, but no inhibition. Patients with fecal incontinence and normal rectoanal inhibitory and excitatory reflexes may be a subgroup of patients with incontinence with the best preserved sphincter function and the least sphincter damage. Abnormalities of the rectoanal reflexes in patients who are incontinent may be the result of masking of the underlying influence of one of the sphincter muscles.

Absence of the rectoanal inhibitory reflex has been noted by other investigators. Sun et al. (18) reported an absence of the rectoanal inhibitory reflex in patients with incontinence and suggested that higher inflation volumes were necessary in such patients. These higher volumes resulted in a rebound increase of pressure on deflation and a positive reflex.

In addition, in patients with fecal incontinence, pudendal neuropathy also appears to result in abnormalities of the rectoanal excitatory reflex. We have studied 15 patients, specifically examining pudendal nerve terminal motor latency (PNTML), abnormalities in the rectoanal excitatory reflex and single fiber density as makers for pudendal neuropathy (19). Pudendal nerve terminal motor latency (PNTML) was prolonged in 10 patients and normal in five patients while increased single fiber density indicated neuropathy in 12 patients and was normal in two patients. The distal RAER was abnormal in 13 patients and normal in two. The three diagnostic modalities were in agreement in ten patients, confirming neuropathy in nine and excluding it in one patient. Ten patients with fecal incontinence had a normal PNTML, but an abnormal distal excitatory reflex; five patients had an abnormal PNTML, but a normal distal excitatory reflex and 15 patients had both PNTML and excitatory reflex that were abnormal. Thus, an abnormal rectoanal excitatory reflex appears to correlate well with neurophysiologic tests used to diagnose pudendal neuropathy.

Assessment of other parameters of the rectoanal inhibitory reflex may yield further information in patients with incontinence. Kaur and colleagues (20,21) found that significantly greater sphincter relaxation was seen at each volume of rectal distention in incontinent patients compared with constipated and healthy control subjects. Similarly, Zbar (22) and colleagues compared parameters of the rectoanal inhibitory reflex in 42 patients with fecal incontinence and with chronic constipation. Excitatory and inhibitory latencies, maximum excitatory and inhibitory pressure, amplitude and slope of inhibition, slope and time or pressure recovery, and area under the inhibitory curve were all measured. The recovery time under the inhibitory curve differed at various sphincter levels and among the patient groups; however, incontinent patients had the most rapid recovery. It was concluded that continence may rely in part on some of these characteristics of rectoanal inhibition and that there may be some parameters that would predict functional results following low anastomosis.

Rectoanal Reflex and Constipation

The rectoanal inhibitory reflex has been studied in patients with constipation and incontinence and compared with healthy control subjects. Kaur et al. (20) studied 55 constipated subjects and 99 incontinent patients. A variety of parameters of the rectoanal inhibitory reflex were studied, including the percentage of sphincter relaxation at each volume. There was no difference in the three groups in the volume of distension required to elicit the rectoanal inhibitory reflex. Greater sphincteric relaxation was seen at each volume in incontinent patients compared with constipated patients. Similarly, other studies have not found significant differences among patients with incontinence, constipation, and normal control subjects with respect to the rectoanal inhibitory reflex. The main role of eliciting the reflex in patients with constipation is to identify those patients with Hirschsprung's disease, which represent a minority of adult patients with chronic constipation.

Hirschsprung's disease is characterized by an absence of ganglion cells in the mucosal and submucosal plexuses. The aganglionic segment may occur for a variable length, at times including the entire colon and rectum. Absence of the RAIR may be the only reliable way of establishing a diagnosis of Hirschsprung's disease, especially in patients with short segment disease (Figure 2.2.3).

In patients with megarectum, sufficient inflation volumes are necessary to elicit the RAIR. In our laboratory, inflation volumes of 180 cubic centimeters are often necessary to elicit the reflex in patients with megarectum. A false-negative reflex may be obtained with low inflation volumes.

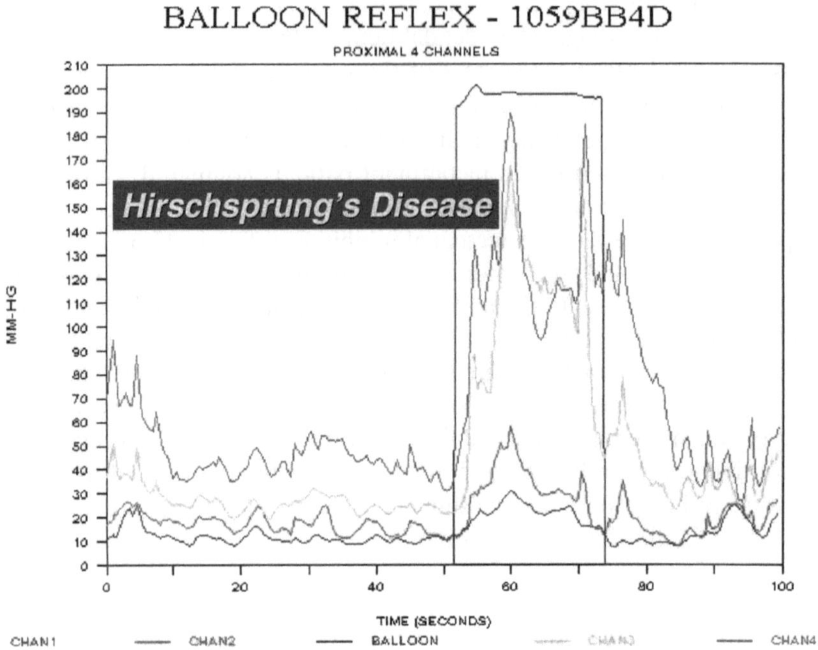

FIGURE 2.2.3. Absence of the RAIR in a patient with Hirschsprung's disease.

RAIR After Pelvic Surgery

The RAIR is generally absent after low anterior resection, coloanal anastomosis, and after ileoanal pouch procedure. Regeneration of the reflex has been demonstrated after both a hand-sewn and stapled anastomosis (7,10). In a study of 46 patients who underwent low anterior resection with stapled anastomosis for carcinoma of the rectum, the reflex was present in 43 preoperatively, but only in eight of 45 patients on the tenth postoperative day (10). Six of 29 patients (21%) studied between six and 12 months after surgery had a RAIR, and the reflex was demonstrated in 17 of 20 patients (85%) studied two years postoperatively. Recovery of anal function after low anterior resection or coloanal anastomosis seems to correlate with recovery of the RAIR. Similarly, in patients who have undergone an ileoanal pouch procedure, the reflex does return with time after operation, and this correlates with the patient's ability to discriminate between feces and flatus (23). In children, the RAIR and continence have been studied in patients with anorectal malformations, particularly high and intermediate imperforate anus, and the presence of the reflex appears to correlate with postoperative continence (24).

Conclusions

The RAIR is a record for the diagnosis of juvenile Hirschprung's disease. Recent analysis of this internal anal sphincter function has shown inherent parametric differences that may subgroup for some patients with fecal incontinence and constipation and that broadly correlates with postoperative functional deficit following low coloanal hand-sutured and stapled anastomosis. At present, it is unknown whether innate differences in preoperative rectoanal inhibition may encode for patients who fare worse following straight coloanal anastomosis and whether these patients may benefit in the short term from colonic pouch reconstruction or coloplasty (25). At present, it also would appear that attempts to use recorded variations in preoperative rectoanal inhibition to assist in decision making and to predict functional outcome in rectal surgery for evacuatory dysfunction have been unsuccessful (26).

References

1. Gowers WR. The automatic action of the sphincter ani. Proc R Soc Lond (Biol). 1877;26:77–84.
2. Denny-Brown D, and Robertson EG. An investigation of the nervous control of defecation. Brain. 1935;58;256–310.
3. Lowry AC, Simmang CL, Boulos P, et al. Consensus statement of definitions for anorectal physiology and rectal cancer. Colorectal Dis. 2001;3:272–5.
4. Duthie, and Bennett RC. The relation of sensation in the anal canal to the functional anal sphincter; a possible factor in anal continence. Gut. 1963; 4:179–82.
5. Miller R, Bartolo DCC, Cervero F, and Mortensen NJM. Anorectal sampling: a comparison of normal and incontinent patients. Br J Surg. 1988;75:44–7.
6. Lubowski DZ, Nicholls RJ, Swash M, and Jordan MJ. Neural control of internal anal sphincter function. Br J Surg. 1987;74:688–90.
7. Lane RH, and Parks AG. Function of the anal sphincters following colo-anal anastomosis. Br J Surg. 1977;64:596–9. Surg. 1980;67:655–7.
8. Williams NS, Price R, and Johnston D. Long term effect of sphincter preserving operations for rectal carcinoma on function of the anal sphincter in man. Br J Surg. 1980;67:203–8.
9. Suzuki H, Matsumoto K, Amano S, Fujioka M, and Honzumi M. Anorectal pressure and rectal compliance after low anterior resection. Br J Surg. 1980; 67:655–7.
10. O'Riordain MG, Molloy RG, Gillen P, Horgan A, and Kirwan WO. Rectoanal inhibitory reflex following low stapled anterior resection of the rectum. Dis Colon Rectum. 1992;35:874–8.
11. O'Kelly TJ. Nerves that say NO: a new perspective on the human rectoanal inhibitory reflex. Ann R Coll Surg Engl. 1996;78:31–8.
12. Rattan S, Sarkar A, and Chakder S. Nitric oxide pathway in rectoanal inhibitory reflex of opossum internal anal sphincter. Gastroenterology. 1992;103:43–50.

13. Coller JA. Clinical application of anorectal manometry. Gastroenterol Clin North Am. 1987;16:17–33.
14. Stein BL, and Roberts PL. Manometry and the rectoanal inhibitory reflex. In: Wexner SD and Bartolo DCC, editors. Constipation: Etiology, evaluation and management. Oxford: Butterworth Heineman; 1995. pp 63–76.
15. Sangwan YP, Coller JA, Barrett RC, Murray JJ, Roberts PL, and Schoetz DJ Jr. Distal rectoanal excitatory reflex: a reliable index of pudendal neuropathy. Dis Colon Rectum. 1995;38:916–20.
16. Sangwan YP,Coller JA, Schoetz DJ Jr, Murray JJ, and Roberts PL. Latency measurement of rectoanal reflexes. Dis Colon Rectum. 199;38:1281–5.
17. Sangwan YP, Coller JA, Schoetz DJ, et al. Spectrum of abnormal rectoanal reflex patterns in patients with fecal incontinence. Dis Colon Rectum. 1996;39:59–65.
18. Sun WM, Read NW, and Donnelly TC. Impaired internal anal sphincter in a subgroup of patients with idiopathic fecal incontinence. Gastroenterology. 1989;97:130–5.
19. Sangwan YP, Coller JA, Barrett RC, Murray JJ, Roberts PL, and Schoetz DJ. Prospective comparative study of abnormal distal rectoanal excitatory reflex, pudendal nerve terminal motor latency, and single fiber density as markers of pudendal neuropathy. Dis Colon Rectum. 1996;39:7894–8.
20. Kaur G, Gardiner A, and Duthie GS. Rectoanal reflex parameters in incontinence and constipation. Dis Colon Rectum. 2002;45:928–33.
21. Kaur G, Gardiner A, Lee PW, Monson JR, and Duthie GS. Increased sensitivity to the recto-anal reflex Is seen in incontinent patients. Colorectal Dis. 1999;Suppl 1:39A–40A.
22. Zbar A, Aslam M, Gold DM, Gatzen C, Gosling A, and Kmiot WA. Parameters of the rectoanal inhibitory reflex in patients with idiopathic fecal incontinence and chronic constipation. Dis Colon Rectum. 1998;41:200–8.
23. Sagar PM, Holdsworth PJ, and Johnston D. Correlation between laboratory findings and clinical outcome after restorative proctocolectomy: serial studies in 20 patients with end-to-end pouch-anal anastomosis. Br J Surg. 1991;78:67–70.
24. Lin CL, and Chen CC. The rectoanal relaxation reflex and continence in repaired anorectal malformations with and without an internal sphincter saving procedure. J Pediatr Surg. 1996;31:630–3.
25. Zbar AP, and Ramesh J. Parameters of the rectoanal inhibitory reflex in different anorectal disorders. Dis Colon Rectum. 2003;46:557–8.
26. Zbar AP, Beer-Gabel M, and Aslam M. Rectoanal inhibition and rectocele. Physiology versus categorization. Int J Colorect Dis. 2001;16:307–12.

Editorial Commentary

The presence of a rectoanal inhibitory reflex (RAIR) has been the hallmark for the exclusion of the diagnosis of Hirschsprung's disease but there is clear evidence that it functions as a subtle anorectal sampling mechanism for flatus/feces differentiation. In this respect, its postoperative return in some discernable form appears to correlate with reported functional improvement after low anterior resection. Moroever, parameter differentiation of its form in some cases, (namely its latency, extent and mode of recovery as well as the presence of rectoanal excitation), although technique dependent, appears to be somewhat disease specific and to offer an explanation for continence maintenance in patients who exhibit sphincter defects. It is unknown at present whether these parameters can preoperatively predict for patients likely to fare badly after procedures which involve prolonged endoanal distraction, deliberate internal anal sphincterotomy (or sphincter ablation) or after straight coloanal anastomosis. What is clear is that there is a recentralization of the importance of the internal anal sphincter in continence maintenance and for its protection where possible in endoanal surgery.

AZ

Chapter 2.3
Vectorvolume Manometry

Andrew P. Zbar

Introduction

Longitudinal pressure profilometry is part of standard practice in urodynamics (1) and in the assessment of the lower esophageal sphincter (2,3), however, its use in the anal canal has been comparatively limited (4). Although combined radial and longitudinal pressures in the anal canal using a pull-through catheter (or automated pull-through) technique have been described (5–7), the value of added three-dimensional (3D) computer-generated sphincter maps in clinical anorectal practice remains unclear (8,9). Few comparisons have actually been performed between computerized and conventional station pull-through anal manometry in health and disease (10). This chapter reviews the physical principles of vectorvolume manometry of the anal canal and available results in the normal anal canal and in different anorectal conditions, offering a personal view concerning its role in coloproctological practice.

The Physical Principles and Analysis of Vectorvolumetry

The variations recorded in radial pressure measurement within the anal canal across the length of functional sphincter represent the summated effects of overlapping internal/external anal sphincters (11,12), and it is difficult to allocate individual components of the anorectal pressure profile to specific correlative anatomical parts (13). Longitudinal pressure asymmetry across the anal canal was first recorded by Taylor and colleagues using a sliding double-lumen catheter, permitting the simultaneous measurement of radial and longitudinal pressures originally designed for use in patients with varying anal sphincter lengths on conventional station technology in men and women (5).

In standard anorectal laboratories, a rough estimation of the anal canal length is made based on the distal extent of recorded pressures and the recognition of the proximal rectal recording as an estimate of canal disposition, usually employing 4-quadrant pressure profiling with delineation of the high-pressure zone (HPZ) length at rest (and during maximal squeeze). This HPZ length is defined as the length of the sphincter where pressures exceed 50% of the maximal pressure recorded, either at rest or during sustained squeeze (14). These estimates are at best crude, providing a sense of median physiological sphincter length and an impression of asymmetry that differs between the sexes in the proximal anal canal and that influences the interpretation of functional anteroanal sphincter defects of clinical importance in patients presenting with postobstetric fecal incontinence (15–17).

The recent introduction of an automated rapid pull-through method for conduct of standardized anorectal manometry minimizes the effect of variations in functional anal sphincter length that otherwise would influence their station measurements to an intrarectal pressure reference of zero (18,19). In vectorvolumetry, the catheter has at least eight radially disposed channels for sectorial averaging where the more lumina used, the more data points obtained during catheter withdrawal and the less mathematical interpolation required by the computer program needed to create a vectorgram. The computer software transfers the data obtained from each catheter into a 3D triplet of coordinates dependent upon the axial position of the probe via vector calculation (Figure 2.3.1).

Here, the x and y coordinates are measured at an angulation away from the center of the anal canal with the z axis point determined vertically from the axial position of the probe. For any given pressure point, a sector pressure polygon results that corresponds to the vector volume where:

$$\text{Vector volume (V V)} = \sum_{i=1}^{8} \text{d.sin}\,(45)\{P_1P_2 + P_2P_3 + P_3P_4 + \ldots P_8P_1\}$$

where I = the level above the anal verge (with recordable pressures), d = the distance between station measurements and P doublets of pressure are the pressure vectors for each sector wedge (Figure 2.3.1). The volume recorded has no parameters as such, representing the total integration of vector polygons given the speed of catheter withdrawal. The personal computer (PC) is interfaced with a high-resolution color monitor equipped with a graded palette for construction of a color-coded vectorgram where sampling occurs at a frequency of 100 hertz (Hz). (For an average sphincter length at a withdrawal speed of one centimeter sec^{-1}, there are an average of 15000 data points) (10,20). Smoothing vectography is then provided by spline–curve interpolation for screen rotation, creating semiquantitative analysis vectography where indentations represent increases in the overall pressure profile (21).

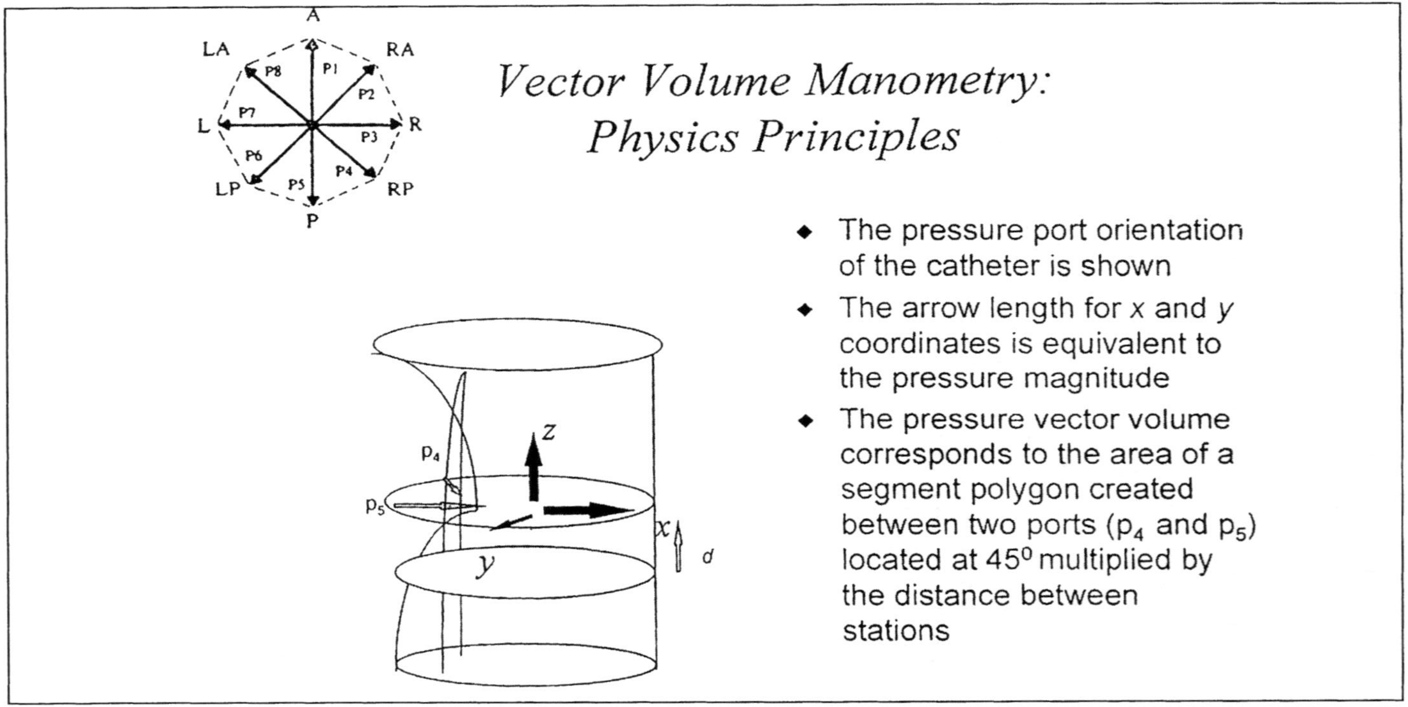

FIGURE 2.3.1. The physical principles of vectorvolume manometry. An eight-channel radially disposed polyethylene catheter is used. At a constant rate of withdrawal this provides sector polygons of summated pressure at 45-degree angles that are integrated to create a vectorvolume measurement and vector diagram by point interpretation. (This diagram is reproduced from Zbar AP, Aslam M, Hider A, Toomey P, and Kmiot WA. Comparison of vector volume manometry with conventional manometry in anorectal dysfunction. Tech Coloproctol. 1998;2:84–90, page 85, with permission from Springer-Verlag, London).

Anal Vectorgraphy in Health and Disease

Work from our group has compared conventional and vectorvolume manometry in normal patients, those with passive fecal incontinence, patients with full-thickness rectal prolapse, and patients with chronic anal fissure (10). Vector manometry was performed in this study as described by Coller et al. (12), utilizing automated pull-through with a custom-made puller (ICSMT [Imperial College School of Medicine and Technology], Hammersmith Hospital Bioengineering, London) and an eight-channel polyethylene catheter with radially disposed ports at 45-degree angles, 4.8 millimeters in diameter (Arndorfer Inc., Greenvale, WI) utilizing data acquisition with Polygram ™ Lower GI edition software (5.05 C4 Version, Synectics Medical Inc., Irving TX).

Parameters measured included mean resting vector volume (MR V V), mean squeeze vector volume (MS V V), HPZ length (rest and squeeze), maximal pressure at rest (MPR), maximal pressure during sustained squeeze (MPS), and percentage asymmetry (rest and squeeze) with manometric runs recorded three times using a mean value for each analysis. The percentage asymmetry of the sphincter was defined as the percent derivation of integrated cross-sections from a perfect circle. Sectorial pressures were reported for pooled analysis, creating left, right, posterior, and anterior mean pressures. Statistical analysis was determined using one-way analysis of variance (ANOVA), where normality of residuals was determined by the Shapiro–Francia test and using the Kruskal–Wallis test for nonparametric data with geometric means ± 95% confidence interval (CI) for log-transformed data, medians and interquartile ranges (IQRs) for non-transformable data, and Pearson's correlation for comparisons.

Normal controls were age-matched where possible with the incontinent and rectal prolapse groups. (Normals mean age 58.9 years, range 29 to 86 years; Incontinent mean 50.4 years, range 22 to 90 years; Chronic Anal Fissure mean 36.2 years, range 22 to 58 years). Tables 2.3-1 and 2.3-2 show the geometric means, medians, and IQR values for all variables of the different groups. As expected, significant differences are evident for maximal resting anal pressure (MRAP) between normal and incontinent patients and with chronic fissure cases, with similar trends of differences in maximal squeeze pressure (MSP) comparing normal controls with incontinent and prolapse patients. These changes are reflected in MRV V where the trends mirror the resting changes between groups using conventional anorectal manometry. Equally, the MS V V differed significantly between incontinent and normal patients with similar differences in recorded MPS values between normal and fissure patients, showing a trend that mirrored the squeeze data in the different subgroups using conventional manometric techniques. In general, MPR values tended to exceed MRAP pressures, with MPS values tending to be, on average, lower than MSP measurements. The explanation for the difference between MPR and MRAP may be that the movement (withdrawal) of the catheter evokes some voluntary reflex

TABLE 2.3-1. A geometric means and 95% confidence intervals for measured variables in the different patient groups.

Variable	Incontinent Geometric mean (CI)*	Prolapse Geometric mean (CI)	Normal Geometric mean (CI)	Fissure Geometric mean (CI)
MSP	114.5[1] (102.4, 128.0)	146.4[5] (124.9, 171.6)	203.9 (171.6, 242.3)	232.8 (184.1, 294.4)
MRW	5787[2] (4006, 8358)	14814 (8127, 27005)	11890 (7152, 19767)	39066[4] (25116, 60764)
% Asymetry (Rest)	34.92 (32.15, 37.92)	32.83 (29.77, 36.19)	31.10 (27.90, 34.70)	31.20 (27.12, 35.89)
% Asymetry (Squeeze)	30.36 (27.73, 33.25)	27.64 (24.68, 30.95)	28.63 (25.46, 32.20)	30.19 (25.20, 36.16)
HPZ length (Squeeze)	16.65 (15.02, 18.46)	16.79 (13.96, 20.16)	15.91 (13.10, 19.33)	17.17 (14.14, 20.85)
MPR	49.20[2] (42.81, 56.55)	70.35 (55.77, 88.76)	68.69 (54.79, 86.12)	127.6[3] (110.3, 147.6)
MPS	76.6[1] (67.6, 86.8)	96.2 (81.0, 114.4)	121.3 (94.7, 155.4)	173.3 (139.4, 215.5)

* CI = Confidence Intervals.
[1] Normal vs Incontinent, $p < 0.001$; [2] Normal vs Incontinent, $p < 0.01$; [3] Normal vs Fissure, $p < 0.001$; [4] Normal vs Fissure, $p < 0.01$; [5] Normal vs Prolapse, $p < 0.01$; MRAP, Maximal resting anal pressure as recorded by conventional manometry (mm Hg); MSP, Maximal squeeze pressure as recorded by conventional manometry (mm Hg); MR V V, Mean resting vectorvolume; MS V V, Mean squeeze vector volume; HPZ(r), High-pressure zone length at rest (cm); HPZ(s), High-pressure zone length during sustained squeeze (cm); MPR, Mean pressure at rest as calculated by vector manometry (mm Hg); MPS, Mean pressure during sustained squeeze as calculated by vector manometry (mm Hg).
Reproduced from Zbor AP, Aslam M, Hider A, Toomey P, and Kmiot WA. Comparison of vector volume manometry with conventional manometry in anorectal dysfunction. Tech Coloproctol. 1998; 2: 84–90, page 86, with permission from Springer-Verlag, London.

sphincter [external anal sphincter (EAS)] contraction and a response to perfusate leakage, whereas the meaning of the latter finding may be that the sustained squeeze required for generation of the MPS is more difficult in some cases where the squeeze command may be met with buttock clenching and thigh contractions rather than a sustained EAS squeeze of acceptable duration. This phenomenon of poor squeeze duration has been found in some neurological disorders such as Parkinson's disease (22), where the phenomenon of squeeze index (area under the squeeze curve) appears to be reduced (23). No basic differences were detected in HPZ lengths or percentage asymmetry at rest or during sustained squeeze between the major patient groups.

Sectorial resting and squeeze differences are shown respectively in tabulated form (Tables 2.3-3 and 2.3-4) and graphically (Figures 2.3.2 and 2.3.3) with an ordering from incontinent → prolapse → normal → fissure, although there is a substantial CI overlap between groups. There was no evidence of inherent sectorial differences for different anorectal conditions

TABLE 2.3-2. Medians and interquartile ranges for variables in the different patient groups.

Variable	Incontinent median (IQR)*	Prolapse median (IQR)	Normal median (IQR)	Fissure median (IQR)
MRAP	40[1] (30, 60)	55 (40, 90)	60 (46, 80)	85[4] (76.25, 90)
MS V V	1633[2] (8753, 40700)	21015 (9818, 95203)	52622 (13291, 91531)	90175 (33098, 198800)
HPZ length (Rest)	14 (11, 17)	13.5 (10.5, 20)	12 (9.5, 28)	14 (12, 16.25)

* I.Q.R. = Interquartile Range.

[1] Normal vs Incontinent, $p < 0.001$; [2] Normal vs Incontinent $p < 0.01$; [4] Normal vs Fissure, $p < 0.01$.

MRAP, Maximal resting anal pressure as recorded by conventional manometry (mm Hg); MSP, Maximal squeeze pressure as recorded by conventional manometry (mm Hg); MR V V, Mean resting vector voiume; MS V V, Mean squeeze vector volume; HPZ(r), High-pressure zone length at rest (cm); HPZ(s), High-pressure zone length during sustained squeeze (cm); MPR, Mean pressure at rest as calculated by vector manometry (mm Hg); MPS, Mean pressure during sustained squeeze as calculated by vector manometry (mm Hg).

Reproduced from Zbar AP, Aslam M, Hider A, Toomey P, and Kmiot, WA. Comparison of vector volume manometry with conventional manometry in anorectal dysfunction. Tech Coloproctol. 1998; 2: 84–90, page 86, with permission from Springer-Verlag, London.

at rest or during squeeze, although there was a trend towards higher anterior sector pressures in the fissure patients. These variations in sectorial pressure differences detected by vectography in incontinence and fissure patients have been shown by others (24–26). In chronic anal fissure, for example, relative anal sphincter hypertonia appears to be global. Our study also appears to confirm a general reduction in maximal squeeze variables

TABLE 2.3-3. Means and 95% confidence intervals by group and sector at rest as determined by vector manometry.

Group	Sector Pressures (mm Hg)			
	Anterior mean (CI)	Right lateral mean (CI)	Posterior mean (CI)	Left lateral mean (CI)
Incontinent	24.2 (20.2, 28.1)	19.3 (15.4, 23.2)	22.8 (18.9, 26.8)	23.6 (19.7, 27.5)
Prolapse	34.9 (28.6, 41.2)	28.3 (22.0, 34.6)	31.9 (25.6, 38.2)	35.7 (29.4, 41.9)
Normal	29.8 (23.2, 36.4)	27.6 (21.0, 34.2)	28.2 (21.6, 34.9)	31.1 (24.5, 37.8)
Fissure	48.3 (41.1, 55.5)	41.7 (34.5, 48.9)	45.3 (38.2, 52.5)	47.0 (39.8, 54.2)

Reproduced from Zbar AP, Aslam M, Hider A, Toomey P, Kmiot WA. Comparison of vector volume manometry with conventional manometry in anorectal dysfunction. Tech Coloproctol. 1998; 2: 84–90, page 87, with permission from Springer-Verlag, London.

TABLE 2.3-4. Means and 95% confidence intervais by group and sector during sustained squeeze as determined by vector manometry.

Group	Sector pressures (mm Hg)			
	Anterior mean (CI)	Right lateral mean (CI)	Posterior mean (CI)	Left lateral mean (CI)
Incontinent	36.1 (31.2, 41.1)	30.5 (25.5, 35.4)	34.8 (29.9, 39.8)	35.9 (31.0, 40.9)
Prolapse	45.5 (37.4, 53.5)	38.3 (30.3, 46.4)	44.2 (36.2, 52.3)	45.2 (37.2, 53.3)
Normal	48.7 (40.5, 56.9)	46.5 (38.3, 54.8)	48.3 (40.0, 56.5)	52.9 (44.7, 61.1)
Fissure	60.6 (51.4, 69.8)	52.1 (42.9, 61.3)	61.0 (51.8, 70.2)	62.5 (53.3, 71.7)

Reproduced from Zbar AP, Aslam M, Hider A, Toomey P, Kmiot WA. Comparison of vector volume manometry with conventional manometry in anorectal dysfunction. Tech Coloproctol. 1998; 2: 84–90, page 88, with permission from Springer-Verlag, London.

with age, particularly in the female (27,28), although more work needs to be done to ascertain specific gender and age variables in vector-derived parameters.

Correlation coefficients between conventional and vectorvolumetric manometry are shown in Tables 2.3-5a and 2.3-5b for rest and squeeze. respectively, with a close correlation between the resting variables (MRAP, MPR, and MR V V) and the squeeze parameters (MSP, MPS, and MS V V).

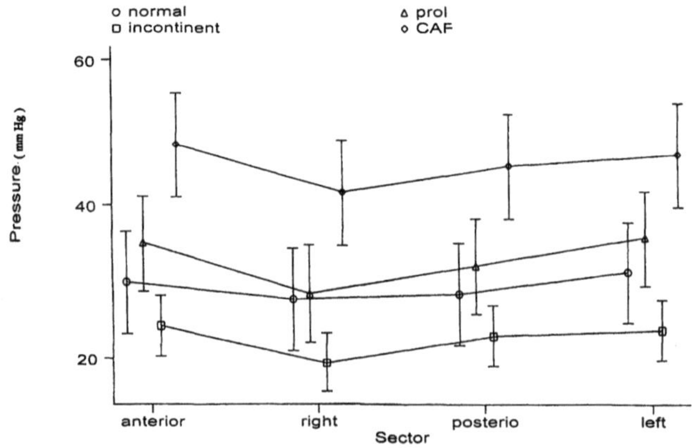

FIGURE 2.3.2. Sectorial pressures *at rest* (means plus 95% confidence intervals) as derived from the vectorvolume manometry program for the different anorectal conditions. (Reproduced from Zbar AP, Aslam M, Hider A, Toomey P, and Kmiot WA. Comparison of vector volume manometry with conventional manometry in anorectal dysfunction. Tech Coloproctol. 1998;2:84–90, page 87, with permission from Springer-Verlag, London).

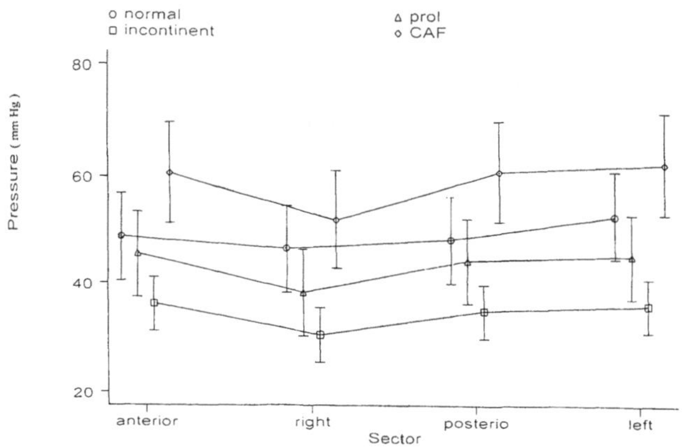

FIGURE 2.3.3. Sectorial pressures *during sustained squeeze* (means plus 95% confidence intervals) as derived from the vectorvolume manometry program for the different anorectal conditions. (Reproduced from Zbar AP, Aslam M, Hider A, Toomey P, and Kmiot WA. Comparison of vector volume manometry with conventional manometry in anorectal dysfunction. Tech Coloproctol. 1998;2:84–90, page 88, with permission from Springer-Verlag, London).

There is also a high resting HPZ length correlation with other vector-derived variables, with somewhat less of a correlation between HPZ length at squeeze and other squeeze vector-calculated parameters. Few studies comparing conventional and vectorvolume manometry are available. There appears to be a close correlation between most of these recorded parameters at rest and during sustained squeeze both in health and disease. No clear correlation was evident from this work (or those of other groups) between sectorial asymmetry and demonstrable sphincter defects, as evident on endoanal ultrasonography (29).

TABLE 2.3-5a. Correlation coefficients (and p values) at rest between vector-derived and conventional manometric measurements.

	MRAP	MR V V	HPZ	MPR
MR V V	0.51 (<0.001)			
hpz(r)	0.17 (0.07)	0.43 (<0.001)		
MPR	0.79 (<0.001)	0.70 (<0.001)	0.19 (0.05)	
%Asymetry	–0.21 (0.027)	–0.24 (0.009)	–0.07 (0.45)	–0.29 (0.003)

TABLE 2.3-5b. Correlation coefficients (and p values) during squeeze between vector-derived and conventional manometric measurements.

	MSP	MS V V	%Asymetry(s)	HPZ(s)
MS V V	0.59 (<0.001)			
%Asymetry(s)	−0.13 (0.18)	−0.24 (0.01)		
HPZ(s)	−0.14 (0.14)	0.26 (0.006)	−0.04 (0.72)	
MPS	0.86 (<0.001)	0.78 (<0.001)	−0.19 (0.05)	−0.11 (0.26)

Reproduced from Zbar A, Aslam M, Hider A, Toomey P, Kmiot WA. Comparison of vector volume manometry with conventional manometry in anorectal dysfunction. Tech Coloproctol. 1998; 2: 84–90, page 88, with permission from Springer-Verlag, London.

Vectormanometry and the Effects of Minor Anorectal Surgery

Few studies have prospectively assessed physiologic function following lateral internal anal sphincterotomy for chronic anal fissure (30–32). In our recent studies, significant differences in vectography have been noted prospectively after lateral internal anal sphincterotomy for percentage resting asymmetry, MR V V, MPR, and HPZ length, as well as for the squeeze variables, MPS and MS V V (33) (Figure 2.3.4). Equally, significant prospective differences have been noted for MPR, MR V V, and MPS between those patients who remained continent after the procedure when compared with those who developed fecal leakage, with significant differences between groups of recordable HPZ length at rest [overall mean preoperative HPZ length = 37.6 millimeters versus mean postoperative HPZ length (incontinent group) = 20.4 millimeters; mean postoperative HPZ length (continent group) = 39.3 millimeters, $P < 0.001$]. Resting asymmetry increased an average of 6.7% after lateral sphincterotomy in those who remained continent compared with a 3.1% fall in the resting asymmetry index in those who became incontinent ($P < 0.001$).

The reasons for impairment of squeeze function, even in those patients who remain continent after lateral sphincterotomy, are unclear. It may be that there are inherent differences in the length of sphincterotomy between these patients, or that there are differences in the mechanism of overall anal

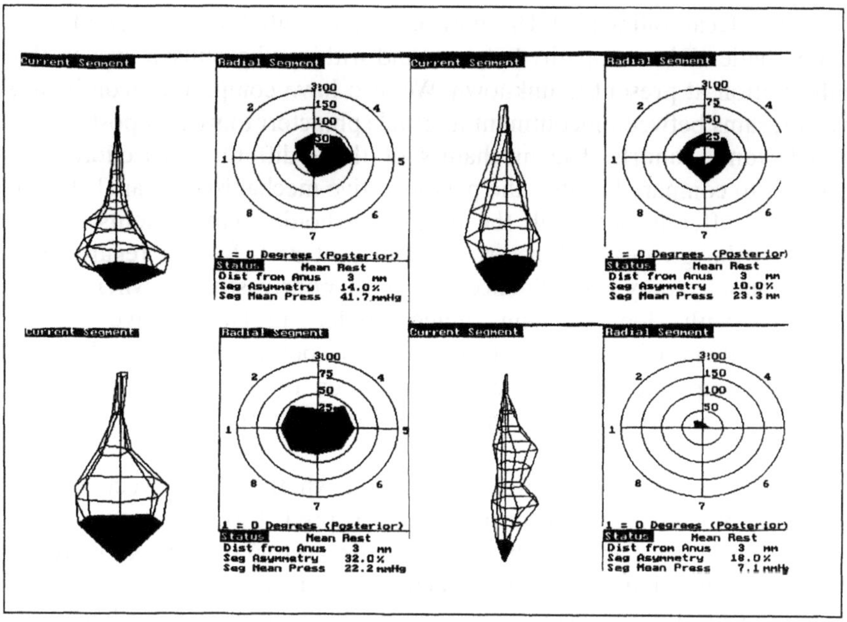

FIGURE 2.3.4. Representative vectorvolumes at rest for patients undergoing lateral internal anal sphincterotomy. Top: Presphincterotomy (left) and postsphincterotomy (right) pattern in a continent patient. Bottom: Presphincterotomy (left) and postsphincterotomy (right) pattern in an incontinent patient. (Reproduced from Zbar AP, Aslam M, and Allgar V. Faecal incontinence after internal sphinctcrotomy for anal fissure. Tech Coloproctol. 2000;4:25–8, with permission from Springer-Verlag, London).

closure (34). There may conceivably be voluntary sphincter reflex activity and fatigue that differs between groups and following operation even in the continent patients after surgery as a herald of impending leakage during the phenomenon of anorectal sampling as contents enter the anal canal following rectal motor activity (35). The causes of postoperative incontinence following this type (and other types) of minor anorectal surgery are, however, multifactorial (36).

The function clearly does not rely entirely on the presence either of an occult preexisting sphincter defect or upon inadvertent intraoperative sphincter injury, for example following hemorrhoidectomy, although these are clearly both important. We have previously shown that chronic anal fissure patients may preoperatively show constitutively shorter subcutaneous EAS lengths that overlap the termination of the internal anal sphincter (IAS) where lateral internal anal sphincterotomy will render the distal anal canal relatively unsupported and that predictably will lead to postoperative fecal soiling (37). This may be supplemented by an inherent associated pudendal neuropathy between and within subgroups; however, this information at present is unknown. We also have compared incontinence vectorgrams between incontinent internal sphincterotomy and posthemorrhoidectomy cohorts. The mechanics of these different procedures are difficult to compare because the postoperative mechanisms of anal closure are very different, although the posthemorrhoidectomy patients appear to show the greatest sphincter asymmetry at rest. In this regard, posthemorrhoidectomy incontinence has been poorly studied where some patients with long-standing hemorrhoidal prolapse have shown substantially impaired anal sphincter pressures before surgery (38,39). This may be compounded by an innate disruption of resting IAS tone during prolonged or excessive endoanal distraction during the procedure (40–42).

It is unclear from our preliminary data whether these vectographic changes noted in specific incontinent cohorts predict for long-term impairment of continence and whether preoperative vectograms are predictive of patients likely to have impaired sphincter function after formal lateral internal sphincterotomy. Recently, because of the concerns regarding post-sphincterotomy functional outcome, there has been a trend towards more tailored (less extensive) internal sphincterotomies in topically resistant chronic anal fissure patients (43–45). Pescatori and colleagues have shown that preoperative manometry can predict some patients who may have poor functional outcomes following standard-length internal sphincterotomy where preoperative normal anal tone (as opposed to hypertonia) may mitigate against standard-length internal sphincter division (46). This issue will only be determined by the conduct of prospective randomized trials to determine if preoperative manometric values (conventional or computerized) define at-risk subgroups for postoperative fecal leakage. Given the anal fissure recidivism rates reported after topical therapies (47), it may well be that the pendulum has swung back towards selective standard (and selective limited) internal sphincterotomy, which may permit the performance of such trials (48).

Conclusions

The role of vectorvolume manometry as part of the routine armamentarium in anorectal physiology for the clinician is unproven. The equipment and software is expensive and not widely available, requiring an automated system of catheter withdrawal, which is an extra expense. Although it has been validated by comparison of resting and squeeze parameters available, its prospective place remains to be determined. It is possible that it may define patients who will benefit from limited sphincterotomy where preoperative values based on sphincter hypertonia may be used in topically resistant chronic anal fissure, where it is known that internal sphincterotomy (particularly in parturient women) may be more extensive than intended (49). With a better definition of the prospective physiologic risk in some patients who present with postobstetric anterior anal fissures, there also will be a more defined role for elective cutaneous advancement anoplasty in this disease (50,51), as well as delineation of subtle and subclinical dysfunction which may predictably respond to directed biofeedback therapies in subgroups left with some forms of incontinence after minor anorectal surgery (52).

References

1. Klopper PJ, de Haas F, and Dijkhuis T. Computerized experimental multichannel urethral pressure profilometry. World J Urol. 1990;8:159–62.
2. Bombeck CT, Vaz O, DeSalvo J, Donahue PE, and Nyhus LM. Computerized axial manometry of the esophagus: a new method for the assessment of antireflux operations. Ann Surg. 1987;206:465–72.
3. Marsh RE, Perdue CL, Awad ZT, Watson P, Selima M, Davis RE, and Filipe CJ. Is analysis of lower esophageal sphincter vector volumes of value in diagnosing gastroesophageal reflux disease? World J Gastroenterol. 2003;9:174–8.
4. Perry RE, Blatchford GJ, Christensen MA, Thorson AG, and Attwood SEA. Manometric diagnosis of anal sphincter injuries. Am J Surg. 1990; 159:112–7.
5. Taylor BM, Beart RW, and Phillips SF. Longitudinal and radial variations of pressure in the human anal sphincter. Gastroenterology. 1984;86:693–7.
6. McHugh SM and Diamant NE. Anal canal pressure profile: a reappraisal as determined by rapid pull-through technique. Gut. 1987;28:1234–41.
7. Williamson JL, Nelson RL, Orsay C, Pearl RK, and Abcarian H. A comparison of simultaneous longitudinal and radial pressure recordings of anal canal pressures. Dis Colon Rectum. 1990;33:201–6.
8. Ho Y-H and Goh HS. Computerized 3-dimensional vector volume analysis—the role of a new method for assessing anal sphincter competence. Ann Acad Med Singapore. 1992;21:263–6.
9. Yang Y-K and Wexner SD. Anal pressure vectography is of no apparent benefit for sphincter evaluation. Int J Colorectal Dis. 1994;9:92–5.
10. Zbar AP, Aslam M, Hider A, Toomey P, and Kmiot WA. Comparison of vector volume manometry with conventional manometry in anorectal dysfunction. Tech Coloproctol. 1998;2:84–90.
11. Hill JR, Kelly ML, Schlegel JF, and Code CF. Pressure profile of the rectum and anus in healthy persons. Dis Colon Rectum. 1960;3:203–9.
12. Coller JA. Clinical application of anorectal manometry. Surg Clin N Am. 1987;16:17–33.
13. Williams AB, Kamm MA, Bartram CI, and Kmiot WA. Gender differences in the longitudinal pressure profile of the anal canal related to anatomical structure as demonstrated on three-dimensional anal sonography. Br J Surg. 2000;87:1674–9. Comments in: Zbar AP, Beer-Gabel M. Br J Surg 2001;88:1015–6.

14. Zbar AP, Aslam M, Gold DM, Gatzen C, Gosling A, and Kmiot WA. Parameters of the rectoanal inhibitory reflex in patients with idiopathic fecal incontinence and chronic constipation. Dis Colon Rectum. 1998;41:200–8.
15. Sultan AH, Kamm MA, Hudson CN, Thomas JM, and Bartram CI. Anal sphincter disruption during vaginal delivery. N Engl J Med. 1993;329:1905–11.
16. Bollard RC, Gardiner A, Phillips K, and Duthie GS. Natural gaps in the female anal sphincter and the risk of post-delivery sphincter injury. Br J Surg. 1999; 86(Suppl 1):50A–1A.
17. Bollard RC, Gardiner A, Duthie GS, and Lindow SW. Anal sphincter injury. Fecal and urinary incontinence: a 34-year followup after forceps delivery. Dis Colon Rectum. 2003;46:1083–8.
18. Coller JA and Sangwan YP. Computerized anal sphincter manometry performance and analysis. In Smith LE, editor. Practical guide to anorectal testing. 2nd ed. New York: Igaku-Shoin; 1995. p. 51–100.
19. Zbar AP and Jonnalagadda R. Parameters of the rectoanal inhibitory reflex in different anorectal disorders. Dis Colon Rectum. 2003;46:557–8.
20. Dijkhuis T, Benidman WA, van der Hulst VPM, and Klopper PJ. Graphical representation of eight-channel pressure profiles on a personal computer. Med Biol Eng Comput. 1990;28:502–4.
21. Waegemaekers CTBJ. Profielmeting van de distale oesophagus sphincter [thesis]. University Amsterdam; 1980.
22. Ashraf W, Pfeiffer RF, and Quigley EMM. Anorectal manometry in the assessment of anorectal function in Parkinson's disease: a comparison with chronic idiopathic constipation. Mov Disord. 1994;6:655–63.
23. Saad LH, Coy CS, Fagundes JJ, Ariyzono MdeL, Shoji N, and Goes JR. Sphincteric function quantification by measuring the capacity to sustain the squeeze pressure of the anal canal. Arq Gastroenterol. 2002;39:233–9.
24. Williams N, Barlow J, Hobson A, Scott N, and Irving M. Manometric asymmetry in the anal canal in controls and patients with fecal incontinence. Dis Colon Rectum. 1995;38:1275–80.
25. Williams N, Scott NA, and Irving M. Effect of lateral sphincterotomy on internal anal sphincter function: a computerized vector manometric study. Dis Colon Rectum. 1995;38:700–4.
26. Keck JO, Staniunas RJ, Coller JA, Bennett RC, and Oster ME. Computer-generated profiles of the anal canal in patients with anal fissure, Dis Colon Rectum. 1995;38:72–9.
27. Loening-Baucke V and Annas S. Effect of age and sex on anorectal manometry. Am J Gastroenterol. 1985;80:50–3.
28. Bannister JJ, Abouzekry L, and Read NW. Effect of ageing on anorectal function. Gut. 1987;28:353–7.
29. Braun JC, Trentner KH, Dreuw B, Klimaszewski M, and Schumpelick V. Vector manometry for differential diagnosis of faecal incontinence. Dis Colon Rectum. 1994;37:989–96.
30. Melange M, Colin JF, Van Wyersch T, and Vanheuverzwyn R. Anal fissure: correlations between symptoms and manometry before and after surgery. Int J Colorectal Dis. 1992;7:108–11.
31. Xynos E, Tzotzinis A, Chrystos E, Tsovaras G, and Vassiakis JS. Anal manometry in patients with fissure in ano before and after internal sphincterotomy. Int J Colorectal Dis. 1993;8:125–8.

32. Garciá-Aguilar J, Belmonte Montes C, Perez JJ, Jensen L, Madoff RD, and Wong WD. Incontinence after lateral internal sphincterotomy – anatomical and functional evaluation. Dis Colon Rectum. 1998;41:423–7.
33. Zbar AP, Aslma M, and Allgar V. Faecal incontinence after internal sphincterotomy for anal fissure. Tech Coloproctol. 2000;4:25–8.
34. Gibbons CP, Trowbridge EA, Bannister JJ, and Read NW. Role of anal cushions in maintaining continence. Lancet. 1986;I:886–7.
35. Miller R, Bartolo DCC, Cervero F, and Mortensen NJM. Anorectal sampling: a comparison of normal and incontinent patients. Br J Surg. 1988;75:44–7.
36. Zbar AP, Beer-Gabel M, Chiappa AC, and Aslam M. Fecal incontinence after minor anorectal surgery. Dis Colon Rectum. 2001;44:1610–23.
37. Zbar AP, Kmiot WA, Aslam M, Williams A, Hider A, Audisio RA, Chiappa A, and deSouza NM. Use of vector volume manometry and endoanal magnetic resonance imaging in the adult female for assessment of anal sphincter dysfunction. Dis Colon Rectum. 1999;42:1411–8.
38. Bruck CE, Lubowski DZ, and King DW. Do patients with haemorrhoids have pelvic floor denervation? Int J Colorectal Dis. 1988;3:210–4.
39. Ho Y-H, Seow-Choen F, and Goh HS. Haemorrhoidectomy and disordered rectal and anal physiology in patients with prolapsed haemorrhoids. Br J Surg. 1995;82:596–8.
40. Leong AF, Husain MJ, Seow-Choen F, and Goh HS. Performing internal sphincterotomy with other anorectal procedures. Dis Colon Rectum. 1994;37:1130–2.
41. Ho Y-H and Tan M. Ambulatory anorectal manometric findings in patients before and after haemorrhoidectomy. Int J Colorectal Dis. 1997;12:296–7.
42. Abbasakoor F, Nelson M, Beynon J, Patel B, and Carr ND. Anal endosonography in patients with anorectal symptoms after haemorrhoidectomy. Br J Surg. 1998;85:1522–4.
43. Littlejohn DRG and Newstead GL. Tailored lateral sphincterotomy for anal fissure. Dis Colon Rectum. 1997;40:1439–42.
44. Hussein AM, Shehata MAS, Zaki Y, and El Seweify MEA. Computerized anal vector manometric analysis in patients treated by tailored lateral sphincterotomy for anal fissure. Tech Coloproctol. 2000;4:143–9.
45. Garcea G, Sutton C, Mansoori S, Lloyd T, and Thomas M. Results following conservative lateral sphincterotomy for the treatment of chronic anal fissures. Colorectal Dis. 2003;5:311–4.
46. Pescatori M, Maria G, and Anastasio G. "Spasm related" internal sphincterotomy in treatment of anal fissure. A randomized prospective study. Coloproctology. 1991;1:20–2.
47. Richard CS, Gregoire R, Plewes EA, et al. Internal sphincterotomy is superior to topical nitroglycerin in the treatment of chronic anal fissure: results of a randomized controlled trial by the Canadian Colorectal Surgical Trials Group. Dis Colon Rectum. 2000;43:1048–58.
48. Zbar AP and Beer-Gabel M. Tailored sphincterotomy or fissurectomy and anoplasty. Authors reply. Dis Colon Rectum. 2002;45:1564.
49. Sultan AH, Kamm MA, Nicholls RJ, and Bartram CI. Prospective study of the extent of internal anal sphincter division during lateral sphincterotomy. Dis Colon Rectum. 1994;37:1031–3.

50. Corby H, Donnelly VS, O'Herlihy C, and O'Connell PR. Anal canal pressures are low in women with postpartum anal fissure. Br J Surg. 1997;84:86–8.
51. Kenefick NJ, Gee AS, and Durdey P. Treatment of resistant anal fissure with advancement anoplasty. Colorectal Dis. 2002;4:463–6.
52. Pucciani F, Rottoli ML, Bologna A, Cianchi F, Forconi S, Cutellè M, and Cortesini C. Pelvic floor dyssynergia and bimodal rehabilitation: results of combined pelviperineal kinesitherapy and biofeedback training. Int J Colorectal Dis. 1998;13:124–30.

Chapter 2.4
Clinical Rectal Compliance Measurement

Robert D. Madoff and Andrew A. Shelton

In order to maintain anal continence, the resistive forces of the anal sphincter must counteract the forces that promote fecal expulsion, including gravity and rectal contractility. Considerable work has been done to elucidate the physiology of anal sphincter function, but far less is understood about normal and abnormal rectal function.

It is widely believed that the rectum serves as a reservoir capable, under normal conditions, of comfortably storing stool until voluntary evacuation is effected. Indeed, the rectum responds to filling by visceral relaxation to accommodate the fecal load (1). Indirect evidence for an advantageous effect of a storage reservoir may be inferred from 1. the absolute need to create a pouch reservoir to avoid incontinence after an ileoanal anastomosis, and 2. the relatively superior function of colon J-pouches and coloplasty reservoirs (as compared with straight coloanal anastomoses) (2–4).

However, if rectal distensibility is universally agreed to be a good thing, there is considerably less agreement on exactly how it should be measured. For the most part, investigators have sought, through a variety of techniques, to determine rectal compliance, defined as the change in rectal volume (or cross-sectional area) per unit change in rectal pressure. It can be seen from this definition that highly compliant rectums distend readily with filling, resulting in little change in rectal pressure; conversely, noncompliant rectums accommodate volume poorly, causing intrarectal pressure to rise substantially. Compliance has been measured in order to describe rectal function in irritable bowel syndrome (5,6), in neurologic disorders (7,8), and after pelvic irradiation (9–11). The effect of surgery on rectal compliance also has been studied after low anterior resection (12), hysterectomy (13), and Delorme's prolapse repair (14). Age and gender differences have been noted in rectal compliance determinations (15). Rectal compliance has been reported to be diminished in patients with fecal incontinence (16).

This clinical approach should be read in conjunction with the chapter on the biomechanical properties of rectal distension [Chapter 2.5(i)] and that on the research laboratory use of impedance planimetry [Chapter 2.5(ii)].

TABLE 2.4-1. Normal rectal compliance.

First author, year (Ref. no.)	Compliance (mL/cm H_2O)
Suzuki, 1982 (39)	15.7
Varma, 1985 (11)	9.0
Roe, 1986 (40)	5.1
Pedersen, 1986 (41)	12.0
Oettle, 1986 (42)	4.5
Rao, 1987 (31)	11.5
Allan, 1987 (43)	5.9
Prior, 1990 (6)	7.3
Sorensen, 1992 (15)	17.0
Alstrup, 1995 (17)	6.5
Felt-Bersma, 2000 (32)	7.0*

*mL/mmHg.

The simplest and most popular technique for measuring rectal compliance utilizes a rectal balloon that is serially inflated as rectal pressure is recorded. More recent innovations include the use of impedance planimetry and the barostat. In addition, endorectal ultrasound has been used to determine changes in the rectal cross-sectional area (17), but these techniques are still somewhat experimental and have not yet gained clinical popularity.

A number of criticisms have been leveled against the current clinical measures of compliance, particularly the balloon inflation technique, which is both technique- and operator-dependent (18). As a practical matter, published compliance values measured in healthy individuals vary as much as 4-fold, a fact that suggests a lack of standardization of technique or of interpretation (Table 2.4-1). Some factors that can influence compliance measurement include the size and nature of the balloon or bag used for inflation (19,20), the type of distension (ramp vs. step) (19,21), the speed of inflation (21,22), and the distending medium (air vs. water) (21). Other potential sources of variability include the feeding status of the patient (fed vs. fasted), the use of cleansing enemas prior to testing, the use of sedation, and the presence or absence of associated discomfort during the procedure (21).

One important area of concern is that a single number cannot accurately describe a nonlinear pressure–volume curve. Even for a given patient, the measured compliance would depend entirely on the region of the curve selected, namely, the steep upslope, the flat mid-portion, or the slope of the median trend-line through the curve (23).

In addition to practical problems, a number of theoretical concerns have been raised regarding determination of compliance based upon pressure–volume determinations (18):

A primary concern is that the technique models the rectum as a closed, rather than an open-ended, cylinder [See Chapter 2.5(ii)]. A balloon is required to prevent reflux of the distending medium into the sigmoid colon. In practice, this technique defines the top of the rectum as the proximal limit of the balloon's axial expansion. Accordingly, balloons of different shapes and sizes result in different measured compliance values (Figure 2.4.1). Indeed, a lead pipe would appear to be highly compliant if a balloon with unlimited axial expansion were used for the test. Krogh et al. demonstrated experimentally that coiling and elongation of compliant rectal balloons were a major source of error in the determination of rectal pressure–volume curves (19). Compliance may be measured more accurately by using a technique such as impedance planimetry, which relies on determination of the rectal cross-sectional area rather than volume (24,25). Alternatively, compliance may be determined by using an inflatable bag secured at either end on a catheter to preclude axial expansion or linear extrusion. Krogh et al. demonstrated that compliance determined by either impedance planimetry or an inflatable bag is more reproducible, as compared with a compliant rectal balloon (19).

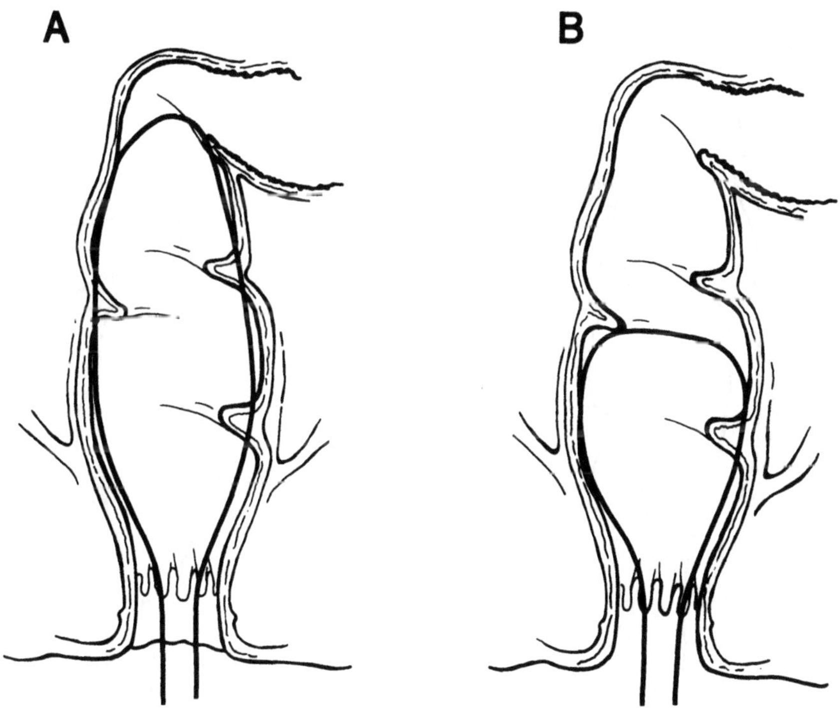

FIGURE 2.4.1. Effect of rectal balloon axial distension on measured rectal compliance. Even if rectums (A) and (B) are mechanically identical, measured compliance in (A) will be greater. Reproduced from Madoff RD, Orrom WJ, Rothenberger DA, and Goldberg SM. Rectal compliance: a critical reappraisal. Int J Colorectal Dis. 1990;5:37–40, page 38, with permission from Springer-Verlag Berlin.

Another concern is that rectal pressure/volume determinations take no account of rectal size. A very large rectum would require a very large infusion volume to initiate rectal wall distension; "normal" volumes would effect no change in pressure and compliance would appear to be high. Conversely, a small rectum would rapidly reach the limit of its physiologic range and would appear to be "noncompliant" in standard testing (Figure 2.4.2). For example, patients with acquired megacolon have high measured rectal compliance (26), a finding seemingly at odds with the thick-walled rectum encountered in this disease. This discrepancy can be explained by the failure to differentiate between rectal capacity and rectal compliance. This problem has been addressed in the lung by pulmonary physiologists, who calculated "specific compliance" normalized to resting lung volume (27). However, this approach has not been adopted by anorectal physiologists. Similarly, colonic J-pouches and coloplasty reconstructions have function superior to that of straight coloanal anastomoses, an observation that has been attributed to

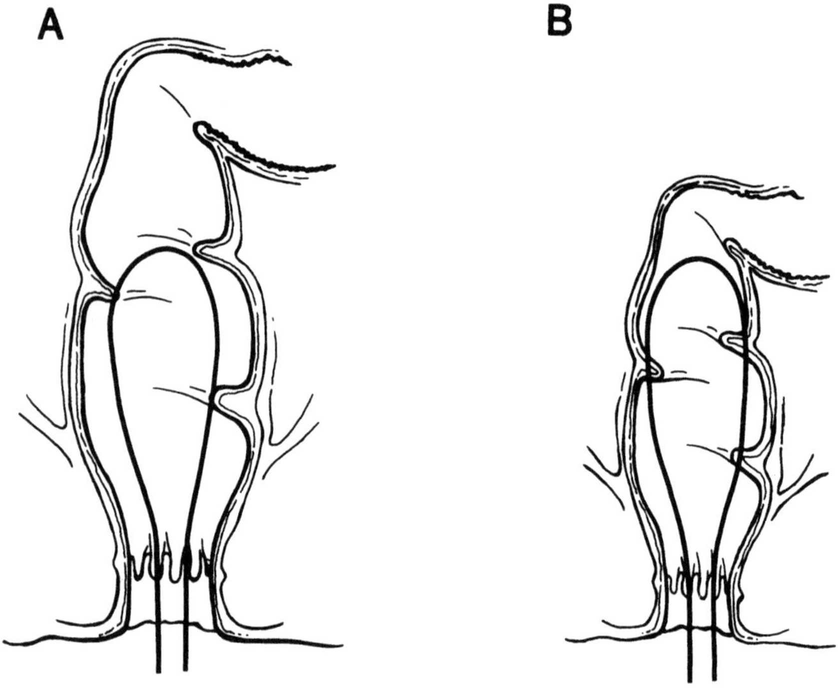

FIGURE 2.4.2. Effect of rectal size on measured rectal compliance. Regardless of its wall stiffness, rectum (A) will have a higher measured compliance than (B). Reproduced from Madoff RD, Orrom WJ, Rothenberger DA, and Goldberg SM. Rectal compliance: a critical reappraisal. Int J Colorectal Dis. 1990;5:37–40, page 38, with permission from Springer-Verlag, Berlin.

improved neorectal compliance (4,28). At least part of the observed improvement is likely due to increased neorectal capacity.

A third concern is that rectal pressure/volume determinations do not account for the contribution of extrarectal tissues. The rectum resides in the bony pelvis surrounded by soft tissue structures. The size of the pelvis and the nature of the surrounding tissue could quite possibly affect rectal compliance measurement. Indeed, in an animal model, the measured compliance of ileal pouches was significantly different when determined in vivo and ex vivo (29).

Still another concern is that the relative contribution of smooth muscle tone to overall compliance is variable and uncertain. No consensus has been reached as to whether compliance is a mechanical property of the rectal wall itself or whether it is the functional sum of both mechanical (passive) and contractile muscle (active) elements. In healthy individuals, substantial differences in rectal compliance measured on different days have been attributed to variability in rectal tone (19). Rapid colonic distension decreases measured compliance by activating neural reflexes (30) and the administration of clonidine (an α_2-agonist) increases colonic compliance.

Alterations in compliance also have been noted within individuals depending on disease status. Rao et al. (31) demonstrated a decrease in rectal compliance in patients with active ulcerative colitis, where compliance normalized when the colitis was in remission. Decreased compliance also has been noted in the presence of rectal inflammation by other investigators (32,33). Again, Rao et al. (31) have demonstrated that the increase in rectal reactivity (pressure increase in response to distension) was higher in patients with active colitis when compared with healthy controls or with patients with quiescent disease. Therefore, abnormal compliance in patients with colitis may be due to reversible increases in rectal tone and spasticity, rather than to fixed alterations in the substance of the rectal wall. This hypothesis is supported by work in our laboratory, where our group has demonstrated a decrease in rectal compliance, as determined in vivo in patients with active inflammatory bowel disease; however, resected rectal specimens from these same patients showed similar tissue elasticity (18).

Rao et al. (22,23) have emphasized the stress–strain relationship rather than compliance in evaluating rectal wall stiffness. Here, stress is defined as force per unit of the cross-sectional area. Strain is defined as deformation produced by the stress. In the case of the rectum, strain can be defined as the ratio of change in the circumference to the original circumference; this relationship can be simplified to the ratio of change in radius to the original radius. A stress–strain curve is then plotted and the rectal wall stiffness is determined by calculating the slope of the tangent to this curve at various strain levels [incremental elastic modulus (IEM)]. The series elastic component (SEC), a measure of the viscous and elastic properties of the rectal wall in the absence of active muscle contraction, also can be determined.

Rao et al. (22) compared IEM and rectal compliance determinations in a series of healthy volunteers. They used a balloon catheter for rectal distension and an endorectal ultrasound transducer to evaluate changes in rectal diameter. Both IEM and SEC were highly reproducible. Incremental elastic modulus had a linear relationship with strain, but compliance did not, with SEC varying inversely with the rate of rectal inflation, suggesting a greater contribution of muscle contraction at higher rates. This group concluded that IEM (or more correctly, the slope of the IEM vs. strain curve) would be a more ideal measure of rectal viscoelasticity. Furthermore, they noted that because impedance planimetry simultaneously measures both rectal pressure and radius, it would lend itself well to clinical IEM determination [See Chapter 2.5(ii)].

The barostat has been used increasingly to investigate rectal compliance. This device maintains a constant pressure in the rectum by varying rectal volume through a feedback mechanism. Recommendations for standardized barostat testing procedures have been published, but they have not yet gained universal acceptance (21). Barostat-determined compliance is higher in men than in women (34) and does not appear to be affected by age (35). Barostat bag volumes decrease after meals (35), suggesting an increase in rectal tone and a decrease in compliance. Increased body mass index decreases compliance (36), an effect presumed to be due to elevated intra-abdominal pressure that is transmitted to the pelvis. Barostat studies have shown normal compliance in incontinent patients (36) and in women with obstructed defecation (37), but decreased compliance in patients with irritable bowel syndrome (38). However, those results must be accepted with caution because confirmatory studies from different laboratories have yet to be carried out.

Conclusions

The concept of rectal compliance as a determining factor for rectal function is appealing. However, several important obstacles must be overcome. First, consensus must be reached on what the term "compliance" means; is it a measure of the viscoelastic properties of the rectal wall, or does it refer to the active and passive elements that define distensibility of an innervated, muscular organ? Second, the overlapping effects of rectal compliance and rectal capacity need to be sorted out. Third, agreement is needed as to the correct technique to measure compliance, and standardized equipment and protocols must be adopted. Once these steps have been taken, we will be in a better position to understand exactly how compliance affects rectal behavior, both in health and in disease.

References

1. Duthie HL. Dynamics of the rectum and anus. Clin Gastroenterol. 1975; 4:467–77.
2. Hallbook O, Pahlman L, Krog M, Wexner SD, and Sjodahl R. Randomized comparison of straight and colonic J pouch anastomosis after low anterior resection. Ann Surg. 1996;224:58–65.
3. Ho YH, Tan M, and Seow-Choen F. Prospective randomized controlled study of clinical function and anorectal physiology after low anterior resection: comparison of straight and colonic J pouch anastomoses. Br J Surg. 1996;83:978–80.
4. Mantyh CR, Hull TL, and Fazio VW. Coloplasty in low colorectal anastomosis: manometric and functional comparison with straight and colonic J-pouch anastomosis. Dis Colon Rectum. 2001;44:37–42.
5. Kendall GP, Thompson DG, Day SJ, and Lennard-Jones JE. Inter- and intraindividual variation in pressure-volume relations of the rectum in normal subjects and patients with the irritable bowel syndrome. Gut. 1990;31:1062–8.
6. Prior A, Maxton DG, and Whorwell PJ. Anorectal manometry in irritable bowel syndrome: differences between diarrhea and constipation predominant subjects. Gut. 1990;31:458–462.
7. Sun WM, Read NW, and Donnelly TC. Anorectal function in incontinent patients with cerebrospinal disease. Gastroenterology. 1990;99:1372–9.
8. Nordenbo AM, Andersen JR, and Andersen JT. Disturbances of ano-rectal function in multiple sclerosis. J Neurol. 1996;243:445–51.
9. Yeoh EK, Russo A, Botten R, et al. Acute effects of therapeutic irradiation for prostatic carcinoma on anorectal function. Gut. 1998;43:123–7.
10. Iwamoto T, Nakahara S, Mibu R, Hotokezaka M, Nakano H, and Tanaka M. Effect of radiotherapy on anorectal function in patients with cervical cancer. Dis Colon Rectum. 1997;40:693–7.
11. Varma JS, Smith AN, and Busuttil A. Correlation of clinical and manometric abnormalities of rectal function following chronic radiation injury. Br J Surg. 1985;72:875–8.
12. Suzuki H, Matsumoto K, Amano S, Fujioka M, and Honzumi M. Anorectal pressure and rectal compliance after low anterior resection. Br J Surg. 1980; 67:655–7.
13. Smith AN, Varma JS, Binnie NR, and Papachrysostomou M. Disordered colorectal motility in intractable constipation following hysterectomy. Br J Surg. 1990;77:1361–5.
14. Plusa SM, Charig JA, Balaji V, Watts A, and Thompson MR. Physiological changes after Delorme's procedure for full-thickness rectal prolapse. Br J Surg. 1995;82:1475–8.
15. Sorensen M, Rasmussen OO, Tetzschner T, and Christiansen J. Physiological variation in rectal compliance. Br J Surg. 1992;79:1106–8.
16. Rasmussen O, Christensen B, Sorensen M, Tetzschner T, and Christiansen J. Rectal compliance in the assessment of patients with fecal incontinence. Dis Colon Rectum. 1990;33:650–3.
17. Alstrup NI, Skjoldbye B, Rasmussen OO, Christensen NE, and Christiansen J. Rectal compliance determined by rectal endosonography. A new application of endosonography. Dis Colon Rectum. 1995;38:32–6.

18. Madoff RD, Orrom WJ, Rothenberger DA, and Goldberg SM. Rectal compliance: a critical reappraisal. Int J Colorectal Dis. 1990;5:37–40.
19. Krogh K, Ryhammer AM, Lundby L, Gregersen H, and Laurberg TS. Comparison of methods used for measurement of rectal compliance. Dis Colon Rectum. 2001;44:199–206.
20. Toma TP, Zighelboim J, Phillips SF, and Talley NJ. Methods for studying intestinal sensitivity and compliance: in vitro studies of balloons and a barostat. Neurogastroenterol Motil. 1996;8:19–28.
21. Whitehead WE and Delvaux M. Standardization of barostat procedures for testing smooth muscle tone and sensory thresholds in the gastrointestinal tract. The Working Team of Glaxo-Wellcome Research, UK. Dig Dis Sci. 1997; 42:223–241.
22. Rao GN, Drew PJ, Monson JR, and Duthie GS. Incremental elastic modulus—a challenge to compliance. Int J Colorectal Dis. 1997;12:33–6.
23. Rao GN. Evaluation of rectal dynamics and viscoelasticity in health and disease [MD thesis]. University of Hull; 1998.
24. Gregersen H and Kassab G. Biomechanics of the gastrointestinal tract. Neurogastroenterol Motil. 1996;8:277–97.
25. Dall FH, Jorgensen CS, Houe D, Gregersen H, and Djurhuus JC. Biomechanical wall properties of the human rectum. A study with impedance planimetry. Gut. 1993;34:1581–6.
26. Varma JS and Smith AN. Reproducibility of the proctometrogram. Gut. 1986; 27:288–92.
27. Comroe JH. Physiology of respiration: An introductory text. Chicago (IL): Year Book Medical Publishers; 1974.
28. Hallbook O, Nystrom PO, and Sjodahl R. Physiologic characteristics of straight and colonic J-pouch anastomoses after rectal excision for cancer. Dis Colon Rectum. 1997;40:332–8.
29. Thayer ML, Madoff RD, Jacobs DM, and Bubrick MP. Comparative intrinsic and extrinsic compliance characteristics of S, J, and W ileoanal pouches. Dis Colon Rectum. 1991;34:404–408.
30. Bharucha AE, Hubmayr RD, Ferber IJ, and Zinsmeister AR. Viscoelastic properties of the human colon. Am J Physiol Gastrointest Liver Physiol. 2001;281:G459–66.
31. Rao SS, Read NW, Davison PA, Bannister JJ, and Holdsworth CD. Anorectal sensitivity and responses to rectal distention in patients with ulcerative colitis. Gastroenterology. 1987;93:1270–5.
32. Felt-Bersma RJ, Sloots CE, Poen AC, Cuesta MA, and Meuwissen SG. Rectal compliance as a routine measurement: extreme volumes have direct clinical impact and normal volumes exclude rectum as a problem. Dis Colon Rectum. 2000;43:1732–8.
33. Loening-Baucke V, Metcalf AM, and Shirazi S. Anorectal manometry in active and quiescent ulcerative colitis. Am J Gastroenterol. 1989;84:892–7.
34. Sloots CE, Felt-Bersma RJ, Cuesta MA, and Meuwissen SG. Rectal visceral sensitivity in healthy volunteers: influences of gender, age and methods. Neurogastroenterol Motil. 2000;12:361–8.
35. Lagier E, Delvaux M, Vellas B, et al. Influence of age on rectal tone and sensitivity to distension in healthy subjects. Neurogastroenterol Motil. 1999;11: 101–7.

36. Salvioli B, Bharucha AE, Rath-Harvey D, Pemberton JH, and Phillips SF. Rectal compliance, capacity, and rectoanal sensation in fecal incontinence. Am J Gastroenterol. 2001;96:2158–68.
37. Gosselink MJ, Hop WC, and Schouten WR. Rectal compliance in females with obstructed defecation. Dis Colon Rectum. 2001;44:971–7.
38. Steens J, Van Der Schaar PJ, Penning C, Brussee J, and Masclee AA. Compliance, tone and sensitivity of the rectum in different subtypes of irritable bowel syndrome. Neurogastroenterol Motil. 2002;14:241–7.
39. Suzuki H and Fujioka M. Rectal pressure and rectal compliance in ulcerative colitis. Jpn J Surg. 1982;12:79–81.
40. Roe AM, Bartolo DC, and Mortensen NJ. Diagnosis and surgical management of intractable constipation. Br J Surg. 1986;73:854–61.
41. Pedersen IK, Christiansen J, Hint K, Jensen P, Olsen J, and Mortensen PE. Anorectal function after low anterior resection for carcinoma. Ann Surg. 1986;204:133–5.
42. Oettle GJ and Heaton KW. "Rectal dissatisfaction" in the irritable bowel syndrome. A manometric and radiological study. Int J Colorectal Dis. 1986;1:183–5.
43. Allan A, Ambrose NS, Silverman S, and Keighley MR. Physiological study of pruritus ani. Br J Surg. 1987;74:576–9.

Chapter 2.5(i)
Impedance Planimetry: Application for Studies of Rectal Function

Hans Gregersen

Editorial Commentary

Chapter 2.5 is divided into two main sections: the physical principles of impedance planimetry and the clinical use of this technology in specialized coloproctological practice. The first part of this chapter is written by Professor Hans Gregersen of Denmark, who first described and utilized this technology in a series of animal models; the second part of the chapter is written by Graeme S. Duthie and A.W. Gardiner of the Colorectal Department of Castle Hill Hospital in Hull, United Kingdom, who have some experience with its research and clinical potential. This chapter should be read in conjunction with Chapter 2.4 on Rectal Compliance, by Robert D. Madoff and Andrew A. Shelton. In essence, to maintain its role in continence, the reservoir capacity of the rectum (or the neorectum) is crucial, and although compliance ($\Delta V \div \Delta P$) is infrequently measured in anorectal laboratories, variation in compliance is likely to affect clinical function in such conditions as pouch (ileal or colonic)–anal anastomoses, the post-irradiated anastomosis, and following coloplasty or rectal augmentation procedures. In most anorectal units, compliance in one form or another is performed with an incremental increase in a balloon size for the creation of a proctometrogram, which describes the rheological pressure/volume changes of the rectum during distension (1).

Because of the asymmetry of the rectum and because it is not closed rostrally during distension, there will be variation in reported compliances in the same patient and between patients. The inherent characteristics of the rectum (mega- or microrectum), the deformability of the extrarectal tissues, and the dynamic nature of rectal sensation and accommodation to expanding volumes will equally affect measured compliance (2,3). Alternatives to this approach, such as impedance planimetry, employ more complicated formulae of stress–strain relationships of the rectum (4) for the objective standardization of the viscoelastic properties of the healthy and diseased rectum. This latter approach aims to determine methods of measurement of rectal wall stiffness, usually based on ramp inflation, where biological tissues may be assessed in their departure from the classical engineering stress–strain relationships as described by Hooke and Young for nonbiological materials (5).

The advantage of impedance plainimetry is that it makes the estimation of biomechanical properties of a distensible organ possible at a specific viscus wall circumference that is able to be determined by cross-sectional area measurement (6) based on a physical principle called the field gradient (7). The technique is as yet effectively untested in humans and requires sophisticated software and custom-made measuring devices and impedance detection equipment (8,9). These probes are capable of simultaneously recording in vivo wall thickness and luminal cross-sectional area with changes in electrical impedance (10). Both the physics and the research characteristics of impedance planimetry are presented. Its clinical role remains to be prospectively determined.

AZ

References

1. Madoff RD, Orrom WJ, Rothenberger DA, and Goldberg SM. Rectal compliance: a critical appraisal. Int J Colorectal Dis. 1990;5:37–40.
2. Bouchoucha M, Denis P, Arhan P, Faverdin C, Devroede G, and Pellerin D. Morphology and rheology of the rectum in patients with chronic idiopathic constipation. Dis Colon Rectum. 1989;32:788–92.
3. Broens PMA, Penninckx FM, Lestár B, and Kerremans RP. The trigger for rectal filling sensation. Int J Colorect Dis. 1994;9:1–4.
4. Rao GN, Drew PJ, Monson JRT, and Duthie GS. Incremental elastic modulus—a challenge to compliance. Int J Colorect Dis. 1997;12:33–6.
5. Fung YCB. Elasticity of soft tissues in simple elongation. Am J Physiol. 1967;213:1532–43.
6. Gregersen H and Djuhuus JC. Impedance planimetry: a new approach to biomechanical intestinal wall properties. Dig Dis. 1991;9:332–40.
7. Lose G, Colstrup H. Saksager K, and Kristensen JK. A new probe for measurement of related values of cross-sectional area and pressure in a biological tube. Med Biol Eng Comput. 1986;24:488–92.
8. Andersen MB, Støkilde-Jørgensen H, and Gregersen H. Versatile software system for analysis of gastrointestinal pressure recordings. Dig Dis. 1991;9:382–8.
9. Jørgensen CS, Dall FH, Jensen SL, and Gregersen H. A new combined high-frequency ultrasound-impedance planimetry measuring system for the quantification of organ wall biomechanics in vivo. J Biomech. 1995;28:863–7.
10. Gregersen H and Andersen MB. Impedance measuring system for quantification of cross-sectional area in the gastrointestinal tract. Med Biol Eng Comput. 1991;29:108–10.

Introduction

Over the past 100 years there has been a lot of interest in the mechanical function of the digestive tract. One might expect that the knowledge base in gastrointestinal mechanics would be large today; however, this is not the case. In general, developments in methodology have been slow and fundamental concepts remain to be investigated so that, in effect, our understanding of "mechanical" disease in the gut has scarcely changed for many years. New multidisciplinary efforts based on bioengineering principles can overcome some of the problems imposed by the complexity of the gut although new methods and concepts in mechanics still remain to be applied to the gastrointestinal tract.

This chapter outlines the physical principles of the impedance planimetric method, its technical aspects of measurement, sources of error and its application to studies of the human rectum, and the derivation of relevant biomechanical parameters. Before going into the detail about impedance planimetry, it is relevant to discuss briefly the visceral distension techniques in general.

Distension Techniques

Distension techniques must be seen in the light of manometry; a technique commonly used to record the mechanical activity of the gastrointestinal tract. Manometry detects the changes in luminal pressure caused by contractions. In nonsphincteric regions, however, the technique only measures occluding phasic contractions from the circular muscle layer, whereas those phasic and tonic contractions that do not reduce the lumen to the diameter of the tiny probe will not be detected.

The distension of a bag placed in the lumen of the gastrointestinal tract is nowadays commonly performed in organs to investigate the force-deformation relationship, tone, and the motor and sensory responses to mechanosensitive receptors. The distension of a viscus also is used in the diagnosis and treatment of various gastrointestinal diseases such as to forcefully open the lower esophageal sphincter during hydrostatic or pneumodilatation in cases of esophageal achalasia.

In research, distension of a viscus often is performed in vivo and in vitro with concomitant measurements of pressure, volume, and cross-sectional area (CSA). The distension can be combined with such imaging techniques as B-mode ultrasonography to obtain objective geometric data on the CSA and wall thickness of a viscus when these are important research data. Visceral distension can be performed in several ways. When the pressure is controlled, the procedure is said to follow an isobaric protocol, and when the volume is controlled, it is called an isovolumetric protocol. The distension test can be done stepwise (or staircase) with each stepwise increase being made either incrementally or to new degrees of distension at random with respect to magnitude. In contrast, a ramp-wise distension consists of the continuous inflation of the bag at a wide range of possible inflation rates. Volume is controlled easily, whereas the control of bag pressure, diameter, CSA, tension, and strain are more difficult to control, requiring specialized techniques. Importantly, although volume is controlled easily by using a pump, it may not provide a uniform and reproducible stimulus of the wall (vide infra). Selection of a proper test protocol basically depends on the purpose of the study where many considerations must be made. The most important considerations in this regard are:

- Reproducibility. This factor often is not considered in studies in vivo. In order to obtain reproducible results, the tissue must be preconditioned, namely, that the test must be repeated until the responses become stable before data actually are collected. The investigators must decide from the initial experience what the criteria for stability are.
- Loading pattern. The duration of loading and the magnitude of loading are important for the definition of physiological processes in the tissue and for determining whether or not reversible or irreversible damage occurs. Stepwise distension can be especially troublesome here because it can impede blood flow to the distended part for considerable time periods. It is also important to know that this sort of distension is most suited to studies where viscoelastic properties of the tissue are of interest because in stepwise distension, the tissue is suddenly strained or stressed. In contrast, ramp distension provides a continuously increasing load where the time-dependent properties of the tissue do not come into play. This approach is of importance in vivo for animal and human rectal studies (1–4), as well as being applied in other visceral sites such as the small intestine (5), the duodenum (6), the esophagus (7), the aorta (8), and the ureter (9).

Consideration of Geometric Factors in Distension Studies

Because most data on the distensibility of various gastrointestinal organs have been obtained mainly in vivo by bag distension methods, such an approach will be considered in greater detail. The most important aspects of this approach relate to:

- the experimental design
- the probe design
- the method of stimulation and measurement
- the geometry and mechanical properties of the bags
- the properties of the tissue and its surroundings
- the assumptions in the analysis

In general, the boundary of a geometrically measurable parameter must be in complete contact with the measurand that is in the process of measuring the CSA of a tube or the volume of an organ of any shape. Here, the whole circumference and surface area of the bag should be in contact with the organ, an ideal that is never completely attained in volume measurements in the intestine. It is important to ensure that the applied pressure is properly transmitted to the tissue; that is, the bag must be large enough so that it does not contribute its own elastic properties to the measurements. In other words, the pressure of the distension must be transmitted entirely to the organ wall itself, which, with a large enough bag, can be a reasonable assumption. Hysteresis of the bag and the infusion system is usually almost negligible, but it should always be looked for and assessed by testing (vide infra).

To avoid difficulties in interpretation of results in studies involving the distension of the intestine, the bag should be rather short in order to provide a localized distension to imitate the size and shape of a bolus in the upper gastrointestinal (GI) tract or feces in the distal part of the large intestine. In some rectal studies, very long bags have been used where the data concerning tone and distensibility may be difficult to interpret because reflex stimulation and inhibition of phasic activity are likely to occur at the same time at the proximal and distal ends of the bag, respectively. When this occurs, the volume and pressure in the bag do not change much despite all the activity in the response. That is, volume measurements in a long bag may show little change even though the shape changes are considerable and conversely, great volume changes may accompany very small shape changes. Therefore, the results depend on the level of phasic contractility in the segment under study. This explains why the definition of specific tone (as opposed to tetanic tone, which is a summation of phasic contractions) does not apply for studies using the barostat (a method for combined pressure–volume measurement) because this technique provides a three-dimensional (3D) measure of tone that is difficult to differentiate from phasic contractility. Thus, barostat reports of rectal distensibility in health and disease are more a representation of a series of summated phasic contractions.

Because of the limitations with these bag techniques, it is necessary that measurements be obtained at one location, necessitating accurate measurement of the luminal CSA rather than the volume. Another significant limitation with pressure–volume measurements is the fact that the bag will inexorably tend to elongate as it fills rather than distend the organ wall by symmetrical radial expansion alone because of the resistance to deformation of the viscus in the radial direction. The magnitude of the elongation will depend on the bag material, but it tends to occur with virtually any bag type (Figure 2.5(i).1). This effect has several important implications, namely:

- Even a small error in volume in the low-pressure range, as shown in Figure 2.5(i).1, will affect the results of a tension–strain analysis because the reference length for the strain measurement is determined in this range.

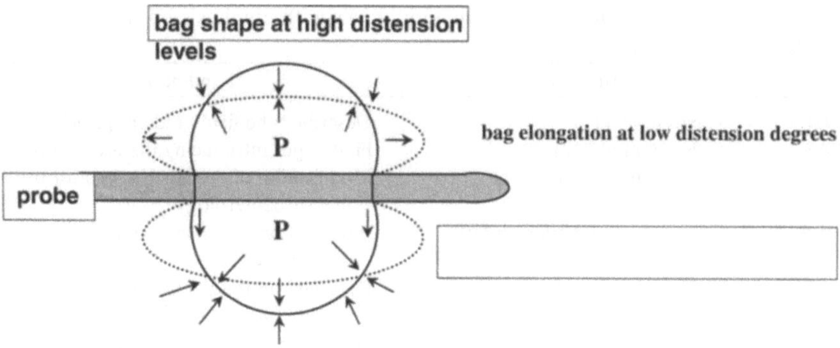

FIGURE 2.5(i).1. A schematic illustration of a bag distending the intestine. High (solid line) and low (dotted line) distension levels are shown for a fairly rigid balloon. The arrows indicate the direction of forces for the balloon pressurized with the lower pressure (top) and for the higher pressure (bottom).

- Parameters such as wall tension and compliance will tend be overestimated.
- The large variation in intestinal size between subjects gives rise to a large variation in the pressure–volume relationship and compliance, particularly using similar bag sizes with variable compliances.
- Elongation will increase the stimulation area so that the receptive field will be larger, provoking possible activation of larger numbers of neural afferents.

Impedance planimetry and endosonographic methods for measurement of luminal CSA have been developed to overcome these invalidating problems where CSA, as a function of pressure, provides important information on luminal dimensions during loading and with further mechanical analysis, provides data on the material properties of the wall itself. Biomechanical analysis of a distensible viscus is dependent on geometric factors; consequently, geometric assumptions must be made to simplify the analysis. For example, the Laplace equation is valid for a thin-walled circular tube or a sphere. In more complex geometries, the mechanical models are more complex and may require numerical analysis. Obviously, this has consequences for the interpretation of data on tone and distensibility, but very few studies consider the proper geometry and estimate the degree to which the tubular sections of the gastrointestinal tract are circular. Current understanding is obtained mainly from pressure–volume measurements rather than more accurate methods to assess more directly the mechanical properties of the gut wall. The following is a description of impedance planimetry, a technique based on fewer assumptions and better validation than the pressure–volume methods.

TABLE 2.5(i)-1. Impedance planimetric landmarks with emphasis on methodological developments and rectum studies.

Year	Authors	Landmark
1971	Harris et al. (11)	Described the field gradient principle
1983	Colstrup et al. (12)	First paper introducing the use of a bag
1988	Gregersen et al. (13)	Modification of the bag method for use in gastroenterology
1991	Gregersen and Andersen (10)	Introduction of the term impedance planimetry
1991	Dall et al. (1)	First data on the porcine rectum
1993	Dall et al. (14)	First data on the human rectum
1999	Gregersen et al. (15)	Development of tensiometer and tensiostat
2001	Andersen et al. (16)	Development of a multi-CSA system for rectum studies
2002	Krogh et al. (17)	Application in rectum of patients with spinal cord lesions
2002	Lundby et al. (18)	Application to an irradiated mouse rectum model
2002	Gregersen et al. (19)	Data on the in vivo length-tension properties of GI tissue
2002	Drewes et al. (20)	Introduction of the multimodal model

Impedance Planimetry

Impedance planimetry is a technique for measurement of the luminal CSA in hollow organs, especially in cylindrical tubes. Other names, such as the field gradient principle and the four-electrode technique, are still in use, especially in the field of urology. The term impedance planimetry, as suggested in 1991 by Gregersen and Andersen (10), denotes a method to measure the size of a plane by the measurement of electrical impedance. Impedance planimetry uses a simple electrical principle based on Ohm's law. However, as with any new technique, the potential sources of error and the static and dynamic properties of the system must be considered. The few sources of error in impedance planimetry can be controlled easily. A description of the major historical landmarks in the development of impedance planimetry is given before introducing the principle of CSA measurement, the sources of error, and system properties in further detail.

The History of the Impedance Planimetry Technique

More than three decades ago, Harris and coworkers described a method using the principles of impedance measurements for the assessment of the CSA in the ureter (11). The measurement system consisted of four or more electrodes placed in a linear array on a thin probe that was passed into the ureter. If a voltage was applied to the two end electrodes, a current flowed between them when a urine bolus passed past the electrodes. During the flow of current, the investigators observed the potential difference between the two detection electrodes. Because an inverse relation exists between CSA and the potential difference in an enclosed volume of a conducting fluid (vide infra), CSA could be deduced from such measurements of potential differences. The system was made usable for measurements of CSA, contraction velocity, and bolus shape, specifically in the ureter.

Colstrup et al. (12) further developed the impedance method for urological use in 1983, whene he introduced a system with the electrodes placed inside a fluid-filled nonconductive latex bag (a balloon) for the measurement of compliance (defined as the change in CSA ÷ the change in bag pressure). This system had the advantage that the flow of current was confined to the fluid in the bag. The system proved sufficient for studies of the active and passive properties of the urethral wall in females presenting with stress incontinence.

In 1988, Gregersen et al. (13) modified Colstrup's bag method for studies of the gastrointestinal tract. The relatively large size of the gastrointestinal tract (especially the size of the large intestine) demanded the further development of this modified measuring system. The modified system was named "impedance planimetry" in 1991 by Gregersen and colleagues (10), the term reflecting the measurement of a two-dimensional (2D) variable based on the recording of electrical impedance. Also in 1991, the first data on the rectum appeared from a porcine model (1), with the method being introduced in healthy volunteers in 1993 (14). In 2001, Andersen et al. (16) developed a multi-electrode system for studying several CSAs in the rectum, providing relevant validation data. In 2002, data appeared on rectal remodeling in irradiated mice (18) and on rectal function in patients with acute and chronic spinal lesions (17). Other major technological developments during recent years have been the development of the:

- Tensiometer—tensiostat. Developed in 1999 by Gregersen, Barlow, and Thompson (15) for the measurement and control of circumferential wall tension and strain in the gastrointestinal tract. The development was facilitated by the need for better control of the distension stimulus because the mechanoreceptors in the intrinsic and extrinsic pathways respond to changes in stress and strain rather than to changes in pressure or volume. In addition to the impedance planimeter, a personal computer (PC) computes tension online and controls a pump that infuses and withdraws fluid from a reservoir into the bag. The system records variations in tension when the bag is inflated to a given pressure, volume, or CSA. In tension control mode, the PC regulates the pump to infuse and withdraw fluid to obtain the selected tension. Gregersen, Barlow, and Thompson (15) have given further details and physiological data related to the use of this technique in the esophagus. The tensiometer has not yet been used in rectum studies.

- Multimodal probe. In 2002, Drewes and coworkers (20) used this system for stimulation of sensory receptors in the intestinal wall, as well as to obtain a better understanding of visceral symptoms and pain. Sensory nerve receptors situated in the gastrointestinal wall respond to several types of stimuli. Multimodal refers to mechanical, chemical, thermal (cold and warm), and electrical stimulation, and the multimodal testing régime must make possible these modes in the same experiment. All modalities can induce pain separately and in combination. Furthermore, central phenomena such as temporal summation and viscerosomatic relations can be studied using this method. This mimics the mechanisms known to be active in clinical diseases of the gastrointestinal tract. The multimodal probe has not yet been used in studies on the rectum.
- In vivo length-tension diagram. Described by Gregersen and coworkers in 2002 (19). This new approach is based on the controlled ramp distension of a bag, along with the continuous determination of tension and strain in the wall of the viscus under-active and passive conditions. The tension is deconstructed into passive and active tension components and is related to the degree of bag distension and the sensory responses.

Impedance planimetry is now at the stage where it is commercially available for experimental animal and clinical human studies (GMC Aps, Hornslet Denmark, GMC@simplanner.dk). The equipment was produced previously by Gatehouse Medical, Denmark and the probes by TensioMed, Denmark.

The Principle of Cross-Sectional Area Measurement

In order to understand the assessment of CSA using changes in electrical impedance, we need to consider a linear array of four electrodes mounted on a catheter as shown in Figure 2.5(i).2, which operate under the principle of Ohm's law. When a constant alternating current (I) is induced in an electrical volume conductor by the two outer (excitation) electrodes, the potential difference (V) between the two inner (detection) electrodes is defined by:

$$V = I\,Z \tag{1}$$

where Z is the electrical impedance.

If the two excitation electrodes are placed sufficiently far from the detection electrodes, a uniform electrical field is created in the vicinity of the detection electrodes. Z (the electrical impedance of the fluid) also can be expressed as $d\ \delta^{-1}\ CSA^{-1}$ with d being the distance between the detection electrodes and δ being the conductivity of the fluid. Thus, the

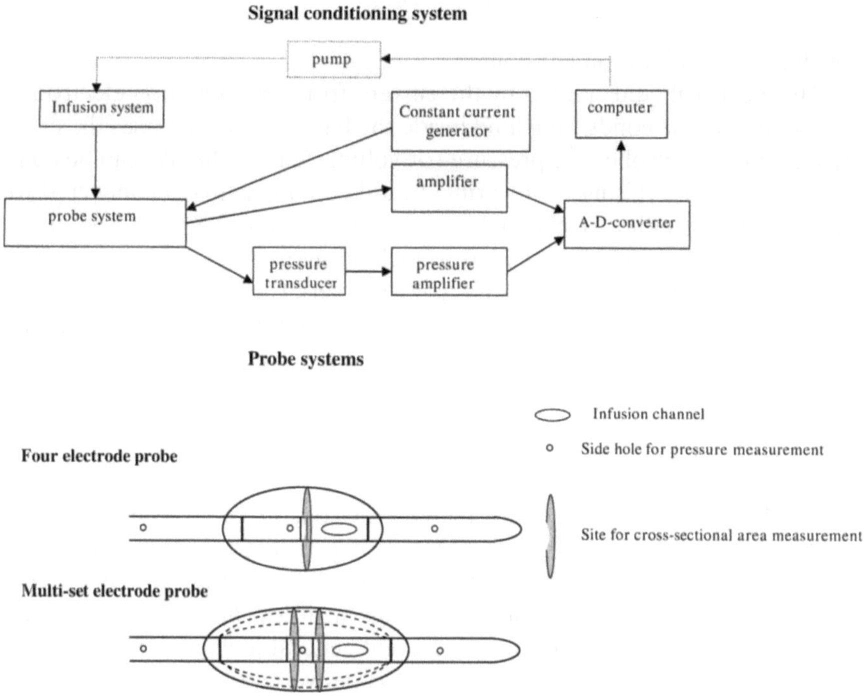

FIGURE 2.5(i).2. Schematics of the impedance planimetry and tensiostat system. Two different probe designs are illustrated. The system renders possible pressure–cross-sectional area measurements, evaluation of peristaltic reflex responses, and standardization of the stimulation stimulus in terms of tension or strain. The group of dashed lines (shown only inside the two bottom balloons) forming a field between the two outer excitation electrodes represent the flow of constant AC current. In the tensiometer system, a computer-controlled pump is added to the system, as shown by the dotted lines. The computer calculates tension in real time from measurements of balloon pressure and CSA and remote controls the pump to infuse/withdraw fluid from the balloon in order to change tension.

potential difference between the detection electrodes can be expressed as:

$$V = I\ d\ \delta^{-1}\ CSA^{-1} \quad (2)$$

This equation is valid for circular, as well as noncircular, cross-sections. I, d, and δ are constant for any given experiment. Thus, V is inversely proportional to the CSA so that:

$$V = k\ CSA^{-1} \quad (3)$$

Direct proportionality between the output V and the CSA can be obtained by means of reciprocating software. After reciprocation, Equation 3 then can be written as:

$$V = k\ CSA \tag{4}$$

where k is a calibration constant.

The electrical field created by the current from the excitation electrodes is confined to the conducting fluid inside the bag that encompasses the electrodes onto the probe. The pressure (or volume) inside the bag can be controlled either by raising or lowering a fluid container that is connected to the bag using either a channel or a pump (Figure 2.5(i).2). The four-electrode system can be extended to include many sets of detection electrodes (multi-electrode systems) so that serial cross-sections can be obtained along the longitudinal axis. This has the advantage that the 3D geometry of the bag can be modeled where the spatial and temporal distribution of contractions can be described in more detail.

The Signal Conditioning System

Each channel in the impedance planimeter consists of an excitation unit with a sine wave generator and an alternating current generator, as well as a signal-processing unit with a differential amplifier, rectifier, and filter. The sine wave generator creates a sine voltage with low harmonic distortion. The signal is fed into the alternating current generator where it is converted into a constant AC current. The current is delivered to the two excitation electrodes that generate an electrical field between them. The potential difference between the two detection electrodes is amplified, filtered, converted (analogue to digital), and then fed to the computer. Figure 2.5(i).2 illustrates two types of probes and the basic setup design of the signal processing system.

The excitation current is 100 microamperes in the clinical impedance planimeters produced by Gatehouse Medical (now GMC, Denmark) and 250 microamperes in the older impedance planimeters designed for animal experimental use. A large current has the advantage that it increases the magnitude of the potential difference, that is, the signal-to-noise ratio is improved. Furthermore, the "linear" range of the calibration curve increases because of patient safety; this obviously puts limitations on the magnitude of the current available. Similar considerations must be made concerning the AC frequency used, where, in general, a high-frequency AC current is less dangerous than a low-frequency current.

Impedance Planimetric Calibration Procedures

Calibrations are made in rigid tubes or in a plastic block with holes of known luminal CSAs. A series of holes increasing in diameter from a few millimeters to 80 millimeters will cover most biological applications, including the large bowel in humans. For a rectal study, it is sufficient to have six to eight calibration tubes covering a range of diameters from one to eight centimeters. The calibration constant depends on the:

- current intensity,
- conductivity of the fluid (that is reliant on the temperature),
- distance between the excitation electrodes.

In large organs, the calibration curves are highly "nonlinear"; therefore a single constant is not sufficient. Previous studies either have used an initial two-point calibration with measurements made only within the "linear" CSA range or have utilized multi-point calibration data with up to 16 calibrations points to render the data more linear. The multi-point calibration has the advantage that it increases the resolution, accuracy, and range of measurement when compared with the two-point calibration system.

Errors and Optimization Procedures

The work by Harris et al. from 1971 on ureteral physiology still stands as one of the most important methodological studies for this basic technique (11). Most of the other works that appeared in the 1970s and 1980s merely provided experimental validation of the sources of error originally pointed out by Harris and colleagues. First, it was demonstrated that Equation 2 is valid for a straight tube as long as the slope of the wall between the detection electrodes is small. Furthermore, an approximation of the potential distribution in a conical tube was provided, leading to an estimation of the error associated with a slope of the wall between the detection electrodes and for the error due to asymmetric probe positioning, (i.e. radial displacement of the probe).

It is advantageous to keep the distance between the detection electrodes small and to keep the probe in a central position. The latter is especially true for a large organ such as the rectum. Several subsequent studies by other authors have added experimental data to this theoretical error analysis as proposed by Harris and coworkers. The probe design also was considered in this work where the authors made the following recommendations:

- The distance between the excitation and detection electrodes must be finite and large enough to provide a uniform current flow in the region of the detection electrodes. The distance should be approximately equal to the radius of the bolus (or bag) at the excitation electrode.
- The distance between the excitation and detection electrodes can be decreased somewhat by using relatively large excitation electrodes. Low-impedance electrodes with a large surface area serve to distribute the current more uniformly than point electrodes.
- The distance between the detection electrodes must be small (< the expected radius) so that the variation in cross-section from one electrode to the next is small compared with the luminal cross-section itself.
- The detection electrodes must be as small as possible. Furthermore, they themselves must be high-impedance elements so as to provide a minimum scattering effect.

Other authors also have dealt with possible sources of error in impedance planimetric measurements (21–24). The errors can effectively be divided into those directly associated with the CSA measurement and those related to the derived biomechanical parameters. The section below considers these sources of error in CSA and pressure measurement and indicates strategies designed to optimize the validity of these recordings using the impedance planimetry technology.

Conductivity of the Fluid, Distance Between Detection Electrodes, and Magnitude of the Current

The distance between the detection electrodes, the conductivity of the fluid, and the current used must all be constant during an experiment according to Equations 2–4. This assumption is valid with the use of a reliable constant current generator, a probe with fixed electrodes, and a bag system where the current is confined to the fluid in the bag. It can be seen from Equation 2 that the potential difference increases when the current increases, when the distance between the detection electrodes increases, or when the conductivity decreases. If the magnitude of the potential difference between the detection electrodes is increased (by placing the electrodes further apart or by increasing the current), the signal-to-noise ratio also will increase. However, a large distance between the detection electrodes may induce errors due to the slope of the wall providing some boundary limits on the magnitude of current safely available. Therefore, the best way to study large organs like the rectum is to increase the potential difference by using a fluid with a low electrical conductance. This usually is obtained by diluting physiological saline a thousand times with distilled water. The conductivity of a fluid also depends on its temperature. Therefore, it is important to maintain the temperature constant both during calibrations and experiments. However, from physics we know that this dependency is linear. Consequently, a correction factor can be introduced if the temperature of the fluid is known.

Electrode Distances and Calibration Curves

The measurements must be within the range of the calibration curve because the curve approaches an asymptotic constant at high CSAs. The calibration curve is highly dependent on the excitation–detection electrode distance (vide supra). Therefore, measurements can be optimized by selecting proper distances between the electrodes. With the current system, the rule of thumb is that the highest measurable CSA corresponds to a diameter of four to five times the distance between the detection and excitation electrodes. However, this is only a guideline because the linearity of the calibration curve also may depend on the electrode materials, electrode size, and current. The range of the calibration curve also depends on the impedance of the fluid and on gain setting in the signal conditioning system.

Irregular (Noncircular) Shape of the Cross-Section

In biological systems, the question naturally arises as to whether the CSA measurement is accurate in an irregular or asymmetric geometry. For example, the intestine is collapsed at rest and at low luminal pressures, and although the lumen may become circular at higher pressures, it is likely that an irregular (noncircular) CSA produces an innate error in measurement as a direct result of luminal asymmetry. As mentioned above, it is not an assumption for Ohm's law that the cross-section is circular as long as the field is uniform. Validation experiments have been done in phantom models where rods have been inserted to make the lumen of a calibration tube irregular, and CSAs obtained by ultrasound and impedance planimetry have been compared within these distorted models. It has been concluded from these studies that noncircular geometry does not cause significant errors (25,26).

Dislocation of the Probe from the Center Axis and Bag Properties

The error due to dislocation of the probe from the center or longitudinal axis of the bag to an eccentric position within the bag can be either calculated from theory or measured experimentally. Experimental validation studies in vitro (where the probe was forced to an eccentric position) have shown that the error can be large. This is especially relevant when studying a large organ like the rectum. The error depends on the electrode distances, the current, the stiffness of the probe, and the bag size. The so-called "dislocation error" can be avoided by using a large bag that unfolds without stretching during distension of the organ under study. Furthermore, the bag must be mounted loosely in the axial direction. A properly mounted bag of sufficient length will straighten the probe and thereby keep it in the middle of the bag; otherwise the probe will bend and shift to an eccentric position with subsequent errors in CSA measurements. This can be evaluated easily by direct vision of the probe position during inflation of the bag. Ultrasonography and X-ray also have been used to validate the position of the probe in studies in vivo (27). The material of the bag is also important here, where a thin, nonstretchable and nonconducting material with low bending rigidity (such as 30 to 50μ thick polyurethane) appears to be optimal. Stretchable materials (such as latex) deform primarily in a longitudinal direction during distension because of the resistance to stretch in the radial direction. The bag elongation with a material such as latex does not directly affect the CSA measurements, but it severely affects any volume measurement and any distensibility measure derived from that volume measurement. Hence, compliance assessments using latex may not be accurate reflections of wall stiffness or visceral biomechanics. Furthermore, any significant elongation of the bag increases the size of the distension area and so a greater number of mechanosensitive receptors will be stimulated.

Slope of the Wall Between the Detection Electrodes and Configuration of the Bag Outside the Detection Area

Harris devised a series of ways to compute the error due to the slope of the wall that exists between the detection electrodes. In theory, this error can be rather large. Experimental validation of the error demands visualization by means of X-rays or ultrasonography. Most gastrointestinal organs studied have been fairly straight so that this source of error often can be neglected.

Dynamic Properties of the Measurement System

The dynamic properties of a measurement system must be characterized in relation to what it is intended to measure. If the upper frequency limit is too low, it will result in phase shift and amplitude reduction. With regard to impedance planimetry, the properties of the CSA measurement system, the pressure measurement system, and the infusion/bag system must all be taken into account. Because the CSA measurements are based on electrical measurements rather than on a mechanical system, the dynamic characteristics of the CSA measuring system are not of any real concern. The upper frequency limit is far higher than the frequency of contraction observed in rectal motility recordings where pressure measurements performed correctly will not result in problems that could be affected by the dynamic properties of the rectum.

The infusion system gives rise to the biggest concerns since we are dealing here with the flow of liquids. This can be overcome by using a pump to control the infusion rate rather than using a pressure-controlled distension protocol based on changing the height of a level container. If recordings of passive tissue properties (i.e., without muscle contractions) are made, the infusion time does not become important; however, if a level container controls pressure, fluid is allowed to move in and out of the bag during the distension. When phasic contractions are present, fluid will flow between the level container and the bag. This fluid flow depends on a number of factors, as determined by Poisseuille's law. To reduce the resistance to flow, the infusion channel should be as short as possible with the largest possible luminal diameter. Reduction also can be obtained by using a fluid with a lower viscosity than physiological saline. Furthermore, the smaller the bag the better (i.e. the length of the bag should be as short as possible to reduce the fluid volume). As a result, fluid mechanics and its flow within the bag and tubing will be a source of error. Hysteresis within the system also must be considered. It is a measure of the difference in pressure–CSA curves between inflation and deflation of the bag. Several validation studies have shown that hysteresis can effectively be neglected with the probes currently in use (28).

Biomechanics

An understanding of biomechanics requires an appreciation of biology, mathematics, mechanics, and statistics. Biomechanics seeks to explain the mechanical behavior of living organisms, and when applied to intestinal biology, it requires a thorough understanding of intestinal structure, anatomy, function, pathophysiology, and symptomatology. The complexity of the intestine demands a multidisciplinary effort through the use of experimental, analytical, and numerical methodology.

Medicine has long disregarded the mechanics of the gut as a matter for serious consideration despite the prominence of disordered mechanics in much of clinical gastroenterology. A degree of disorder in motor function characterizes many (if not most) of our patients with gastrointestinal complaints. Nearly all patients with rectal disease, for example, exhibit some abnormality in mechanical function, and mechanical dysfunction often complicates the connective tissue disorders, diabetes, and neurological diseases.

An important concept in biomechanics is the basic relation between stress and strain. The complexity of the gastrointestinal tract makes the mechanical analysis of the gut wall much more difficult than that of structures made of the usual engineering materials. Simple and rudimentary measures such as compliance (the slope of the pressure–volume curve) often are used to describe the mechanical properties of the rectum. In mechanics, however, a compliance measure alone is insufficient where reliance on this single value actually can lead to wrong conclusions about the behavior of the material being studied.

Application of Biomechanics in the Intestine

In the partially self-regulated intestinal system, distension can elicit both inhibition and excitation of motility by way of intrinsic and extrinsic reflex circuits. Distension also evokes sensations such as pain through the central nervous connections of the gut. The sensing elements are afferent neurons activated by mechanoreceptors and by pain receptors (nociceptors) in the gut wall (these receptors are hypothetical constructs rather that identifiable morphological structures).

Biomechanical and bioengineering principles can be applied to almost any problem related to intestinal function and pathophysiology. A mechanical analysis of the operation of the intestine can be important in advancing our understanding of such a wide-ranging set of interrelated matters as:

- the passive viscoelastic properties of the gut wall,
- the motor and sensory responses of the gut wall to mechanoreceptor stimulation,
- the mechanics of fecal transport,

- the nature and origin of tone in smooth muscle,
- the growth and development of the gut,
- the origin of intestinal diseases characterized by mechanical dysfunction,
- the development of new clinical tests for mechanical dysfunction in the gut.

Definitions of Terms

One principal objective in tissue biomechanics is to determine the stresses and strains in biological tissues when forces are acting upon them. The fact that forces applied to solids deform them demands a study of the force–deformation relationship. Soft biological tissues such as the gastrointestinal tract express mechanical properties that are intermediate between solids and fluids; that is to say, anisotropy prevails due to their heterogeneous structure where ultimately the deformation is finite, the stress–strain relation is nonlinear, and where viscoelastic behavior is pronounced. Due to the high water content of biological tissues, they possess the mechanical properties of both an elastic solid and a viscous fluid. These mechanical properties are time dependent in that the stress–strain response does not occur instantly. When the material is suddenly strained and the strain is kept constant, the corresponding stresses induced in the wall actually decrease with time—a phenomenon called "stress relaxation." If the material is suddenly stressed and the stress is maintained constantly, the material continues to deform; this is a second phenomenon called "creep." If the material is subjected to a cyclic loading, the stress–strain relationship in the loading process is different from that in the unloading process, and this is a third phenomenon referred to as "hysteresis." Stress relaxation, creep, and hysteresis are all features of viscoelasticity. Knowledge about these viscoelastic features is useful when designing rectal distension protocols (Table 2.5(i)-2).

Stress

Mechanical stress is force per unit CSA $\left(\sigma = \frac{F}{A}\right)$ with units of Pa or $N\ m^{-2}$ (the SI unit for force is the Newton, being the force required to give a mass of one kilogram an acceleration of $1\ ms^{-2}$). The force may be applied perpendicular to the surface, representing the bolus pressure (normal stress) exerted on the wall, or parallel to the surface, representing the force exerted by the fluid flow (shear stress) on the wall. Normal stresses may be either compressive or tensile. In a cylindrical tube, we deal with radial, circumferential, and longitudinal components of stress in the respective directions. In tubular organs, the major tensile stress induced by distension is in the circumferential direction. Therefore, only circumferential stress and tension will be considered in the following.

TABLE 2.5(i)-2. Some terms often used in mechanics.

Compliance	The ratio between volume change and pressure change
Constitutive equation	In mechanics, a constitutive equation describes the mechanical properties of a material (the stress-strain relation)
Elastic modulus	The proportionality constant between stress and strain
Membrane tension	Multiplying the uniform stress with wall thickness gives the membrane tension, expressed as force per unit length
Preconditioning	In mechanical testing of living tissues in vitro, loading and unloading are repeated for a number of cycles until the stress–strain relation becomes stabilized so that repeatable results are obtained
Strain	Forces applied to solids cause deformation or strain. It is useful to describe the change by dimensionless ratios such as the length divided by a reference length since it eliminates the absolute length from consideration (where initial length L_0 E and stretched length L result in ratios such as L/L_0 or $(L - L_0)/L_0$. Elongation causes tensile (positive) strain whereas shortening causes compressive (negative) strain
Stress	The force per unit surface area. A normal stress (τ_{11}, τ_{22}, and τ_{33}) is perpendicular to the surface while shear stress (τ_{12}, τ_{13}, and τ_{23}) is parallel to the surface.
Viscoelasticity	Time dependence of the response to stress or strain. Stress relaxation, creep, and hysteresis are features of viscoelasticity (vide supra).

Circumferential Stresses in Thin-Walled Tubular Organs

First, we will assume that the gastrointestinal tract is a thin-walled cylindrical pressure vessel and that the weight of the gastrointestinal segment and its contents can be neglected. During luminal pressure loading, the equilibrium condition requires that the force in the intestinal wall in the circumferential direction be balanced by the force in the intestinal lumen contributed by the inflation pressure. When the geometry is cylindrical, it can be shown that the average circumferential wall stress is

$$\tau_\theta = \frac{pr_i}{h} \tag{5}$$

where p, r_i, and h are the transmural pressure, internal radius, and wall thickness, respectively. This formula is commonly known as Laplace's law. This law can be derived from consideration of equilibrium. It should be noted that the stress in Equation 5 is averaged over the thickness of the segment and does not describe any regional distribution of stress across the wall thickness. Furthermore, the Laplace stress may refer to either the wall thickness in the undeformed state (h_0) (named the engineering stress) or to the thickness in the deformed state (true stress).

Because of its simplicity, the law of Laplace has been used extensively in gastrointestinal and cardiovascular physiology to explain why rupture occurs when segments of viscera are excessively distended. An important implication of the law is that wall stress is related to pressure and to the wall thickness-to-radius ratio.

It is important to recognize the assumptions on which Laplace's law is based. It was originally developed to describe the features of a homogeneous material with a simple geometry, the relationship between pressure, surface tension, and the curvature of a liquid surface. Despite the fact that it was probably never meant to be used in physiology, it receives frequent attention from many investigators in gastrointestinal motor physiology. For any tubular organ, the following assumptions apply in respect to the law of Laplace: the segment must be a circular cylinder with a uniform thickness along the circumference, and a static equilibrium of forces is required (i.e., acceleration must not occur). These conditions are virtually never met in physiology.

Stress (Tension) in a Membrane

Perhaps many readers more readily recognize the formulas expressed below as Laplace's law. In this case, the organ is considered to be very thin walled (a membrane). Hence, membrane theory must be considered rather than the shell theory presented above, and tension is computed rather than stress. This approach often is used in physiology when the wall thickness is immeasurable.

Laplace's law originally refers to the relationship between the pressure difference, the wall tension, and the curvature of the membrane surface. Consider a thin-walled membrane surface and assume that the wall tension is constant everywhere. Then the law of Laplace reads:

$$T = \Delta P\left(\frac{1}{r_1}+\frac{1}{r_2}\right)^{-1} \tag{6}$$

where r_1 and r_2 are the principal radii of curvature of the surface, T is the total tension per unit length of the mid surface of the membrane, and ΔP is the transmural pressure difference. ΔP often is assumed to be equal to the pressure inside the membrane with the assumption that the external pressure is zero. The equation reduces to $T = \Delta P\, r$ in the case of a cylinder because one of the radii tends to infinity, and to $T = \Delta P \frac{r}{2}$ for a sphere because the two radii in that case are equal. Laplace's law often is used for bag distension studies in tubular organs if the wall thickness cannot be measured. More general equations have to be considered if the luminal CSA is elliptical rather than circular.

Equation 6 is valid as long as the membrane is so thin that bending rigidity can be neglected. Furthermore, there are several underlying assumptions such. Although the isotropy assumption is not really valid for many biological tissues, the parameter has proved to be useful. The analysis requires a static equilibrium of forces and, consequently, zero inertial forces. The circumferential tension is equal to the product of the average circumferential stress (Equation 5) and wall thickness. Tension also is called the membrane stress resultant.

The tension measured in vivo [total tension (T_{total})] often will be composed of active and passive components. The total tension during distension can be determined from a distension test without the use of muscle-relaxant drugs. The passive tension ($T_{passive}$) that results from passive components such as the extracellular collagen is obtained from distension testing with muscle relaxants. Assuming, as a first approximation, an additive relationship, the active tension (T_{active}) contributed by smooth muscle activity then can be computed using the equation

$$T_{total} = T_{active} + T_{passive}$$

The three tensions can be plotted as functions of strain (vide infra) to yield information about muscle function and tissue stiffness.

Strain and Strain Rate

The term "deformation" refers to a change in the shape of a continuum (a continuous distribution of matter in space) between some initial (undeformed) configuration and a subsequent (deformed) configuration. Deformation can take many forms; for example, when we pull on a strip of tissue, it stretches, and if we inflate a tubular organ, it distends. To be able to describe such deformations quantitatively, strain measures must be introduced. Strain rate refers to a change in strain as a function of time (i.e. the derivative of the strain–time curve).

Strain Measures

For a continuum subjected to deformation, strains can be defined in several different ways in relation to the deformation gradient. For simplicity, consider a tissue strip of initial length L_0 that when stretched becomes the length L such that the change in length can be described by several dimensionless ratios where:

Stretch ratio
$$\lambda = \frac{L}{L_0} \tag{7}$$

Cauchy strain
$$\epsilon = \frac{L - L_0}{L_0} \tag{8}$$

Green's strain
$$E = \frac{L^2 - L_0^2}{2L_0^2} \tag{9}$$

Thus, for a continuum subjected to finite deformation, strains can be defined in several different ways in relation to the deformation gradient.

The selection of the proper strain measures is dictated primarily by the stress–strain relationship. The strains can be computed for all surfaces or interfaces between layers where the geometric data can be obtained, and as such, the measures are dimensionless. This is advantageous because it eliminates the absolute length and any system of units from consideration, making comparison possible between specimens of various sizes. In Equations 7 through 9, the strain measures are expressed as a fraction of the initial length (so-called Lagrangian strains); however, they also may be expressed as a fraction of the final length (so-called Eulerian strains). Either one of these strain measures is useful. In infinitesimal elongations, the strain measures are equal; however, in finite elongations, they differ. The Cauchy strain is especially useful in the linearized theory of elasticity, which is valid when ε is infinitesimal. Hence, it usually is called the "infinitesimal strain" or "engineering strain." For finite deformations, strain, as defined by Green, is more conveniently related to stress. One strain measure can readily be transformed into another as shown below, where:

$$\varepsilon = \lambda - 1 \quad \text{and} \quad E = \frac{(\epsilon + 1)^2 - 1}{2} \tag{10}$$

In some cases, one strain measure may have advantages over others. As stated above, Green strain and Kirchhoff stress are commensurate measures that are useful in strain energy functions. On the other hand, the stretch ratio is a more convenient measure when the tissue can be considered incompressible. In the case of incompressibility, the product of the stretch ratios in the three principal directions equals one. Thus, if two stretch ratios are known, it is possible to compute the final unknown value.

It is characteristic for soft biological tissues to undergo large deformations with a very low degree of compressibility—what we have traditionally referred to as compliance. However, the issue is more complex than this traditional view because these tissues resist changes in volume much more strongly than changes in shape. For the majority of practical applications within the physiological range, soft tissues can be considered relatively incompressible. This idea has been verified for arterial tissue, but it remains an assumption in tissues of the gastrointestinal wall (1,29).

The strain measures readily can be used for the study of organs of complex configuration so long as the geometric data can be obtained. In the case of the gastrointestinal tract, let us, for simplicity, consider a straight circular cylindrical tube of homogenous material. We may refer to radial, circumferential, and longitudinal components of strain in their respective directions, as defined before. These are the normal components of strain in the wall of the cylinder. During luminal pressure loading (distension), the circumferential length increases (tensile circumferential strain), the wall thickness decreases (compressive radial strain), and compression or elongation may occur in the longitudinal direction (dependent on the material properties). During contraction of the circumferential muscle layer, the circumferential strain will be compressive (negative) and the wall will become thicker. It is important to notice that impedance planimetry can be used to quantitate the length of the inner circumference. Thus, the strain derived is at the mucosal surface in the circumferential direction.

One issue that has not been touched upon yet is the determination of the initial (so-called reference) length. It is apparent from Equations 7 through 9 that the strain measure depends upon the correct determination of the initial length. This is a difficult task for several reasons. First, it may be difficult to suppress smooth muscle activity, and second, strain may vary throughout the intestinal wall.

In the case where the geometry of the zero-stress state cannot be obtained (i.e., the tissue configuration where no stress is present), other methods are needed. For the comparison of strains (and tension–strain relations) in different segments or before and after an intervention, r_0 can be determined at the same level of tension rather than at the same pressure level, in accordance with Laplace's law. Thus, a plot of tension versus radius for each set of data can be extrapolated to give the lowest tension value. At this specific tension, it is easy to determine the reference radius graphically for the different specimens. For ease of measurements, circumferences can be used instead of radii; then some kind of curve fitting usually is used. In this respect, it is important to obtain numerous valid measurement points as close to the unloaded state as possible; however, it is equally important to realize that the curves may be translated from a curve referring to the true zero-stress state onto the strain axis. It also is emphasized that, in determining average stress–strain relations such as Cauchy strain and Cauchy stress (according to Laplace's law), the mid-wall radius should be determined. This often is impossible in vivo; therefore the luminal radius is used in many studies.

Constitutive Equations and Material Constants

The properties of materials are specified by constitutive equations. A constitutive equation in solid mechanics relates stress and strain through a set of material constants. The proportionality constant between stress and strain is called the elastic modulus, and for a linear "Hookean" material, it is called Young's modulus. For such material, the mechanical properties are elastic and the constitutive equation is simplified to Hooke's law (vide infra). In biological tissues, however, the relation between stress and strain is nonlinear and the strain is usually large (finite deformation). The nonlinear (usually exponential-like) mechanical behavior, which likely reflects the mechanical properties of collagen, facilitates stretch in the physiological pressure range and prevents overstretch and damage to the tissue at higher stress levels. Overstretch can induce a plastic deformation in which the tissue can no longer return to its original state when unstressed. Due to this nonlinearity, it is necessary to compute an incremental elastic modulus, as has been performed in the human rectum (30).

Material constants often are derived with the use of exponential or polynomial laws. The stress–strain data are plotted and then fitted using a least-square method with an exponential stress–strain relationship such as of the form:

$$\sigma = \beta[\exp(\alpha\varepsilon) - 1] \tag{11}$$

for the circumferential direction. Because the strain is referred to the zero-stress state, we must have $\sigma = 0$ when $\varepsilon = 0$, as satisfied by Equation 11. A least-square fit is used to determine the values of α and β for the circumferential direction. The tangent modulus, E, is the slope of the stress–strain relationship (a measure of tissue stiffness) and can be computed analytically from Equation 11, where:

$$E = \frac{d\sigma}{d\varepsilon} = \alpha[\sigma + \beta] \tag{12}$$

In the linear stress–strain range, the tangent modulus is equivalent to Young's modulus. Normally, a linear relationship will be found between the tangent modulus and the stress as a result of the exponential nature of the stress–strain relation.

The Biomechanical Meaning of Compliance

Many simplistic estimates of stiffness are made unsound by the neglect of such well-defined and fundamental characteristics of the gastrointestinal wall, such as anisotropy, nonlinear behavior, finite deformation, and viscoelasticity. In fact, the mechanics of the gut wall are so complex that even techniques with far better resolution than those currently available would not permit the complete characterization of the 3D mechanical behavior of the gastrointestinal tract in vivo. However, an ideal characterization is not required for clinical purposes. Only a general but validated means to express overall stiffness is useful and necessary. Commonly used parameters in rectal physiology such as compliance and tone are defined and discussed below.

Compliance is defined as the change in luminal dimension (volume or CSA) divided by the corresponding change in pressure where:

$$C = \frac{\Delta V}{\Delta P}, \quad \text{or} \quad C = \frac{\Delta CSA}{\Delta P} \tag{13}$$

and where V = volume and P = pressure, respectively. Thus, in this formulation, compliance is the reciprocal of stiffness. Usually, it is given either as a single averaged value or as a function of pressure. The compliance parameter merely expresses the differences in luminal dimensions between pressure steps; hence, this parameter does not take into account the actual degree of stretch that occurs under luminal pressure loading, the variations in the unstressed basal luminal diameter, or the wall thickness (31). The measurement of the volume of a distending bag, as represented by the CSA or diameter in a cylindrical viscus, is invalid because the volume also reflects the (unmeasured) elongation of the bag that must take place as the pressure rises within it during inflation. Consequently, the measurement of compliance as an index of wall stiffness has almost no true meaning in terms of the mechanics of the gut wall despite the fact that many coloproctological articles have reported this proctometrogram approach, particularly following the construction of a neorectum (32). Moreover, there is considerable debate about the reproducibility of this simplistic technique because the measures are never really standardized (33). More direct methods to measure (or estimate) CSAs and circumferences are available using various experimental approaches. In this regard, it is often advantageous to express the distensibility rather than stiffness in terms of CSA and transmural pressure where the distensibility is defined as the ratio of fractional change of CSA to the change in transmural pressure (P_{tm}), such that:

$$D = \left(\frac{1}{CSA_0} \frac{\Delta CSA}{\Delta P_{tm}} \right) \tag{14}$$

where CSA_0 is the reference cross-sectional area. This parameter can be computed directly from a *P-CSA* curve (34).

By contrast, tone is dependent upon phasic contraction defined by the temporal contraction characteristics observed. The time between the onset and the offset of rhythmic contractions is measurable in terms of seconds, with little variability, and such events recur at a reasonably constant frequency in any particular location. In contrast, the duration of the contractions involved in the generation and maintenance of tone can be measured in minutes or hours, where tonic contractions may show no obvious pattern or regularity. Tone importantly contributes to the fundamental diameter of the conduit in gastrointestinal viscera. Therefore, the capacity to generate tone is a crucial property of gastrointestinal muscle, especially in sphincters and in the parts of the gut that serve as reservoirs, allowing pooling to occur such as the gastric fundus, the terminal ileum, the cecum, and the colon.

In relation to the anorectal region, it is obvious that the internal anal sphincter (IAS) exhibits tone because it is characterized by a sustained muscle contraction (see Chapter 4). In general, the sphincter muscle exhibits myogenic tone; however, not all tone in the gut is myogenic. Hormones and excitatory nerves also modify the force of contraction in sphincters and elsewhere. Tone also can be described as specific and tetanic in nature, where specific tone is characterized as a sustained contraction at one locus and tetanic tone represents fused phasic (or rhythmic) contractions measurable at any given point. The smooth muscle outside sphincteric regions also is capable of developing tonic contractions. Tone in such regions is more difficult to detect and to measure than tone in the sphincter areas. In intestinal manometry, tonic contractions can occur without an apparent elevation of baseline pressure at the same time that phasic contractions (lasting a few seconds) are recognized. These tonic events may happen because the small rise in intraluminal pressure generated by the tonic contraction of the muscle is reasonably stable and because the pressure dissipates into regions adjacent to the site of the recording when there is nothing to keep it confined. This occurrence is now widely termed the "common-cavity" phenomenon. For this reason, tone, in most of the gastrointestinal tract, cannot even be detected by means of ordinary perfusion manometry, although many reports define resting sphincter pressure as a measure of basal IAS tone (35).

Extensive work has been done on tone in the rectum, but the measurements have been almost exclusively by the evaluation of volume variations in a bag held at a constant low intraluminal pressure—the so-called barostat technique (36,37). The limitations of this method are considerable for reasons already provided in this chapter. Because the gastrointestinal tract, in some parts, is a reasonably uniform cylinder, it makes geometric sense to define tone as a sustained active stress tending to produce strain that leads to a reduction in luminal CSA and circumference or surface area. This stress represents the activation of the smooth muscle. Most studies of tone in vivo define it in terms of changes in "strain" (volume at a constant predefined pressure or a change in the slope of the compliance curve $\Delta V/\Delta P$) without knowledge of the nature of the active or passive stresses involved. Naturally, such a definition leads to much confusion because the relationship between stress and strain is complicated. The definition and measurement of tone in terms of stress, rather than as strain or deformation, gives rise to the need for the knowledge of forces in both the active and the passive components of the stress induced.

Preconditioning Behavior

Many investigators give insufficient consideration to the experimental protocol used in the assessment of rectal distension where it often is unrecognized that a specific loading pressure may be reached at different volumes depending upon the "history" of the loading. The investigator must take into account the two forms of history-dependent mechanical behavior, namely time-dependent viscoelasticity and load-dependent strain softening during repeated distension protocols. It also is important to consider carefully the reproducibility of the results in these distension protocols, to design them specifically for the purpose intended, and to create a coefficient of variation for each laboratory based upon that reproducibility.

In mechanical testing of living tissues, preconditioning is absolutely necessary to obtain repeatable results. In preconditioning, the loading and unloading processes are repeated for a number of cycles until the stress–strain relationship becomes reproducible. The rationale for preconditioning is that the tissues need to adapt to new loads. In most gastrointestinal tissues, the curves in mechanical studies are not repeatable before 3 to 10 cycles have been carried out. Figure 2.5(i).3 shows data obtained in

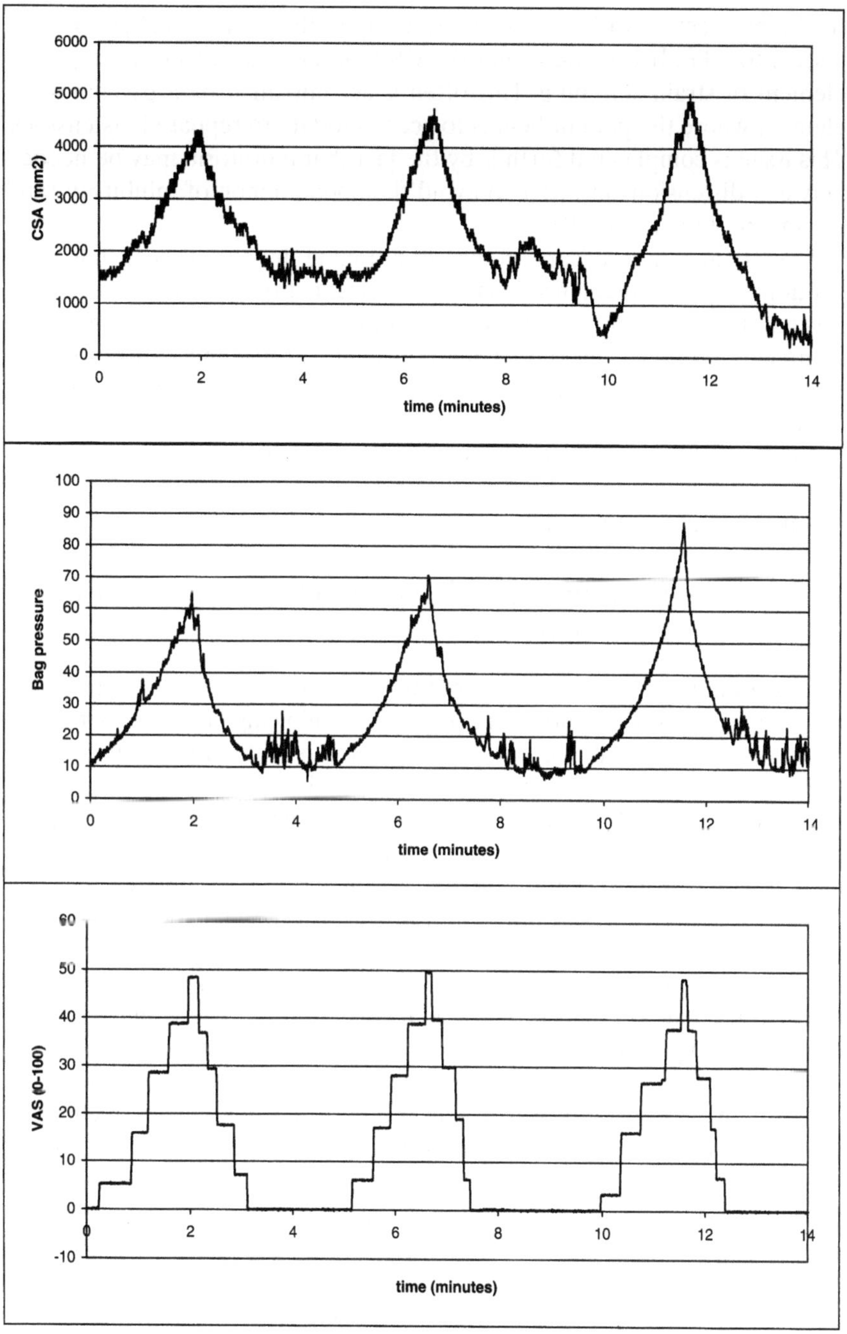

FIGURE 2.5(i).3. Bag CSA (top), bag pressure (middle), and VAS (bottom) from a distension in a subject where the distension was stopped at VAS = 5 (shown as 50 in the figure).

the human rectum with three distensions up to the pain level (VAS = 50 on a scale to 100). It is evident that the CSA became larger, indicating some element of strain softening. This often is accompanied by a psychological element where the patient begins to accommodate to repeated distensions. This issue is complicated further by the fact that moratoria may be needed between distensions in order to avoid the phenomenon of inhibitory (and excitatory) fatigue (38,39).

The change that occurs in preconditioning in soft tissues has conventionally been recognized as a viscoelastic property, like creep and relaxation. However, a different strain-history dependence has been demonstrated in certain rubber materials and cardiac and gastrointestinal tissues, and it is now believed that some of the history dependence in soft tissues that previously has been attributed to viscoelasticity is, in fact, the result of strain softening, a phenomenon in itself that probably serves as a protective mechanism that reduces stresses during repeatedly high stretching of the viscus or tissue (19).

Procedures Related to Studying the Human Rectum with Impedance Planimetry

This section describes the most common procedures used for human rectal measurements. Rectal studies are performed following emptying with a 0.3 to 0.5 meters long and five to twelve millimeters wide probe that contains side holes for pressure measurements, both distal and proximal to and inside the bag. The bag must be up to eight centimeters in maximal diameter in order not to contribute its own elastic properties to the measurements. After proper calibration of the impedance planimeter at body temperature and calibration of the pressure sensors, the probe is passed through the anal canal into the rectum with the patient lying on a bed in the left lateral position during the entire conduct of the study. The side holes distal to the bag are placed in the anal canal and the bag is placed in the rectum starting just above the puborectalis sling. Determination of the rectal resting pressure (abdominal) must be done as it serves as the reference for the distension series. Using the perfused manometry technique, this is normally determined as the difference between the pressure measured before bag distension minus the atmospheric pressure. Ideally, the pressure should be determined during infusion of smooth muscle relaxants to ensure that tone does not affect the reference pressure. The distension series can be performed as a stepwise test where the pressure is changed, equilibrating the pressure in the bag by changing the height of the fluid container above the zero level or by infusion of a certain volume for a specified time. Usually, the pressure is changed stepwise up to five kilopascal (kPa) (1 kPa = 10 cmH_2O). A different method of distension is the ramp test, where the pressure or volume rate is controlled and where 100 milliliters per minute may be infused until the pain level is reached. Perception data during infusion normally are obtained using visual analogue scales or scores of referred pain, with most data being displayed online during the study. Following bag inflation, the bag then is deflated to a pressure below zero for one to two minutes in order to complete the emptying process. Passive rectal properties then can be studied by carrying out distensions during infusion of a smooth muscle relaxant, and data handling can be performed offline after the study is terminated to determine the tone and mechanical properties of the organ.

Data Obtained in the Human Rectum Using Impedance Planimetry—Available Early Results

Most data obtained in the gastrointestinal tract have been from the duodenum and esophagus (40–42). Impedance planimetric data on the rectum is relatively sparse despite the obvious potential of the method in rectal physiology and clinical work (4). Data on the normal human rectum were first provided by Dall et al. in 1993 (4), where distensions were performed using pressures up to 40 cmH_2O above baseline rectal pressure. It was found that steady-state rectal CSA values had a nonlinear relation to increasing distension pressure. Despite the significant methodological development and the encouraging results, it took several more years to expand this work with clinical studies by Rao et al. (30) and Krogh et al. (43) on incremental elastic modulus during ramp inflation at variable rates in normal volunteers. This area recently has been expanded to the diseased rectum and, specifically, disorders such as fecal incontinence and evacuatory dysfunction (44–46) and with acute and chronic spinal cord injury (47).

The purpose of this last study reported by Klaus Krogh (47) in his thesis was to observe rectal wall properties and the rectoanal inhibitory reflex following spinal cord damage where 25 patients with spinal cord injury (14 with supraconal lesions and 11 with conal/cauda equina lesions) were studied one to four weeks after injury and 17 patients were studied again between six and fourteen months following their injury. It was found that rectal tone was higher than normal in patients with acute and chronic supraconal lesions, but significantly lower in patients with acute and chronic conal/cauda equina lesions. The proportion of subjects with single giant rectal contractions was also significantly higher than normal after acute supraconal spinal cord injury, but not following acute conal/cauda equina lesions. Rectal tone and the number of giant rectal contractions did not change significantly from the acute to the chronic phase of spinal cord injury. From this work it was concluded that rectal tone is stimulated by the sacral spinal cord, but inhibited by supraspinal centers within the central nervous system. Likewise, rectal contractility is inhibited by supraspinal centers, and the rectoanal inhibitory reflex is stimulated by the sacral spinal cord. Alterations caused by either type of spinal cord lesion were present after one to four weeks and did not appear to change significantly within the first year following spinal cord injury.

Similar studies by Petersen et al. using this new technology studied sensory and biomechanical responses to distension of the normal human rectum and sigmoid colon (48). The relation between pain intensity and pressure, CSA, and tension–strain relations of the rectum and sigmoid colon were assessed in this study in normal subjects following standardized distension using impedance planimetry where it was found that the tension–strain relation did not differ between the normal rectum and the sigmoid colon. The VAS score for every modality (air, defecation, and pain) revealed an increase in intensity as a function of pressure whereas the VAS score in the rectum and the sigmoid colon as a function of tension and strain did not show any significant differences. It was concluded that the biomechanical properties in the sigmoid colon and rectum were alike where, for a given wall tension and circumferential strain, the sensibility was equivalent in the two sites and where, in effect, the observed differences in perception between the two segments were more related to the greater CSA developed in the rectum. This approach has been used by the same group to assess differential sensitivity and distensibility of the rectum and sigmoid colon in patients with irritable bowel syndrome (IBS) where patients were studied with electrical and mechanical stimuli. The calculated pressures at the pain-detection threshold in the sigmoid colon were generally lower in the IBS patients; otherwise no differences were seen in sensation rating to the different distension pressures. The CSA was slightly higher in controls for the different pressures, whereas no differences between the groups were seen in strain and tension of the rectum and sigmoid colon. From these data it was concluded that the visceral hypersensitivity in IBS is more related to alterations in the nervous system rather than to intrinsic biomechanical parameters such as the tension and strain of the gut wall.

These types of studies are still early, but they constitute a beginning for impedance planimetry in functional bowel disorders and its use as a tool for the relation of parameters to function following the construction of neorectal reservoirs and as an objective measure of objective rectal wall stiffness in such conditions as inflammatory bowel disease. The latter has a long history of measurement with methodology that is probably somewhat simplistic (49–51); however, given the success of impedance planimetry studies in other parts of the gastrointestinal tract, it is likely that it will become important in future studies of rectal mechanics and mechanotransduction.

Conclusions

This chapter has highlighted the research approach towards the physiological assessment of distensibility of the rectum using compliant bags, discussing the inherent errors in the determination of compliance as it pertains to biological systems. Because of the anisotropy of the human gut, which is composed of a heterogeneous range of tissues with different deformabilities, the presence of a neurohumoral tone, the nonlinear effects on the stress–strain relationship, and the viscoelastic properties of isolated and repeated distension stresses on the intestine, no model of compliance will define the real relationship of deforming stress and strain. Moreover, this clinical assessment is dependent upon many assumptions concerning gut geometry, directional distension, luminal size, and wall stiffness and thickness that cannot be measured accurately in vivo or that are either wrongly assumed to be constant or are neglected in manometric practice. The use of impedance planimetry for the electrical determination of cross-sectional area during distension has provided a means in the rectum for the determination of a nonlinear incremental elastic modulus that, to some extent, defines rectal wall stiffness in health and disease. It remains to be seen whether this can be used as an objective marker of rectal damage in ulcerative or radiation proctitis, or whether it will assist in the postoperative estimation of the biomechanical properties of constructed neorectal reservoirs.

References

1. Dall FH, Jørgensen CS, Djurhuus JC, and Gregersen H. Biomechanical wall properties of the porcine rectum: A study using impedance planimetry. Dig Dis Sci. 1991;9:347–53.
2. Arhan P, Faverdin C, Persoz B, et al. Relationship between viscoelastic properties of the rectum and anal pressure in man. J Applied Physiol. 1976;41:677–82.
3. Akervall S, Fasth S, Nordgren S, Oresland T, and Hulten L. Rectal reservoir and sensory function studied by graded isobaric distension in normal man. Gut. 1989;30:496–502.
4. Dall FH, Jorgensen CS, Houe D, Gregersen H, and Djurhuus JC. Biomechanical wall properties of the human rectum. A study with impedance planimetry. Gut. 1993;34:1581–6.
5. Duch BU, Petersen JAK, Vinter-Jensen L, and Gregersen H. Elastic properties in the circumferential direction in isolated rat small intestine. Acta Physiol Scand. 1996;157:157–63.
6. Gregersen H, Kassab G, Pallencaoe E, Lee C, Chien S, Skalak R, and Fung YC. Morphometry and strain distributiuon in guinea pig duodenum with reference to the zero-stress state. Am J Physiol. 1997;273(36):G865–74.
7. Villadsen GE, Petersen JAK,Vinter-Jensen L, Juhl CO, and Gregeresen H. Impedance planimetric characterization of the normal and diseased esophagus. Surg Res Commun. 1995;17:225–42.
8. Storkholm JH, Frøbert O, and Gregersen H. Static elastic wall properties of the abdominal porcine aorta in vitro and in vivo. Eur J Vasc Endovasc Surg. 1997;13:31–6.
9. Gregersen H, Knudsen L, Eika B, Frokiaer J, and Djurhuus J. Regional differences exist in elastic wall properties in the ureter. Scand J Urol Nephrol. 1996;30:343–8.

10. Gregersen H and Andersen MB. Impedance measuring system for quantification of cross-sectional area in the gastrointestinal tract. Med Biol Eng Comput. 1991; 29:108–10.
11. Harris JH, Therkelsen EE, and Zinner NR. Electrical measurement of ureteral flow. In: Boyarsky S, Tanagho EA, Gottschalk CW, and Zimskind PD, editors. Urodynamics. London: Academic Press; 1971. p. 465–72.
12. Colstrup H, Mortensen SO, and Kristensen JK. A probe for measurements of related values of cross-sectional area and pressure in the resting female urethra. Urol Res. 1983;11:139–43.
13. Gregersen H, Stodkilde-Jorgensen H, Djurhuus JC, and Mortensen SO. The four-electrode impedance technique: a method for investigation of compliance in luminal organs. Clin Phys Physiol Meas. 1988;9:61–4.
14. Dall FH, Jorgensen CS, Houe D, Gregersen H, and Djurhuus JC. Biomechanical wall properties of the human rectum. A study with impedance planimetry. Gut. 1993;34:1581–6.
15. Gregersen H, Barlow J, and Thompson DG. Development of a computer-controlled tensiometer for real-time measurements of tension in tubular organs. Neurogastroenterol Motil. 1999;11:109–18.
16. Andersen IS, Gregersen H, Buntzen S, Djurhuus JC, and Laurberg S. New probe for measurement of dynamic changes in rectum. Neurogastroenterol Motil 2004;16:99–105.
17. Krogh K, Mosdal C, Gregersen H, and Laurberg S. Rectal wall properties in patients with acute and chronic spinal cord lesions. Dis Colon Rectum. 2002;45(5):641–9.
18. Lundby L, Dall FH, Gregersen H, Overgaard J, and Lauerberg S. Distensibility of the mouse rectum: application of impedance planimetry for studying age-related changes. Colorectal Dis. 2001;1:34–41.
19. Gregersen H, Lundby L, and Overgaard J. Early and late effects of irradiation on morphometry and residual strain of mouse rectum. Dig Dis Sci. 2002;47: 1472–9.
20. Drewes AM, Petersen P, Rossel P, Gao C, Hansen JB, and Arendt-Nielsen L. Sensitivity and distensibility of the rectum and sigmoid colon in patients with irritable bowel syndrome. Scand J Gastroenterol. 2001;36:827–32.
21. Mortensen SO, Djurhuus JC, and Rask-Andersen H. A system for measurements of micturition urethral cross-sectional areas and pressures. Med Biol Eng Comput. 1983;21:482–8.
22. Lose G, Colstrup H, Saksager K, and Kristensen JK. A new probe for measurement of related values of cross-sectional area and pressure in a biological tube. Med Biol Eng Comput. 1986;24:488–92.
23. Gregersen H and Djurhuus JC. Impedance planimetry: a new approach to biomechanical intestinal wall properties. Dig Dis. 1991;9:332–40.
24. Gregersen H and Kassab G. Biomechanics of the gastrointestinal tract. Neurogastroenterol Motil. 1996;8:277–97.
25. Fung YC. Biomechanics. Mechanical properties of living tissues. New York: Springer-Verlag; 1993.
26. Hammer HF, Phillips SF, Camilleri M, and Hanson RB. Rectal tone, distensibility, and perception: reproducibility and response to different distensions. Am J Physiol. 1998;274:G584–90.

27. Villadsen GE, Petersen JAK, Vinter-Jensen L, Juhl CO, and Gregersen H. Impedance planimetric characterisation of the normal and diseased oesophagus. Surg Res Comm. 1995;17:225–42.
28. Fung YC, Perrone N, and Anliker M, editors. Biomechanics: its foundations and objectives. Englewood Cliffs, New Jersey: Prentice-Hall; 1972.
29. Storkholm JH, Villadsen GE, Krogh K, Jørgensen CS, and Gregersen H. Dimensions and mechanical properties of porcine aortic segments determined by combined impedance planimetry and high-frequency ultrasound. Med Biol Engineer Comput. 1997;35:21–6.
30. Rao GN, Drew PJ, Monson JRT, and Duthie GS. Incremental elastic modulus—a challenge to compliance. Int J Colorectal Dis. 1997;12:33–6.
31. Madoff RD, Orrom WJ, Rothenberger DA, and Goldberg SM. Rectal compliance: a critical appraisal. Int J Colorectal Dis. 1990;5:37–40.
32. Ho Y-K, Seow-Choen F, and Tan M. Colonic J-pouch function at six months versus straight coloanal anastomosis at two years: randomized controlled trial. World J Surg. 2001;25:876–81.
33. Varma JS and Smith AN. Reproducibility of the proctometrogram. Gut. 1986;27:288–92.
34. Gregersen H and Christensen J. Gastrointestinal tone. Neurogastroenterol Motil. 2000;12:501–8.
35. Zbar AP and Kmiot WA. Anorectal investigations. In: Phillips RKS, editor. A companion to specialist surgical practice. Colorectal surgery. 1st ed. London: WB Saunders Company Limited; 1997. p. 1–33.
36. Bell A, Pemberton JH, Hanson R, and Zinsmeister AR. Variations in muscle tone of the human rectum: recordings with an electromechanical barostat. Am Physiol Soc. 1991;260(23): G17–25.
37. Brilliant P and Pemberton JH. Rectal compliance. In: Smith LE, editor. Practical guide to anorectal testing. 2nd ed. New York: Igaku-Shoin; 1995. p. 227–34.
38. Zbar AP, Aslam M, Gold DM, Gatzen G, Gosling A, and Kmiot WA. Parameters of the rectoanal inhibitory reflex in patients with idiopathic fecal incontinence and chronic constipation. Dis Colon Rectum. 1998;41:200–8.
39. Kaur G, Gardiner A, Lee PW, Monson JR, and Duthie GS. Increased sensitivity to the recto-anal reflex is seen in incontinent patients. Colorectal Dis. 1999; Suppl 1:39A–40A.
40. Andersen MB, Gregersen H, Kraglund K, and Stodkilde-Jorgensen H. Radial analysis of duodenal motility recordings in humans. Scand J Gastroenterol. 1991;26:843–51.
41. Gregersen H, Orvar KB, and Christensen J. Biomechanical properties of the duodenal wall and tone during phase I and phase II of the MMC. Am J Physiol. 1992;263:G795–G801.
42. Juhl CO, Vinter-Jensen L, Djurhuus JC, Gregersen H, and Dajani EZ. Biomechanical properties of the oesophagus damaged by endoscopic sclerotherapy. Motil Clin Perspect Gastroenterol. 1997;40:867–73.
43. Krogh K, Ryhammer AM, Lundby L, Gregersen H, and Laurberg TS. Comparison of methods used for measurement of rectal compliance. Dis Colon Rectum. 2001;44:199–206.

44. Felt-Bersma RJ, Sloots CEJ, Poen AC, Cuesta MA, and Meuwissen SGM. Rectal compliance as a routine measurement. Extreme volumes have a direct clinical impact and normal volumes exclude rectum as a problem. Dis Colon Rectum. 2000;43:1732–8.
45. Salveoli B, Bharucha AE, Rath-Harvey D, Pemberton JH, and Phillips SF. Rectal compliance, capacity and rectoanal sensation in fecal incontinence. Am J Gastroenterol. 2001;96:2158–68.
46. Gosselink MJ, Hop WCJ, and Schouten WR. Rectal compliance in females with obstructed defecation. Dis Colon Rectum. 2001;44:971–7.
47. Krogh K. Colorectal function in patients with spinal cord lesions [thesis]. Aarhus University, Denmark; 2000.
48. Petersen P, Gao C, Rossel P, Qvist P, Arendt-Nielsen L, Gregersen H, and Drewes AM. Sensory and biomechanical responses to distension of the normal human rectum and sigmoid colon. Digestion. 2001;64:191–9.
49. Farthing MJG, and Lennard-Jones JE. Sensibility of the rectum to distension and the anorectal distension reflex in ulcerative colitis. Gut. 1978;19:64–9.
50. Suzuki H, and Fujioka M. rectal pressure and rectal compliance in ulcerative colitis. Jpn J Surg. 1982;12:79–81.
51. Broens PMA, Penninckx FM, Lestár B, and Kerremans RP. The trigger for rectal filling sensation. Int J Colorect Dis. 1994;9:1–4.

Chapter 2.5(ii)
Impedance Planimetry: Clinical Impedance Planimetry

GRAEME S. DUTHIE and Angela B. GARDINER

Background

Rectal dynamics traditionally have been assessed using the construct of "rectal compliance" measurement, assessing the change in volume with changes in rectal pressure. Various studies have reported "normal control" results over a wide range of measurements (1–7), reflecting the relative lack of reproducibility of the technique where there are differing amounts and speeds of rectal distension and variable biomechanical rectal properties (Figure 2.5(ii).1). This reported range has effectively limited the clinical and research usefulness of the technique.

Impedance planimetry [determination of cross-sectional area (CSA) of a hollow viscus] in relation to pressure variation with distension offers a more reliable investigation of rectal dynamics, and although its measurement would mirror that of standard rectal compliance assessment, in theory its recording would have several clinical advantages.

Impedance planimetry (IP) is a technique first described for determining CSA measurement, contraction velocity, and bolus shape (8). It is based on the field gradient principle and is performed using a thin probe with four electrodes attached. The technique was developed further in 1976, being performed using a probe with two electrodes attached for the investigation of ureteric peristalsis and urine flow in pigs (9,10). Further developments allowed the addition of manometry recording devices, and in the 1990s, IP was used in the human esophagus for bolus velocity and clearance assessments employing eight and twenty electrode systems, respectively (11).

In 1983, Colstrup et al. developed the technique for the measurement of active forces by the addition of an expanding, non-conducting latex balloon to the probe (12). This enabled the measurement of passive biomechanical wall properties because the current that facilitated the recording was restricted to the balloon. This method has since been applied in esophageal and duodenal (13) studies and in limited anorectal work (14).

The system originally was designed for use in small diameter lumens, so it was necessary to develop a system capable of recording larger diameters

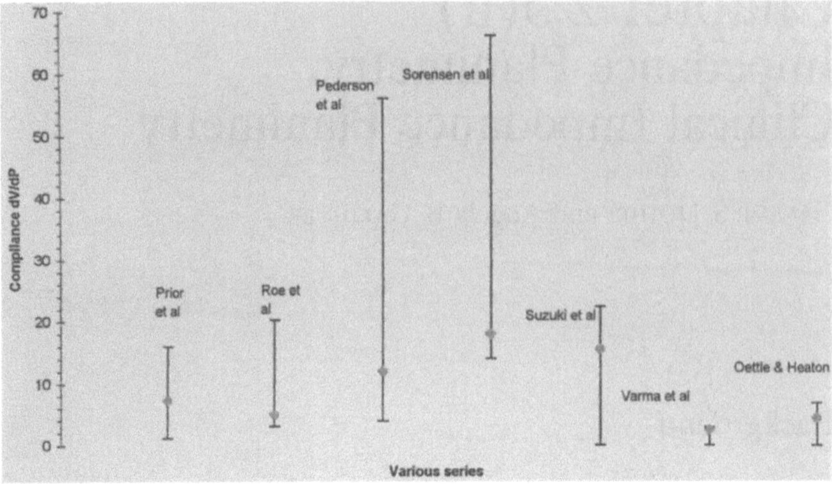

FIGURE 2.5(ii).1. Reported normal compliance values in the available current literature.

such as those found in the gastrointestinal (GI) tract. This was achieved in 1990 by the use of a larger current, a current amplifier, and an improved reciprocal generator enabling the distance between electrodes to be reduced, permitting a decrease in the probe length (15).

Measurement of CSA [see Chapter 2.5(i)]

The catheters used for IP often are constructed with hollow silicone tubing (around five to ten millimeters in diameter), allowing for the addition of a pressure transducer that measures anal and/or rectal pressure during conduction of the study. In addition, four copper ring drive electrodes are mounted onto the exterior of the catheter at approximately 65 millimeter spacings, with the sensing electrodes positioned some two millimeters apart. For successful recording, low-concentration saline solution is the only suitable medium with which to inflate the balloon while recording CSA. The ring electrodes and pressure transducer(s) are attached to a recording device, and the recorder is connected to a personal computer (PC) by a serial lead. A real-time recording usually is observed on the PC during the study.

The cross-sectional area is measured according to the field gradient principle where the impedance of a fluid inside a balloon is measured. A current is introduced from the outer electrodes within the balloon, and the difference in voltage between the two inner electrodes is $V = I \times R$ (Ohm's law), with R being equivalent to the electrical impedance of the saline solution within the balloon. The latter parameter also can be derived using the formula $d \times c^{-1} \times \text{CSA}^{-1}$, where d is the distance between the inner electrodes and c is the conductivity of the saline solution. Hence, the voltage difference can be calculated from $V = I \times d \times c^{-1} \times \text{CSA}^{-1}$, where if I, d, and c are constant, then V will be inversely proportional to the measured CSA. The addition of a reciprocal generator in the circuit provides the CSA measurement (15). There have been [as has been discussed extensively in the Chapter 2.5(i)] a number of significant sources of error that also have been discussed by various authors and that are either related to CSA measurement or to biomechanical errors and assumptions (16–19). Cross-sectional area measurement is dependent on correct positioning of the probe, constant temperature of the conducting fluid, and stability and reproducibility of the conductivity. These errors are reduced if the temperature and conductivity are kept constant for the duration of the study.

Measurements also must not exceed the maximum CSA of the non-stretched balloon and also must be found to be within the calibration curve of the system. The placing of the electrode should be such that the balloon is positioned above the anal canal where balloon distension does not cause anal canal distortion.

Methods

The catheter system is attached to a recording device and the manufacturer's guidelines for calibration and zeroing are followed (GMC Aps; Hornslet, Denmark). A noncompliant polythene balloon/bag should be used as the fluid reservoir, and the balloon must be purged of *all* air because any air within the system will yield errors in the recordings. A condom may be attached over the catheter for sterility purposes if desired. Figure 2.5(ii).2 illustrates a typical catheter that is available for the assessment of impedance planimetry.

Upon completion of the calibration and the zeroing of the pressure transducer(s) where applicable, various diameters of plastic tubing should be measured for bench testing. Very small diameters are not easily measured due to the enfolding of the polythene bag that is used as the balloon, but it is recognized that small diameters are quite rare in clinical practice. Recommendations have been made by the manufacturer that detail, if necessary, any requirements for performing recalibration of internal settings in the advent of non-reproducible results or errors obtained during real-time recordings.

The catheter complex may be positioned within a condom for the duration of the test and for purposes of sterility because the addition of the condom should ensure that none of the catheter complex comes into contact with the subject. The condom should overlap the balloon set-up by approximately four to five centimeters and therefore can be seen externally

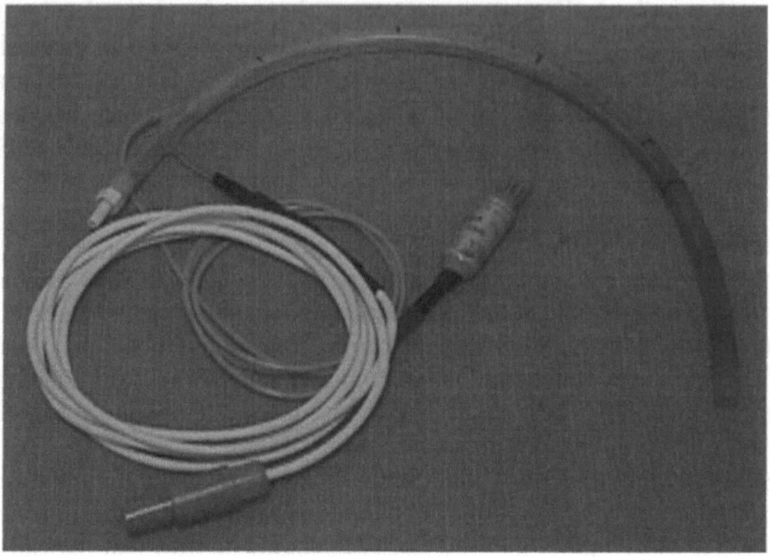

FIGURE 2.5(ii).2. Impedance planimetry catheter for clinical human use.

while the catheter is in position. A glycerin suppository and instructions for its home use prior to the appointment may be given, depending on laboratory practice, and tends to aid clearance of the rectum prior to the investigation.

With the subject in the left lateral position, the catheter is introduced into the anal canal with the aid of lubricating jelly. The catheter complex is inserted up to a depth that ensures adequate clearance of the anal canal by the balloon. It is important for the balloon on the catheter complex to be clear of the anal canal so as to avoid distortion of the rectal filling mechanism and artifact production during the investigation. The procedure is explained to the subject, who signs an informed consent for its conduct and performance. This should include instruction to express a feeling of initial movement/filling, the desire to pass flatus, the urge to defecate, and then finally at the point of maximum tolerance, which is similar to data recorded for a rectal compliance study as performed in association with conventional anorectal manometry. The catheter complex is attached to an infusion pump that has been previously purged of all air and primed with the diluted saline solution. It is essential to ensure the tubing used in the pump is completely primed with the saline because the further dilution of the saline will inhibit the measurement of the CSA by the copper ring electrodes. The real-time recording for the procedure is activated and allowed to stabilize as recognized on the PC screen.

The filling method used is very similar to that of methods utilized for assessing rectal compliance. The infusion pump is switched on to infuse at a known constant rate where 60 milliliters of fluid per minute is generally sufficient. At the onset of the saline infusion, a note should be made of the time at the start of the procedure, which enables identification during the procedural analysis. This can either be done on paper or on the recording, if the software program permits. When the initial sensation is observed by the subject, the time should again be noted. The same procedure then should be followed at the sensations of desire to pass flatus and urge to defecate. The subject is then asked to continue to hold on for as long as possible in an attempt to try and postpone defecation. This is continued until the point where the subject expresses that they are no longer able to postpone defecation. At this point, the infusion pump is switched off and a marker is added to the tracing. Then the fluid is allowed to drain from the catheter complex.

Once the fluid has been drained completely from the balloon, the recording is stopped and saved to disk. The catheter complex is removed from the subject, then cleaned and sterilized as per the manufacturer instructions and hospital disinfection guidelines. The tracings obtained are analyzed along similar lines to the standard methods of manometric analysis. Figure 2.5(ii).3 highlights a typical tracing obtained during a recording of CSA and rectal pressure measurement. Rectal (and anal canal, if available) pressures and CSAs are obtained from the tracings as the basic measurements. These

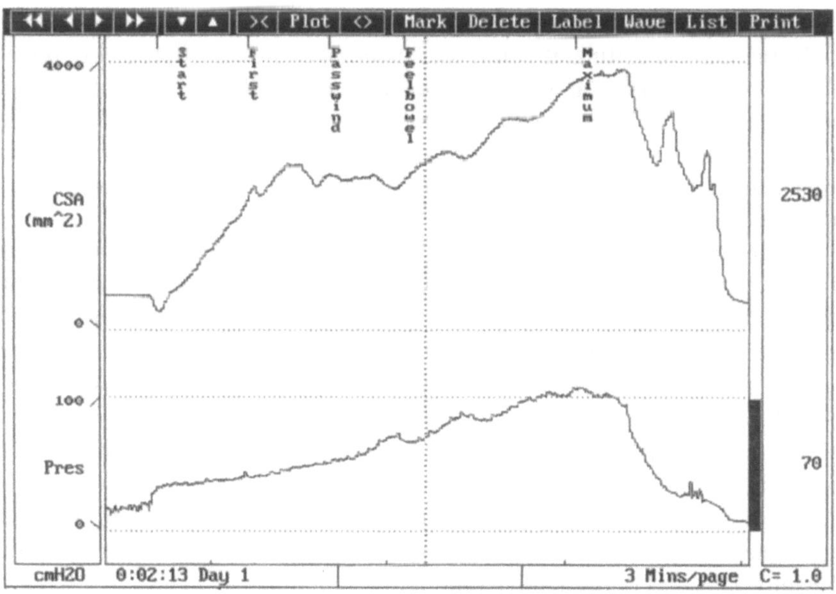

FIGURE 2.5(ii).3. Combined simultaneous CSA and pressure measurement trace during clinical IP.

tracings are generally visible throughout the procedure. Various analytical techniques can be employed on the tracing as required.

This method also facilitates the measurement of a compliance-type procedure, which is of benefit to the user in the laboratory because both procedures can be employed at the same time. The volumes can be calculated at the onset of the various sensations described by the subject, along with changes in rectal (and anal, where available) pressures at each sensory level.

Other methods of performing IP have described the stepwise inflation of a rectal balloon with increasing amounts of conducting fluid. This generates rectal pressures that are recorded at five centimeter H_2O intervals from five centimeters H_2O up to forty centimeters H_2O, and then the volume at each pressure increment is calculated.

Results and Discussion

Results have shown that impedance planimetry has the ability to give a much more detailed picture of rectal dynamics during distension of the rectal wall. *When simply comparing planimetry tracings to that of those obtained from rectal compliance, there are obvious differences.* With a broader knowledge of rectal function dynamics, it would follow that the planimetry trace follows a more expected pattern of what is understood to occur within the rectum, whereas compliance traces do not always appear to correspond to what would be expected to be seen during "normal" rectal distension (16–18).

In the clinical setting, it is important to have an indication of the rectal function of a particular subject when considering their treatment. From what has been observed in some studies, it can be said that the technique of IP provides valuable additional information regarding rectal function that cannot be generated by the traditional method of rectal compliance (19).

Where a low rectal capacity may be assumed for a subject, it is important to have knowledge of the elasticity/dynamics of the rectal wall during the study and also what properties it displays at the maximum tolerated volume (MTV). From what is understood of normal rectal dynamics, one would expect that the recorded rectal pressure at the MTV would be elevated because increasing rectal wall distension will, at some point, reach near-maximal distension and result in defecation. However, this is not always demonstrated in the traditional method of rectal compliance. This may not be a true reflection of the subject's rectal capacity, but this may be an indication of the balloon distorting, which can be due to an inelastic rectal wall (20,21) or a highly compliant balloon.

For impedance planimetry to be of benefit in the measurement of rectal wall distension, it is necessary to fully distend the rectal wall, which does result in an elevation of the rectal pressure. The elevation of rectal pressure eventually will reach a peak at the point of maximum tolerated volume, resulting in an immediate desire for defecation.

Rectal pressures demonstrated during rectal compliance often are found to be lower than what has been demonstrated using impedance planimetry; however, it could be questionable as to whether or not a substantial increase in rectal pressure will be observed during standard compliance because the balloon may be distorting without truly stretching the rectal wall to its maximum (22). Dall et al. (18) referred to a study performed within the porcine rectum in which stepwise pressure increases are made from 10 centimeters H_2O to eighty centimeters H_2O, where the maximum possible CSA that could be measured was 1590 square millimeters.

The feature of CSA measurement increases the capacity of the investigations over what is currently available. By connecting rectal activity with CSA, it is possible to obtain a true indication of rectal capacitance and how it corresponds to rectal activity (i.e. does the MTV correspond to an elevated rectal pressure, and if so, to what degree?). Moreover, is the rectal pressure increase at a steady uniform rate, or is there a rapid increase over a short period of time? The latter parameter is likely to vary with increasing rectal wall stiffness.

Overall, the establishment of this method for anorectal physiological assessment will undoubtedly and valuably increase the knowledge that is currently obtained. The practical planimetry procedure does not differ substantially from traditional compliance measurement with the exception of the balloon set-up, and once mastered, the IP technique is quite straight forward. Undoubtedly, there is the scope to further improve the procedure as more research is undertaken to define catheter design and capability. It would be advantageous to be able to increase the CSA measurement capacity, but not to a degree that would reduce the sensitivity of the catheter (23,24). It is recognized, however, that there always exists the possibility that certain subjects will have rectal diameters that are not measurable reliably, as in, for example, cases of megarectum. For these types of subjects, this method would not offer much more information than that already obtained from standard anorectal physiological assessment.

The ability to record anal canal pressure simultaneously with rectal pressure also would be of huge benefit in the routine laboratory setting. This then could allow for the current standard method of rectal compliance to be replaced. Such an approach would be of use when looking at anorectal coordination during rectal distension and may further expand our knowledge of sampling and the rectoanal inhibitory reflex.

Impedance planimetry does appear to have increased the potential knowledge that can be obtained from anorectal physiological assessment. It is a simple and reliable technique that improves upon the current method used by many in the assessment of the biomechanical properties of the healthy and diseased rectum during distension. Its place in the assessment of the capacity of neorectal reservoirs and the correlation with symptomatology in cases of small capacitance, dysfunction, or sepsis remains to be determined.

References

1. Prior A, Maxton DG, and Whorwell PJ. Anorectal manometry in irritable bowel syndrome: differences between diarrhea and constipation predominant subjects. Gut. 1990;31:458–62.
2. Roe AM, Bartolo DC, and Mortensen NJ. Diagnosis and surgical management of intractable constipation. Br J Surg. 1986;73:854–61.
3. Pedersen IK, Christiansen J, Hint K, Jensen P, Olsen J, and Mortensen PE. Anorectal function after low anterior resection for carcinoma. Ann Surg. 1986; 204:133–5.
4. Sorensen M, Rasmussen OO, Tetzschner T, and Christiansen J. Physiological variation in rectal compliance. Br J Surg. 1992;79:1106–8.
5. Suzuki H and Fujioka M. Rectal pressure and rectal compliance in ulcerative colitis. Jpn J Surg. 1982;12:79–81.
6. Varma JS and Smith AN. Reproducibility of proctometrogram. Gut. 1986; 27:288–92.
7. Oettle GJ and Heaton KW. "Rectal dissatisfaction" in the irritable bowel syndrome. A manometric and radiological study. Int J Colorectal Dis. 1986;1:183–5.
8. Harris JH, Therkelsen EE, and Zinner NR. Electrical measurement of ureteral flow. In: Urodynamics. London: Academic Press; 1971. p. 465–72.
9. Djurhuus JC, Constantinou CE. Assessment of pyeloureteral function using a flow velocity and cross sectional area measurement. Invest Urol. 1979;17:103–7.
10. Rask-Andersen H and Djurhuus JC. Development of a probe for endoureteral investigation of peristalsis by flow measurement and cross sectional area measurement. Acta Chir Scand. 1976;472:59–65.
11. Fass J, Silny J, Braun J, Heindrichs U, Dreuw B, Schumpelick V, and Rau G. Ein neues verfahren zur quantitiven bestimmung oesophagealer motilitatsmuster mittels einer vieffachen impedanzmessung. Chirurgisches Forum 1989 fur experimentelle und klinische forschung. Berlin: Springer; 1989.
12. Colstrup H, Motensen SO, and Kristensen JK. A probe for measurements related values of cross sectional area and pressure in the female urethra. Urol Res. 1983;11:139–43.
13. Gregersen H, Kraglund K, and Djurhuus JC. Variations in duodenal cross sectional area during the interdigestive migrating motor complex. Am J Physiol. 1990;259:G26–31.
14. Gregersen H, Sorensen S, Sorensen SM, Rittig S, and Andersen AJ. Measurement of anal cross sectional-area and pressure during anal distension in healthy volunteers. Digestion. 1991;48:61–9.
15. Gregersen H and Djurhuus JC. Impedance planimetry: a new approach to biomechanical intestinal wall properties. Dig Dis. 1991;9:332–40.
16. Arhan P, Faverdin C, Persoz B, Devroede G, Dubois F, Dornic C, and Pellerin D. Relationship between viscoelastic properties of the rectum and anal pressure in man. J Appl Physiol. 1976;41(5 pt 1):677–82.
17. Dall FH, Jorgensen CS, Houe D, Gregersen H, and Djurhuus JC. Biomechanical wall properties of the human rectum. A study with impedance planimetry. Gut. 1993:34:1581–6.

18. Dall FH, Jorgensen CS, Djurhuus JC, and Gregersen H. Biomechanical wall properties of the porcine rectum: a study using impedance planimetry. Dig Dis. 1991;9:347–53.
19. Frobert O, Storkholm JH, Gregersen H, and Bagger JP. In vivo assessment of luminal cross sectional areas and circumferential tension-strain relations of the porcine aorta. Scand J Thorac Surg. 1996;30:11–9.
20. Gregersen H and Andersen MB. Impedance measuring system for quantification of cross sectional area in the gastrointestinal tract. Med Biol Eng Comput. 1991;29:108–10.
21. Krogh K, Ryhammer AM, Lundby L, Gregerson H, and Laurberg S. Comparison of methods used for measurement of rectal compliance. Dis Colon Rectum. 2001;44:199–206.
22. Madoff RD, Orrom WJ, Rothenberger DA, and Goldberg SM. Rectal compliance: a critical reappraisal. Int J Colorectal Dis. 1990;5:37–40.
23. Rao GN, Drew PJ, Monson JRT, and Duthie GS. Physiology of rectal sensations: a mathematic approach. Dis Colon Rectum. 1997;40:298–306.
24. Rao SS, Hayek B, Summers RW. Impedance planimetry: an integrated approach for assessing sensory, active and passive biomechanical properties of the human oesophagus. Am J Gastroenetrol. 1995;90:431–8.

Chapter 2.6
Ambulatory Manometry

Andrew P. Zbar

Introduction

Ambulant recordings from the lower gastrointestinal (GI) tract first utilized capsule radiotelemetry although, because radiofrequency was used, much of the signal was disrupted (1). Newer capsules have pressure-sensitive microtransducers for fixed-frequency radiosignaling (2,3). Systems for the assessment of continuous anorectal pressure measures for prolonged periods were developed independently by Miller et al. (4) and Kumar and colleagues (5); the latter group devised a methodology for the assessment of sleep-patterned anorectal continuous monitoring. This chapter discusses the technical aspects and suggested indications for this largely experimental technique and its use in the coloproctology laboratory.

Technical Aspects of Continuous Ambulatory Anorectal Manometry

Short-course ambulatory anorectal manometry (AARM) provides an understanding of anorectal function during provocative maneuvers such as changes in posture, straining, and coughing, as well as assessing the effects of sleep, anorectal sampling, and micturition. The recording system consists of a probe housing the pressure-sensitive sensors with a battery-driven amplification unit and a portable cassette recorder for continuous monitoring. The data is interpreted by pulse interval modulation recorded on magnetic tape that is marked with a one-minute automated marker where the interval between pulses is proportional with pressure recorded on a pulse train. The magnetic tape may be decoded for production of an analogue chart record, which then can be matched to a patient diary of events (6). Digital assessment may be used, filtering peak findings and smoothing the trace with a smoothing filter designed to remove high- and low-frequency artifacts. The anorectal recording probe, encoding box, and portable tape recorder are shown in Figure 2.6.1.

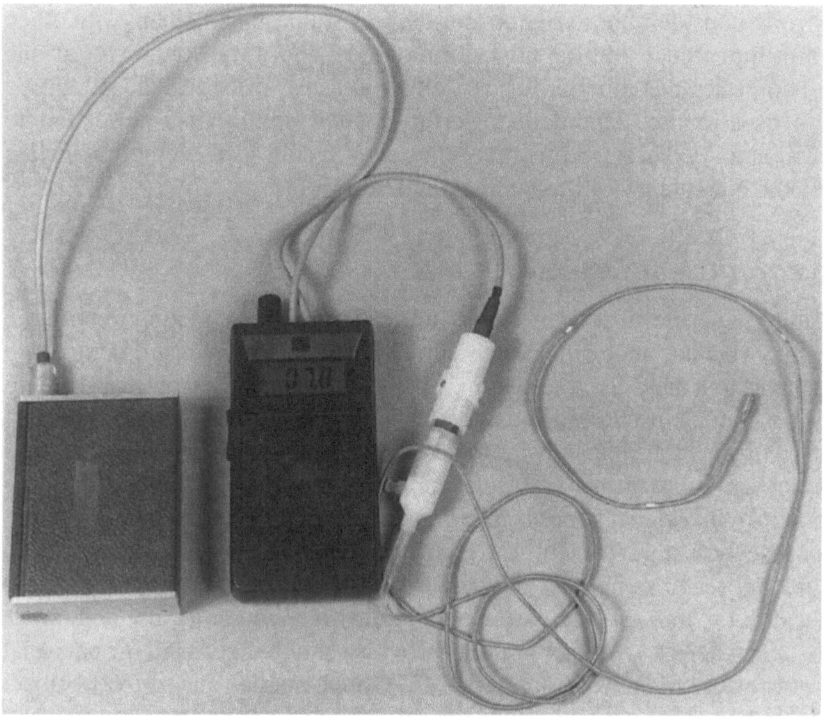

Figure 2.6.1. Ambulatory recording hardware. (With permission, D Kumar, RI Hallan, NR Womack, PR O'Connell, R Miller. Measurement of anorectal function. Chapter 3. In Clinical Measurement in Coloproctology. D Kumar, DJ Waldron, NS Williams Eds. Springer-Verlag, London 1991. p. 40)

This technique has been supplemented by a portable hand-held anal manometric device consisting of an air-filled microballoon system and a microtransducer (7–9). This area has been reviewed recently by Duthie and colleagues (10), where hand-held manometry has been shown to be repeatable for resting, squeeze, and cough pressure analyses.

Findings

Recordings in Normal Controls

The rectum contracts normally at five to ten cycles per minute, with slow postprandial phase cycles at three cycles per minute running every 20 to 30 minutes and with observed periodic rectal motor complexes every 90 minutes at night and during the day. These rectal complexes are slow propagated contractions resembling the phase III contractions of the migratory motor complex (MMC) seen in the small bowel (11,12). In the anal canal, there is considerable variation during wakefulness and sleep, with sleep motor quiescence and the imposition of slow and ultra-slow waves at one to two cycles per minute during waking and just prior to defecation and with occasionally exhibited powerful isolated contractions unrelated to rectal activity. These factors are definitely affected by the emotional state and the consistency of the luminal content (13,14).

Recordings in Disease

Studies have shown slowed activity in slow-transit constipation in both the rectum and the anal canal when compared with age-matched controls in response to a meal. Such studies may prove beneficial when patients present with a history of chronic constipation and where there is borderline evidence of slow transit in conventional marker studies (15). Equally, this technique has been shown to display impaired anorectal sampling in some patients with relatively poor initial functional outcome following low anterior resection as part of a postoperative "anterior resection syndrome" (16). Here, anorectal sampling (attributed to distinguishing between flatus and faucal entry into the rectum or neorectum) is manometrically defined as the time when the rectal pressure rises with a simultaneous fall in anal canal pressure for content discrimination (17). Such studies may provide objective data in some patients about the role of neorectal reservoir reconstruction and about the importance of preservation of the anal transition zone (18,19) although the issues after low anterior resection (in particular urgency) are complex, involving pouch design and capacity, the absence of pouch anastomotic sepsis (which may affect compliance), preoperative sphincter integrity, and avoidance of intraoperative sphincter damage during either stapled or hand-sewn anastomosis.

In these early small studies, normal sampling slow-wave activity of the rectum disappears with evidence of moderately high neorectal pressures and a reduced anorectal pressure gradient. This finding has translated into the more widespread use of colonic pouch (and more recently, coloplasty) reconstructions in selected cases where initial functional outcome appears superior (20–22). However, there is little evidence to suggest that the delayed function of patients undergoing some form of neorectal reservoir is superior to those having a coloanal anastomosis (23). This issue is somewhat complex because the J pouch is not just a pelvic colonic conduit or "transplant." It has an antiperistaltic component coupled with interposition of a denervated segment, which often can result in considerable evacuatory difficulty (see Chapter 9.1) (21).

In ileoanal pouch procedures (performed for ulcerative colitis and familial polyposis), sampling responses are initially poor, with reported episodes of nocturnal soiling correlating with increased pouch motor activity when the pouch is normally quiescent (24). Improved understanding of pouch physiology may have therapeutic implications for the design of pouch construction in some patients (25).

Chronic pruritis ani patients have been shown to have intermittent internal anal sphincter (IAS) relaxation associated with unrecognized episodes of fecal soiling (26), a finding that mirrors the physiological disturbance in fecally incontinent patients presenting with passive incontinence (27). Here, transient IAS relaxation is arbitrarily defined as a two to three cycle inhibition of IAS electromyogram (EMG) activity associated with a fall in anal canal pressure exceeding five centimeters H_2O, which tends to occur at four cycles per minute during wakefulness and which is not preceded by an increase in rectal pressure. Studies in some patients following hemorrhoidectomy where there is reported fecal soiling have shown lower ambulatory recorded pressures with reduced slow wave activity, although these changes appear to correlate poorly with observed episodes of incontinence (28).

Conclusions

In theory, ambulatory anorectal manometry may improve our understanding of continence and may be suitable for monitoring the dynamic variations in pressure over prolonged periods of time, providing information about rectoanal differential pressure coordination in health and in disease. At the present time, it must remain an experimental tool (29–31), however, it may have a current clinical place in those patients presenting with normal or low-normal resting manometry and fecal soiling (particularly after anorectal surgery) in the face of a normal endoanal ultrasound, in some patients who have essentially normal colonic transit and chronic constipation, and in the delineation of those with poor function following construction of a neorectal reservoir. The latter group is currently part of anorectal research, although preoperative parameters may shed light on patients who predictably are likely to perform poorly after straight coloanal anastomosis.

References

1. Connell AM, McCall J, Misiewicz J, and Rowlands E. Observation of the clinical use of radiopills. Br Med J. 1963;ii:771–4.
2. Browning C, Valori R, Wingate DL, and Maclachlan D. A new pressure sensitive ingestible radiotelemetric capsule. Lancet. 1981;ii:509–15.
3. Womack NR, Williams NS, Holmfield JHM, Morrison JFB, and Simpkins KC. New method for the dynamic assessment of anorectal function in constipation. Br J Surg. 1985;72:994–8.
4. Miller R, Lewis GT, Bartolo DCC, Cervero F, and Mortensen NJ. Sensory discrimination and dynamic activity in the anorectum: evidence using a new ambulatory technique. Br J Surg. 1988;75:1003–7.

5. Kumar D, Waldron D, Williams NS, Browning C, Hutton MRE, and Wingate DL. Prolonged anorectal monitoring and external anal sphincter electromyography in ambulant human subjects. Dig Dis Sci. 1990;35:641–8.
6. Browning C, Valori RM, and Wingate DL. Receiving, decoding and noise-limiting systems for a new pressure sensitive, ingestible radio-telemetric capsule. J Biomed Eng. 1983;5:262–6.
7. Dent JA. A new technique for continuous sphincter pressure measurement. Gastroenterology. 1976;71:263–7.
8. Miller R, Bartolo DCC, James D, and Mortensen NJM. Air-filled microballoon manometry for use in anorectal physiology. Br J Surg. 1989;76:72–5.
9. Orrom WJ, Williams JG, Rothenberger DA, and Wong WD. Portable anorectal manometry. Br J Surg. 1990;77:876–7.
10. Bollard RC, Gardiner A, and Duthie GS. Outpatient hand held manometry: comparison of techniques. Colorectal Dis. 2001;3:13–6.
11. Szurszewski JH. A migrating electric comp-lex of the canine small intestine. Am J Physiol. 1969;217:1757–63.
12. Kumar D, Williams NS, Waldron D, and Wingate DL. Prolonged manometric recording of anorectal motor activity in ambulant human subjects; evidence of periodic activity. Gut. 1989;30:1007–11.
13. Whitehead WE, Engel BT, and Schuster MM. Irritable bowel syndrome: physiological and psychological differences between diarrhea-predominant and constipation-predominant patients. Dig Dis Sci. 1980;25:404–13.
14. Wilgan P, Mishkinpour H, and Becker M. Effect of anger on colon motor and myoelectric activity in irritable bowel syndrome. Gastroenterology. 1988;94: 1105–6.
15. Ferrara A,Pemberton JH, Grotz RL, and Hanson RB. Prolonged ambulatory recording of anorectal motility in patients with slow-transit constipation. Am J Surg. 1994;167:73–9.
16. Williamson MER, Lewis WG, Holdsworth PJ, Finan PJ, and Johnston D. Decrease in the anorectal pressure gradient after low anterior resection of the rectum: a study using continuous ambulatory manometry. Dis Colon Rectum. 1994;37:1228–31.
17. Miller R, Bartolo DC, Cervero F, and Mortensen NJ. Anorectal sampling: a comparison of normal and incontinent patients. Br J Surg. 1988;75:44–7.
18. Miller R, Bartolo DCC, Cervero F, and Mortensen NJM. Does preservation of the anal transition zone improve sensation after ileal-anal anastomosis for ulcerative colitis? Clinical controversies in inflammatory bowel disease. Bologna: Topografia Negri SRC; 1987. p. 205.
19. Lewis WG, Holdsworth PJ, Stephen B, Finan PJ, and Johnston D. Role of the rectum in the physiological and clinical results of colo-anal and colorectal anastomosis after anterior resection for rectal carcinoma. Br J Surg. 1992;79:1082–6.
20. Romanos J, Stebbing JF, Smilgin Humphreys MM, Takeuchi N, and Mortensen NJM. Ambulatory manometric examination in patients with colonic J pouch and in normal controls. Br J Surg. 1996;83:1744–6.
21. Ho Y-H, Tan M, Leong AFPK, and Seow-Choen F. Ambulatory manometry in patients with colonic J-pouch and straight coloanal anastomosis. Randomized controlled trial. Dis Colon Rectum. 2000;43:793–9.
22. Furst A, Suttner S, Agha A, Beham A, and Jauch KW. Colonic J-pouch vs. coloplasty following resection of distal rectal cancer: early results of a prospective, randomized pilot study. Dis Colon Rectum. 2003;46:1161–6.

23. Ho Y-H, Seow-Choen F, and Tan M. Colonic J-pouch function at six months versus straight coloanal anastomosis at two years. World J Surg. 2001;25:876–81.
24. Miller R, Orrom WJ, Duthie G, Bartolo DCC, and Mortensen NJM. Ambulatory anorectal physiology in patients following restorative proctocolectomy for ulcerative colitis: comparison with normal controls. Br J Surg. 1990;77:895–7.
25. Nicholls RJ and Pezim ME. Restorative proctocolectomy with ileal reservoir for ulcerative colitis and familial polyposis: a comparison of three reservoir designs. Br J Surg. 1985;72:470–4.
26. Farouk R, Duthie GS, Pryde A, and Bartolo DCC. Abnormal transient internal sphincter relaxation in idiopathic pruritis ani: physiological evidence of ambulatory manometry. Br J Surg. 1994;81:603–6.
27. Sun WN, Read NW, Miner PB, Kurgan DD, and Donnelly TC. The role of transient internal anal sphincter relaxation in faecal incontinence. Int J Colorect Dis. 1990;5:31–6.
28. Ho YH and Tan M. Ambulatory anorectal manometric findings in patients before and after haemorrhoidectomy. Int J Colorectal Dis. 1997;12:296–7.
29. Duthie GS. Ambulatory monitoring in anorectal disease [thesis]. University of Aberdeen; 1992.
30. Farouk R and Bartolo DCC. The clinical contribution of an integrated laboratory and ambulatory anorectal physiology assessment in faecal incontinence. Int J Colorectal Dis. 1993;8:60–5.
31. Ronholt C, Rasmussen OO, and Christiansen J. Ambulatory manometric recording of anorectal activity. Dis Colon Rectum. 1999;42:1551–9.

Chapter 2.7
The Use of Colonic Motility and Transit Studies

NANCY BAXTER and JOHN H. PEMBERTON

Introduction

Colonic motility is poorly understood. Techniques for measurement of motility in the colon are relatively rudimentary when compared with other parts of the gastrointestinal (GI) tract, perhaps because of the relative inaccessibility of much of the colon and the relatively slow progression of its contents. In addition, there is substantial variation in transit between normal individuals. Despite this, however, motility disturbances are common, particularly in patients presenting to specialized colorectal units with an interest in evacuatory dysfunction.

Constipation is the most common digestive complaint, with up to 20% of the population reporting this symptom (1). A thorough understanding of the assessment of colonic motility and transit is essential to the management of many of these patients. Controlled transit of contents through the colon enables fluid, electrolyte, and short-chain fatty acid absorption. Transit also allows the controlled excretion of the waste products of digestion in an infrequent and socially acceptable fashion. Different areas of the colon assume various roles, with the right side having a greater role in absorption and the left side a greater role in storage and elimination.

Movement of stool content through the colon requires a complex neuromuscular coordination of segmental and mass muscular contraction. It is affected in turn by stool content and the underlying needs of the host. Ordinarily, colonic transit time ranges from 36 to 48 hours, where seemingly disorganized motor complexes and contractions achieve relatively slow propulsion. Segmental contractions dominate and facilitate mixing and absorption, and material is moved forward and backward, eventually being propelled slowly in an antegrade fashion. Mass movements (Giant Migratory Complexes) occur infrequently in the colon, but are essential for the distal propulsion of bowel contents and for defecation. This second major pattern results from distension in the transverse and descending colon propelling the contents forward effectively for relatively long distances. Mass movements occur only one to two times daily in healthy states.

Detailed information regarding colonic motility may be useful in the evaluation of a variety of patients. Motility studies are essential in the evaluation of severe idiopathic constipation. Many patients present with the symptom of constipation; however, the threshold for this complaint is variable (1), and given the wide spectrum of normal bowel movement frequency between individuals, this is not surprising. In fact, patients may interpret hard stool consistency as constipation, even if stool frequency and volume are not problematic. Therefore, as a symptom, constipation is complex and a more reliable method of evaluation is necessary (2). Certainly, stool frequency does not necessarily correlate with colonic transit. A number of patients presenting with the complaint of severe constipation with infrequent stools may have no demonstrable abnormality on transit studies (3). In contrast, patients passing pebble-like small volume stools with "normal" frequency may have distinctly abnormal colonic motility. Stool frequency is at best a poor surrogate measure of motility or transit.

Even in patients with established constipation, determining the principal cause(s) will influence recommended treatment. Severe constipation may result from slow transit, obstructed defecation, or a combination of the two, as well as having no underlying explanation (see Chapter 6.2). Diagnosis is essential for the planning of therapy where patients with slow transit constipation are unlikely to benefit from pelvic floor retraining, and where patients with pelvic floor dysfunction may be spared a major surgical procedure. Moreover, colonic motility and transit studies have not been used widely in the study of diarrheal illness, but they may have some role, particularly in the evaluation of individuals with diarrhea-predominant irritable bowel syndrome or in those presenting with fecal urgency.

The ideal transit study should be reliable, valid, and simple to perform, with little specialized equipment required. The test itself should be minimally invasive and not influence transit. In addition, the test must be highly acceptable to patients, particularly when there is a possibility that, over time, it might be repeated. Unfortunately, no single study fulfills all these criteria. The tests that are available may be divided into two broad categories: tests of colonic transit (using radiopaque markers or scintigraphy) and tests of colonic pressure and activity (manometry and barostat measurements). Transit measures will be described in detail, as they are used clinically. The use of measures of colonic pressure and activity is largely restricted to research use only.

Transit Studies

As early as 1902, Cannon had made observations on the movement through the feline colon of bismuth subnitrate, noting that there was a differential effect of colonic entry and exit of substrate (4). An objective evaluation of colonic transit is generally one of the first steps in the assessment of a severely constipated patient. Prior to such studies, a thorough history and physical examination is performed, as many common causes of constipation can be determined in this fashion. In many cases, particularly if symptoms were new, mechanical obstruction should be ruled out through colonoscopy, computed tomography (CT) colography, or by barium enema. In these specialized cases, the unit may have decided, for the purposes of objective follow-up and reporting, to employ some form of scaled constipation questionnaire (5,6) rather than the adoption of the simpler Rome criteria where symptoms exceed three months in duration, where there is one reported bowel movement every four days, and/or if more than 25% of these movements are accompanied by excessive straining (7,8).

Very early studies showed the movement of glass beads of different colors in humans (9), where a range of different markers have been used historically, including knotted cellulose thread and small pieces of silver and gold (10). The movement of particulate matter is complex and partly depends on material density (heavier contents moving slower than light ones), the level of mixing, mass propulsions, interhaustral shuttling function, and retropulsion (11,12). Cinefluorography outlines the mass movement of material, but it is only qualitative, and the use of markers permits the bowel to be divided into segments where mathematical calculation can be performed in a constructed way. Such an approach permits the oral or cecal administration of the marker for the assessment of the mouth-to-anus time or for segmental transit determination. The administration of many markers or markers over time should help minimize the sampling errors induced by day-to-day variations in bowel function and effective transit. Other markers that traditionally have been (and no longer are) used include barium, a range of dyes (such as carmine red), and chemicals, including chromium sesquioxide, and cupric thiocyanate (13).

Radiopaque Marker Studies

Radiopaque markers have been used for over 30 years in the evaluation of constipation (14). These markers are ingested and move through the colon along with bowel contents. Initially, transit was estimated by evaluation of the expelled markers in the stool using radiography of the stool itself. The feasibility and acceptability of the study was improved with substitution of abdominal radiography.

Administration

For the test, markers are ingested and their passage through the colon recorded. In the most commonly performed test, 20 radiopaque markers are ingested on a single day. Patients should maintain their normal diet, but avoid the use of laxatives for the duration of the test. Other forms of the test involve ingestion of markers on a number of consecutive days; however, this increases the complexity of the test, yet does not appear to improve the reliability. Radiographs do not need to be taken on a daily basis. Abdominal X-rays, including the pelvis, generally are taken at three and five days and continued until all markers are expelled or to seven days after marker ingestion. This assessment of whole gut transit originally used solid two- to five-millimeter polyethylene pellets impregnated with barium sulphate 20% (W/W) and small 2.7 to 4.5 millimeter diameter particles of radiopaque polythene tubing, which have a specific gravity similar to stool. The main refinements in this comparatively simple technique have been in the definition of regional normal values in reducing X-ray exposure and in minimizing the inconvenience of the test (14,15). These techniques generally depended upon the regular appearance of markers within the stool using a basic mathematical formula that converted the number of markers to time (hours) between the time of ingestion and that of recovery. When daily administration had "equilibrated" with daily excretion, a whole colonic transit time was calculated (16).

Evaluation of segmental colonic transit may be important in some individuals, particularly those with abnormalities isolated to the distal colon or with outlet obstruction. To evaluate segmental transit, serial X-rays can be taken to follow the movement of the markers. Alternatively, 20 markers per day can be ingested for three days, assuming that a steady state of ingestion and elimination has been reached within three days and that segmental transit over this time period is consistent. Using this technique, a single radiograph can be taken at four days, minimizing exposure to ionizing radiation, which is particularly important in the pediatric population.

Interpretation

There is substantial variation in the excretion of markers among normal individuals (Table 2.7-1) (17). The mean transit for normal individuals is 36 hours, and the majority will have expelled all markers within four to five days (17,18). However, at three days, most normal individuals would be expected to have excreted over 80% of all markers. Because of the wide normal variation, only individuals with retention of more than 20% of markers beyond five days would be considered to definitely have abnormal transit (Figure 2.7.1). Patients with severe constipation may not excrete all markers even after ten days. Basically, right and left colonic, sigmoid and rectal differentiation is made by drawing a line between bony landmarks of the vertebral column and pelvis, as described by Arhan et al. (19) and Smith (20). After two days, markers may be located over all of the colonic segments (as defined), with movement beyond this period of time from the right to the left colon, where they are lost in an exponential fashion. This method of calculation, where there is a mathematical expression based on the time interval between films, involves considerable radiation exposure,

TABLE 2.7-1. Maximum "normal" transit time through the large bowel (mean + 2 SD in hours).[1]

Adults	Chaussade et al., 1986 (6)	Chaussade et al., 1990 (7)	Metcalf, 1990 (8)	Arhan et al., 1981 (9)	Hinds et al., 1989 (10)	Bouchoucha et al., 1992 (11)	Bouchoucha et al., 1992 (11)*
Markers Technique		Multiple Ingestion				Single Ingestion	
Right Colon	24	24	32	38	24	37	20
Left Colon	30	31	39	37	32	26	14**
Rectosigmoid	44	33	36	34	45	41	25
Colon and Rectum	67	67	68	93	76	88	43**

* Stress-free controls.

** $p < 0.01$ as compared with other controls.

[1] Adapted from Devroede G. Radiopaque markers and transit. In: Schuster MM, Crowell MD, and Koch KL, editors. Schuster atlas of gastrointestinal motility in health and disease. Hamilton, Canada: BC Decker Inc.; 2002. Table 19.5. p. 275.

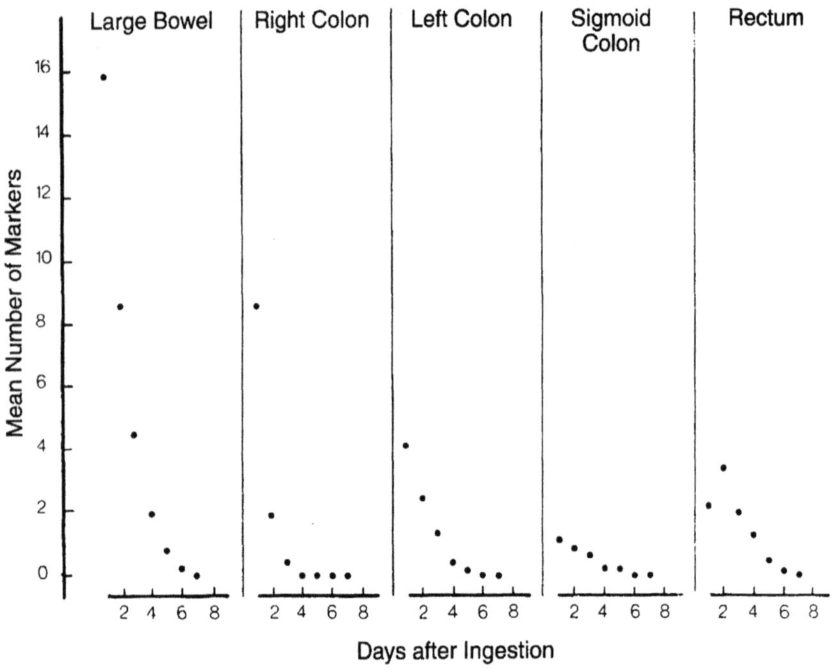

FIGURE 2.7.1. Average transit of radiopaque markers through the large intestine. (Reproduced with permission from Prather CM, Chapter 20 in Schuster MM, Crowell MD, and Koch KL, editors. Schuster atlas of gastrointestinal motility in health and disease. Hamilton, Canada: BC Decker Inc.; 2002. Figure 19.17. p. 277.)

which has been modified by Metcalf into single-film technology on Day 4 (21). Both these techniques rest on the assumption that the colon handles all markers in the same way on each day and that a 24-hour sampling method is an accurate approximation of continuous observation (22,23). Interpretation also is complicated in those patients with very rapid or extremely delayed transit times.

In Metcalf's original work, she stressed the use of pretest barium studies (if they had been performed), which can be useful in the determination of segmental colonic components. In general, markers located to the right of the vertebral spinous processes above a line from the fifth lumbar vertebra to the pelvic outlet are assigned to the right colon, and markers to the left of the vertebral spinous processes and above an imaginary line drawn from the fifth lumbar vertebra to the anterior superior iliac crest are defined as left colonic (Figure 2.7.2). All markers that are inferior to the line drawn from the pelvic brim (right) and the crest (left) are rectosigmoid/rectal, where any pelvic lying cecum or transverse colon are reassigned in accordance with the basic gas patterns observable. All calculations are based on the technique as described by Arhan and colleagues (19), where:

$$\text{Mean transit} = 1/N\sum_{i=1}^{j}\frac{n_i(i+1)-t(i-1)}{2} \qquad (1)$$

such that N is the number of markers ingested, n is number of markers present on the film taken at time t_i, $t(i+1)-(i-1)/2$ is time interval between successive films, and j is the number of films taken.

Using these techniques, three main variants of delayed transit may be identified by the use of markers. In classic slow transit constipation, movement of markers is delayed; however, all segments appear to be affected (Figure 2.7.2) Conversely, in a number of patients, abnormal transit may be localized to a single segment of the colon, most commonly the sigmoid and rectum. Abdominal radiographs at three and five days in such patients will reveal an abnormal number of markers in the rectum, with the remainder of the colon cleared of markers. More rarely, abnormal transit may be localized to the right colon. In such cases, once markers have passed this segment, transit normalizes. Moreover, a number of constipated patients will also have normal transit studies. In some cases, noncompliance may be suspected and a repeat study will need to be made, with a radiograph taken immediately after marker ingestion to document compliance of marker ingestion. In some cases where markers are still present on the last available radiograph, the "transit time" calculated will be less than the real transit time, and additional X-rays may be required to define the presence of rectosigmoid holdup.

Advantages/Disadvantages

The test is simple, relatively inexpensive to perform, and is widely available. It is the most commonly performed test of colonic motility, and therefore

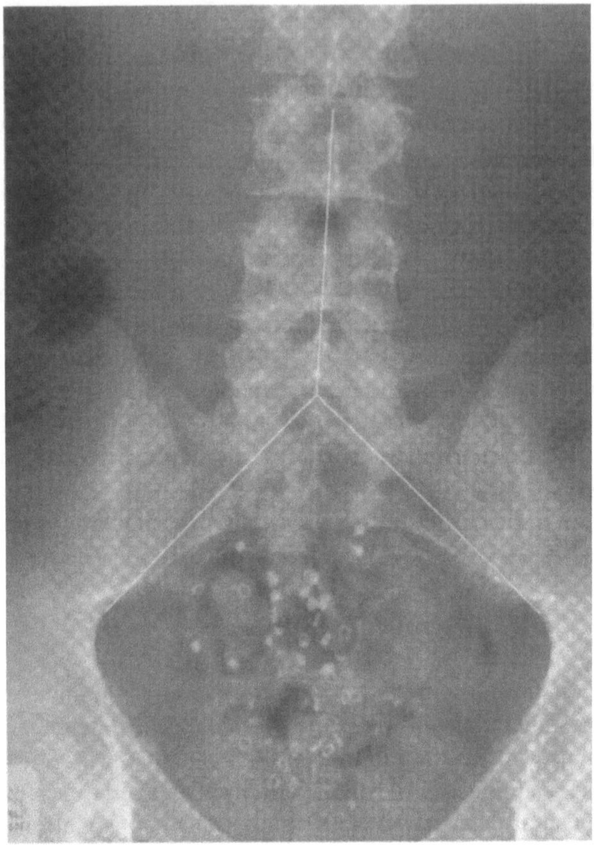

FIGURE 2.7.2. Transit study showing retention of markers in the rectosigmoid. The film has been marked to show the right and left colons and the rectosigmoid. (Reproduced with permission from Arhan P, Devroede G, Jehannin B, et al. Segmental colonic transit time. Dis Colon Rectum. 1981;24:625–9.)

has the most accepted norms. However, the test is relatively long, taking up to seven days. In addition, it is largely qualitative and does not provide reproducible whole or segmental transit times.

Colonic Scintigraphy

Colonic scintigraphy shares many principles with radiopaque marker studies; however, it enables a more quantitative evaluation of transit. If different isotopes are used, both solid and liquid transit can be assessed, which can be linked to inert, poorly absorbed agents like diethylenetriamine pentaacetic acid (DTPA), where the principles that have been applied to the assessment of gastric emptying may in part be translated to the colon. This issue is complex, however, since one must take into account the oral-to-cecal transit time, and areas that overlie the duodenojejunal flexure may confuse the determination of colonic transit. The former may be obviated by the more invasive technique of colonic intubation (24), or by the novel use of carrier pH-sensitive polymers, which dissolve in the ileum so that the entry into the cecum (25,26) is the effective zero-time of the study.

Administration

To perform colonic transit studies using scintigraphy, patients ingest a radioactive isotope. The movement of the isotope through the intestinal tract is followed with a gamma camera linked to a computerized processing unit, where more continuous observation of the passage of the radioisotope is possible. Several isotopes have been used to assess transit, including ^{99m}Technetium, ^{111}Indium, and ^{131}Iodine. Although technetium is relatively cheap and widely available, the half-life of this isotope is six hours, and this limits its usefulness in the evaluation of the colon. Indium (with a half-life of almost three days) is the most commonly used isotope for this type of study. Most authors describe administering 2 MBq ^{111}Indium orally for the study, although other dosages have been reported. Anterior and posterior images are then taken using a gamma camera with a medium energy parallel hole collimator. Although different authors have reported varying schedules, transit is probably best evaluated with images taken at 10 to 12 hours, 24 hours, and 48 hours (28). The test performs similarly in men and women (27).

Interpretation

Approaches here vary, but the colon is divisible into regions of interest. Many authors recommend the use of a geometric center with a weighted average of counts in the colonic segments for the interpretation of colonic scintigraphy. To calculate a geographic center (GC), the colon is divided into five segments (Figure 2.7.3) (28, 29). The ascending colon is represented in Segment 1, the transverse colon in Segment 2, the descending colon in Segment 3, the sigmoid and rectum in Segment 4, and excreted stool in Segment 5. The number of counts in each segment is then determined. The isotope count in the stool is assumed to be the total count administered minus the amount remaining in the colon. The GC is calculated by multiplying the percentage of the total number of counts in a given segment by the segment number, adding the result for each segment and dividing by 100 where:

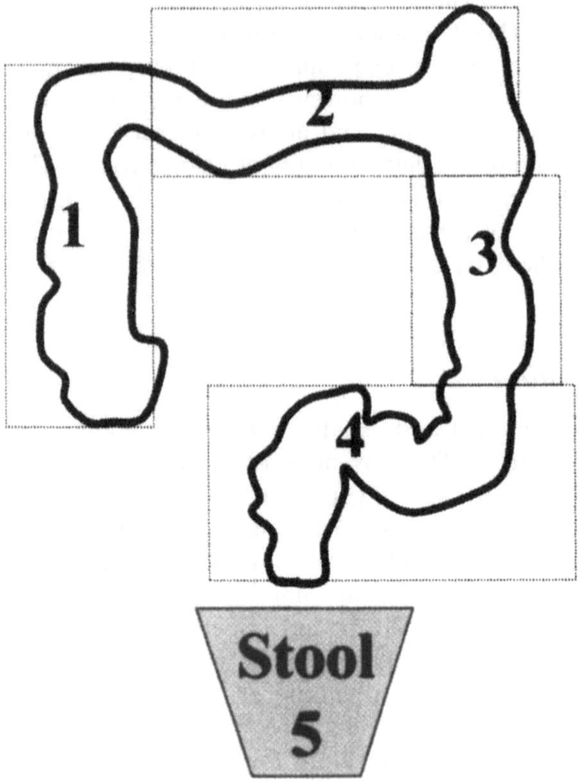

FIGURE 2.7.3. Landmarks for dividing colon into segments to calculate the geometric center. (Reproduced with permission from Prather CM, Chapter 20 in Schuster MM, Crowell MD, and Koch KL, editors. Schuster atlas of gastrointestinal motility in health and disease. Hamilton, Canada: BC Decker Inc.; 2002. Figure 20.4. p. 285.)

$$GC = \begin{pmatrix} \%\text{Counts in Segment } 1 \times 1 + \%\text{ Counts in Segment } 2 \times 2 \\ +\%\text{Counts in Segment } 3 \times 3 + \%\text{Counts in Segment } 4 \times 4 \\ +\%\text{Counts in Segment } 5 \times 5 \end{pmatrix} / 100 \quad (2)$$

Corrections generally are made for isotope decay. Normal values for the GC are presented in Table 2.7-2. Of note, the geometric center at 48 hours has been demonstrated to be more reproducible than measurement at 24 hours (30,31). Interpretation of the study requires visual inspection of the image to differentiate global slow transit from outlet obstruction, as well as calculation of the geometric center (Figure 2.7.4); however, if the distribution of the isotope in the colon is non-uniform, the progression of the GC may be artifactually distorted. The issue is complicated further by the physicodynamics of radioisotopic use where decay, tissue attenuation, and

TABLE 2.7-2. Normal values for scintigraphic transit.[2]

Author	Technique	Subjects	# Colonic Regions	4-Hour GC	24-Hour GC	48-Hour GC
Krevsky et al. (29)	Cecal instillation	7	7	4.8 (5 h)	5.3	6.3
Burton et al. (30)	Coated capsule —charcoal	10	5	1.1	2.7	NA
Notghi et al. (33)	Coated capsule —pellets	8	5	1.4	2.8	4.1
Krevsky et al. (36)	PO liquid isotope	15	7	NA	4.2	6.2
Camilleri et al. (37)	Coated capsule —pellets	22	5	1.1	2.8	NA

[2] Adapted from Prather CM. Scintigraphy. In: Schuster MM, Crowell MD, and Koch KL, editors. Schuster atlas of gastrointestinal motility in health disease. Hamilton, Canada: BC Decker Inc.; 2002. Table 20.2. p. 286.

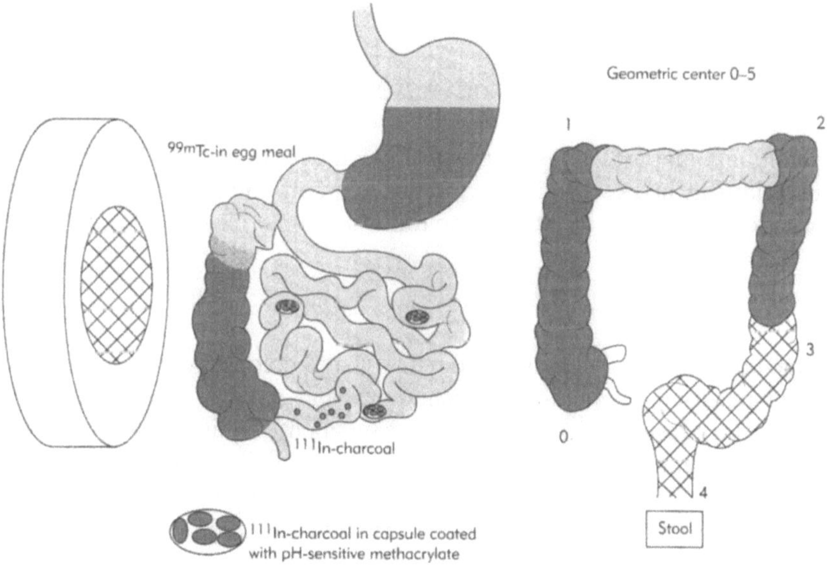

FIGURE 2.7.4. Scintigraphic method to evaluate gastric, small bowel, and colon transit. A delayed-release, pH-sensitive capsule delivers isotopically labeled solid particles to the colon to estimate colon transit. Geometric center refers to the weighted average of counts in four regions of colon and stool. (Reproduced with permission from von der Ohe MR and Camilleri M. Measurement of small bowel and colonic transit: Indications and methods. Mayo Clin Proc. 1992;67:1169–79.)

isotopic overlap must be taken into consideration (32). Cut-off points for abnormal values should be standardized for each laboratory, as they may vary with differing methods of evaluation and different times of evaluation. Abnormal cut-off points typically are selected at more than two standard deviations from the normal values. Constipation related to diffuse delay or right-sided delay may be identified using this geometric center technique, although left-sided delay may result in a normal value for the GC in some rare cases where a visual inspection of the image is essential (33).

Advantages/Disadvantages

Colonic scintigraphy allows a quantitative assessment of colonic motility, and in this way it has advantages over radiopaque markers. However, the technique requires the active participation and interest of the Department of Nuclear Medicine. The standardization required likely precludes all but centers with a specialized interest from relying on this modality. Images may be taken at many time intervals without increasing the total radiation exposure. This may be particularly useful in assessing motility in children.

Research Methods in the Assessment of Colonic Transit

Additional methods of assessment of colonic motility exist; however, they are relatively invasive and labor intensive, largely limiting application to the research setting. These include the following.

Colonic Manometry

Pancolonic and segmental manometry of the colon have been described using perfused or solid-state technology and may be performed in an ambulatory fashion (34). Pancolonic assessment requires colonoscopy for the placement of transducers. Although the clinical application of this technique is currently limited, highly useful information regarding normal colonic contraction is being gathered (Figure 2.7.5) (35). In addition, this may be an ideal way to evaluate the effect of drugs on colonic motility in a research setting (36). Limited information is available regarding alterations in manometry in patients with disease, even in the research setting (37).

The original techniques have advanced from open-ended air-filled tubes to more sophisticated strain gauges and high-fidelity electronic transducers with the facility for long temporal recordings (38). In humans, intermittent contractile activity of the colon has been poorly studied, with evidence of short cycle bursts of activity in both the right and the left colon (39,40). The role of these phasic contractions in motility and mass movement, as well as

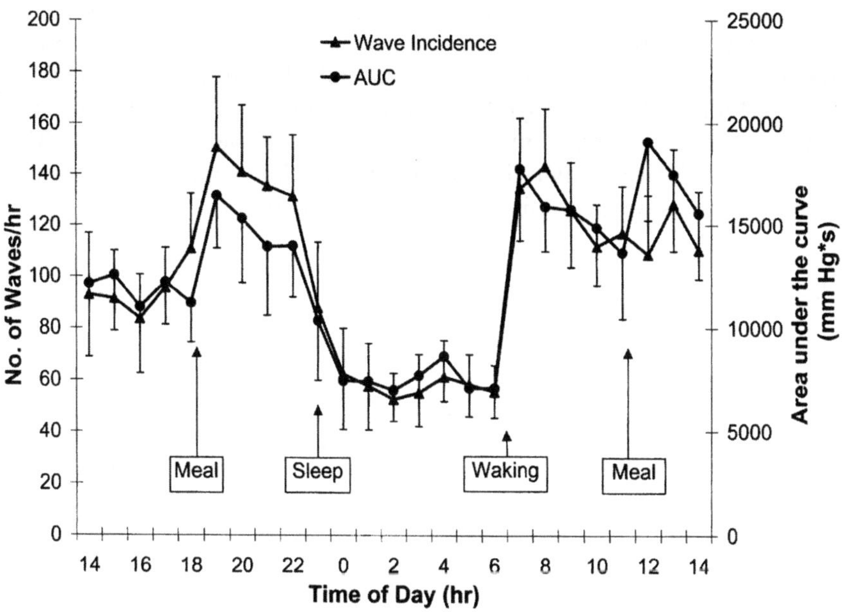

FIGURE 2.7.5. A 24-h profile of incidence and intensity of pressure waves in healthy humans. (Reproduced with permission from Rao SC, Sadeghi P, Beaty J, Kavlock R, and Ackerson K. Ambulatory 24-h colonic manometry in health humans. Am J Physiol Gastrointest Liver Physiol. 2001;280:G629–39. Figure 1. pp G631.)

in colonic absorptive capacity, is not understood, nor is the gastrocolic reflex mechanism (41–43). These activities are accompanied by diurnal variation in isolated but propagated high amplitude waves moving at one centimeter sec^{-1} just after waking and meals (44) in the absence of true peristaltic waves, which may be secondarily affected by the pH and osmolarity of the luminal content and by colonic distension. The issue is complex because there may be retrograde and long-lasting powerful contractions that are not distally propulsive, even in the normal state (45).

This approach has been supplemented by colonic electromyography, which appears to be an extremely complex phenomenon where there is much interspecies difference (46). Interpretation has been assisted by Fast Fourier and spike pattern recognition analysis of *in vivo* recordings of human colonic myoelectric activity, although the results have been very variable with phasic and continuous slow wave activities demonstrated. These are dependent to some extent on the methodology used, whether that be by serosal bipolar electrodes or by mucosal monopolar measurements and by the colonic position of the electrode (47–51).

The role of these methods is still experimental, with little understanding of what represents normal data, let alone what is pathological and disease related. Computerized electronic integration may provide colonic motility pattern indices that will define pathological periodicity of propagating and non-propagating pressure waves that may be disease specific (52). In diseased states, for example, colonic EMG has failed to produce recognizable patterns for irritable bowel syndrome, although there is a characteristic long spike pattern for diarrhea-predominant irritable bowel syndrome (IBS), whereas paradoxical activity has been seen in colonic manometric studies in some patients with chronic intractable constipation (53).

Barostat Measurements

The colonic barostat device is a bag inserted into the colon. It is filled with air and maintained at a constant pressure. Changes in colonic tone therefore produce increases or decreases of the volume of the bag, and using this principle, the barostat device may be used to evaluate colonic contraction and relaxation. The barostat device has been used to evaluate colonic tone in physiologic conditions (54). The barostat may allow colonic sensitivity to be evaluated in a quantitative fashion, and in addition, this device may be useful in assessing colonic compliance in diseased states and after pharmacologic intervention. The device has been used only for a short time and further understanding of normal physiology is required before this test is used more widely, even in research settings.

Conclusions

Although problems with colonic motility and transit are a common cause of patient complaints, accurate assessment of these complaints remains limited by available assessment tools. Transit studies, including radiopaque markers and colonic scintigraphy, are able to provide a gross assessment of transit and are highly useful in the clinical management of the constipated patient. However, many symptomatic individuals will appear "normal" using one or all of these tests. In addition, these tests do not evaluate the underlying mechanisms for abnormal transit. Further information from research studies using measures of colonic pressure and activity hopefully will improve our understanding of both normal and pathologic colonic motility and transit and the clinical role of these specialized investigations in coloproctological practice.

References

1. Walter S, Hallbook O, Gotthard R, Bergmark M, and Sjodahl R. A population-based study on bowel habits in a Swedish community: prevalence of faecal incontinence and constipation. Scand J Gastroenterol. 2002;37:911–6.
2. Koch A, Voderholzer WA, Klauser AG, and Muller-Lissner S. Symptoms in chronic constipation. Dis Colon Rectum. 1997;40:902–6.

3. Glia A, Lindberg G, Nilsson LH, Mihocsa L, and Akerlund JE. Clinical value of symptom assessment in patients with constipation. Dis Colon Rectum. 1999; 42:1401–8.
4. Cannon WB. The movements of the intestines studied by means of roentgen rays. Am J Physiol. 1902;6:251–77.
5. Agachan F, Chen T, Pfeifer J, Reissman P, and Wexner SD. A constipation scoring system to simplify evaluation and management of constipated patients. Dis Colon Rectum. 1996;39:681–5.
6. Knowles CH, Eccersley AJ, Scott SM, Walker SM, Reeves B, and Lunniss PJ. Linear discriminant analysis of symptoms in patients with chronic constipation. Validation of a new scoring system (KESS). Dis Colon Rectum. 2000;43: 1419–26.
7. Whitehead WE, Chaussade S, Corazziari E, and Kumar D. Report of an international workshop on management of constipation. Gastroenterol Int. 1999;4: 99–113.
8. Koch A, Voderholzer, Klauser AG, Müller-Lissner S. Symptoms in chronic constipation. Dis Colon Rectum. 1997;40:902–6.
9. Alvarez WC and Freedlander BL. The rate of progress of food residues through the bowel. JAMA. 1924;83:576–80.
10. Hoelzel F. The rate of passage of inert materials through the digestive tract. Am J Physiol. 1930;92:466–97.
11. Ritchie JA, Truelove SC, Ardran GM, and Tuckey MS. Propulsion and retropulsion of normal colonic contents. Dig Dis. 1971;16:697–704.
12. Steadman CJ and Phillips SF. Measurement of colonic motor function. In: Kumar DS, Waldron DJ, and Williams NS, editors. Clinical measurement in coloproctology. London: Springer-Verlag; 1991. p. 19–36.
13. Manousos ON, Truelove SC, and Lumsden K. Transit times of food in patients with diverticulosis or irritable colon syndrome and normal subjects. Br Med J. 1967;iii:760–2.
14. Hinton JM, Lennard-Jones JE, and Young AC. A new method for studying gut transit times using radioopaque markers. Gut. 1969;10:842–7.
15. Cummings JH and Wiggins HS. Transit through the gut measured by analysis of a single stool. Gut. 1976;17:219–23.
16. Cummings JH, Jenkins DJ, and Wiggins HS. Measurement of the mean transit time of dietary residue through the human gut. Gut. 1976;17:210–8.
17. Devroede G. Radiopaque markers and transit. In: Schuster MM, Crowell MD, and Koch KL, editors. Schuster atlas of gastrointestinal motility in health and disease. Hamilton, Canada: BC Decker Inc.; 2002. Table 19.5. p. 265–82.
18. Bouchoucha M, Devroede G, Arhan P, et al. What is the meaning of colorectal transit time measurement? Dis Colon Rectum. 1992;35:773–82.
19. Arhan P, Devroede G, Jehannin B, et al. Segmental colonic transit time. Dis Colon Rectum. 1981;24:625–9.
20. Metcalf A. Transit time. In: Smith LE, editor. Practical guide to anorectal testing. New York/Tokyo: Igaku-Shoin; 1990. p. 17–22.
21. Metcalf AM, Phillips SF, Zinsmeister AR, MacCarty RL, Beart RW, and Wolff BG. Simplified assessment of segmental colonic transit. Gastroenterology. 1987;92:40–7.

22. Chaussade S, Roches H, Khyari A, Couturier D, and Guerre J. Mesure du temps de transit colique (TTC): description et validation d'une nouvelle technique. Gastroenterol Clin Biol. 1986;10:385–9.
23. Chaussade S, Gosslein A, Hostein J, Leman M, and Ponsot P. Determination du temps de transit colique (TTC) global et segmentaire dans une population de 96 sujet solontaires sains. Gastroenterol Clin Biol. 1990;14:95–7.
24. Krevsky B, Malmud LS, D'Ercole FF, Maurer AH, and Fisher RS. Colonic transit scintigraphy. A physiologic approach to the quantitative measurement of colonic transit in humans. Gastroenterology. 1986;91:1102–12.
25. Hardy JG, Healey JNC, Lee SW, and Reynolds JR. Gastrointestinal transit of an enteric-coated delayed-release 5-aminosalicylic acid tablet. Aliment Pharmacol Ther. 1987;1:209–16.
26. Proano M, Camilleri M, Phillips SF, Brown ML, and Thomforde GM. Transit of solids through the human colon: regional quantification in the unprepared bowel. Am J Physiol. 1990;258:G856–62.
27. Hinds JP, Stoney B, and Wald A. Does gender or the menstrual cycle affect colonic transit? Am J Gastroenterol. 1989;84:123–6.
28. Notghi A, Hutchinson R, Kumar D, Tulley N, and Harding LK. Use of geometric center parametric images in scintigraphic colonic transit studies. Gastroenterology. 1994;107:1270–7.
29. Krevsky B, Malmud LS, D'Ercole F, Maurer AH, and Fisher RS. Colonic transit scintigraphy. A physiologic approach to the quantitative measurement of colonic transit in humans. Gastroenterology. 1986;91:1102–12.
30. Burton DD, Camilleri M, Mullan BP, Forstrom LA, and Hung JC. Colonic transit scintigraphy labeled activated charcoal compared with ion exchange pellets. J Nucl Med. 1997;38:1807–10.
31. Cremonini F, Mullan BP, Camilleri M, Burton DD, and Rank MR. Performance characteristics of scintigraphic transit measurements for studies of experimental therapies. Aliment Pharmacol Ther. 2002;16:1781–90.
32. Collins PJ, Horowitz M, Shearman DJC, and Chatterton BE. Correction for tissue attenuation in radionuclide gastric emptying studies: a comparison of a lateral image method and a geometric mean method. Br J Radiol. 1984; 57:689–95.
33. Notghi A, Hutchinson R, Kumar D, Smith NB, and Harding LK. Simplified method for the measurement of segmental colonic transit time. Gut. 1994;35: 976–81.
34. Hagger R, Kumar D, Benson M, and Grundy A. Periodic colonic motor activity identified by 24-h pancolonic ambulatory manometry in humans. Neurogastroenterol Mot. 2002;14:271–8.
35. Rao SC, Sadeghi P, Beaty J, Kavlock R, and Ackerson K. Ambulatory 24-h colonic manometry in health humans. Am J Physiol Gastrointest Liver Physiol. 2001;280:G629–39.
36. Krevsky B, Maurer AH, Niewiarowski T, and Cohen S. Effect of verapamil on human intestinal transit. Dig Dis Sci. 1992;37:919–24.
37. Camilleri M and Zinsmeister AR. Towards a relatively inexpensive noninvasive, accurate test for colonic motility disorders. Gastroenterology. 1992;103:36–42.
38. Soffer EE, Scalabrini P, and Wingate DL. Prolonged ambulant monitoring of human colonic motility. Am J Physiol. 1989;257:G601–6.
39. Sarna S, Latimer P, Campbell D, and Waterfall WE. Electrical and contractile activities of the human rectosigmoid. Gut. 1982;23:698–705.

40. Kerlin P, Zinsmeister A, and Phillips S. Motor responses to food of the ilerum, proximal colon and distal colon of healthy humans. Gastroenterology. 1983;84:762–70.
41. Holdstock DJ, Misiewicz JJ, Smith T, and Rowlands EN. Propulsion (mass movements) in the human colon and its relationship to meals and somatic activity. Gut. 1970;11:91–9.
42. Snape WJ, Wright SH, Battle WM, and Cohen S. The gastrocolic response: evidence for a neural mechanism. Gastroenterology. 1979;77:1235–40.
43. Misiewicz JJ. Human colonic motility. Scand J Gastroenterol. 1984;19 Suppl: 43–51.
44. Narducci F, Bassotti G, Gaburri M, and Morelli A. Twenty four hour manometric recording of colonic motor activity in healthy man. Gut. 1987;28:17–25.
45. Chauve A, Devroede G, and Bastin E. Intraluminal pressures during perfusion of the human colon in situ. Gastroenterology. 1976;70:336–40.
46. Huizinga JD and Daniel EE. Control of human colonic motor function. Dig Dis Sci. 1986;31:865–77.
47. Taylor I, Duthie HL, Smallwood R, and Linkens D. Large bowel myoelectric activity in man. Gut. 1975;16:808–14.
48. Sunshine AG, Perry R, Reynolds JC, Cohen S, and Ouyang A. Colonic slow-wave analysis: limitations of usefulness of fast Fourier transform (FFT). Dig Dis Sci. 1989;34:1173–9.
49. Schang JC, Hemond M, Herbert M, and Pilote M. Myoelectrical activity and intraluminal flow in human sigmoid colon. Dig Dis Sci. 1986;31:1331–7.
50. Parker R, Whitehead WE, and Schuster MM. Pattern recognition program for analysis of colon myoelectric and pressure data. Dig Dis Sci. 1987;32:953–61.
51. Dapoigny M, Trolese JF, Bommelaer G, and Tournut R. Myoelectric spiking activity of right colon, left colon and rectosigmoid of healthy humans. Dig Dis Sci. 1988;33:1007–12.
52. Rogers J and Misiewicz JJ. Fully automated computer analysis of intracolonic pressures. Gut. 1989;30:634–41.
53. Waldron D, Bowes KI, Kingma YJ, and Cote KR. Colonic and anorectal motility in young women with severe idiopathic constipation. Gastroenterology. 1988;95:1388–94.
54. Whitehead WE and Delvaux M. Standardization of barostat procedures for testing smooth muscle tone and sensory thresholds in the gastrointestinal tract. The Working Team of Glaxo-Wellcome Research, UK. Dig Dis Sci. 1997;42: 223–41.

Editorial Commentary

Professors Nancy Baxter and John Pemberton outline in their expert fashion not only the currently available methods for colonic transit assessment, but the newer methods now under development. Unfortunately as they note "although problems with colonic motility and transit are a common cause of patient complaints, accurate assessment of these complaints remains limited to available assessment tools." Despite this shortcoming, they have succinctly, yet in a comprehensive manner, outlined methods of transit assessment. Certainly, as they also note, the most common currently acceptable method of transit assessment is pancolonic assessment using a single radioopaque marker containing either 20 or 24 rings with a single xray taken on the 5th postingestion day. Although segmental transit and newer forms of transit assessment such as the barostat and radioisotope scintigraphy are under development, none of them are ever commonly used. The most important facet of all of these studies is that, regardless of the method of performance, the result will undoubtedly be the key feature in determining the therapy for constipation. Specifically, patients with colonic inertia with normal pelvic floor function may well be offered a colectomy for constipation whereas patients with pelvic outlet delay with normal transit would not be offered surgery. Thus, the largest and most morbid procedure offered to patients with constipation will be determined by this single study. It is therefore somewhat reassuring to recognize that a colonic transit study is, in its simplest and most commonly used form, reproducible. Specifically, one study from Cleveland Clinic Florida concluded that not only is colonic transit time reproducible, but the success rate of colectomy for colonic inertia is significantly higher in patients who undergo repeat transit study than in those who undergo colectomy based on a single study.

SW

Chapter 2.8
Anorectal Sensitivity

Richelle J.F. Felt-Bersma

Anorectal sensitivity plays a role in the defecation process and in maintaining fecal continence. Variation in anorectal sensibility is also important in pain syndromes, such as irritable bowel syndrome, proctalgia fugax, and chronic anal pain. Although the anus and rectum are closely related, their functions differ; therefore, aspects pertaining to the sensitivity of each are discussed separately.

Rectal Sensitivity

Introduction

In 1960, Duthie and Gairns (1) were the first to describe the significance of nerve endings in the anorectum although their presence had been noted independently by Sotolo (2) and Fan (3) in the 1950s. These have greatest profusion at the anal transitional zone above the anal valves, where they include Meissner's touch corpuscles, Krause end-bulbs (necessary for the acute sensation of cold), specialized genital friction corpuscles, Golgi-Mazzoni bodies required for local pressure, and Pacinian corpuscles for distension (4). Rectal sensitivity is dependent upon mechanoreceptors that are situated in the superficial and deep layers of the rectal wall. The superficial receptors are situated in the mucosal layer and travel to the autonomic presacral ganglia, whereas the deep receptors have their fields in the muscular layers, serosa, and mesentery, projecting to the lumbar cord. Sensory afferents travel with the pelvic splanchnic nerves to the S2/3 junction. Nociceptive pathways travel in both parasympathetic and sympathetic systems via the inferior and superior hypogastric plexus to L1/2 since these are abolished during spinal anesthesia and diminished after pudendal nerve blockade.

Thus, some primary afferents fire action potentials in response to stretch or tension in the gut wall, whereas others are activated by chemical or mechanical stimuli directed at the mucosa. These mucosal stimuli probably work, at least in part, by activating specialized enteroendocrine cells in the mucosal epithelium, such as the serotonin-containing enterochromaffin cells. The primary afferent neurons then release synaptic transmitters to excite other classes of enteric neurons in nearby ganglia (5). Next, some fibers run up to the brain, where only a part of the sensations are represented on the frontal cortex for perception.

The feeling of rectal filling is the preliminary event at the onset of the defecation process. A bowel movement consists of colonic contractions that proceed distally and increase rectal pressure and awareness. Simultaneously, the anal sphincters relax with the onset of the colonic contractions. When the location is suitable, defecation will occur. Otherwise, the external sphincter contracts voluntarily and the rectum relaxes by increasing its compliance.

Measuring Technique

Different methods have been used to measure visceral perception and rectal compliance. Initially, latex balloons on a catheter connected with a syringe were used to perform volume-controlled distension. Later on, roller pump and intraballoon pressure measurement were used to slowly distend the balloon and calculate compliance. In 1985, Azpiroz and Malagelada (6) introduced the barostat, which consisted of a highly compliant polyethylene bag mounted on a catheter connected to a computer-controlled distension pump. With this system, volume-, pressure-, or wall tension-controlled distension can be performed in an intermittent or continuous distension manner. The subject of compliance and its measurement is discussed in Chapters 2.4 and 2.5.

Mucosal electrosensitivity (see "Anal Sensitivity" section) measures sensitivity of the rectal mucosa for a low electrical current. It has limited use outside of research facilities. When performing studies, it is very important to describe the methods used for rectal visceral sensitivity and compliance measurement because the results may differ accordingly. Additionally, the normal values should be well established for each anorectal laboratory.

Latex Balloon Measurement: The Triggers for Rectal Filling Sensation

Patients typically are asked to report a threshold for the feeling of rectal filling in which most anorectal laboratories ask about the first perceived volume, the urge volume, and the maximal tolerated volume. These recorded volumes are assumed to represent rectal capacity and to give some overall impression of rectal compliance although they are unable to define real aspects of rectal distensibility or rectal wall stiffness (7). Moreover, it needs to be recognized that an overall perception of the weight of the rectal contents is completely different to the phenomenon of sensation induced by rectal filling, where these sensations may be determinants of variations in rectal pressure and not volume. These, in effect, represent components of the receptive and elastic properties of the rectum and the rectal ampulla

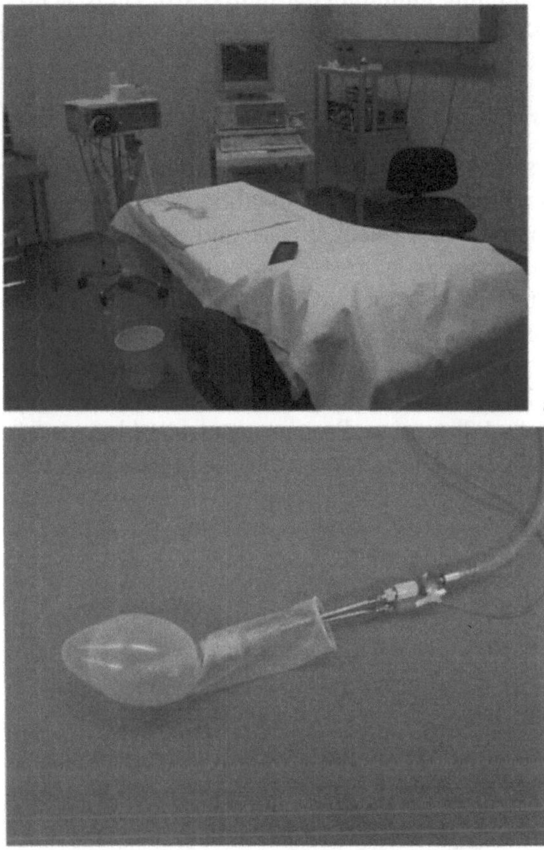

a b

FIGURE 2.8.1. Roller pump configuration. (a) Set up; (b) Latex balloon.

without reflecting anything to do with mucosal sensibility or the activity of tension-activated stretch receptors.

For the determination of these values, latex balloons are used in combination with a water pump or with a syringe filled with air or water (8) (Figure 2.8.1). The use of water or gas to distend the balloon does not seem to influence the measured compliance or sensation. Latex, because of its stiffness, influences the results of pressure, volume, and compliance measurement. Therefore, the intraballoon pressure values have to be corrected in order to obtain the real rectal pressures and compliance measurements. Measurement points for sensitivity are the moment of first sensation, urge volume (UV), and the maximum tolerated volume (MTV). Generally, in the literature, normal values of first sensation vary between 40 and 90 milliliters with a pressure between 10 and 30 mmHg, urge at about 140 milliliters with a pressure between 20 and 40 mmHg, and MTV between 200 and 300 milliliters with a pressure of 50 to 95 milliliters. Compliance ranges between five and nine milliliters per mmHg (8). There is no clear evidence that this approach of altered basic rectal sensibility correlates with disease type (9,10).

Barostat Measurements

A barostat system consists of a highly compliant polyethylene bag and a feedback-controlled computerized inflation device (Figure 2.8.2). Visceral perception, compliance, tonic response, and phasic contractility can all be investigated using this system. The distension protocol may considerably affect the results of visceral perception studies. The pressure or volume defining a sensory threshold, and subsequently the concept of hyperreactivity or hypersensitivity to distension, will be influenced by the distension method (11,12). Luminal distension can be achieved by pressure- or volume-controlled distension. Pressure-controlled inflation is preferable to volume-controlled or wall tension-controlled techniques because pressure-

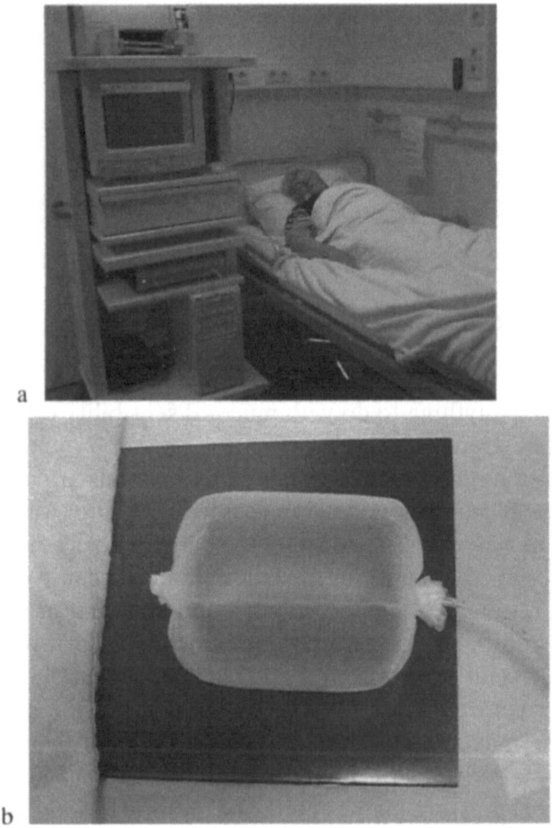

FIGURE 2.8.2. Barostat configuration. (a) Set up with patient; (b) Polyethylene balloon.

controlled methodology is independent of the shape of the bag or of the bowel. Different protocols have been described, such as intermittent or continuous distension techniques. In addition, increasing (incremental) or randomly chosen stimuli may be used because anticipation may play a role in sensory awareness, as observed elsewhere in the body. Whether it is possible to measure distinct sensations with these two different types of distension remains to be seen; however, there is a fairly good correlation between the volumes recorded for first sensation and urge and volumes and pressures recorded at MTV with the latex and the polyethylene balloon measurement (8). However, the polyethylene balloon tends to have a higher maximal toleration threshold than the latex balloon in any given patient.

The compliance curve (volume/pressure curve) derived from this data is an S-shaped curve that is indicative of the viscoelasticity of the gut, as well as the surrounding anatomy [see Chapter 2.5(i)]. Sensory thresholds should always be looked at in relation to measured compliance—a feature that is indicative of the starting rectal volume (and hence the likelihood of a megarectum in the patient) and the intrinsic wall stiffness and thickness. Changes in the threshold level can be misinterpreted if there is also a change in compliance, and equally, similar compliance values may be obtained in very different rectal pathologies when the rectum is over distended. Barostat measurements have been reported to have a variable reproducibility where results are affected by gender, age, and body mass index. Age tends to increase sensory thresholds, where men have larger rectal volumes, but the same rectal sensitivity pressure thresholds (8). Brain imaging during rectal distention tests has demonstrated some difference in cerebral representation between the sexes (5).

Certain drugs will also influence visceral sensitivity, where, for example, Somatostatin, 5-HT_3 antagonists, and κ-opioid agonists increase sensory thresholds. Rectal tone is measured by setting a standardized pressure. The inflation device aspirates or inflates air into the bag so that the set pressure will be maintained; these volume alterations reflect the intrinsic tone of the bowel wall. Rectal tone measurements have been shown to generally increase after a meal in healthy controls (13,14) and often are found to be diminished in multiparous women.

Rectal Sensitivity in Clinical Syndromes

Many studies have been performed in different patient groups and controls. Because methods differ between centers, results are not always easily comparable. In addition, in all patient groups, there is an overlap with controls where only extreme values have some clinical consequence (8).

Irritable Bowel Syndrome (IBS)

Patients with irritable bowel syndrome (IBS) are generally hypersensitive to balloon distension (15). This occurs in both diarrhea-predominant and constipation-predominant IBS patients (16). In addition, rectal sensitivity is influenced by the menstrual cycle in women (17); however, these differences are only indicative of IBS since there is an overlap with controls. Because rectal compliance is not different in patients with IBS when compared with controls (14), and because patients with colonic irritation due to mild ulcerative colitis do not report comparable hypersensitivity (18), it suggests that the hypersensitivity registered in IBS patients is due to an abnormal perception in the visceral afferents. The level of this abnormality has not yet been defined. Irritable bowel syndrome patients tend to label visceral stimuli in negatively affected terms and score higher on anxiety ratings in psychological tests, particularly when they show hypersensitivity (16,19).

Chronic Constipation

Visceral sensitivity can be decreased in patients with longstanding severe idiopathic constipation, especially those with slow transit constipation (20). There is no correlation between pelvic floor dysfunction, physiology and rectosigmoid transit, total colon transit, or any other basic physiological parameters (21). Depending on the definition of constipation, 25 to 60% of the constipated patients show rectal hypersensitivity or sigmoid hypersensitivity and also could be classified as constipation-predominant IBS (21).

Fecal Incontinence and Rectal Prolapse

Patients with fecal incontinence can have a normal or disturbed rectal sensitivity when compared with controls (8,22), and no difference has been noted between idiopathic and traumatic incontinence (8). Patients with fecal incontinence also can have a lowered or normal rectal compliance. Some incontinent patients with normal anal sphincter function have a lower rectal compliance when compared with incontinent patients with sphincter dysfunction. A low rectal compliance causes urgency, being most prominent when the capacity of the rectum is lower than 100 milliliters—a feature also detected in proctitis (8). A capacity of 60 milliliters almost invariably leads to fecal incontinence (8) and should be considered a strong contraindication for re-anastomosis or an indication to propose a stoma to the patient. A capacity larger than 500 milliliters is only seen in constipated patients and should be an indication to better regulate defecation. Reduced compliance generally is associated with a reduced rectal sensitivity and urgency (22) where disturbed sensitivity has implications for the close relationship between the perception of rectal distension, attendant external anal sphincter (EAS) contraction, and transient internal sphincter relaxations (23). In this regard, rectal sensitivity and compliance are only of importance when extreme low values are found (8), and it has been recommended that perineal approaches such as Altemeier's proctosigmoidectomy (where there may be excessive or prolonged endoanal distraction and manipulation) are ill advised in full-thickness rectal prolapse if there is grossly impaired rectal sensitivity or an absent preoperative rectoanal inhibitory reflex (RAIR) (24). Here, it has been suggested in part that continence may return in some patients where manometry is deranged, correlating with improved rectal mucosal sensitivity following the return of the mucosa to a more normal position (24–26).

Rectocele

In patients with a rectocele, rectal visceral sensitivity is decreased, but rectal compliance is not different when compared with healthy controls (27). Compliance curves and rectal sensitivity do not change after transvaginal repair or only temporarily vary following transanal repair with recovery after a year (28). Possibly, the decrease in MTV can be explained from direct plication of the rectal wall during transanal surgery in contrast to the vaginal approach.

Solitary Ulcer Syndrome

Patients with solitary rectal ulcer have lower rectal sensitivity thresholds, urge volumes, and MTVs when compared with controls, which may be due to alterations in compliance and/or perception where similar findings have been found in those patients presenting with full-thickness rectal prolapse (29).

Inflammatory Bowel Disease

Patients with ulcerative colitis with mild inflammation of the distal colon have higher discomfort thresholds than do controls (18). In contrast, patients without endoscopic abnormalities in the rectum tend to have an increased first sensation with attendant disturbances in rectoanal inhibition (30). Rectal compliance tends to be decreased in both the active and the quiescent colitic phases (8).

Radiation Proctitis

Patients with chronic proctitis usually have a reduction in rectal compliance, especially in those presenting with fecal urgency (31). Histology suggests that smooth muscle hypertrophy and myenteric plexus damage are both contributory.

Proctalgia Fugax

In the resting state, patients with proctalgia fugax have normal anorectal function and morphology; however, they may exhibit a motor abnormality of the anal smooth muscle during an acute attack (32).

Anal Sensitivity

Introduction

The anal canal is sensitive to touch, pain, temperature, and movement. This enables discrimination between flatus, fluid, and feces, although the responses of the anal canal are greater than those achievable by local touch impulses that are transmitted by the regional somatic nervous system (33). The anocutaneous sensations in the perianal area and in the anal canal below the dentate line are conveyed by afferent fibers to the pudendal nerve (S2-4). Several factors play a role in the awareness of anal sensitivity: an intact mucosa, a submucosa with its hemorroidal plexus, nerve endings in the mucosa and submucosa, afferent fibers in the pudendal nerve, and the central nervous system connections within the spinal cord and brain (Figure 2.8.3).

Measuring Technique

Historically, Duthie and Gairns utilized von Frey hairs, pinpricks, and metal plates of varying temperatures to objectively assess anal sensation (1), although the data provided was qualitative at best. Several methods have been developed to more quantitatively measure anal sensitivity. Perianal sensitivity can be neurological, as measured by means of a needle; however, measuring in the anus is difficult and the method is very subjective. Infu-

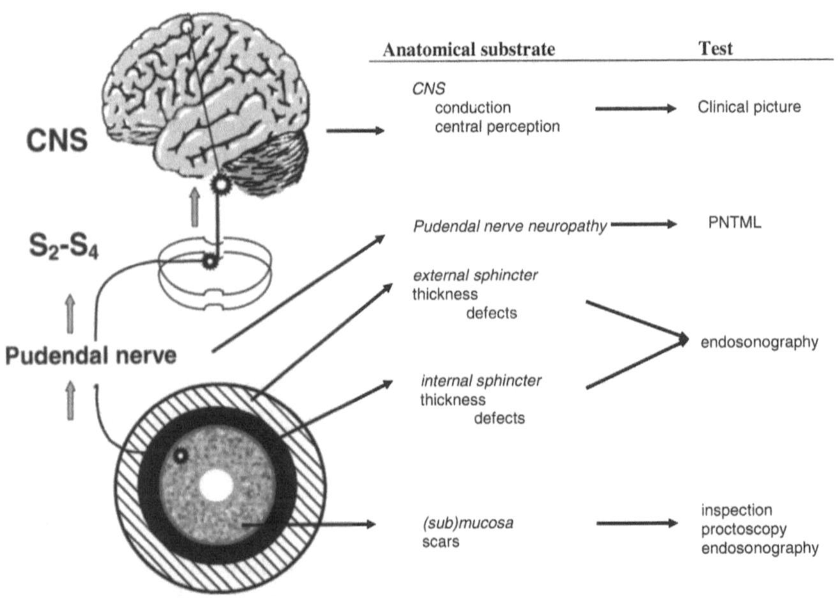

FIGURE 2.8.3. Anal sensitivity: Model of causative factors and testing.

sion with water at different temperatures also has been performed, but it is cumbersome and does not reveal more information than other measurements. The standard techniques used include the determination of mucosal electrosensitivity (10) and temperature sensation assessment (34,35).

Anal Mucosal Electrosensitivity (MES)

Roe et al. (10) used two electrodes with a constant square wave current with variable intensity to objectify anal sensitivity, although the original technique using a square wave electrical current was introduced by Siegel (36). This is a very easy and reliable tool to measure anal sensitivity and has been used by many centers with anorectal laboratories. The modality by which MES works is not clear, as it may stimulate many different types of receptors (37). A specially constructed 10 Fr Dover catheter with a diameter of five millimeters on which two platinum wire electrodes are mounted one centimeter apart is used. The probe is introduced into the anal canal, where a constant current (square wave stimulus 100 milliseconds at five pulses per second) is serially increased from one to twenty milliamperes until the threshold of sensation is indicated by the patient as a tingling or pricking sensation. This system is best utilized following the determination of the functional anal canal length using conventional anorectal manometric equipment. The system uses a custom-made constant current generator with a reference electrode placed on the thigh (38). The system used for the anal canal mirrors that also used to investigate urethral sensory thresholds that employed an electrode doublet hitched to a urethral catheter (39,40). Measurements can be performed, if desired, at several levels in the anal canal (high, middle, low). A high MES threshold reflects a decreased anal sensitivity. Normal values for MES vary between two and seven milliamperes where it has been found that increasing age is associated with a diminishing MES value. The reproducibility of the test has been shown to be satisfactory (41).

Anal Sensitivity in Clinical Syndromes

Many patient groups have been evaluated. There are two studies that have examined several patient subgroups using this technology (10,41), although many other studies have included MES measurements in their patient workup. Incontinent patients invariably have a high MES. In patients with anal sphincter defects, with or without fecal incontinence, MES tends to be increased, with the highest values found in patients with a combined sphincter defect. In incontinent patients, however, our group has found no difference between those with or without a sphincter defect (41), and it may be that concomitant neuropathy is part of the explanation for this finding. Following vaginal delivery, MES also increases, although it also tends to recover by six months (42). Only women with a persistent sphincter tear had an increased MES after six months in this study, although no pudendal nerve terminal motor latency (PNTML) measurements were made. Women with IBS have increased MES recordings both before and after delivery, and it is postulated that these patients are at risk for delayed fecal incontinence, although prospective data is not yet available (43).

Low perineal position and obstructed defecation also is related to a high MES (41,44), whereas patients with constipation have been reported by some to have an unaltered (10) or even a higher MES (41) value than normal. Patients with diabetic neuropathy show higher MES recordings (45), with proctitis patients generally having a normal MES (41). Patients with anal fissures have a low MES (10,41), whereas those with hemorrhoids have an increased MES (10,41), and excising them appears to increase the MES even further.

Mucosual electrosensitivity has prospectively been assessed after anorectal surgery. Here, rectopexy, independent of the procedure used, either leaves MES unaltered (41) or actually improves anal sensitivity (25,46). Sphincter repair (and post-anal repair) do not change MES (47). Proctocolectomy, including transitional zone excision, diminishes anal sensitivity (48), and although there is much speculation regarding the altered physiology following restorative proctectomy (and restorative proctocolectomy for ulcerative colitis and familial polyposis) and the preservation or excision of the anal transitional zone (49,50), it generally is suggested that its preservation and the avoidance of any form of mucosal proctectomy is associated with better clinical outcome in terms of fluid and flatus differentiation (and its physiological equivalent—anorectal sampling) and reports by the patient of nocturnal urgency (51–53). Transanal endoscopic microsurgery (TEMS) does not appear to alter MES (54).

The use of MES has been compared with other anorectal function tests in our large study (41), where no clear relationship has been demonstrated between anal sensitivity and other neurophysiologic measurements, such as electromyography or PNTML, and where there was little correlation between attendant distal pudendal neuropathy and mucosal electrical insensitivity. Weak correlations existed between measured MES and anorectal pressures and rectal or measured submucosal thickness on endosonography. Looking at an anatomical model that could possibly determine anal sensitivity measured by MES (Figure 2.8.3) in a multivariate analysis, only age, internal anal sphincter thickness, and submucosal thickness were independent factors in determining MES, although these factors only accounted for 10% of the recorded MES variance.

Temperature Sensation

The anal canal in a broad sense is no different from other sensitive areas of the body in the discrimination of different thermal conductivities (55). Hot and cold stimuli specifically designed for the anal canal have been constructed (34) using water-perfused thermodes incorporated into anal probes whereby heated water of different temperatures are pumped using thermostatically controlled baths for rapid temperature change. Using continuous recording via a thermocouple with patient-directed event changes, the researcher can record the minimum detectable temperature change with variation from normal to hot (or cold) and the reverse direction for the calculation of a median value. There is some evidence that there is blunted sensation as determined in this way in patients presenting with fecal incontinence when compared with normal controls, and there is a moderate correlation between this testing and MES estimates (2). Because continence is preserved after mucosal proctectomy, there is much that is unknown concerning this area, and its recording remains a research tool. It may be that sensory perception assessment in patients with postdefecatory leakage (particularly following minor anorectal surgery) may provide more insight into specialized dysfunction (56).

Conclusions

Rectal sensitivity and compliance can be measured with a latex balloon connected with a syringe and/or water pump or with a polyethylene balloon filled with air connected to a barostat. Rectal tone can only be measured with a barostat where hypersensitivity can be found in patients with IBS and relative hyposensitivity may be found in several patient groups like fecal incontinence, constipation, rectocele, and rectal prolapse. The assessment of rectal sensation is not readily reproducible, relying on sensibility to balloon distension with the recording of a threshold rectal distension volume, a constant sensation volume, an urge volume, and a maximal tolerated volume. These values give a broad idea concerning rectal capacity and the suggestive diagnosis of megarectum in some patients presenting with evacuatory dysfunction. The assumptions concerning the clinical and manometric assessment of rectal compliance have been outlined in Chapters 2.4 and 2.5, and they are inherently representative of the differences between these physical and engineering measurements in solid cylindrical distensible "vessels"' and their determination and translation to the biomechanical properties of living systems.

Anal sensitivity can be measured easily with MES. Many patients with anal abnormalities with or without complaints can have a disturbed anal sensitivity. In addition, there is an overlap with controls. Only patients with fissures or proctitis seem to have a normal anal sensitivity. Aging, internal anal sphincter defects, and submucosal thickening are the most important determinants of anal sensitivity. Anal sensitivity measurement is not a crucial tool in daily clinical management, but a sophisticated test incorporated in anorectal function testing for selected patients in a research setting. Although it is clear that patients with abnormal sensation may report normal continence (and equally that those with normal anal canal sensibility may present with fecal leakage), it is still believed that an integrity of sensory function in the anal canal plays an important role in continence maintenance. Here it has been suggested that some patients with fecal incontinence require impairment of both motor and sensory function where there may be very high recorded sensory thresholds to balloon distension (57)—an abnormality more often seen in patients with chronic idiopathic constipation where there may be an attendant sensory abnormality detectable in the upper anal canal that by itself may not be sufficient to result in reported fecal leakage. In these patients, there is a poor perception of rectal distension and fullness.

References

1. Duthie HL and Gairns FW. Sensory nerve endings and sensation in the anal region of man. Br J Surg. 1960;67:585–9.
2. Sotolo JR. Nerve endings of the walls of the descendent colon and rectum. Z Zellforsch. 1954;41:S101–11.
3. Fan WW. Histological studies of sensory nerves in the sigmoid and rectum. Arch Fur Jap Chir. 1955;24:567–74.
4. Rogers J, Hayward M, Henry M, and Misiewicz JJ. Temperature gradient between the rectum and anal canal: evidence against the role of temperature sensation as a sensory modality in the anal canal of normal subjects. Br J Surg. 1988;75:1083–5.
5. Cook IJ and Brooks SJ. Motility of the large intestine. In: Sleisenger and Fordrans. Gastrointestinal and liver diseases. 7th ed. Philadelphia, PA: Saunders; 2002.
6. Azpiroz F and Malagelada JR. Physiologic variations in canine gastric tone measured by electronic barostat. Am J Physiol. 1985;248:G229–37.
7. Broens PMA, Penninckx FM, Lestar B, and Kerremans RP. The trigger for rectal filling sensation. Int J Colorect Dis. 1994;9:1–4.
8. Felt-Bersma RJF, Sloots CEJ, Poen AC, Cuesta MA, and Meuwissen SGM. Rectal compliance as a routine measurement: extreme volumes have clinical importance. Dis Colon Rectum. 2000;43:1732–8.
9. Buchman P, Mogg GAG, Alexander-Willams J, Allan RN, and Keighley MRB. Relationship of proctitis and rectal capacity in Crohn's disease. Gut. 1980;21: 137–40.
10. Roe AM, Bartolo DCC, and Mortensen NJM. New method for assessment of anal sensation in various anorectal disorders. Br J Surg. 1986;73:310–2.
11. Whitehead WE and Delvaux M. Standardization of barostat procedures for testing smooth muscle tone and sensory thresholds in the gas-trointestinal tract. Dig Dis Sci. 1997;42:223–41.
12. Delvaux MM. Barostat measurements. In: Schuster MM, editor. Schuster atlas of gastrointestinal motility in health and disease. 2nd ed. Hamilton, Canada: BC Decker Inc.; 2002. p. 253–64.
13. SlootsCEJ, Felt-Bersma RJF, Cuesta MA, and Meuwissen SGM. Visceral sensitivity in rectal distension with the barostat in healthy volunteers. Neurogastroenterol Motil. 2000;12:361–8.

14. Steens J, Van Der Schaar PJ, Penning C, Brussee J, and Masclee AA. Compliance, tone and sensitivity of the rectum in different subtypes of irritable bowel syndrome. Neurogastroenterol Motil. 2002;14(3):241–7.
15. Ritchie J. Pain from distension of the pelvic colon by inflating a balloon in the irritable bowel syndrome. Gut. 1973;14:125–32.
16. Prior A, Maxton DG, and Whorwell PJ. Anorectal manometry in irritable bowel syndrome: differences between diarrhea and constipation predominant subjects. Gut. 1990;31:458–62.
17. Houghton LA, Lea R, Jackson N, and Whorwell PJ. The menstrual cycle affects rectal sensitivity in patients with irritable bowel syndrome but not healthy volunteers. Gut. 2002;50:471–4.
18. Chang L, Munakata J, Mayer EA, Schmulson MJ, Johnsons TD, Bernstein CN, Saba L, Naliboff B, Anton PA, and Matin K. Perceptual responses in patients with inflammatory and functional bowel disease. Gut. 2000;47:497–505.
19. Naliboff BD, Munakata J, Fullerton S, Gracely RH, Kodner A, Harraf F, and Mayer EA. Evidence for two distinct perceptual alterations in irritable bowel syndrome. Gut. 1997;41:505–12.
20. Penning C, Steens J, van der Schaar PJ, Kuyvenhoven J, Delemarre JB, Lamers CB, and Masclee AA. Motor and sensory function of the rectum in different subtypes of constipation. Scand J Gastroenterol. 2001;36:32–8.
21. Mertz H, Naliboff B, and Mayer EA. Physiology of refractory constipation. Am J Gastroenterol. 1999;94:609–15.
22. Salvioli B, Bharucha AE, Rath-Harvey D, Pemberton JH, and Phillips SF. Rectal compliance, capacity, and rectoanal sensation in fecal incontinence. Am J Gastroenterol. 2001;96:2158–68.
23. Sun WN, Read NW, Miner PB, Kerrigan DD, and Donnelly TC. The rolc of transient internal sphincter relaxation in faecal incontinence. Int J Colorectal Dis. 1990;5:31–6
24. Zbar AP, Takashima S, Hasegawa T, and Kitabayashi K. Perineal rectosigmoidectomy (Altemeier's procedure): a review of physiology, technique and outcome. Tech Coloproctol. 2002;6:109–16.
25. Deen KI, Grant E, Billingham C, and Keighley MRB. Abdominal resection rectopexy with pelvic floor repair versus perineal rectosigmoidectomy and pelvic floor repair for full thickness rectal prolapse. Br J Surg. 1994;81:302–4.
26. Siproudhis L, Bellissani E, Juguet F, Mendier M-H, Allain H, Bretagne J-F, and Gosselin M. Rectal adaptation to distension in patients with overt rectal prolapse. Br J Surg. 1998;85:1527–32.
27. Sloots CEJ, Meulen AJVD, and Felt-Bersma RJF. Rectocele repair improves evacuation and prolapse complaints independent of anorectal function and colonic transit time. Int J Colorectal Dis. In press.
28. Van Dam JH, Huisman WM, Hop WCJ, and Schouten WR. Fecal incontinence after rectocele repair: a prospective study. Int J Colorectal Dis. 2000;15:54–7.
29. Sun W-M, Read NW, Carmel Donelly T, Bannister JJ, and Shorthouse AJ. A common pathophysiology for full thickness rectal prolapse and solitary rectal ulcer. Br J Surg. 1989;76:290–5.
30. Muller MH, Kreis ME, Gross ML, Becker HD, Zittel TT, and Jehle EC. Anorectal functional disorders in the absence of anorectal inflammation in patients with Crohn's disease. Br J Surg. 2002;89:1027–31.

31. Broens P, Van Limbergen E, Penninckx F, and Kerremans R. Clinical and manometric effects of combined external beam irradiation and brachytherapy for anal cancer. Int J Colorectal Dis. 1998;13:68–72.
32. Eckardt VF, Dodt O, Kanzler G, and Bernhard G. Anorectal function and morphology in patients with sporadic proctalgia fugax. Dis Colon Rectum. 1996;39:755–62.
33. Rogers J. Rectal and anal sensation. In: Swash M and Henry MM, editors. Coloproctology and the pelvic floor. Oxford: Butterworth Heinemann; 1992. p. 54–60.
34. Miller R, Bartolo DCC, Cervero F, and Mortensen NJM. Anorectal temperature sensation: a comparison of normal and incontinent patients. Br J Surg. 1987;74:511–5.
35. Miller R. The measurement of anorectal sensation. In: Kumar D, Waldron D, and Williams NS, editors. Clinical measurement in coloproctology. London: Springer-Verlag; 1991. p. 60–6.
36. Siegel H. Cutaneous sensory threshold stimulation with high frequency square wave current. J Invest Dermatol. 1951;18:441–5.
37. Vierck CJ, Greenspan JD, Ritz LA, and Yeomans DC. The spinal pathways contributing to the ascending conduction and descending modulations of pain sensation and reactions. In: Yaksh TL, editor. Spinal afferent processing. New York: Plenum Press; 1986. p. 275–329.
38. Kiesswetter H. Mucosal sensory thresholds of urinary bladder and urethra measured electrically. Urol Int. 1977;32:437–48.
39. Powell PH and Feneley RCC. The role of urethral sensation in clinical urology. Br J Urol. 1980;52:539–41.
40. Zbar AP and Kmiot WA. Anorectal investigation. In: Phillips RKS, editor. A companion to specialist surgical practice: colorectal surgery. London: WB Saunders; 1998. p. 1–33.
41. Felt-Bersma RJF, Poen AC, Cuesta MA, and Meuwissen SGM. Anal sensitivity test: what does it measure and do we need it? Dis Colon Rectum. 1997;40: 811–6.
42. Cornes H, Bartolo DC, and Stirrat GM. Changes in anal canal sensation after childbirth. Br J Surg. 1991;78:74–7.
43. Donnely VS, O'Herlihy C, Campbell DM, and O'Connell PR. Postpartum fecal incontinence is more common in women with irritable bowel syndrome. Dis Colon Rectum. 1998;41:586–9.
44. Solana A, Roig JV, Villoslada C, Hinojosa J, and Lledo S. Anorectal sensitivity in patients with obstructed defecation. Int J Colorectal Dis. 1996;11:65–70.
45. Aitchison M, Fischer BM, Carter K, McKee R, MacCuish AC, and Finlay IG. Impaired anal sensation and early diabetic fecal incontinence. Diabetic Med. 1991;8:960–3.
46. Duthie GS and Bartolo DC. Abdominal rectopexy for rectal prolapse: A comparison of techniques. Br J Surg. 1992;79:107–13.
47. Orrom WJ, Miller R, Cornes H, Duthie G, Mortensen NJ, and Bartolo DC. Comparison of anterior sphincteroplasty and postanal repair in the treatment of idiopathic fecal incontinence. Dis Colon Rectum. 1991;34:305–10.
48. Holdsworth PJ and Johnston D. Anal sensation after restorative proctocolectomy for ulcerative colitis. Br J Surg. 1988;75:993–6.

49. Komatsu J, Oya M, and Ishikawa H. Quantitative assessment of anal canal sensation in patients undergoing low anterior resection for rectal cancer. Surg Today. 1995;25:867–73.
50. Yamana T, Oya M, Komatsu J, Takase Y, Mikuni N, and Ishikawa H. Preoperative anal sphincter high pressure zone, maximum tolerable volume, and anal mucosal electrosensitivity predict early postoperative defecatory function after low anterior resection for rectal cancer. Dis Colon Rectum. 1999;42:1145–51.
51. Deasy JM, Quirke P, Dixon M, Lagopoulos M, and Johnston D. The surgical importance of the anal transitional zone in ulcerative colitis. Br J Surg. 1987;74:533.
52. Johnston D, Holdsworth PJ, Nasmyth DG, Neal DE, Primrose JN, Womack N, and Axon ATR. Preservation of the entire anal canal in conservative proctocolectomy for ulcerative colitis: a pilot study comparing end-to-end ileoanal anastomosis without mucosal resection with mucosal proctectomy. Br J Surg. 1987;74:940–4.
53. Miller R, Bartolo DCC, Cervero, and Mortensen NJM. Does preservation of the anal transitional zone influence sensation after ileo-anal anastomosis for ulcerative colitis? Clinical Controversies in Inflammatory Bowel Disease Bologna: Tipografia Negri S.R.L. 1987:205A.
54. Kennedy ML, Lubovski DZ, and King DW. Transanal endoscopic microsurgery excision: is anorectal function compromised. Dis Colon Rectum. 2002;45:601–4.
55. Hyndman OR and Wolkin J. Anterior chordotomy. Arch Neurol Psychiatry. 1943;50:129–48.
56. Zbar AP, Beer-Gabel M, Chiappa AC, and Aslam M. Fecal incontinence after minor anorectal surgery. Dis Colon Rectum. 2001;44:1610–23.
57. Lubowski DZ and Nicholls RJ. Faecal incontinence associated with reduced pelvic sensation. Br J Surg. 1988;75:1086–8.

Editorial Commentary

The clinical importance of anorectal sensitivity testing as part of laboratory assessment is debatable. Although it is clear that altered rectal and anal sensitivity is a feature of some poor outcomes after procedures such as perineal mucosectomy (Délorme's procedure) and perineal rectosigmoidectomy (the Altemeier procedure) in full-thickness rectal prolapse, these do not appear to be preoperative predictive factors in the definition of the correct operative approach. Extended mucosectomy, however, does appear to correlate with impaired anorectal sensitivity and discrimination in low anterior resection and ileal pouch-anal anastomosis, correlating with nocturnal urgency and reported episodes of leakage in many cases. In cases of pelvic sepsis due to anastomotic dehiscence following either coloanal or ileoanal anastomosis, (an adverse event in about 12%) some amount of fibrotic tissue impairs an effective contact between the bowel wall distended by the faecal bolus and the spindle nerve receptors surrounding the levator muscle, thus affecting rectal sensation and the conscious awareness of impending evacuation.Reduced preoperative rectal sensation during anal manometry has also been shown to be a predictive factor for postoperative anal incontinence in male patients following fistulectomy.

MP

Chapter 2.9
Neurophysiology in Pelvic Floor Disorders

Guillermo O. Rosato and Carlos M. Lumi

Introduction

Colorectal surgeons, gastroenterologists, gynecologists, and urologists have gained a growing interest in the neuroanatomy and neurophysiology of the pelvic floor, which is driven by an increased knowledge of the pathophysiology of pelvic floor disorders. Pelvic disorders of defecation and micturition are common, but the true prevalence of pelvic floor disorders is still not well known.

Several diagnostic procedures have been developed to assess pelvic floor function. Some still remain as experimental tools, whereas others have gained more widespread clinical application. Neurophysiology applied to pelvic floor disorders (i.e., constipation and incontinence) has been used routinely as a diagnostic and therapeutic tool (1).

Diagnostic neurophysiology of pelvic floor muscle disorders includes three main procedures: 1) Concentric needle electromyography (CNEMG), 2) single fiber electromyography (SFEMG), and 3) pudendal nerve terminal motor latency (PNTML).

Sacral reflex latencies and somatosensory-evoked potentials have less general clinical application. Nerve conduction and electromyography (EMG) studies measure the efferent or motor innervation, whereas afferent fiber injury is more difficult to characterize and quantify. Sensory thresholds studies are also available. These studies stimulate a distal site (i.e., the anal mucosa) and determine the sensory limits of perception (anal electrosensitivity) (see Chapter 2.8). The sensory threshold is carried by afferent somatic and visceral nerve fibers to the central nervous system (probably through the pudendal nerve and pelvic plexus), whereas sacral reflexes regulate rectal sensitivity and contractility (2). Sacral reflexes measure the integrity of the afferent and efferent limbs by stimulating a distal site and measuring the time it takes for the reflex contraction of the superficial perineal muscles. After synapsing in the central nervous system by a polysynaptic pathway, efferent fibers (through the pudendal nerve) carry the response to the skeletal muscle being studied. Sensory thresholds usually are low, and sacral reflexes usually require stimulation using three times the sensory threshold current with latencies measuring less than 100 milliseconds. The bulbocavernosus reflex is the most explored sacral reflex.

Somatosensory-evoked potentials assess the integrity of the afferent branches of the pelvic nerves. They are measured by applying a distal stimulus, such as electric stimulation or balloon distension of the rectum or anal mucosa, and recording evoked potentials from the central nervous system, such as the brain or lumbar spine. The latter can be performed with transcutaneous stimulation at L1 and L4 using saline-soaked pad electrodes delivering 500 to 1500 volt single impulses. Central stimulation may be performed with magnetic brain stimulation and has been described for use in patients with spinal or central neurological disorders affecting the pelvic floor and in patients with polyneuropathy/myopathy syndromes. The results are less than satisfactory and not readily applicable or reproducible (3,4). Electrophysiology tests can distinguish between the integrity of the nerve, muscle, and neuromuscular junction, where they can identify the level of nerve injury, determine if it is recent or old, and whether it is acute, chronic, or ongoing.

Concepts in Electromyography and Basic Neurophysiology

The precise measure of neuromuscular integrity is achieved through EMG, which relies on the recording of electrical activity generated by muscle fibers (5,6). Anal sphincter EMG was first recorded by Beck in 1930 (7) with a concentric needle as originally described by Adrian and Bronck in 1929 (6).

A motor unit consists of a single anterior horn cell within the central nervous system, all its peripheral nerve fibers, motor end plates, and the muscle fibers it innervates. This is the basic functional element of a skeletal muscle. One muscle fiber (MF) is innervated by one motoneuron (MN), but one MN may supply many MFs. The motor unit is important not only for the motor control of the MF, but also in maintaining a neuromuscular trophic effect. The composition of a muscle by MF types (Table 2.9-1) depends in part on the functional demands on that muscle. Striated muscles are classified into two types—Types I and II. Type I muscle units are slow tonic fibers, and Type II muscle units are fast phasic muscle fibers. The majority of the muscle fibers of the levator ani are slow twitch fibers (Type I), which maintain constant tone. Type II fibers are more densely distributed on perianal and periurethral muscles. As an example, the gastrocnemius, which has more of a role in static postural maintenance, has predominantly Type I (S-slow twitch, fatigue resistant) alpha MNs (Table 2.9-1). In contrast, the first dorsal interosseous muscle of the hand partici-

TABLE 2.9-1. Types of alpha motoneurons and their corresponding muscle fiber type.*

Relative Characteristics	Alpha Motoneuron Types I (S = slow twitch, fatigue resistant)	II (FR = fast twitch, resistant to fatigue)	II (FF = fast twitch, fast to fatigue)
Neuronal cell body size	Smaller	—	Larger
Axon diameter	Smaller	—	Larger
Axon conduction velocity	Slow	Fast	Faster
Firing rate	Slow and regular on minimal effort	Intermediate	Fast on stronger effort
Relative excitability threshold	Lower	Intermediate	Higher
Twitch tension	Low, longer	Intermediate, long	High, brief
Contraction time	>99 milliseconds	Intermediate	<85 milliseconds
Fatigability	Slow	Relatively slow	Fast
Force generated	Low	Moderately high	High

* Modified from Barkhaus PE, Nandekar SD, Quan D, Talavera F, Busis NA, Benbadis SR, Lorenzo N. EMG Evaluation of the Motor Unit: The Electrophysiologic Biopsy. eMedicine J. 2002;3(1): section 2–11.

pates in more rapid, phasic movements and has more Type II-FF (fast twitch, fast to fatigue) MNs (8).

The motor unit territory (MUT) is defined as "the area in a muscle over which the muscle fibres (MFs) belonging to an individual motor unit (MU) are distributed" (9). In humans, motor unit territories (MUTs) vary in size in different muscles. In a larger proximal limb muscle such as the biceps bracchi, the MUT has an estimated diameter of five to ten millimeters (i.e., cross section) based on scanning EMG studies (10). Experimental studies in animals have suggested greater dispersion of the MUT within a muscle that might change in size along the length of the muscle (11,12).

The motoneurons exert a trophic influence on the MFs. Cross-innervation experiments have demonstrated that MFs may change their histochemical type. "Fast" MUs also may be changed experimentally to "slow" MUs by constant electrical stimulation; thymectomy, castration, and aging also may produce effects on the MU. In elderly individuals, decrease in muscle bulk typically is observed, consequent upon generalized atrophy of individual MFs rather than a decrease in the total number of MFs themselves.

There is electrophysiologic evidence of MU remodeling in elderly individuals. The concentric needle (CN) motor unit action potential (MUAP) has shown an increase in duration with increased age, although not to any significant degree until the individual is older than 60 years of age. The fiber density (as measured in SFEMG) also increases after the sixth decade (13).

During voluntary contraction of individual units within a muscle, the contracting units summate to form a motor unit potential (MUP) (Figure 2.9.1). The MUP has three variables: amplitude, shape, and duration. Amplitude is determined by the algebraic summation of each single fiber potential and the distance of the recording electrode to the fiber. Shape depends on the number of muscle fibers discharging simultaneously. Duration depends on the distribution and surface extent of muscle fibers that correspond to the axon of a motor unit. Duration is the time interval between the first deflection from the base line to the point at which the deflection ultimately returns.

Normally, MUPs are biphasic or triphasic. A potential with more than four phases is referred to as polyphasic. Buchthal et al. (8) defined a "phase" as the part of the MUP that lies between two crossings of the base line.

Electromyography recordings from muscle activity can be performed by the use of: (a) Surface electrodes, (b) CN electrodes, (c) single fiber electrodes, and (d) wire electrodes.

Current Indications for Electromyography

The indications for EMG in the assessment of anorectal disease are diminishing where EMG mapping of the sphincter is unnecessarily invasive in

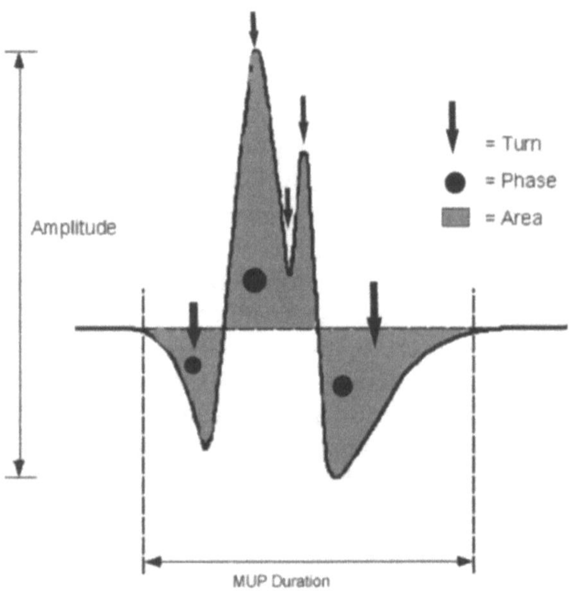

FIGURE 2.9.1. Motor unit potential.

the age of endoanal ultrasonographic imaging of sphincter integrity. Puborectalis EMG may be more accurate than cinedefecography in the delineation of non-relaxing puborectalis syndrome. Electromyography assessment for pelvic floor and anal sphincter muscles is mainly indicated in order to determine: (a) Denervation of muscle fibers, (b) reinnervation of muscle fibers (single fiber density), (c) sphincter integrity, and (d) adequate contraction or relaxation during squeeze or straining (5,6). There still may be a place for serial conventional EMG in some patients with complex perineal injuries in an effort to determine when to reverse fecal diversion or in cases where total anorectal reconstruction (with coloperineal anastomosis) is contemplated after abdominoperineal resection. In the pediatric age group, as well, there may be a case for its use in redo surgery where patients have had a poor functional outcome after surgery for a high anorectal anomaly (14,15).

Concentric Needle EMG Technique

Concentric needle EMG evaluates spontaneous activity, recruitment pattern, and MUAP waveform. A concentric needle electrode (CNE) consists of a fine platinum wire mounted inside a larger diameter metal cannula (65 mm). The inner wire is insulated from the needle cannula, which ends with a 15 degree cut point, exposing the wire electrode surface. Its recording surface is 0.07 square millimeters.

Optimal recording requires an amplifier frequency range of 10 hertz to 10 kilohertz and a sensitivity of 100 to 500 microvolts per centimeter with a usual set of the screen visualization to 100 microvolts per duration and a sweep speed of 20 milliseconds per duration for rest, squeeze, and strain and 500 milliseconds per duration for cough. This set-up can be modified in order to have a better view or analysis of waveforms. All patients receive a full detailed explanation about the examination to be performed. They are placed in the left lateral position, with a metal ground electrode fixed to one of the legs by a Velcro device.

The perianal skin is cleansed with a cotton swab soaked with an antiseptic reducing noise. The concentric needle electrode is introduced through the skin in both the left and the right sides with no anesthetic. This is done at one to one and one half centimeters from the anal verge. The introduction of this needle electrode (NE) is followed by a reactive discharge of MUPs, which is more evident in anxious patients. It is necessary to distinguish this activity from that known as "insertion activity" (IA), due to the mechanical stimulation of the muscle fibers. This is a reaction of the muscle fibers, not from a MUP discharge, and disappears very rapidly as the patient relaxes.

In order to avoid conceptual confusion, we prefer to use the term "reactive activity" to discriminate from IA. It is very difficult to see or register this IA at the anal sphincter because of the reactive activity of the MUP.

The insertion activity in skeletal muscles is a parameter, which in clinical EMG leads one to know the state of excitability and contractile capacity of the muscle fibers.

In the external anal sphincter (EAS) and the puborectalis (PR), MUP discharges also provide information concerning the contractile capacity of the muscle fibers. In cases of fibrosis, there is a loss of contractile capacity of these muscle fibers, and subsequently no MUP or fibrillation is recognized. In the case of denervation, MUP activity is replaced by fibrillation of the denervation potentials. The NE is then advanced four to five centimeters, where electrical activity is detected. The NE having arrived at the PR level, the patient is asked to squeeze, cough, and strain (simulating rectal evacuation), and each of these events is registered on a print-out EMG paper (Figure 2.9.2).

Thereafter, the NE is withdrawn, passing across a zone where no electrical activity is registered, until the examination reaches another area with myoelectrical potentials, assumed to be at the EAS level. Here, again, recordings are made of the "reactive activity" and the same procedure as for the PR is repeated with squeeze, cough, and strain provocation; each registered as events on a print-out EMG paper (Figure 2.9.3).

The response to these different maneuvers in healthy individuals shows an increase in activity (recruitment of MUAPs) during squeeze and cough and a significant decrease or eventual electrical silencing during strain (8,16–18).

Any change in the number of functional muscle fibers in a MU will show an abnormal waveform of MUAP. After nerve damage, the adjacent preserved axons will attempt to reinnervate the muscle fibers that have been denervated, resulting in one ME innervating more muscle fibers as part of the healing process. Therefore, MUAPs tend to have larger amplitudes, longer durations, and more phases (polyphasic or evidence of prior denervation injury). This typical feature is seen in neuropathic conditions. In myopathic pathology, there is a reduction of the number of MFs per MU, resulting in low amplitude and low duration of the waveform.

Pathological patterns are seen, for example. in: (a) Paradoxical contraction of the puborectalis (increased activity during strain as compared with rest or squeeze) (19,20) (Figure 2.9.4), (b) decreased or absent activity during squeeze in traumatic lesions of the sphincter muscles, and (c) spontaneous activity during rest (fibrillation) in denervated muscle fibers, which is difficult to recognize in sphincter muscle due to their smaller fiber size. Under these circumstances it is easier to hear the characteristic noise produced by fibrillation rather than to look at the trace on the screen of the oscilloscope. (d) Localized myoclonia of the anal sphincter (21,22).

Single Fiber EMG (23,24)

This technique is complementary to CNEMG, where additional information can be acquired. In the early 1960s, Stälberg and Trontelj described a

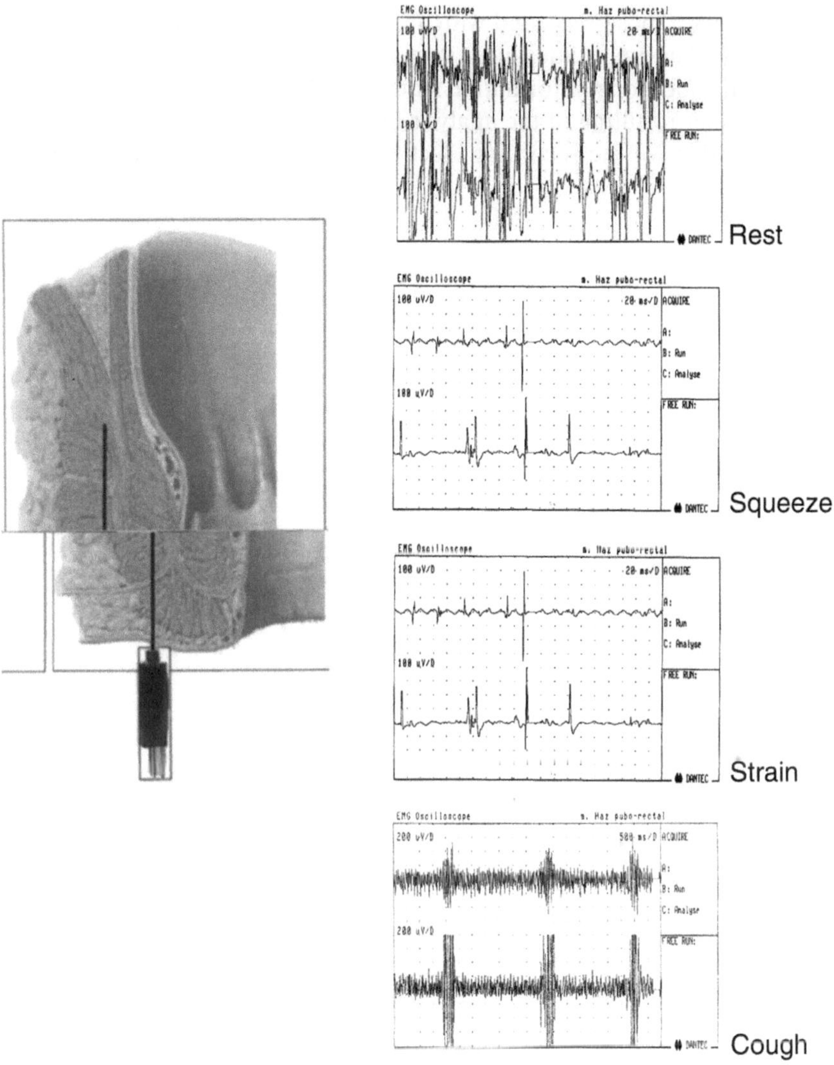

FIGURE 2.9.2. Needle electrode recordings at the puborectalis (PR) for rest, squeeze, strain, and cough.

method to record individual muscle fiber action potentials (24). Patients are examined in the same position as used in CNEMG.

A special electrode (needle electrode), smaller in diameter than the CNE, is utilized. The recording element consists of a central wire that opens laterally near the tip of the needle electrode with a surface of 25 micrometers and that picks up the electrical signals over a recording surface of 0.0003 square millimeters. A reference electrode is placed in a zone of electrical quiescence. The characteristics of single fiber potentials (SFPs) as compared with those recorded with a CN are that the SFPs have a shorter duration, higher amplitude, and a very fast rise time.

The main additional information from SFEMG is fiber density. This is the mean number resulting of the analysis of single muscle potentials in 20 different positions of the recording electrode within the same muscle. Poten-

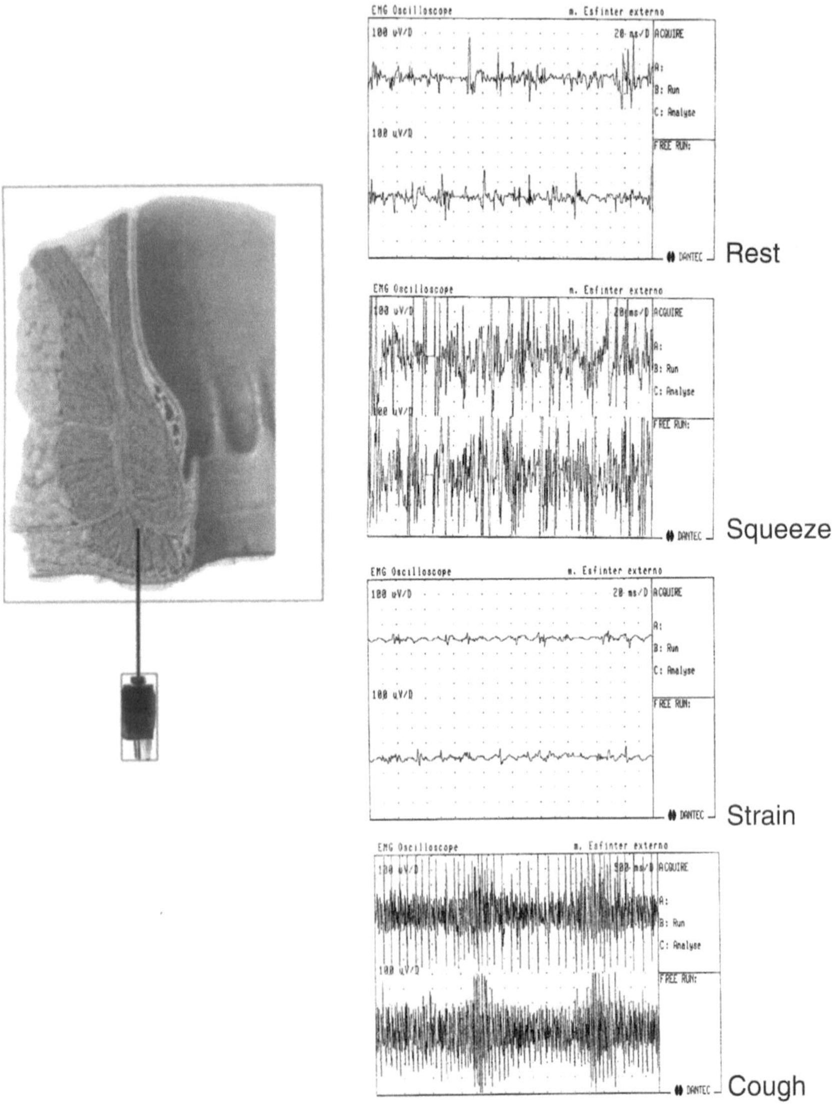

FIGURE 2.9.3. Needle electrode recordings in the external anal sphincter (EAS) for rest, squeeze, strain, and cough.

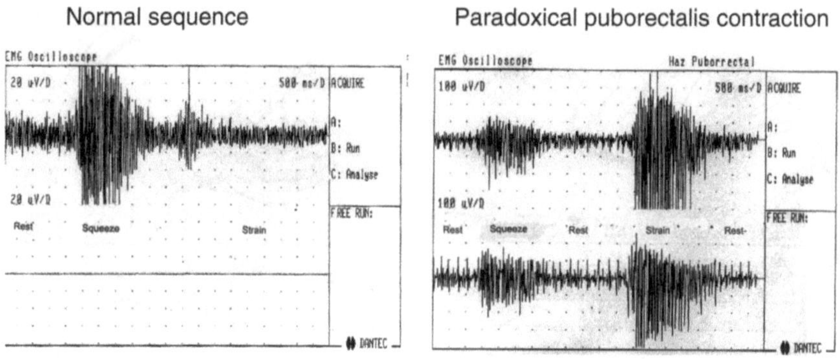

FIGURE 2.9.4. EMG activity record in paradoxical puborectalis contraction (anismus) syndrome.

tials accepted for analysis should be greater than 100 microvolts. The increase in fiber density reflects reinnervation due to nerve sprouting, implying that there are more muscle fibers innervated by an individual axon, and therefore that there are more fibers closer to the uptake area of the electrode (often corresponding to polyphasic action potentials in the EMG).

The fiber density values are increased before any definitive signs of abnormality are found on CNEMG recording. The normal fiber density is 1.5 ± 0.16, but tends to increase after the age of 60 years (13).

Pudendal Nerve Terminal Motor Latency (25,26)

Pudendal nerve stimulation technique assesses the distal motor innervations of the pelvic floor muscles. Pudendal latency measures the time interval between the nerve stimulus and the muscle response. Latency reflects the integrity of the nerve's insulation with myelin, but can indicate damage to the health of the largest and fastest conducting fibers within the nerve. Terminal motor latencies are prolonged in demyelinating diseases and in conditions in which many fast-firing nerve fibers have been damaged.

To perform this test, the patient is positioned in the left lateral decubitus position, with the knees flexed and the hips close to the edge of the examination table. A flat, self-adhesive, disposable electrode is used. This device was developed at the St. Mark's London Hospital (Dantec Electronic, Tonsbakken 16-18 DK-2740, Skovlunde, Denmark), and it is attached to the volar aspect of the index finger, covered initially by a latex glove. It consists of a bipolar stimulating electrode, with the recording electrode placed a standardized distance on the base of the finger. The electrode is attached to the connector cable with an input for EMG recording and an output for nerve stimulation. The examining finger is lubricated with a special gel that

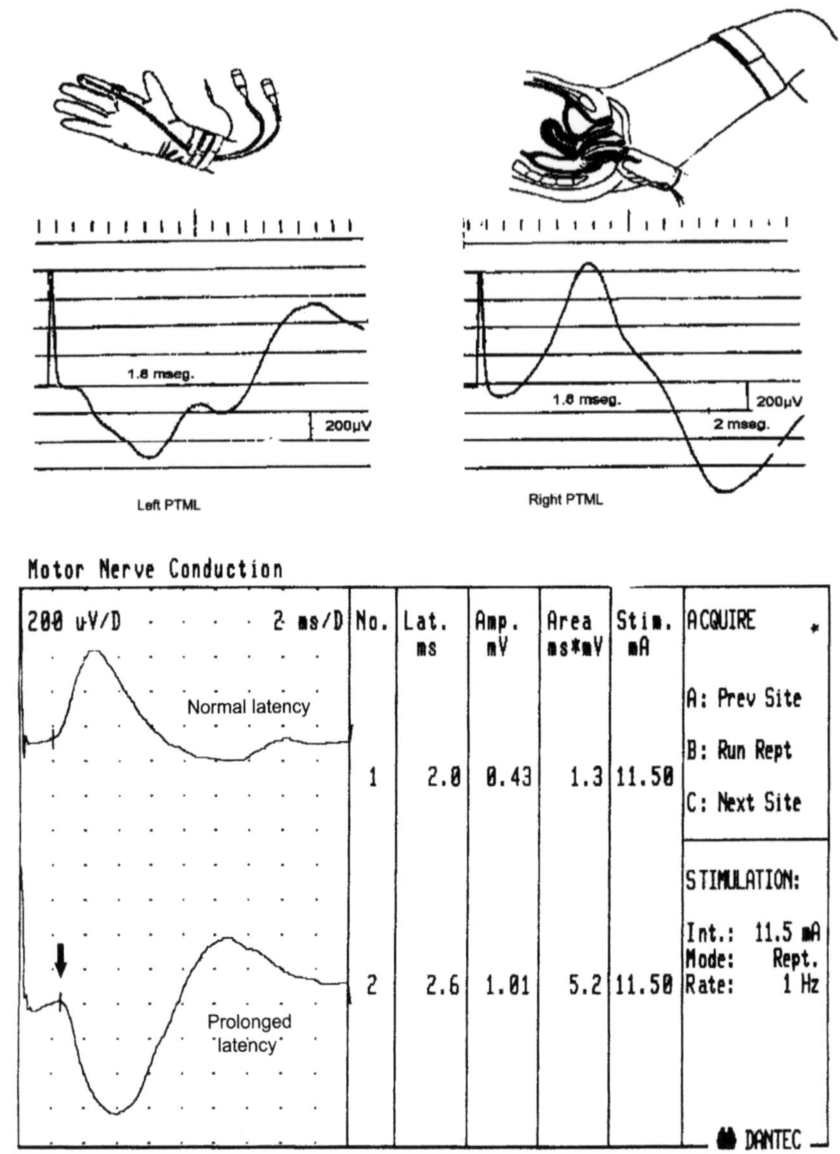

FIGURE 2.9.5. Pudental Nerve Terminal Motor Latency.

improves electric transmission and is introduced into the anal canal, directing it towards the ischial spine (right and left side) (27).

A square stimulus of 0.1 or 0.2 milliseconds in duration (at one-second intervals) is delivered up to the individual threshold, usually not exceeding 15 milliamperes. The response to this stimulus is a palpable EAS contraction and monitor detection of a motor potential on the oscilloscope screen, with the examiner looking for the maximal response and a reproducible wave form. This action potential then is registered and can be printed out, and the maneuver is similar for both right and left pudendal nerves. Measurement of the latency is calculated from the onset of the stimulus to the site of onset of the response.

The normal latency reference value is 2.0 ± 0.2 milliseconds on each side (Figure 2.9.5). Prolongation of PNTML is not unusual after vaginal delivery, rectal prolapse, and with ageing (13,28,29). Pudendal neuropathy has been controversial as a predictor of the functional results after anal sphincteroplasty. The experience of the authors is summarized in Table 2.9-1, which appears to confirm that the presence of pudendal neuropathy does not correlate with incontinence severity (incontinence score), and as a result, sphincteroplasty is not denied to patients with some degree of pudendal neuropathy because many cofactors may influence suboptimal results after sphincteroplasty (e.g., incomplete internal sphincter plication, partial or complete plication disruption, etc.) (30–34).

Unit Experience

Between June 1991 and August 2004, 281 pelvic floor neurophysiologic evaluations were performed in our unit. All patients were submitted for PNTML study, concentric EMG, and SF EMG.

One hundred and ninety seven patients had incontinence as their main complaint, 59 presented with chronic constipation (Rome II criteria), and 25 were referred because of anal or rectal pain, anal fissure, anal stenosis, or anorectal trauma. In the incontinent group, 171 were female and 26 were male, with a mean age of 58.53 years (8–86). The constipation group had 48 female patients and 11 males, with a mean age of 43.69 years (11–86). In the incontinent group of patients, statistical analysis of the means of the recorded PNTML, SF, and recruitment of motor unit potentials (MUP) during voluntary contraction (being 5 for full recruitment of MUPs and 0 for no response) at the level of puborectalis and external sphincters was performed.

The mean incontinence score was 13/20 (0/20–20/20) (17). The findings are summarized in Table 2.9-2.

A correlation analysis was performed between the left and right pudendal motor unit potentials recordings and the incontinence score showing no correlation, with an r value of –0.05039642 (R^2 = 0.0025398) for the left side (A) and an r value of –0.074529894 (R^2 = 0.005554705) for the right side (B). The same procedure was carried on between SF EMG and the incontinence score, and again there was no correlation: r = 0.05969207 (R^2 = 0.00356314) (C).

However, we did find a correlation between the incontinence score and recruitment of MUPs at the PR and the EAS muscles ($p < 0.01$) with an r

TABLE 2.9-2. The mean incontinence score summary of findings.

	Right pudendal motor unit potential	Left pudendal motor unit potential	Single fiber	Right puborectalis motor unit potentials	Left puborectalis motor unit potentials	Right external anal sphincter motor unit potentials	Left external anal sphincter motor unit potentials
Mean	2.32	2.36	2.04	3.46	3.49	2.71	2.75
SD	1.07	1.12	0.436	1.40	1.33	1.51	1.48
Maximum	7.8	9.2	3.5	5	5	5	5
Minimum	0	0	1.06	0	0	0	0

value of –0.386747407 (R^2 = 0.149573556) for the right PR (D), an *r* value of –0.33056617 (R^2 = 0.10927399) for the left PR (E), an *R* value of –0.460363364 (R^2 = 0.211934427) for the right EAS (G), and an *R* value of –0.38729309 (R^2 = 0.14999594) for the left EAS (F).

In our series, a prolonged PNTML and an abnormal SF EMG does not necessarily correspond to a greater degree of incontinence and a decrease in MUP recruitment at the PR and/or the EAS correlates with a greater severity of incontinence (Figure 2.9.6).

This same analysis was used in symptomatically chronically constipated patients. Emphasis was applied on recruitment of MUP regarding the ability of patients to relax the sphincter mechanism while straining and was

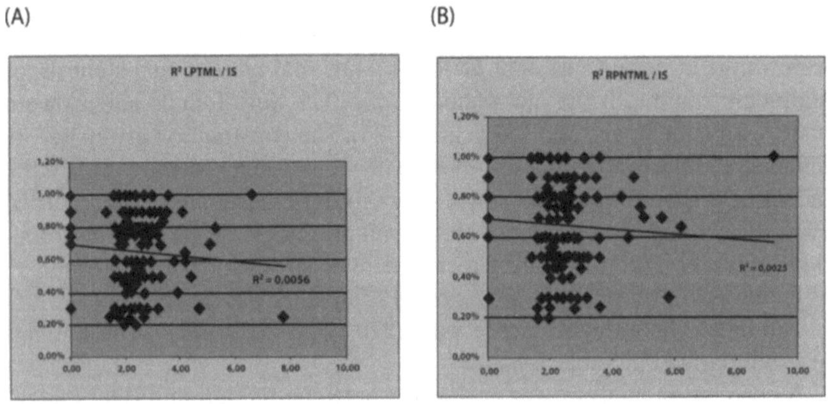

FIGURE 2.9.6. Correlation coefficients between left and right PNTML, incontinence score, and SF EMG recordings and for MUP recruitment versus incontinence score for the left and right PR and EAS musculature. (A)Left PNTML versus incontinence score; (B) right PNTML versus incontinence score; (C) SF EMG recordings versus incontinence score; (D) incontinence score versus MUP recruitment potentials (PR—right side); (E) incontinence score versus MUP recruitment potentials (PR—left side); (F) incontinence score versus MUP recruitment potentials (EAS—left side); (G) incontinence score versus MUP recruitment potentials (EAS—right side).

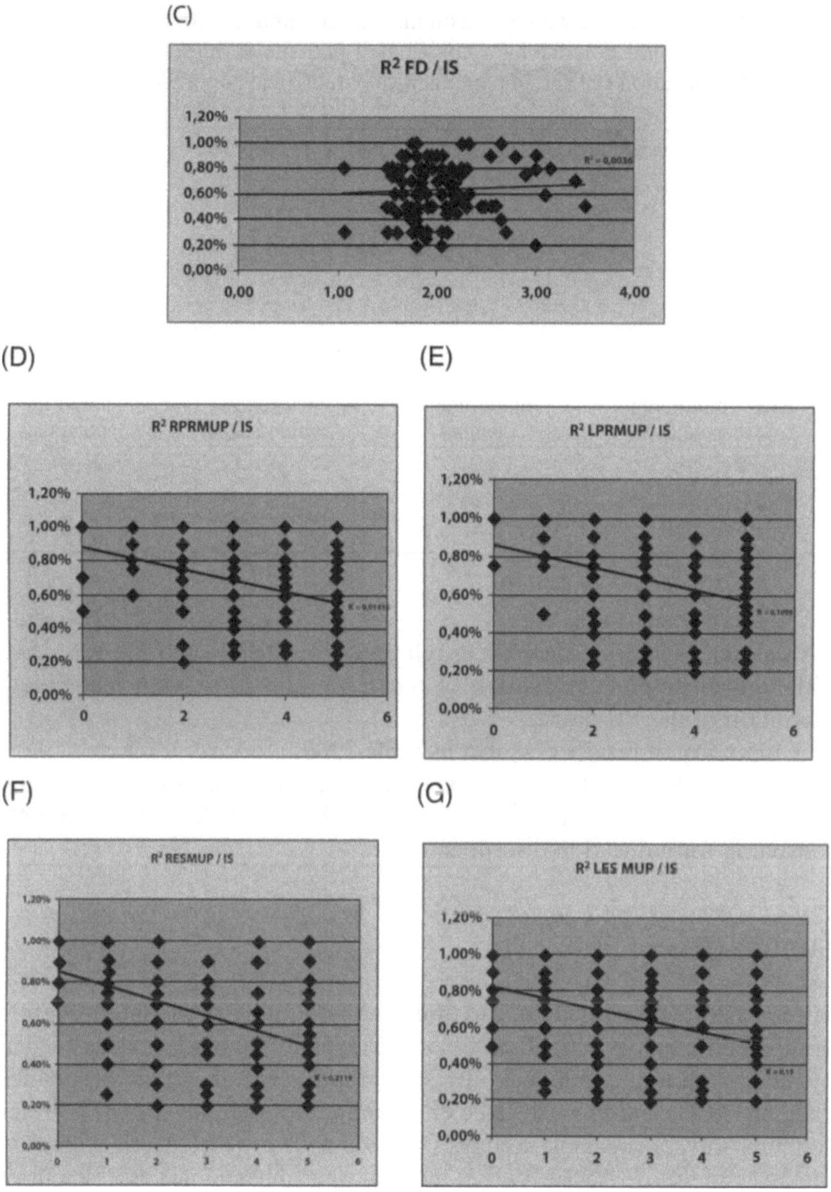

FIGURE 2.9.6. *Continued*

classified as total relaxation (r), incomplete relaxation (ir), and paradoxical contraction (pc); each being compared with MUP recruitment during rest.

In this group, CNEMG diagnosed 10 patients as having PPRC (Paradoxical Puborectalis Contraction) alone, 13 as having PR and EAS paradoxical contraction, 11 patients as having paradoxical contraction of the

TABLE 2.9-3. Recordings for right and left pudendal motor unit potential and SF EMG (means, standard deviation, maximum, and minimum) with right and left PR and EAS motor unit potentials for constipated patients during relaxation (r) and incomplete relaxation (ir) and in patients with paradoxical puborectalis contraction (pc) syndrome.

	Right pudendal motor unit potential	Left pudendal motor unit potential	Single fiber
Means	2.52	2.34	1.81
SD	1.50	1.31	0.48
Maximum	9	8.2	2.8
Minimum	1.3	1.31	1

	Right puborectalis motor unit potentials	Left puborectalis motor unit potentials	Right external anal sphincter motor unit potentials	Left external anal sphincter motor unit potentials
r	25	25	22	22
ir	11	11	13	13
pc	23	23	24	24

EAS alone, eight with incomplete relaxation of the PR and the EAS, five with sole incomplete relaxation of the EAS, and three with incomplete relaxation of the PR alone.

A summary of results is shown in Table 2.9-3.

This procedure contributed to the diagnosis of paradoxical contraction or incomplete relaxation of the sphincter mechanism in 75% of the patients consulting for defecation disorders.

Summary

In the past, EMG was one of the principal modalities in the determination of sphincter injury potentially amenable to repair. This has been superceded by high-resolution endoanal ultrasonography and magnetic resonance imaging (MRI) and reconstructed endoluminal sonography. Its use is either confined to very specialist settings (as discussed) or to research such as in the assessment of IAS EMG (35). Formal neurophysiologic assessment of the pelvic floor in constipated patients is still occasionally a useful complement to other physiology testing where non-relaxing paradoxical PR contraction is suspected, but unclear using defecography or manometry, and when transit studies are difficult to interpret. There is no clear evidence that EMG parameters predict for successful biofeedback outcomes in these complex cases. Pudendal latency must still remain an experimental tool, often included with manometric data in many reports without confident evidence base that abnormal prolongation of the PNTML precludes successful sphincteroplasty outcomes. Its value may be of use to document in these patients who experience delayed deterioration in their functional result. Although a normal PNTML does not indicate an absence of nerve injury (in the same way that an abnormal PNTML is not indicative of abnormal muscle function), SF EMG is an objective marker of muscle reinnervation and may be useful in patients with failed sphincteroplasties or in the context of total anorectal reconstruction.

References

1. Rosato GO, Lumi CM, and Miguel AM. Anal sphincter electromyography and pudendal nerve terminal motor latency assesment. Sem Colon Rectal Surg. 1992;3(2):68–74.
2. Malouf AJ, Vaizey CJ, Nicholls RJ, and Kamm MA. Permanent sacral nerve stimulation for fecal incontinence. Ann Surg. 2000;232:143–8.
3. Olsen AL and Rao SS. Clinical neurophysiology and electrodiagnostic testing of the pelvic floor. Gastoenterol Clin. 2001;30(1):33–54.
4. Speakman CTM, Kamm MA, and Swash M. Rectal sensory evoked potentials: an assessment of their clinical value. Int J Colorectal Dis. 1993;8(1): 23–8.
5. Snooks SJ and Swash M. Nerve stimulation techniques. In: Henry MM and Swash M, editors. Coloproctology and the pelvic floor: Pathophysiology and management. London, UK: Butterworths; 1985. p. 184–206.
6. Adrian ED and Bronk DW. The discharge of impulses in motor nerve fibers: II. The frequency of discharge in reflex and voluntary contractions. J Physiol. 1929;67:119–51.
7. Beck A. Electromyographische untersuchungen am sphinkter ani. Arch Physiol. 1930;224:278–92.
8. Buchtal F. The general concept of the motor unit: Neuromuscular disorders. Res Publ Assoc Res Nerv Ment Dis. 1961;38:3–30.
9. Stälberg E and Antoni L. Electrophysiological cross section of the motor unit. J Neurol Neurosurg Psych. 1980;43(6):469–74.
10. Nomenclature Committee. AAEE glossary of terms in clinical electromyography. Muscle Nerve. 1987;10(8 Suppl):G1–60.
11. Barkhaus PE, Nandekar SD, Quan D, Talavera F, Busis NA, Benbadis SR, and Lorenzo N. EMG evaluation of the motor unit: the electrophysiologic biopsy. eMedicine Journal. 2002;3(1).
12. Monti RJ, Roy RR, and Edgerton VR. Role of motor unit structure in defining function. Muscle Nerve. 2001;24(7):848–66.
13. Lauberg S and Swash M. Effects of ageing on anorectal sphincters and their innervation. Dis Colon Rectum. 1989;32:737–42.
14. Iwai N, Kanida H, Taniguchi H, Tsuto T, Yanagihara J, and Takahashi T. Postoperative continence assessed by electromyography of the external sphincter in anorectal malformations. Z Kinderchir. 1985;40:87–90.
15. Kubota M and Suita S. Assessment of sphincter muscle function before and after posterior sagittal anorectoplasty using a magnetic spinal stimulation techynique. J Pediatr Surg. 2002;37:617–22.

16. Buchthal F, Pinelli P, and Rosenfalck P. Action potentials parameters in normal human muscle and their physiological determinants. Acta Physiol Scand. 1954; 32:219–29.
17. Buchthal F, Guld C, and Rosenfalck P. Multielectrode study of the territory of a motor unit. Acta Physiol Scand. 1957;39:83–104.
18. Buchthal F. Electromyography in evaluation of muscle disease. Method Clin Neurophysiol. 1991;2:25–51.
19. Wexner SD, Cheape JD, Jorge JMN, Heymen S, and Jagelman DG. A prospective assessment of biofeedback for the treatment of paradoxical puborectalis contraction. Dis Colon Rectum. 1992;35:145–50.
20. Jorge LMN and Wexner SD. Etiology and management of fecal incontinence. Dis Colon Rectum. 1993;36:77–97.
21. Fowler CJ. Pelvic floor neurophysioloy. Method Clin Neurophysiol. 1991;2:1–20.
22. Goodgold J and Everstein A. Electrodiagnosis of neuromuscular disease. 2nd ed. Baltimore, MD: Williams & Wilkins; 1977. p. 210
23. Swash M and Snooks SJ. Electromyography in pelvic floor disorders. In: Henry MM and Swash M, editors. Coloproctology and the pelvic floor: pathophysiology and management. London, UK: Butterworths; 1992. p. 184–196.
24. Stälberg E and Trontelj J. Single fiber electromyography. Old walking. Surrey, UK: Mirvalle; 1979.
25. Snooks SJ and Swash M. Nerve stimulation techniques. In: Henry MM and Swash M, editors. Coloproctology and the pelvic floor: pathophysiology and management. London, UK: Butterworths; 1985. p. 196–206.
26. Wexner SD, Marchetti F, Sarlanga V, Corredor C, and Jagelman DG. The neurophysiological assessment of the anal sphincters. Dis Colon Rectum. 1991;34: 606–12.
27. Kiff ES and Swash M. Normal proximal and delayed distal conduction in the pudendal nerves of patients with idiopathic (neurogenic) faecal incontinence. J Neurol Neurosurg Psych. 1984;47:820–3.
28. Ryhammer AM, Laurberg S, and Hermann AP. Long-term effect of vaginal deliveries on anorectal function in normal perimenopausal women. Dis Colon Rectum. 1996;39:852–9.
29. Swash M and Snooks SJ. Electromyography in pelvic floor disorders. In: Henry MM and Swash M, editors. Coloproctology and the pelvic floor: pathophysiology and management. London, UK: Butterworths; 1992. p. 252–6.
30. Shu-Hung Chen A, Luchtefeld MA, Senagore AJ, MacKeigan JM, and Hoyt C. Pudendal nerve latency—does it predict outcome of anal sphincter repair? Dis Colon Rectum. 1998;41:1005–9.
31. Malouf AJ, Norton CS, Engel AF, Nicholls RJ, and Kamm MA. Long term results of overlapping anterior anal sphincter repair for obstetric trauma. Lancet. 2000;355:260–5.
32. Karoui S, Leroi AM, Koning E, Menard JF, Michot F, and Denis P. Results of sphincteroplasty in 86 patients with anal incontinence. Dis Colon Rectum. 2000;43:813–20.
33. Lauberg S, Swash M, and Henry MM. Delayed external sphincter repair for obstetric tear. Br J Surg. 1988;75:786–8.
34. Setti-Carraro P, Kamm MA, and Nicholls RJ. Long-term results of postanal repair for neurogenic faecal incontinence. Br J Surg. 1994;81:140–4.

35. Sorensen M, Nielsen MB, Pedersen JF, and Christiansen J. Electromyography of the internal anal sphincter performed under endosonographic guidance. Description of a new method. Dis Colon Rectum. 1994;37:138–43.

Editorial Commentary

Electromyography and pudendal nerve terminal motor latency assessment are very important facets in the evaluation of pelvic floor function. Electromyography is the most useful test as a complementary examination to an ultrasonography in patients with fecal incontinence. A helpful way of viewing these two tests is to consider ultrasonography as the assessment of "gross" anatomy and electromyography as the method of analyzing "microscopic" anatomy. Specifically, anal ultrasonography may show what is thought to be a defect in the anterior portion of the external anal sphincter, but electromyography has found scar tissue or defunctioned muscle. Conversely, ultrasonography may find what is thought to be intact muscle, but by electromyography, a determination can be made that the muscle is injured. Therefore, these should be used together rather than individually for those patients with fecal incontinence. When both of these studies are combined with the physical examination, then the optimal determination can be made as to the method of treatment for such patients. In addition, measurement of pudendal nerve latency is quite possibly the single most important prognosticator for postoperative function following overlapping sphincter repair. Therefore, electromyography is generally performed combined with pudendal nerve terminal motor latency assessment. Alternatively, there is little reason to perform the uncomfortable needle electromyography in patients with constipation. In this group of individuals, surface electromyography is as reliable, (if not more reliable), than defecography in the diagnosis of paradoxical puborectalis contraction. Regardless of the method of study, electromyography with pudendal nerve terminal motor latency assessment remain important cornerstones within the anorectal physiology laboratory.

SW

Chapter 3
Anorectal Imaging

Chapter 3.1(i)
Evacuation Proctography

Philip J. Shorvon and Michelle M. Marshall

Editorial Commentary

Defecography is still the gold standard for the morphological assessment of the rectum and for the objective determination of its emptying efficiency. It would appear that radiological measurements (at rest, during squeeze and following attempted evacuation/strain), provide no real clinical advantage although they may be justified in the validation of newer comparative techniques. Current evidence shows that the vast majority of these patients have complex multicompartmental problems which relate to the middle and anterior pelvic and perineal viscera (and soft tissues). This highlights the need for a multidisciplinary clinical approach by urogynecologists with an interest in evacuatory difficulty assessing these patients in collaboration with the coloproctologist. Urinary difficulties, gynaecological problems and sexual dysfunction need a greater prospective evaluation in many of these cases. Such a view suggests that in some cases where defaecography forms a central diagnostic plank for surgical decision-making that an extended technique of colpocystography and even defecoperitoneography may be required in specialized centres geared for this approach. The consequence is that there will be increased radiation exposure (often in young females) and that some of these investigations will be relatively poorly tolerated despite their clinical utility. Modern approaches will need to test the efficacy of the newer investigation in an algorithm approach comparing these (such as dynamic magnetic resonance imaging and transperineal ultrasonography) with conventional and extended defecography.

AZ

Introduction

Evacuation proctography (EP) is a relatively new technique. The balloon proctogram, a similar fluoroscopic technique that attempts to characterize anorectal dysfunction by using a barium-filled balloon to simulate a soft stool, has since been superceded (1). Although some rectal evacuation studies had been performed for a number of years (2), the study in 1984 by Mahieu and colleagues popularized the technique, probably because of a burgeoning interest in anorectal surgery for functional evacuatory problems (3). The radiologic criteria for normal evacuation of the rectum was further defined in 1988 by Shorvon et al. and Bartram et al. (4,5), and was variously labeled as defecography, videoproctography, and dynamic rectal examination. Because physiologic defecation is a result of colonic contraction and reflex anorectal accommodatory changes, some of these terms may be relatively misleading since only rectal evacuation is examined; hence, the term evacuation proctography generally is preferred. Several different protocols of EP have been considered, but most are similar to the initial technique described by Mahieu et al. EP—the radiologic visualization of the act of defecation—is, of course, not an exact simulation of defecation since the physical properties of the contrast medium differ from normal fecal content, as does the method of rectal filling and content expulsion.

Initial work in this area concentrated on the evaluation of patients with idiopathic chronic constipation and attempted to separate patients with anorectal dysfunction (so-called "outlet disorders") from those with delayed colonic transit. Despite little scientific data to confirm the inherent diagnostic (and therapeutic) value of EP in primary evacuation difficulty, it has achieved a central place in the investigation algorithm as performed by specialized pelvic floor clinics for patients presenting with these disorders. This is partly a testament to the ease of performing the examination and the fact that no other investigation (up until recently) gave a visual overview of what actually happened during the act of defecation. It should be remembered that EP is an examination of function and not a technique to identify subtle structural or mucosal abnormalities. Of and by itself, defecographic findings are not relied upon solely for operative decision making and should at all times be taken into account with the whole patient picture of history and clinical examination findings (6,7).

During the late 1980s and early 1990s, there were many reported attempts designed to characterize defecographic patterns of rectal and pelvic floor movement during EP that were thought to identify specific structural and physiologic disorders and correlate with specific symptom/examination findings. A complex set of measurements and maneuvers evolved for an extended technique of EP; however, several of these added procedures are now considered unnecessary. More recently, EP has been considered to have a role in the selection of patients presenting with primary evacuatory dysfunction for surgical therapies and approach (such as in rectocele) and for the biofeedback treatment in cases of anismus (8–11).

Indications for EP

Like many investigations, EP is useful only where it is predicted to be helpful in influencing patient management. Many patients with anorectal dysfunction are complicated without clear-cut treatment options and the information obtained by proctography needs to be considered carefully along with clinical and physiological data. Our unit has had extensive experience in its use in the following patient groups.

Constipation

The main indication for EP is in the investigation of refractory constipation. It particularly should be considered in those patients with symptoms suggestive of outlet obstruction (obstipation) or possible prolapse, which is not clinically evident, and it is useful in understanding the mechanisms by which patients manage to enhance defecation where there is reported rectal and/or vaginal digitation or other aiding maneuvers such as perineal pressure, to enhance defecation. Patients presenting with intractable constipation who also fall into this category for defecographic investigation may include patients with suspected rectoanal intussusception, those cases where an enterocele also is suspected in association with a symptomatic rectocele and in those presenting with solitary rectal ulcer syndrome (12–14).

Incontinence

Its value in fecal incontinence is less evident. In patients with major incontinence, it is particularly limited as they are unlikely to be able to retain the barium inserted before getting onto the proctography commode. In patients with soiling, there can be some benefit in performing EP, especially when digital examination, endosonography, or manometry indicate a normal or near-normal sphincter. It also should be remembered that incontinence is a principal symptom in up to one third of patients presenting with evacuatory dysfunction and what is thought to be a clinically significant rectocele (15).

Postoperative Assessments

EP also can be performed in a modified manner to assess dynamic evacuatory function (and capacity) in patients with an ileal pouch (pouchography) and following some other types of reconstructive anorectal surgery—in particular, after some specific reconstructions for anal atresia (16) and in the assessment of post-rectopexy evacuation difficulty (17).

Miscellaneous

EP can be performed in some patients presenting with intractable perianal or rectal discomfort where there is little that is clinically evident to explain their symptomatology, although its yield is low in this group and there is poor correlation with the types of pathology detected and the need for surgical intervention. This patient group may include the constellation of symptoms expressed in the solitary rectal ulcer syndrome, where such defecographic abnormalities as rectoanal intussusception and anismus may be recognized (18).

Contraindications for EP Use

There are no specific contraindications to EP other than its avoidance in pregnancy. Because the radiation dose to the ovaries is considerable (19), EP should be reserved for those women who subsequently are unlikely to have children and only in those for whom it is essential for management. As the testicular dose may be considerable, the technique is also best avoided in young men whenever possible, with a consideration of use of other dynamic tests such as dynamic transperineal ultrasonography (see Chapter 3.2) and dynamic magnetic resonance imaging (MRI) (see Chapter 3.3).

Technique

Although simple in concept and performance, EP requires a very sensitive approach on the part of the investigator and careful reporting in the context of the patient's symptoms and age. Patients often are embarrassed by the procedure. Time taken to take a history prior to the examination is always helpful in gaining the patient's confidence, as patients often will relay information that hitherto they had kept to themselves because of the difficulty of discussing such personal information in an outpatient clinic.

The Screening Room

The screening room should be kept under subdued lighting during the procedure, with as few staff members present as possible. The examination is performed using a standard fluoroscopic unit, preferably with an overcouch tube. In general, patients do not need any prior preparation, although some units give a glycerin suppository or disposable enema to empty the rectum prior to the procedure. Although there is no evidence that an empty rectum alters broad diagnostic interpretation, it does help to standardize the procedure and perhaps make it more pleasant for patients and staff alike.

Female patients are given 150 to 300 milliliters of oral radiographic contrast media at least half an hour before the examination to outline the pelvic small bowel loops and to aid in the identification of coincident enteroceles. Water-soluble contrast media or a mixture of this with barium passes through the small bowel faster than barium alone.

Rectal Contrast

When the oral contrast has passed sufficiently through the bowel, the patient is asked to lie on their left side. In women, a contrast agent is then inserted into the vagina to be able to identify this structure radiographically. In the past, a contrast-soaked tampon was used, but it was soon realized this would splint the vagina to some extent and prevent the formation of rectoceles. In addition, there is limited interpretation of the rectal wall morphology with a tampon in situ, and some authors have suggested that this may diminish the diagnosis of multiple pelvic floor anomalies by the creation of a "crowded-pelvis" syndrome if the rectum is over distended during the procedure (20,21). Contrast-soaked gauze can be used, but the easiest method is to insert a contrast and gel mixture. Our unit uses about 20 milliliters of 50% Aquagel™ with 50% nonionic intravenous (IV) contrast (300 milligrams iodine per 100 milliliters) mixed in a bladder syringe and injected into the vagina with a soft 10F catheter, as this tends not to leak out of the vagina (without distension) as easily as does liquid contrast. With regard to the nature of the rectal contrast used, several authors have suggested that high-viscosity barium, which mimics the characteristics of feces, should be used—most notably, barium sulphate mixed with potato starch. This may be of advantage in those unlikely to readily retain the rectal contrast either by virtue of age or with a preexisting weak anal sphincter and in those cases where it is preferred to scroll the proctogram in an ortho- and antegrade fashion to assess transiently observable anomalies that are not visualized when the contrast is expelled too quickly.

Originally, stiff pastes were made that were inserted with a caulking gun (22). This is time consuming and unpopular with those who have to prepare it, and most now use a pre-made barium paste that originally was designed as an esophageal paste for chest X-Rays (EZ paste™, EZ-EM). One hundred to 150 milliliters is inserted directly into the anal canal with the nozzle of a standard 50-milliliter bladder syringe. Alternatively, the first 30 milliliters could be standard liquid barium to coat the mucosa and, if possible, opacify the distal sigmoid colon. Ikenberry (23) compared examinations using liquid barium, E-Z paste, and a high-viscosity specially prepared paste and found no significant difference in pelvic floor descent or in the demonstration of rectoceles. Various other mixtures have been tried, including "FECOM," which is said to closely simulate normal stool (24). As the syringe inserting the paste is withdrawn, a small amount of barium is placed in the anal canal and a dollop of paste is left at the external anal orifice so these structures also are identifiable on the images.

The Commode

Once the rectal contrast has been inserted, a specially designed commode is placed in front of a vertically placed fluoroscopy table. The commode should incorporate additional filtration (equivalent to 4 mCi) (5,25) in order to obtain a uniform radiographic density at the level of the anal canal and to minimize "flare," which can limit defecographic measurements because of its effect on bony landmarks. (26) The commode should be comfortable and permit adequate lateral fluoroscopy with an even visible radiographic density above and below the top of the commode. Radiation filtration is necessary given the different X-ray absorptions of bone, soft tissue, and barium and the high scatter production encountered particularly above the commode.

The Procedure

The patient sits on the commode and is imaged fluoroscopically in the lateral position. The patient then is asked to perform a number of simple maneuvers such as "squeeze" (contraction of the pelvic floor muscles and anal canal), "strain" (pushing down without evacuation), "cough," and finally "evacuate." For the latter activity, the patient is asked to empty out the rectum as rapidly as possible; a good incentive is to tell the patient that the quicker they do this, the less radiation they will receive (as many patients may feel particular embarrassment during this time). It often is helpful to ask the patient to strain particularly hard at the end of defecation if prolapse is suspected, as sometimes no intussusception or prolapse will occur until the rectum is empty. The advantage here of the sitting defecogram is that it constitutes a more physiological position for the act of defecation than any of the other more sophisticated dynamic imaging technologies, such as conventional dynamic MRI or dynamic real-time ultrasound (27,28). The whole procedure is videotaped on SVHS format tapes and frame-grab images can be taken at any time. Images at rest, squeeze, and during different phases of evacuation are normally captured. With some equipment and with large patients, the frame-grab images can be of too low a resolution, and in these patients, additional spot films are taken. This is only really possible with good quality digital screening equipment or with conventional equipment with 100-millimeter film capability, as changing cassettes is too slow. An image of a radiopaque ruler in the same sagittal plane as the patient's midline is taken with the patient no longer on the commode to allow direct measurements.

The examination can be considered in three phases; resting, evacuation, and recovery (5). At rest, the rectum is angled posteriorly, parallel to the presacral space, where its axis forms an angle with the anal canal of approximately 90 degrees (2). With the anal canal closed, the anorectal junction (ARJ) is identified easily [Figure 3.1(i).1 (a,b)]. Its angulation is due to the puborectalis muscle, which forms a sling posteriorly at the junction of the rectal ampulla and anal canal. The inferior aspect of the ischial tuberosity is used to define the level of the pelvic floor (since this lies along the line of the pubococcygeal ligament) and the ARJ should lie at or just above this level at rest. Although the anorectal angle initially was considered important in maintaining continence, subsequent studies have shown a large overlap between normal patients and those with anorectal dysfunction (4,5,29) and it is no longer considered a discriminatory measurement. The pubococcygeal line is difficult to draw because of glare and identifying the bony landmarks, and the plane of the ischial tuberosities is generally preferred (5).

The simple "squeeze" maneuver raises the pelvic floor, decreasing the anorectal angle and lengthening the anal canal, which gives an indication

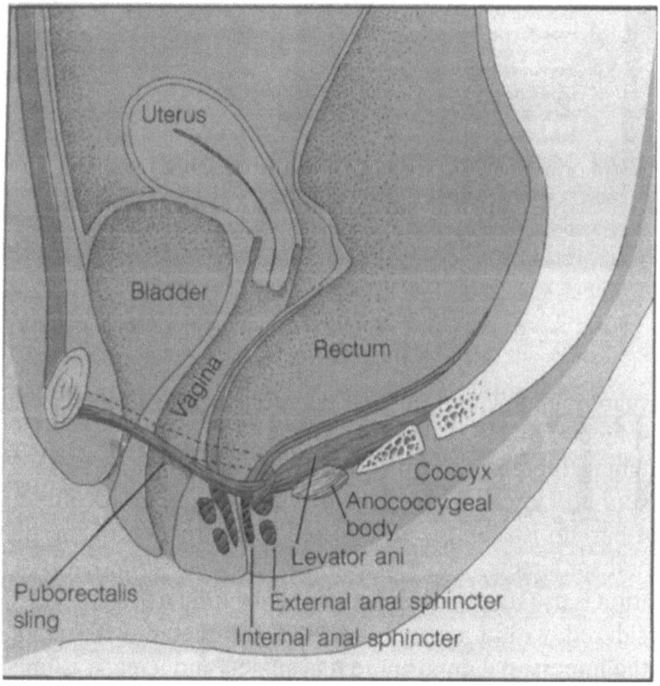

a

FIGURE 3.1(i).1. (a) Line drawing of the rectal and pelvic floor anatomy. (Printed with permission from Shorvon PJ and Stevenson GW. Defaecography: setting up a service. Br J Hosp Med. 1989;41:460). (b) Normal resting and evacuation phases at EP showing placement of a ruler in the position of the patients mid saggital plane, allowing direct measurements to be calculated.

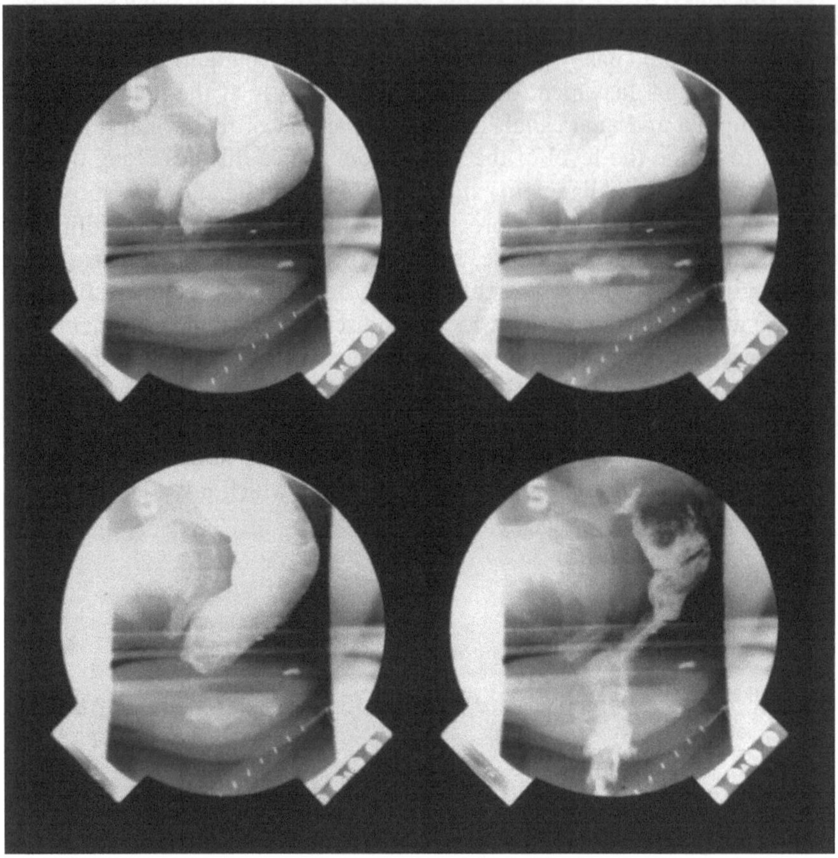

b

FIGURE 3.1(i).1. *Continued*

of pelvic diaphragmatic and puborectalis contraction, as well as that of the external sphincter.

On coughing, there is a sharp rise in intra-abdominal pressure. In normal subjects, very little movement of the pelvic floor and no involuntary incontinence of barium is seen because of reflex contraction of the pelvic floor and external sphincter.

Evacuation is usually rapid and completed within a few seconds, although it is considered within normal limits if completed within 30 seconds. Because the impersonal environment is anxiety inducing, it is important to use pelvic floor descent as a marker of the onset of evacuation. The puborectalis impression is effaced as the canal opens, with an increase in the anorectal angle of approximately 20 degrees, where the rectum and the anal canal together form a "cone shape." Generally, only the distal rectum beyond the main fold is emptied, with some contrast remaining in the rectosigmoid segment (30).

Once the patient stops straining, the anal canal closes and the puborectalis contracts, elevating the ARJ to its resting position.

Modifications and Variations of Technique

Left Lateral Position

When a suitable commode is unavailable, the entire examination may be performed in the left lateral position. The resting position of the pelvic floor is higher than when seated (31), and the lack of any effects of gravity limit the usefulness of this approach.

Area Postrema (AP) Views

The normal proctographic view is a true lateral view. This is a two-dimensional (2D) representation of a three-dimensional (3D) subject, and abnormalities outside the midline will be projected onto this view. Intra-anal intussusception can be demonstrated more easily on an area postrema (AP) view, with widening of the anal canal during straining after evacuation. An occasional radiographic finding is a posterior rectocele or posterolateral pouch/herniation. This is due to a herniation of the rectal wall through the pelvic diaphragm. It is to one side of the midline, where its precise position is best demonstrated by an AP view (32). Similarly, the "concertina" type of rectal movement during evacuation—although not a true intussusception—may contribute to obstructed defecation and is recognizable in the coronal plane. This can only be suspected on the lateral view, needing an AP view for confirmation. The AP view is often difficult to obtain using conventional undercouch fluoroscopic equipment because of the lack of space between the explorator and the table, and patients may actually have to stand up to demonstrate an abnormality.

Failure to Evacuate

Occasionally, patients will be unable to evacuate, and although this may be due to their outlet obstruction, it often is due to embarrassment. To avoid excessive radiographic screening, the investigation staff can place themselves "out of sight" and the patient can be given the fluoroscopy pedal to press when evacuation begins. Additionally, encouragement by explaining that the quicker the examination is performed, the less radiation is received often shortens the procedure. It should be remembered that the average skin dose of radiation during conventional defecography is about 0.02 to 0.66 cGy (centigray) when compared with a barium enema (0.22–0.64 cGy), where the ovarian dose is about 0.036 to 0.053 cGy compared with that of a barium enema of 0.32 to 0.42 cGy (5,7). Patients who "aid" evacuation (e.g., by transvaginal or perineal pressure on a rectocele, or anal digitation to overcome a spastic puborectalis) are encouraged, wherever possible, to demonstrate these actions while screening in order to understand their mechanism.

EP with Concurrent Peritoneography

Peritoneography is a diagnostic technique occasionally used for identifying hernias. It involves injection of non-ionic water-soluble contrast media into the peritoneum. The technique can be used as an addition in defecography in order to visualize the peritoneal cavity, particularly the Pouch of Douglas (33–35). This is useful for demonstrating deep recesses that have the potential for hosting enteroceles, even if these are not evident on the study—in effect, a classification of peritoneoceles (36,37).

Digital Subtraction EP and Computer Analysis

Subtraction techniques in radiology are a well-established means of illustrating the differences between two images; in conventional subtraction radiography, an image is taken prior to contrast administration, then a reversed image (or mask) is superimposed on the radiograph containing contrast so that all non-contrast detail is subtracted and a final image of only the contrast-enhanced structures is seen. This is a slow process, but digital subtraction has since speeded the process to almost real time and allowed a variety of postprocessing computerized enhancements. Similarly, digital subtraction defecography can show just the changes occurring in the rectum and anal canal during defecation, the subtracted images allowing easy analysis for area measurement via planimetry (and therefore assumptions on volume changes) in assessing the rapidity and completeness of rectal emptying (38,39). Although this creates numeric data that is invaluable in further analysis and correlation, it is not considered to add significantly to patient management, and furthermore, such data is probably more accurately achieved with isotope techniques. Moreover, subtracted images actually hindered the visualization of morphological abnormalities in five of 18 patients in one study (40), and hence, digital subtraction is currently little used.

Dynamic Cystoproctography

There is increasing recognition that the different compartments in the pelvic floor (posterior or rectal, middle or vaginal and uterine, and anterior or bladder and urethra in females) are interrelated and that disease processes in one can affect others. Pelvic floor prolapse can affect all compartments at once or be largely confined to one or two compartments only. Many patients undergoing defecography also will have micturating cystography in their diagnostic work-up. For these reasons, there is more interest in the development of multidisciplinary pelvic floor teams and management. It is possible to perform cystography at the same time as EP rather than at a separate investigation. While this has the advantage of seeing the interrelations of the two compartments, the difficulty for both the patient and the investigator is increased. Furthermore, cystography traditionally has been performed by careful pressure measurements taken in the bladder using a rectal catheter to obtain subtracted detrusor pressures from the bladder, and this is difficult to do when defecation is also being assessed. The combined technique is good for showing anatomical abnormalities such as bladder neck problems, cystocele, and prolapse. The concept of "competition for space" within the pelvis has been elaborated by this technique. It has been shown that either a cystocele or an enterocele may be demonstrated, but not both at the same time. Similarly, a rectocele and enterocele may inhibit one another. As a consequence of this, a sequential approach often is used, opacifying the bladder first to demonstrate the degree of cystocele, emptying the bladder, and then opacifying the rectum to perform a standard EP (41).

MRI EP

A number of groups have investigated the use of MRI defecography (42,43) (see Chapter 3.3). The advantage of this technique is the avoidance of ionizing radiation and the visualization of all the organs of the pelvis at the same time. Patient preparation is easier, multiplanar views can be obtained, and perhaps surprisingly, bony landmarks are easier to identify using MRI. The technique also has been shown to be extremely accurate in the delineation of attendant enteroceles, which can be missed in conventional defecography in up to 20% of cases. These are vital for diagnosis where a rectocele may be repaired for evacuatory difficulty and where the preoperative definition of an enterocele prevents residual evacuatory problems (36,44). Studies have been performed with the patients lying supine in a conventional scanner, but others have used open magnets with the patients sitting on specially constructed commodes similar to conventional radiographic defecography. With the former method, both non-evacuation (straining only) and evacuation studies have been performed (27,42,45,46).

There are inherent problems with this approach when compared with defecography. Most MRI studies tend to image only in the midline sagittal plane and are at risk of missing changes outside this plane. Studies without evacuation will miss many morphological abnormalities that only progress as the rectum empties (such as rectoanal intussusception and rectal prolapse), and any such study generally is considered incomplete (47). Supine studies with evacuation are likely to under-represent the true degree of descent and prolapse, although this may be less than initially thought. In many ways, proctograms with the patient sitting in open magnets are the ideal, as not only do they mirror normal evacuation, but all the pelvic organs can be visualized at one time. However, to date, relatively low field magnets

(0.5 Tesla) have been used, and only T1-weighted sequences with a maximum of two images per second have been achieved. It also has required gadolinium rectal paste to be inserted in order for the rectal contents to be visualized. The examination is expensive and the bladder views appear to be sub-optimal on T1-weighted images. Moreover, some proctographic changes can be missed when images are only taken at two-second intervals.

Magnetic resonance imaging studies clearly have many advantages and considerable potential; however, the difficulties with performing these studies, particularly in conventional magnets, are significant. Furthermore, MRI is relatively expensive and currently has somewhat limited availability in most hospitals, particularly for allocation for pelvic floor functional disorder evaluation.

Radioisotope EP

Some centers have performed EP using radioisotopes and a gamma camera (48,49). A potato starch "paste" mixed with Technetium 99^{m} is utilized. The use of isotopes facilitates quantification. By drawing areas of interest around the rectum, rates of emptying, completeness of emptying, and pelvic floor descent are measured. Rectoceles can be diagnosed and the percentage trapping of isotope can be calculated. The technique is useful for the quantification of the effectiveness of surgery for rectal emptying problems. However, the anatomical detail that can be assessed using this method is very limited and morphological abnormalities of the rectum are easily overlooked. The technique has not achieved wide acceptance.

EP in Evacuation Disorders

The significance of structural abnormalities demonstrated by EP is greatly debated because they are found in many normal subjects undergoing this investigation (4). Because there is always a tendency to attribute symptoms to a radiographically demonstrated abnormality, it is important to both consider the incidence of that abnormality in asymptomatic patients and also to try to correlate the finding (as mentioned above) with the patient's symptoms.

Rectocele

This term is used to describe the anterior bulge of the rectal wall that occurs in females during evacuation (4,11). In normal individuals, including nulliparous females, this may be up to two centimeters in depth (3), as measured from the anterior anal canal to the most anterior part of the rectocele. When large (Figure 3.1(i).2), the rectocele acts as a pressure, as well as a volume, reservoir where anal canal opening may be delayed, a phenomenon particularly evident on real-time MRI scanning. Some patients will support the rectovaginal septum during straining in order to counteract this effect, either by digital pressure on the anterior perineum or trans-vaginally. This information, however, is uncommonly volunteered and is best obtained by direct inquiry. Asking the patient to demonstrate this often will confirm the mechanism by which their "aiding" of defecation is effective.

Posterior rectoceles occur fairly rarely, but they are better termed posterior perineal hernias resulting from a defect in the levator ani. The orientation of this will be shown on an AP view during defecography (50). These are often transitory during straining early on, but will become permanent "pouches" with time.

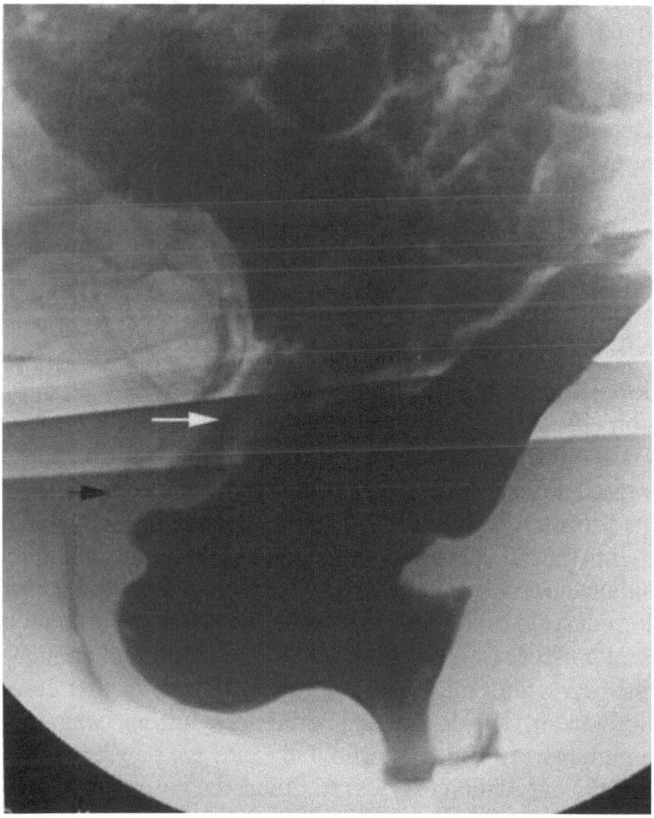

FIGURE 3.1(i).2. Large anterior rectocele. A black arrow delineates the vaginal marker and a white arrow a small enterocoele.

Neither the size of the rectocele or trapping of contrast within it following evacuation has been shown to correlate with symptoms (51,52), and on postoperative EP after rectocele repair, there is no correlation between the radiological appearances and the symptomatic response. A study comparing constipated, incontinent, and asymptomatic patients found a similar prevalence and size of rectoceles in all groups (52). Barium trapping within a rectocele is a not uncommon finding, which could account for symptoms if stool becomes sequestrated or if elevation of intrarectal pressures is inadequate for complete evacuation. In order to examine this postulate, Halligan and Bartram (52) looked for differences in intrarectal pressure during evacuation and the ability to expel a non-deformable balloon between patients with documented barium trapping and those without contrast retention. The presence or absence of a rectocele, its size, or barium trapping had no effect on the patients' ability to expel the balloon, but a marked fall in intra-rectal pressure was seen when the manometer entered the rectocele in seven of 12 patients with barium trapping. This finding suggests that trapping is due to sequestration in the anterior wall of the rectum in an extraperitoneal position, isolating part of the rectocele from differential changes in intra-rectal pressure (53).

The presence of a rectocele or trapping within it should not be taken as a primary sign of impaired evacuation. However, if patients aid evacuation by compressing or splinting the rectocele, it is more likely to be of functional importance. Rectoceles often are found in association with anismus, which may account for poor symptomatic relief if rectocele repair is performed, although this remains controversial (54,55).

Pelvic Floor Descent

Pelvic floor descent of up to three centimeters can be seen during normal evacuation (19). Excessive pelvic floor descent is a common finding (Figure 3.1(i).3), although its significance is still uncertain. While some studies have demonstrated differences between controls and constipated patients, others have failed to show significant differences between constipated or incontinent patients (56,57). Chronic straining has been implicated in the etiology of pudendal neuropathy, but there is no correlation between neuropathy and pelvic floor descent on EP (58). Reduced descent implies a poor increase in intra-rectal pressure (59), but in the elderly or incontinent patient, the position of the pelvic floor may be low at rest, with little further descent during evacuation (56,60). The descending perineum syndrome was a term applied to those patients, often elderly, who had excessive pelvic floor descent and difficultly with evacuation (61). On straining, the perineum balloons and the abdominal pressure appears to "spread" the rectum in a globular fashion with only poor evacuation; in effect, the raised abdominal pressure appears to be "wasted" in creating this rectal configuration rather than directing intra-rectal contents in a cone shape towards the anal canal.

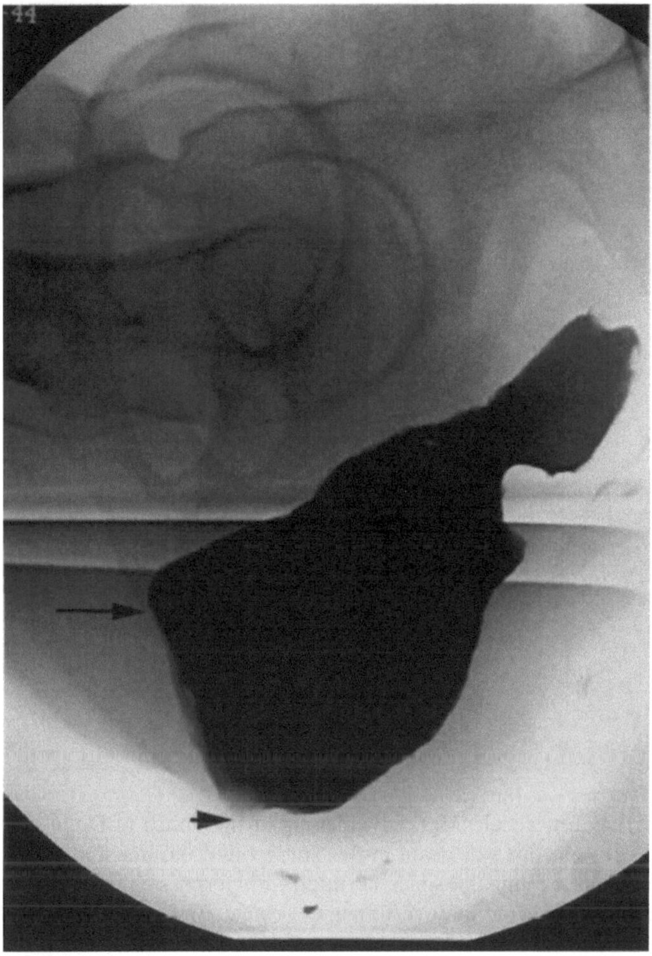

FIGURE 3.1(i).3. Excessive pelvic floor descent. The upper arrow indicates the position of the ischial tuberosities and the lower arrow the anorectal junction in this patient with marked descent.

Enterocele, Sigmoidocele, and Peritoneocele

Herniation of bowel, bladder, or uterus into a deep rectogenital space may occur during evacuation. When the small bowel herniates, this is called an enterocele, whereas a sigmoidocele contains sigmoid colon. This is common following hysterectomy and cystopexy, where enteroceles can be present in up to two-thirds of patients following hysterectomy and a quarter following cystopexy. Enteroceles usually descend between the vagina and rectum, but can invaginate into the vagina itself (Figure 3.1(i).4). While this may be inferred during EP from widening of the rectovaginal distance or compression of the anterior rectal wall, it is best demonstrated when the vagina and small bowel contain contrast. A sigmoidocele, although much less

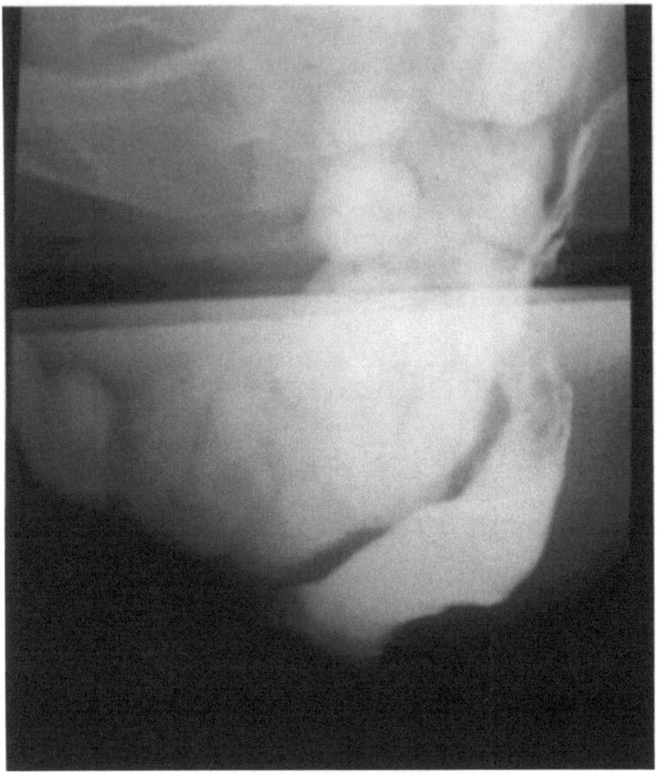

FIGURE 3.1(i).4. Enterocele. Marked widening of the Pouch of Douglas with evacuation. No oral contrast was given in this study, but a barium study later confirms the large enterocele filling this space. (Printed with permission from Shorvon PJ and Stevenson GW. Defaecography: setting up a service. Br J Hosp Med. 1989;41:464).

common, is often easily demonstrated as a herniating soft tissue mass containing fecal residue if no rectal contrast has entered the sigmoid (Figure 3.1(i).5). Enteroceles most commonly are seen on straining at the end of evacuation, and indeed, some units advocate a "post-toilet" image, as patients can sometimes complete evacuation in private when unable to do so on the EP commode.

An enterocele or sigmoidocele requires a deep peritoneal pouch or cul-de-sac, and these may be present without any bowel within. In this situation, they will only be shown on EP if peritoneography is performed at the same time, but recognition is felt to be important as, if overlooked, it may compromise the success of other pelvic floor operations (62).

Intussusception

Various degrees of infolding of the rectal mucosa ranging from anterior mucosal prolapse to full-thickness rectal prolapse or "procidentia" may occur during evacuation. Intussusception has been graded on a seven-point scale (3), although recently there has been a trend towards more simple stratification based on the likely contribution to symptoms. Classification into high- or low-grade intussusception is possible with assessment based on the rectal appearance at the end of evacuation. It is termed intra-rectal when confined to the rectum and intra-anal if the apex enters the anal canal. Generally, low-grade intussusception is defined as circumferential infolding of rectal mucosa, which is less than three millimeters thick and confined to the rectum (3). Full-thickness prolapse defines high-grade intussusception where the prolapsing fold is greater than three millimeters thick and impacts on the anal canal [Figure 3.1(i).6 (a,b)]. It may stop at the internal anal orifice or progress down the anal canal level [Figure 3.1(i).7 (a,b)].

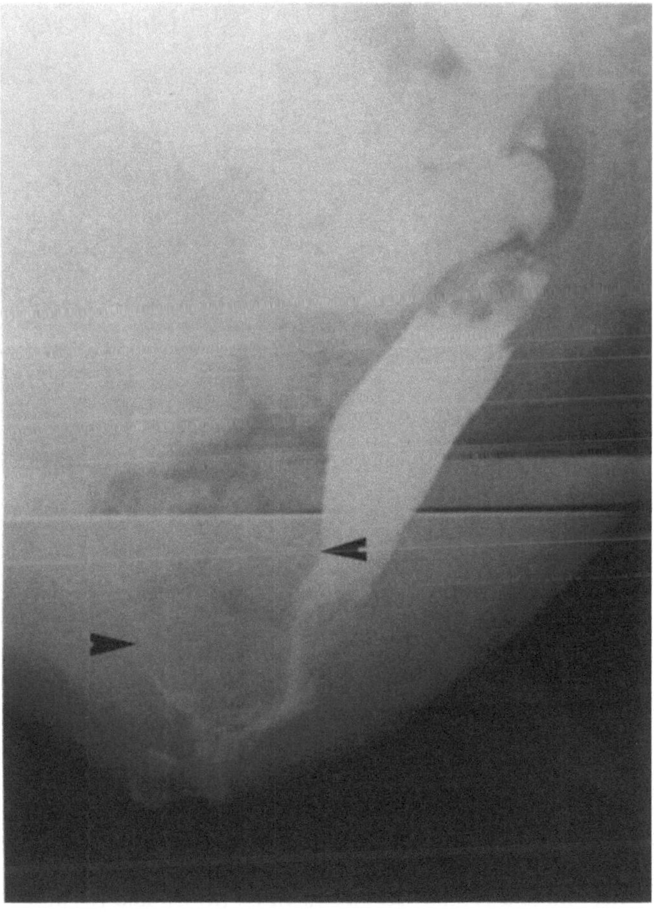

FIGURE 3.1(i).5. Sigmoidocele. Arrowheads indicate the posterior vaginal wall and the anterior rectal wall with a sigmoidocoele projecting between them.

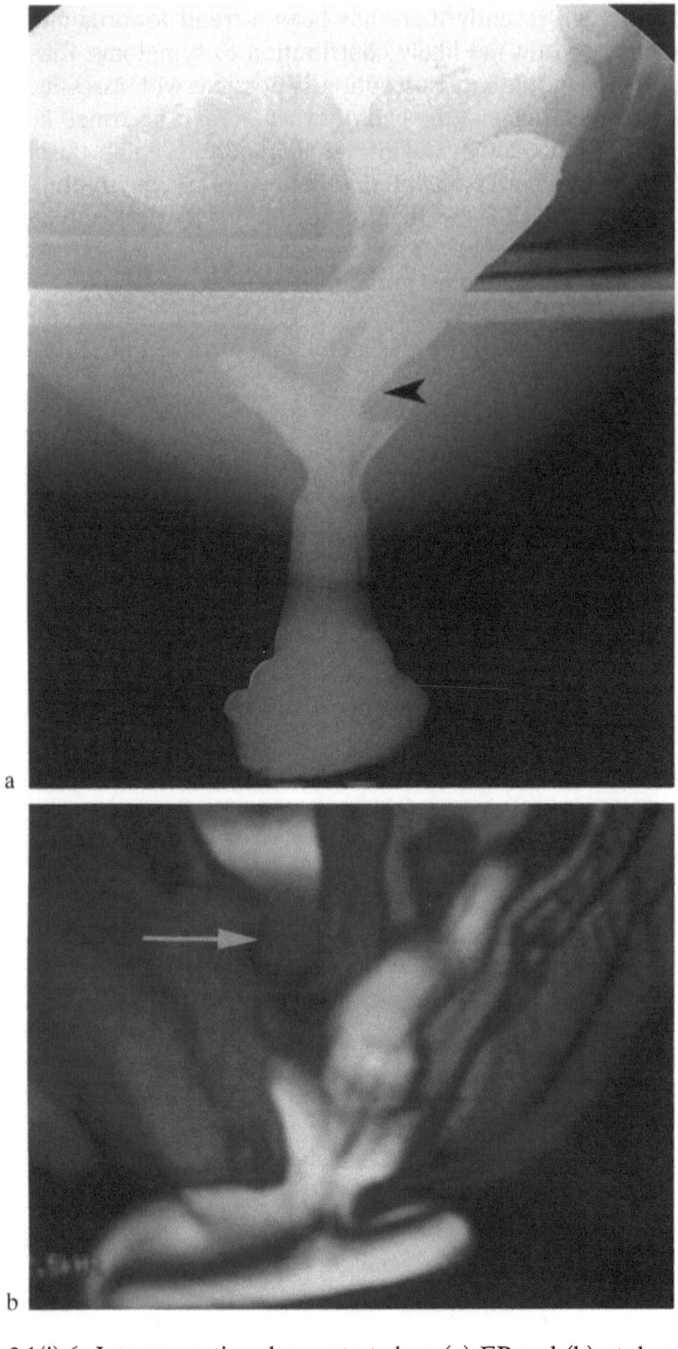

FIGURE 3.1(i).6. Intussusception demonstrated on (a) EP and (b) at dynamic MR proctography in an open magnet. Magnetic resonance also demonstrates a small cystocele (arrow).

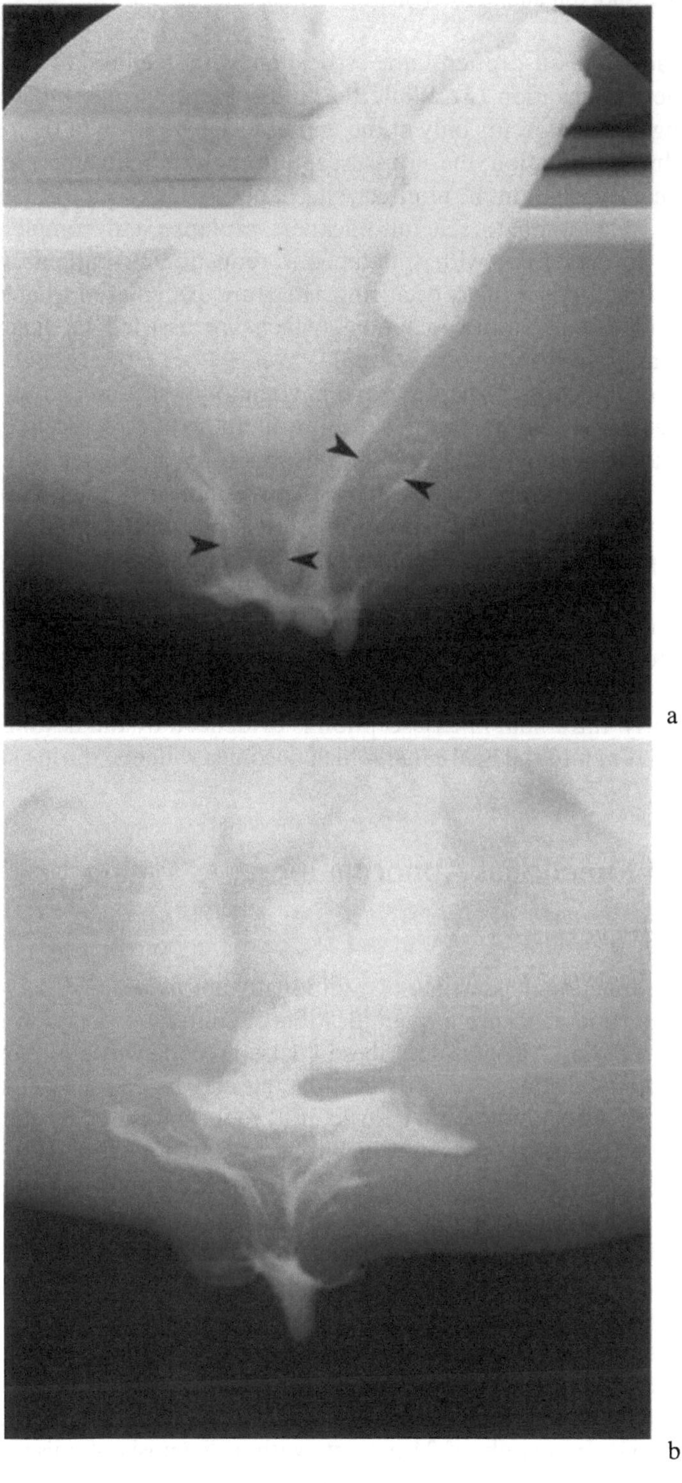

FIGURE 3.1(i).7. Intra-anal intussusception—lateral (a) and AP (b) views. Note enterocele on lateral view.

High-grade intussusceptions are associated with feelings of difficult or incomplete evacuation (4). While the intussusception may impede rectal emptying, it often occurs only at the end of evacuation when the rectum is empty. In this situation, the intussusceptum may be inducing a feeling of incomplete evacuation as, in effect, the patient tries to pass it per anum. It is not uncommon to see full-thickness prolapse and complete rectal prolapse (procidentia) with spontaneous reduction in patients who are unaware that this is actually occurring. These are examples of what has been labeled as "occult" intussusceptions, which are assisted in diagnosis by defecography in suspicious cases (63).

Anterior mucosal prolapse is seen commonly in association with a rectocele, where that part of the rectal wall above the rectocele descends towards the anal canal as the rectum collapses, often associated with barium trapping within the rectocele. There is no established relationship with rectal intussusception (64); however, EP is indicated if anterior wall mucosal prolapse is detected clinically but more significant intussusception is suspected (65).

Asymmetric collapse of the rectal tube during evacuation is often over-interpreted as intussusception. When screening in the AP projection, the valves of Houston, which in part govern the process of rectal collapse, are seen clearly. Intra-anal intussusception is evidenced by the advance of the folded rectum into the anal canal, which becomes widened during straining.

EP and Functional Abnormalities

Anismus

Although functional assessments traditionally are performed in the physiology department, accurate quantification of contrast evacuation is possible using EP (66). Anismus describes impaired rectal evacuation secondary to a functional disturbance of defecation and may be demonstrated in isolation or in association with a structural abnormality. Many alternative terms have been used (some of which reflect postulated etiologies), including spastic pelvic floor syndrome, rectal dyschezia, non-relaxing puborectalis syndrome, and paradoxical sphincter contraction. Failure of the anorectal angle to efface and a prominent puborectalis impression during attempted evacuation are cited frequently in the literature as signs of anismus (Figure 3.1(i).8).

Considerable inter-observer error has been documented in measuring the anorectal angle (ARA) (67), but more importantly, no correlation has been produced between the ARA and the anorectal physiologic criteria for anismus (68). In a study of 24 patients with a diagnosis of anismus based on multiple criteria, only measurements indicating delayed rectal emptying were able to differentiate patients from controls (69). Confounding results

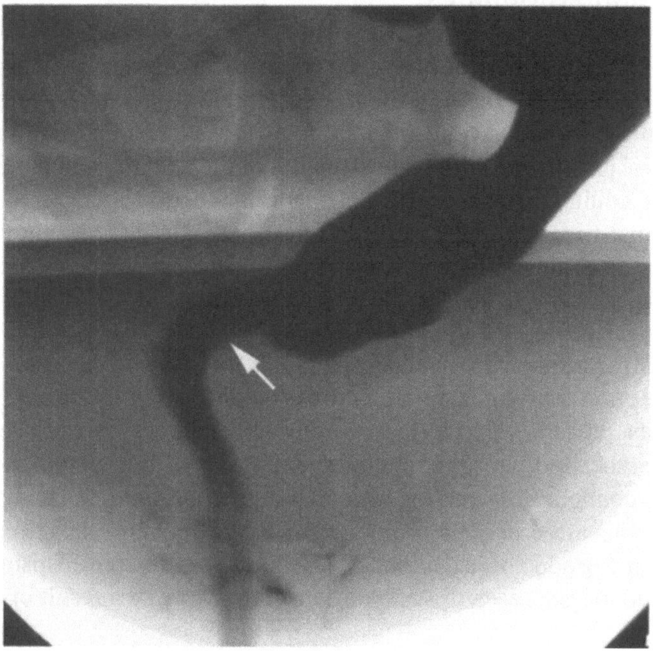

FIGURE 3.1(i).8. Non-relaxing puborectalis muscle.

exist, however, where patients with electromyographic criteria for anismus can demonstrate normal evacuation on EP (70,71). Further confusion has arisen from the results of ambulatory physiology studies, suggesting that some of the signs of anismus may even be a laboratory-observed phenomenon (71–73). In general, patients who evacuate rapidly and completely are unlikely to have anismus; those who cannot do so *may* have anismus, but the finding may be artifactual due to psychological inhibition.

Solitary Rectal Ulcer Syndrome (SRUS)

This condition is normally associated with either overt rectal prolapse or lesser degrees, including rectal intussusception and pronounced anterior rectal wall mucosal prolapse. EP usually identifies one of these abnormalities in patients with solitary rectal ulcer syndrome (SRUS). These patients often strain excessively, and first-line treatment for those without marked prolapse is behavioral, as surgical correction of these various types of prolapse only has moderate success. Endoanal ultrasound can identify thickening of internal sphincter, although the reason for this is unknown (74–76).

Congenital Anomalies

Imperforate anus is part of the spectrum of rectal agenesis. There may be an almost normal distribution of striated muscle from which the external anal sphincter should have formed. In many cases, a colonic "pull through" operation is performed, with reconstruction of the anal canal and perineum. As young adults, varying degrees of incontinence are a common sequel. Resting anal tone is usually reduced due to the absence of any properly developed internal sphincter. Additionally, there may be an ineffective external sphincter (or levator plate) due to either an incomplete muscle ring or misplacement of the anorectum in an eccentric position alongside the malformed sphincter mechanism (77,78). However, because chronic intussusception may cause or exacerbate incontinence, EP is indicated to exclude its presence. There may be varying degrees of sacrococcygeal agenesis associated with high rectal agenesis. Here, the rectum is usually vertical in configuration and the normal puborectalis impression is partially effaced. Evacuation may be prolonged and puborectalis relaxation can be intermittent, producing a "milking" effect on the rectum. Anismus may coexist, and in such cases, disordered evacuation may be a result of a mixed neuropathy.

Post Surgical Appearances

Many surgical procedures have been described for the treatment of rectal prolapse and patients may present postoperatively with recurrent symptoms of evacuatory difficulty or incontinence after these surgeries (79). While recurrent intussusception is not uncommon (reported at between 3 and 17% following perineal procedures and closer to 10% following rectopexy), proctography is indicated to exclude other causes of obstructed evacuation such as a sigmoidocele, anismus, or proximal rectal stenosis.

Abdominal Rectopexy

Here, the rectum is mobilized and the posterior wall elevated and fixed to the presacral fascia with nonabsorbable sutures or mesh. Several modifications to the technique have been described, ranging from alternative fixation techniques to resection rectopexy where the prolapsing rectum and any redundant sigmoid colon are excised (80). Theoretically, this protects against recurrence and sigmoidocele, but because chronic constipation is common in patients with intussusception, the colon alters its configuration over time and new redundant loops may develop.

At EP, there may be widening of the presacral space and a vertical configuration to the rectum, the apex of which is normally angulated and closely approximated to the sacral promontory.

Delorme's Procedure

Rectal prolapse is common in elderly women, many of whom may be unfit for major abdominal surgery. Delorme's procedure (using a perineal approach to excise the prolapsing mucosa and reef the muscularis propria) can be carried out under local or regional anesthetic where necessary. The muscle layers in this segment of bowel are stitched together in a concertina fashion, forming a ring of plicated redundant muscle at the anorectal junction. Resultant decreased rectal capacity and compliance are thought to be important factors implicated in the low incidence of evacuation problems following this procedure, although the post-Delorme's physiology is complex (81). The EP features can reflect the decreased rectal capacity and the plicated muscle at the anorectal junction, which may become stenosed.

Colo Anal Anastomosis

Rectal excision with a colo-anal anastomosis may be performed as part of anterior resection for a low rectal carcinoma. Although remodeling of the neorectum will occur with time, a J-pouch is sometimes created to act as a reservoir and avoid problems of frequency postoperatively. Again, findings at EP will reflect the surgery, with widening of the presacral space and a somewhat vertical configuration to the pouch (82). The most common structural abnormality that may present with evacuatory difficulty is stricture formation, which may result from pouch ischemia or an isolated anastomotic leak.

Pouchography

Panproctocolectomy for ulcerative colitis usually involves formation of an ileal reservoir in an attempt to reduce stool frequency. Several pouch configurations are described, and it is not uncommon to encounter patients with pouch dysfunction, although presentation may be late. Dynamic evaluation of evacuation is similar in principle to EP, although it is sensible to use less-viscous barium. Evacuatory difficulty may be functional or structural. Structural abnormalities include stenosis at the anal anastomosis or of the afferent limb. Dilatation of the distal small bowel is a normal finding after a few months, as it adapts to provide additional reservoir function. Where a long distal segment is present, this may be effaced by the distended pouch as intra-abdominal pressure is raised and the pouch descends inferiorly with the pelvic floor, creating a true outlet obstruction that lies away from the anastomosis (83).

An unsuspected anastomotic leak and chronic presacral sepsis are other causes for long-standing pouch dysfunction. Presacral widening is usually present and a leak or cavity may be demonstrated at EP. If no cavity is seen at EP, it may be worth considering further imaging of the presacral space to exclude sepsis. Obstructive problems with long-standing pouches may be due to adhesions or stricture formation, especially related to the covering ileostomy; here a formal small bowel study often is helpful (84).

Conclusions

EP has been shown to assist our clinical understanding and management in a setting where symptoms and clinical signs often may be confounding (4,5). EP studies are best reported in multidisciplinary meetings alongside clinical and laboratory data. Care must be taken to not always attach clinical significance to morphological radiologic findings, as the range of normality in EP is wide, particularly in females. Correlation of symptoms to visualized abnormalities and the demonstration of the action of patient "aiding maneuvers" often will help in the correct interpretation of studies.

Acknowledgments. We are grateful to Professor C.I. Bartram and Professor W. Gedroyc for their contributions to the figures.

References

1. Preston DM, Lennard-Jones JE, and Thomas BM. The balloon proctogram. Br J Surg. 1984;7:29–32.
2. Burhenne HJ. Intestinal evacuation study: a new roentgenologic technique. Radiol Clin N Am. 1964;33:79–84.
3. Mahieu P, Pringot J, and Bodart P. Defecography: I. Description of a new procedure and results in normal patients. Gastrointest Radiol. 1984;9:247–51.
4. Shorvon PJ, McHugh S, Diamant NE, Somers S, and Stevenson GW. Defecography in normal volunteers: results and implications. Gut. 1989;30:1737–49.
5. Bartram CI, Turnbull GK, and Lennard-Jones JE. Evacuation proctography: an investigation of rectal expulsion in 20 subjects without defecatory disturbance. Gastrointest Radiol. 1988;13:72–80.
6. Marti MC and Mirescu D. Utilité du défécogramme en proctologie. Ann Gastroenterol Hepatol (Paris). 1982;18:379–84.
7. Kuijpers HC. Defaecography. In: Wexner SD and Bartolo DC, editors. Constipation. Etiology, Evaluation and Management. London: Butterworth Heinemann; 1995. p. 77–86.
8. Jones HJ, Swift RI, and Blake H. A prospective audit of the usefulness of evacuating proctography. Ann R Coll Surg Engl. 1998;80:40–5.
9. Harvey CJ, Halligan S, Bartram CI, Hollings N, Sahdev A, and Kingston K. Evacuation proctography: a prospective study of diagnostic and therapeutic effects. Radiology. 1999;211:223–7.
10. McKee RF, McEnroe L, Anderson JH, and Finlay IG. Identification of patients likely to benefit from biofeedback for outlet obstruction constipation. Br J Surg. 1999;86:355–9.
11. Zbar AP, Lienemann A, Fritsch H, Beer-Gabel M, and Pescatori M. Rectocele: pathogenesis and surgical management. Int J Colorect Dis. 2003;18:369–84.

12. Ekberg O, Hjelmqvist B, Leandoer L, et al. Rectal prolapse and internal intussusception, the role of defaecography in pre- and postoperative evaluation. J Med Imaging. 1988;2:88–92.
13. Sadry F, Mirescu D, and Marti M-C. L'exploration radiologique des troubles de la défécation. In: Bessler W, et al., editors. Neue aspekte radiologischer diagnostik und therapie. Huber, Bern: Jahrbuch; 1986. p. 8–91.
14. Rafert JA, Lappas JC, and Wilkins W. Defecography: techniques for improved image quality. Radiol Technol. 1990;61:368–73.
15. Boccasanta P, Venturi M, Calabrò G, Trompetto M, Ganio E, Tessera G, Bottini C, Pulvirenti D'Urso A, Ayabaca S, and Pescatori M. Which surgical approach for rectocele? A multicentric report from Italian coloproctologists. Tech Coloproctol. 2001;5:149–56.
16. Mulder W, de-Jong E, Wanters I, Kinders M, Heij HA, and Vos A. Posterior sagittal anorectoplasty: functional results of primary and secondary operations in comparison to the pull-through method in anorectal malformations. Eur J Paediatr Surg. 1995;5:170–3.
17. Halligan S, Nicholls RJ, and Bartram CI. Proctographic changes after rectopexy for solitary rectal ulcer syndrome and preoperative predictive factors for a successful outcome. Br J Surg. 1995;82:314–17.
18. Goei R, Beaten C, and Arends JW. Solitary rectal ulcer syndrome: findings at barium enema study and defaecography. Radiology. 1988;168:303–6.
19. Hare C, Halligan S, Bartram CI, Gupta R, Walker AE, and Renfrew I. Dose reduction in evacuation proctography. Eur Radiol. 2001;11(3):432–4.
20. Low VH, Ho LM, and Freed KS. Vaginal opacification during defecography: direction of vaginal migration aids in diagnosis of pelvic floor pathology. Abdom Imaging. 1999;24:565–8.
21. Dietz HP and Clarke B. the influence of posture on perineal ultrasound imaging parameters. Int Urogynecol J Pelvic Floor Dysfunct. 2001;12:104–6.
22. Bernier P, Stevenson GW, and Shorvon P. Defecography commode. Radiology. 1988;166:891–2.
23. Ikenberry S, Lappas JC, Hana MP, and Rex DK. Defecography in healthy subjects: comparison of three contrast media. Radiology. 1996;201(1):233–8.
24. Pelsang RE, Rao SS, and Welcher K. FECOM, a new artificial stool for evaluating defecation. Am J Gastroenterol. 1999;94:183–6.
25. Ginai AZ. Evacuation proctography (defecography). A new seat and method of examination. Clin Radiol. 1990;42(3):214–16.
26. Beer-Gabel M, Teshler M, Barzilai N, Lurie Y, Malnick S, Bass D, and Zbar A. Dynamic transperineal ultrasound in the diagnosis of pelvic floor disorders. Pilot study. Dis Colon Rectum. 2002;45:239–48.
27. Schoenenberger AW, Debatin JF, Guldenschuh I, Hany TF, Steiner P, and Krestin GP. Dynamic MR defecography with a superconducting, open-configuration MR system. Radiology. 1998;206:641–6.
28. Beer-Gabel M, Teshler M, Schechtman E, and Zbar AP. Dynamic transperineal ultrasound vs. defecography in patients with evacuatory difficulty: a pilot study. Int J Colorectal Dis. In press 2003.
29. Selvaggi F, Pesce G, Scotto Di Carlo E, Maffettone V, and Canonico S. Evaluation of normal subjects by defecographic technique. Dis Colon Rectum. 1990; 33(8):698–702.

30. LeSaffer LPA. Defecography—Update 1994. The model of expulsion, digital subtraction cysto-colpo-enter-defecography and the perineal support device [thesis]. Belgium: ASZ Aalst Belgium Story-Scientia Gent.
31. Poon FW, Lauder JC, and Finlay IG. Technical report: evacuating proctography—a simplified technique. Clin Radiol. 1991;44(2):113–6.
32. Chen HH, Iroatulam A, Alabaz O, Weiss EG, Nogueras JJ, and Wexner SD. Associations of defecography and physiologic findings in male patients with rectocele. Tech Coloproctol. 2001;5:157–61.
33. Halligan S and Bartram CI. Evacuation proctography combined with positive contrast peritoneography to demonstrate pelvic floor hernias. Abdom Imaging. 1995;20(5):442–5.
34. Bremmer S, Mellgren A, Holmstrom B, and Uden R. Peritoneocele: visualization with defecography and peritoneography performed simultaneously. Radiology. 1998;202:373–7.
35. Bremmer S. Peritoneocele: a radiologic study with defaeco-peritoneography. Acta Radiol. 1998;413 (Suppl):1–33.
36. Lienemann A, Anthuber C, Baron A, and Reiser M. Diagnosing enteroceles using dynamic magnetic resonance imaging. Dis Colon Rectum. 2000;43:205–13.
37. Karlbom U, Nilsson S, Pahlman L, and Graf W. Defecogaphic study of rectal evacuation in constipated and control subjects. Radiology. 1999;210:103–8.
38. LeSaffer LPA. Digital subtraction defecography. In: Smith LE, editor. Practical guide to anorectal testing. 2nd ed. New York: Igaku-Shoin; 1995. p. 161–84.
39. Brady AP, Somers S, Hough D, and Stevenson GW. Digital subtraction in defecography. Abdom Imaging. 1995;20:245–7.
40. Kelvin FM, Hale DS, Maglinte DD, Patten BJ, and Benson JT. Female pelvic organ prolapse: diagnostic contribution of dynamic cystoproctography and comparison with physical examination. AJR Am J Roentgenol. 1999;173:31–7.
41. Healy JC, Halligan S, Reznek RH, Watson S, Bartram CI, Phillips R, and Armstrong P. Dynamic MR imaging compared with evacuation proctography when evaluating anorectal configuration and pelvic floor movement. AJR Am J Roentgenol. 1997;169(3):775–9.
42. Lamb GM, de Jode MG, Gould SW, Spouse E, Birnie K, Darzi A, and Gedroyc WM. Upright dynamic MR defaecating proctography in an open configuration MR system. Br J Radiol. 2000;73(866):152–5.
43. Lienemann A, Anthuber C, Baron A, Kohz P, and Reiser M. Dynamic MR colpocystorectography assessing pelvic floor descent. Eur Radiol. 1997;7:1309–17.
44. Lienemann A. An easy approach to functional magnetic resonance imaging of pelvic floor disorders. Tech Coloproctol. 1998;2:131–4.
45. Law PA, Danin JC, lamb GM, Regan L, Darzi A, and Gedroyc WM. Dynamic imaging of the pelvic floor using an open-configuration magnetic resonance scanner. J Magn Reson Imaging. 2001;13:923–9.
46. Bertschinger KM, Hetzer FH, Roos JE, Treiber K, Marincek B, and Hilfiker PR. Dynamic MR imaging of the pelvic floor performed with patient sitting in an open-magnet unit versus with patien t supine in a closed-magnet unit. Radiology. 2002;223:501–8.
47. Healy JC, Halligan S, Reznek RH, Watson S, Bartram CI, Phillips R, and Armstrong P. Dynamic MR imaging compared with evacuation proctography when evaluating anorectal configuration and pelvic floor movement. AJR Am J Roentgenol. 1997;169:775–9.

48. Wald A, Jafri F, Rehder J, and Holeva K. Scintigraphic studies of rectal emptying in patients with constipation and defecatory difficulty. Dig Dis Sci. 1993; 38(2):353–8.
49. Hutchinson R, Mostafa AB, Grant EA, Smith NB, Deen KI, Harding LK, and Kumar D. Scintigraphic defecography: quantitative and dynamic assessment of anorectal function. Dis Colon Rectum. 1993;36:1132–8.
50. Kenton K, Shott S, and Brubaker L. The anatomic and functional variability of rectoceles in women. Int Urogynecol J Pelvic Floor Dysfunct. 1999;10:223–9.
51. Ting KH, Mangel E, Eibl-Eibesfeldt B, and Muller-Lissner SA. Is the volume retained after defecation a valuable parameter at defecography. Dis Colon Rectum. 1992;35:762–8.
52. Halligan S and Bartram CI. Is barium trapping in rectoceles significant? Dis Colon Rectum. 1995;38:764–8.
53. Marti MC, Roche B, and Deleval J. Rectoceles: value of video-defecography in selection of treatment policy. Colorectal Dis. 1999;1:324–9.
54. van Dam JH, Schouten WR, Ginai AZ, Huisman WM, and Hop WC. The impact of anismus on the clinical outcome of rectocele repair. Int J Colorectal Dis. 1996;11:238–42.
55. Tjandra JJ, Ooi BS, Tang CL, Dwyer P, and Carey M. Transanal repair of rectocele corrects obstructed defaecation if it is not associated with anismus. Dis Colon Rectum. 1999;42:1544–50.
56. Pinho M, Yoshioka K, Ortiz J, Oya M, and Keighley MR. The effect of age on pelvic floor dynamics. Int J Colorectal Dis. 1990;5:207–8.
57. Skomorowska E, Hegedus V, and Christiansen J. Evaluation of perineal descent by defaecography. Int J Colorectal Dis. 1988;3:191–4.
58. Jorge JM, Wexner SD, Ehrenpreis ED, Nogueras JJ, and Jagelman DG. Does perineal descent correlate with pudendal neuropathy? Dis Colon Rectum. 1993;36:475–83.
59. Halligan S, Thomas J, and Bartram C. Intrarectal pressures and balloon expulsion related to evacuation proctography. Gut. 1995;37:100–4.
60. Pinho M, Yoshioka K, and Keighley MR. Are pelvic floor movements abnormal in disordered defecation? Dis Colon Rectum. 1991;34:1117–19.
61. Parks AG, Porter NH, and Hardcastle J. The syndrome of the descending perineum. Proc R Soc Med. 1966;59:477–82.
62. Mellgren A, Johansson C, Dolk A, Anzen B, Bremmer S, Nilsson BY, and Homstrom B. Enterocele demonstrated by defecography is associated with other pelvic floor disorders. Int J Colorectal Dis. 1994;9:121–4.
63. Cuthbertson AM. Concealed rectal prolapse. Aust N Z J Surg. 1980;50:116–17.
64. Allen-Mersh TG, Henry MM, and Nicholls RJ. Natural history of anterior mucosal prolapse. Br J Surg. 1987;74:679–82.
65. Pescatori M and Quondamcarlo C. A new grading of rectal internal mucosal prolapse and its correlation with diagnosis and treatment. Int J Colorectal Dis. 1999;14:245–9.
66. Halligan S, McGee S, and Bartram CI. Quantification of evacuation proctography. Dis Colon Rectum. 1994;37:1151–4.
67. Penninckx F, Debruyne C, Lestar B, and Kerremans R. Intraobserver variation in the radiological measurement of the anorectal angle. Gastrointest Radiol. 1991;16:73–6.
68. Halligan S, Bartram CI, Park HJ, and Kamm MA. Proctographic features of anismus. Radiology. 1995;197:679–82.

69. Felt-Bersma RJ, Luth WJ, Janssen JJ, and Meuwissen SG. Defecography in patients with anorectal disorders. Which findings are clinically relevant? Dis Colon Rectum. 1990;33:277–84.
70. Halligan S, Malouf A, Bartram CI, Marshall M, Hollings N, and Kamm MA. Predictive value of impaired evacuation at proctography in diagnosing anismus. AJR Am J Roentgenol. 2001;177:633–6.
71. Jorge JM, Wexner SD, Ger GC, Salanga VD, Nogueras JJ, and Jagelman DG. Cinedefecography and electromyography in the diagnosis of nonrelaxing puborectalis syndrome. Dis Colon Rectum. 1993;36:668–76.
72. Borstad E, Skrede M, and Rud T. Failure to predict and attempts to explain urinary stress incontinence following vaginal repair in continent women by using a modified lateral urethrocystography. Acta Obstet Gynecol Scand. 1991;70:501–6.
73. Savoye G, Leroi AM, Bertot-Sassigneux P, Touchais Y, Devreoede G, and Denis P. Does water-perfused catheter overdiagnose anismus compared to balloon probe. Scand J Gastroenterol. 2002;37:1411–16.
74. Duthie GS and Bartolo DC. Anismus: the cause of constipation? Results of investigation and treatment [review]. World J Surg. 1992;16:831–5.
75. Marshall M, Halligan S, Fotheringham T, and Bartram CI. Predictive value of internal anal sphincter thickness for diagnosis of rectal intussusception. Br J Surg. 2002;89:1281–5.
76. Sitzler PJ, Kamm MA, Nicholls RJ, and McKee RF. Long-term clinical outcome of surgery for solitary rectal ulcer syndrome. Br J Surg. 1998;85:1246–50.
77. deSouza NM, Gilderdale DJ, MacIver DK, and Ward HC. High resolution magnetic resonance imaging of the anal sphincter in children: a pilot study using endoreceiver coils. AJR Am J Roentgenol. 1997;169:201–6.
78. Zbar AP and deSouza NM. The Anal Sphincter. In: deSouza NM, editor. Endocavitary MRI of the pelvis. Australia: Harwood Academic Publishers; 2001. p. 91–109.
79. Senapati A. Rectal prolapse. In: Phillips RKS, editor. A companion to specialist surgical practice colorectal surgery. 2nd ed. London: WB Saunders; 2001. p. 251–71.
80. Husa A, Sainio P, and von Smitten K. Abdominal rectopexy and sigmoid resection (Frykman–Goldberg operation) for rectal prolapse. Acta Chir Scand. 1988;154:221–4.
81. Zbar AP, Takashima S, Hasegawa T, and Kitabayashi K. Perineral rectosigmoidectomy (Altemeier's procedure): a review of physiology, technique and outcome. Tech Coloproctol. 2002;6:109–16.
82. Hida J, Yasutomi M, Maruyama T, Yoshifuji T, Tokoro T, Wakano T, Uchida T, and Ueda K. Detection of a rectocele-like prolapse in the colonic J pouch using pouchography: cause or effect of evacuation difficulties. Surg Today. 1999;29:1237–42.
83. Seggerman RE, Chen MY, Waters GS, and Ott DJ. Pictorial essay. Radiology of ileal pouch-anal anastomosis surgery. AJR Am J Roentgenol. 2003;180:999–1002.
84. Jarvinen HJ and Luukkonen P. Comparison of restorative proctocolectomy with and without covering ileostomy in ulcerative colitis. Br J Surg. 1991;78:199–201.

Chapter 3.1(ii)
Defecography: A Swedish Perspective*

Annika López, Jan Zetterström, and Anders F. Mellgren

Introduction

The dynamics of rectal evacuation may be displayed by defecography (evacuation proctography). The technique has gained importance as an investigatory tool in patients with anorectal disorders, and the method has been evaluated in a series of studies. During recent years, variants of the technique have been described, opening up the possibility to investigate patients with other pelvic floor symptoms primarily located in other pelvic compartments.

Historical Background

The first publications using cineradiographic techniques for studying the mechanism of defecation were published in the 1960s (1–3). However, the technique was not widely spread until the work of Mahieu et al. (4,5) and Ekberg et al. (6), who increased the global interest in defecography. Defecography is useful in studying anorectal functional and detecting anatomic abnormalities as possible causes of defecation disturbances. Rectocele, enterocele, rectal intussusception, and rectal prolapse can be visualized, and several authors have found defecography useful as a complement to the clinical examination (7,8). Kelvin et al. (9) reported that "evacuation proctography" has a useful role in enterocele detection prior to surgery for pelvic prolapse.

Hock et al. (10) introduced colpo-cysto-defecography of the female pelvis, and Altringer et al. (11) described "four-contrast defecography" with contrast medium in the small bowel, rectum, vagina, and urinary bladder, finding the method helpful in the planning of prolapse surgery. Administration of contrast medium intraperitoneally has been used to study normal

*Ed note: This chapter should be read in conjunction with Chapter 3.1(i)

anatomy and in the evaluation of patients with obscure symptoms in the groin or pelvis (12). The use of intraperitoneal contrast medium in combination with defecography is advocated by some authors (13,14). With this technique, the peritoneal outline is directly visualized and a deep pouch of Douglas can be demonstrated for enhanced diagnosis of peritoneocele and enterocele.

Indications

The most common indication for defecography is constipation presenting as difficult or infrequent evacuation. This issue is extensively discussed in the sections of Chapter 6. Some authors have stressed the role of defecography in incontinent patients with intact sphincters. Defecography may then diagnose a rectal intussusception or identify patients with an obtuse anorectal angle suitable for post-anal repair, as well as patients with large rectoceles who present with a combination of evacuatory dysfunction and incontinence.

A clinical examination, including rectal palpation and rigid proctoscopy or flexible sigmoidoscopy, should be performed before defecography. In several patients, a full colonoscopy also is indicated. A gynecological examination is recommended in female patients. Defecography may be useful in patients with symptoms such as pelvic heaviness or discomfort due to a vaginal protrusion. It is important to assess the pelvic floor as one unit because several symptoms may be present and combinations of anatomical weaknesses are common (15).

Technical Aspects

The techniques of defecography are by no means standardized. Contrast filling of the rectum is universal and contrast medium in the vagina is used by a majority of institutions. Opacification of the small bowel is used only by a few (16), and bowel preparation prior to the investigation is preferred by some (17), but not by others (18–20).

If contrast in the small bowel is used, it is administered orally one to two hours prior to the investigation. Oral contrast is recommended to enable detection of an enterocele, especially when no contrast medium is instilled intraperitoneally (2,4–6). Rectal contrast media of varying consistencies are used and both regular barium enema contrast medium and thick barium paste are employed. Some mix the contrast medium with potato starch, potato flakes, or cellulose to achieve a consistency similar to that of feces. The contrast medium usually is injected with a pistol injector with the patient in the left lateral position. The injected amount varies; some investigators instill contrast medium until a strong urge to defecate is provoked, whereas others use the same volume in all cases. Sometimes liquid contrast is administered prior to the paste to opacify the sigmoid colon in order to detect a sigmoidocele.

Contrast medium in the vagina enhances the possibilities for studying enterocele and rectocele. A contrast medium gel or a tampon soaked with contrast medium is used. The use of a gel is preferable, as a tampon might obscure important diagnostic information (21). Some authors place gauze at the introitus to avoid leakage of contrast medium from the vagina in order to improve the image (22).

After instillation of contrast medium, the patient is seated on a plastic commode in front of a fluoroscopic unit, and the investigation usually is performed in the lateral view. The patient is asked to strain and empty the rectum. As the investigation is rapid and dynamic, it is documented best with video. Spot films sometimes are added to the investigation; these films usually are taken at key points of the study (e.g., at the start, during straining, and after completion of "defecation"). At some centers, an anterior–posterior spot film is added to reveal the coronal configuration of the rectum to help diagnose intussusception (23) and to lateralize a prolapsed organ (15). To minimize the dose exposure, imaging should be intermittent if rectal evacuation is prolonged. Newer digital systems allow substantial reduction in dose.

The procedure usually is not painful for the patient, but it can be stressful, and therefore it is important to explain the procedure thoroughly to the patient beforehand and provide maximal privacy and reassurance for the patient during the procedure.

Radiographic Analysis

Although defecography is a well-established method, there are no standard definitions of the radiographic findings. Studies with asymptomatic volunteers have revealed a range of normal values, and some overlap with pathological states (24). Therefore, it is important to evaluate the findings at defecography in relation to the patients' symptoms, clinical findings, and other functional tests because the anatomical changes found may not always be the cause of the patient's problems.

Rectal Emptying and the Anal Canal

Rectal emptying can be studied by defecography. At the start, before straining is initiated, there should be no leakage of contrast medium. Constipated patients often empty the rectum slowly and incompletely. An emptying time of more than 30 seconds is considered pathological. The anal canal should open during emptying of the rectum, close after emptying, and remain closed at rest.

Rectal Intussusception and Rectal Prolapse

A rectal intussusception starts six to eleven centimeters above the anal verge by formation of a circular indentation, which progressively deepens. Its apex descends towards the anal verge on straining. It sometimes is difficult to differentiate between rectal intussusception and "normal" mucosal folds of the rectum at straining. The size of the intussusception can be graded in different ways, but a commonly used system has the following three grades. When the intussusception remains within the rectum, it is called recto-rectal; when the apex penetrates the anal canal, it is referred to as recto-anal; and an external rectal intussusception that protrudes through the anal verge is equivalent to a rectal prolapse (Figures 3.1(ii).1 and 3.1(ii).2).

Mucosal Prolapse

Defecography usually can differentiate between a mucosal prolapse and a full-thickness rectal prolapse. However, sometimes the differentiation can be difficult, even on defecography. According to Ekberg et al. (6), mucosal

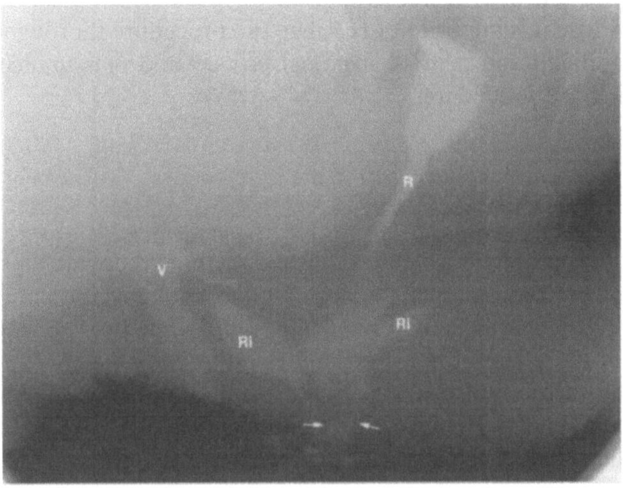

FIGURE 3.1(ii).1. A 56-year-old woman previously operated for a lumbar disc herniation with persistent minor loss of sensitivity in her legs. The patient suffers from anal incontinence and rectal emptying difficulty with excessive straining and a need for digital assistance by pressing on the perineum during defecation. Defecography with contrast medium in the rectum, vagina, and small bowel was performed and the examination demonstrates a rectal intussusception reaching down into the anal canal during straining. V, vagina; R, rectum; Ri, rectal intussusception; arrow, the base of the intussusception.

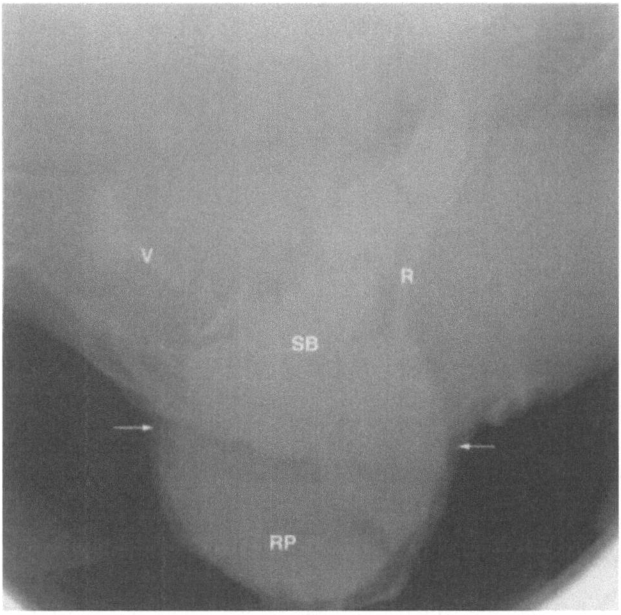

FIGURE 3.1(ii).2. A 44-year-old woman with a two-year history of a rectal prolapse. Defecography was performed with contrast medium in the rectum, vagina. and small bowel and demonstrates a rectal prolapse during straining. V, vagina; R, rectum; RP, rectal prolapse; SB, Small bowel.

prolapse starts three to four centimeters above the anal verge containing only the mucosa [see Figure 3.1(ii).5(b)] (25).

Enterocele

In females, an enterocele usually is diagnosed as a bowel-filled peritoneal sac located between the posterior vaginal wall and the anterior rectal wall, descending below the upper third of the vagina. It often contains small bowel, but sigmoid colon is sometimes evident. In males, it is diagnosed as bowel within a rectal intussusception or a rectal prolapse (Figure 3.1(ii).3).

Rectocele

A rectocele is seen at defecography as a bulge outside the projected line of the anterior rectal wall during straining. The size of the rectocele is measured as the distance between the extended line of the anterior border of the anal canal and the tip of the rectocele (Figure 3.1(ii).4).

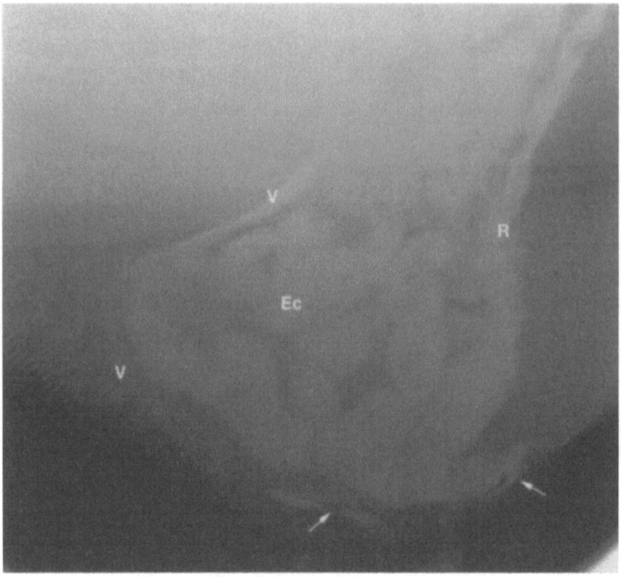

FIGURE 3.1(ii).3. A 66-year-old woman previously operated on with hysterectomy after which there were worsening symptoms of constipation with infrequent bowel emptying about two times a week. Defecography was performed with contrast medium in the rectum, vagina, and small bowel and demonstrates a rectal intussusception reaching into the anal canal and a large enterocele during straining. V, vagina; R, rectum; arrows, rectal intussusception; Ec, enterocele.

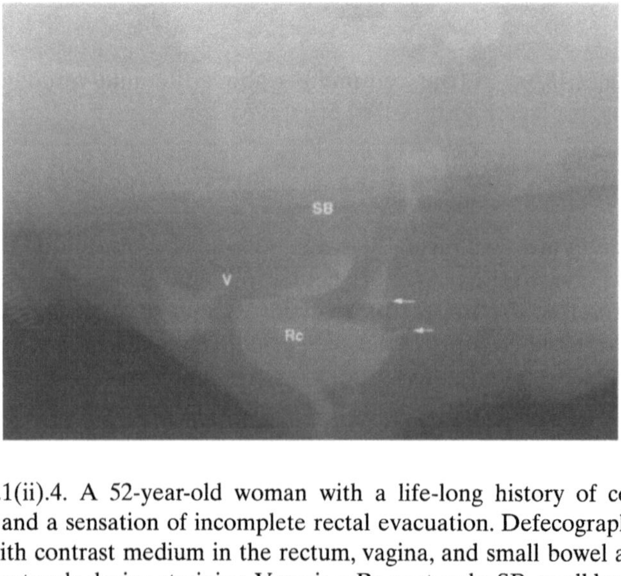

FIGURE 3.1(ii).4. A 52-year-old woman with a life-long history of constipation, straining, and a sensation of incomplete rectal evacuation. Defecography was performed with contrast medium in the rectum, vagina, and small bowel and demonstrates a rectocele during straining. V, vagina; Rc, rectocele; SB, small bowel; arrows, normal mucosal folds.

Perineal Descent

The level of the pelvic floor is estimated on defecography by measuring the distance between the anorectal junction (ARJ) and a fixed structure, such as the ischial tuberosity, the coccyx, or the pubococcygeal line (a line drawn from the lower point of the pubic symphysis and the coccyx). In general, it is accepted that defecography provides the most accurate estimate of perineal descent. However, it is defined in different ways by different authors. Excessive perineal descent can be defined at the start of the examination as a resting anorectal junction positioned more than three centimeters below the ischial tuberosity. It also can be defined as anorectal junction descent of more than three and a half centimeters during maximal straining (26) (Figure 3.1(ii).5).

The Anorectal Angle

The anorectal angle (ARA) can be studied on straining, after the completion of defecation, during squeezing, and at rest (Figure 3.1(ii).6). It can be determined either by estimating a straight line along the posterior border of the rectum or by using the central longitudinal axis (the areas above and below the axis are equal) of the lower rectum and the anal canal (Figure 3.1(ii).6). The range of values for the ARA in asymptomatic subjects is quite wide, but the mean values are rather consistent (27). The ARA is normally wider during straining than at rest due to the relaxation of the puborectalis muscle. Signs of paradoxical sphincter reaction (anismus, paradoxical pelvic floor contraction) can be seen at defecography as an increased impression of the puborectalis muscle or as a reduction of the ARA at straining. Measurement of the ARA or ARJ descent appears to be of little clinical value (28), but it assists in providing some validation of new techniques such as dynamic transperineal sonography [see Chapter 3.2(ii)] (29).

Rectovaginal Space

The space between the contrast medium in the vagina and the contrast medium in the rectum. The width of the rectovaginal space is normally less than one centimeter in the middle portion and assists in the diagnosis of peritoneocele.

Interpretation

After studying 56 asymptomatic patients, Mahieu et al. (4) described a normal defecogram in which several conditions were almost always present. An increase in ARA at the beginning of defecation is seen due to an

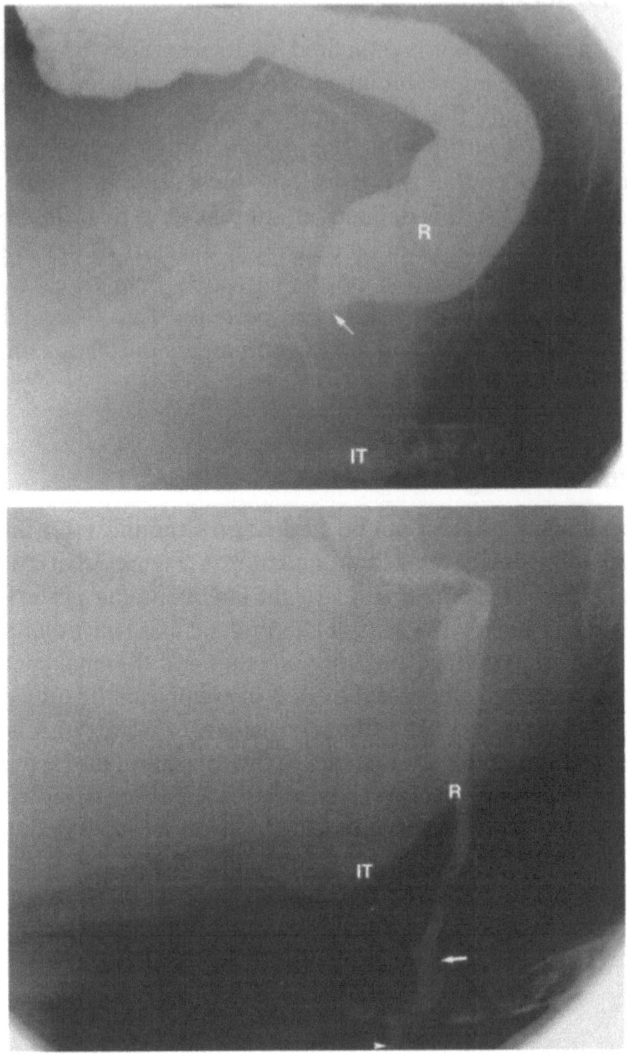

a

b

FIGURE 3.1(ii).5. A 40-year-old man with constipation and excessive straining at stool. During the last year the patient noticed a prolapse with spontaneous repositioning after defecation. Defecography was performed with contrast medium in the rectum and small bowel. (a) Defecography at rest. The anorectal junction is above the ischial tuberosities. (b) Defecography during straining. An extreme case of perineal descent is seen with the anorectal junction significantly below the ischial tuberosities. A mucosal prolapse also is seen. R, rectum; IT, ischial tuberosities; arrow, anorectal junction; arrowhead, mucosal prolapse.

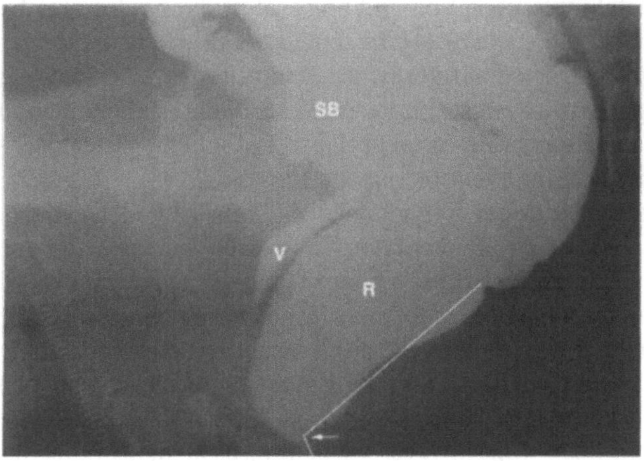

FIGURE 3.1(ii).6. A 45-year-old woman. Defecography with contrast medium in the rectum, vagina, and small bowel was performed and is normal. The anorectal angle (ARA) is indicated at rest, estimating a straight line along the posterior border of the rectum and the anal canal. V, vagina; R, rectum; SB, small bowel; arrow, ARA.

increase in intra-abdominal pressure. The increase in ARA is a consequence of the relaxation of the puborectalis sling, whose impression obliterates the posterior wall of the distal part of the rectal ampulla at rest. The anal canal opens widely to permit passage of rectal content until evacuation is complete, without excessive straining. The pelvic floor shows good resistance, not allowing an excessive descent.

Even though there is an overlap between normal values and pathologic states, there is a broad agreement with the description by Mahieu et al. (4) regarding these normal findings. Concerning the anorectal angle, subsequent studies have shown considerable interobserver variation in estimating the ARA (30); this reflects the degree of difficulty in this interpretation. The correlation between measurement of the ARA and clinical symptoms has been poor, and therefore its clinical value is controversial.

On defecography, a paradoxical sphincter reaction (anismus, paradoxical pelvic floor contraction) is suspected when the puborectalis impression is increased and the ARA is decreased during straining (see Chapter 6.4). Most authorities, however, prefer to study this phenomenon with electromyography (EMG), whereas some authors recommend a combination of EMG, defecography, and manometry (31–33). The clinical significance of paradoxical sphincter reaction (PSR) in constipated patients is debated, as PSR also may be found in nonconstipated patients (34). However, several reports have demonstrated success in treating patients with PSR using biofeedback (35).

Both rectal intussusception and mucosal prolapse also may be found in asymptomatic subjects (20,24). In some studies where the rectal intussusception was corrected surgically, the symptoms of constipation persisted, suggesting that intussusception is a secondary phenomenon (36,37). However, in patients with rectal prolapse and solitary rectal ulcer syndrome (SRUS), surgical intervention may be successful (38).

Rectocele is a frequent finding in patients with defecation disorders. However, rectoceles are common in women because the rectovaginal septum is relatively weak, and a minor bulge of the anterior rectal and posterior vaginal wall are likely to be a normal variant. At defecography, a rectocele usually is not seen at rest, but is visualized during straining. The size can be estimated and barium trapping in the rectocele may be seen. According to some authors, these findings may be used in selecting patients for rectocele repair (8,39–42). However, we believe, as do many other authors, that the main value of defecography is its objective demonstration of the rectocele and concomitant pathology (43,44). There is not always a correlation between the patient's symptoms and the size of the rectocele or the amount of barium trapping. At defecography, it is important to study the video film because a rectocele is sometimes only seen in the beginning of defecation, and it then may be pushed away at the end of defecation in patients with a concomitant enterocele. Therefore, the rectocele may not be seen and is missed on a spot film taken at the end of defecation.

It has been shown in several studies that it is difficult to detect an enterocele on clinical examination (45). On defecography, an enterocele is visualized when opacified bowel descends down into the rectovaginal space. Enteroceles can be large in size, influencing both the vaginal and/or rectal contour, and may sometimes reach deep down towards the perineal body (Figure 3.1(ii).4). An enterocele usually is demonstrated on defecography during rectal evacuation or when evacuation is completed. Some authors recommend a post-toilet film, (a spot film taken when the patient has emptied the bowels in the privacy of a bathroom) because it may sometimes be difficult for the patient to empty the rectum in the study situation where enteroceles can then be missed (46). It is well accepted that an enterocele may cause symptoms of pelvic pressure or heaviness, but the influence of an enterocele on rectal emptying is unclear (47).

Perineal descent is best estimated on defecography. Whether perineal descent is a "syndrome" (48) or a sign of an underlying functional disorder of evacuation is debated. We believe that it is a sign of weakness of the voluntary muscles of the pelvic floor and that an underlying cause needs to be considered (Figure 3.1(ii).5).

Variants of the Defecography Technique

Anorectal symptoms often are combined with other symptoms of the pelvic floor as pelvic heaviness, discomfort due to a vaginal protrusion, or functional symptoms including urinary difficulty, incontinence, or dyspareunia. To obtain a global view of the pelvic floor on radiological investigation, several authors have suggested variants of the basic defecographic technique. Hock et al. (10) introduced colpo-cysto-defecography of the female pelvis and suggested that the uterus and the pouch of Douglas could be recognized by negative contrast where an enterocele was diagnosed when a broadening of the rectovaginal space was evident. Altringer et al. (11) described "four-contrast defecography" with contrast medium also in the small bowel. The use of small bowel contrast to identify an enterocele is preferred because, in patients who have previously undergone pelvic floor surgery, a broad rectovaginal space may consist of scar tissue or fat.

The use of intraperitoneal contrast medium in combination with defecography is advocated in some institutions (13,49,50). Intraperitoneal contrast medium is instilled by puncture of the abdominal wall in the midline one to two centimeters below the umbilicus under fluoroscopic control. It is important to be aware that this is an invasive technique, however, with the advantage that the peritoneal outline can be directly visualized and a deep pouch of Douglas can be demonstrated at rest or during straining. A deep pouch of Douglas reaching below the upper third of the vagina has been named by us as a peritoneocele (51) (Figure 3.1(ii).7), and a peritoneocele may predispose to enterocele formation. When repeated defecographies using concomitant intraperitoneal contrast medium have been performed, it has been noted that bowel is not present in the peritoneocele at all times, which explains why an enterocele can be missed when intraperitoneal contrast medium is omitted. Visualization of the peritoneal outline also is possible with magnetic resonance imaging (MRI), and this is a less invasive method [see Chapter 3.3(iii)].

Contrast medium in the urinary bladder visualizes the bladder base and the changes in bladder configuration during straining. With a catheter, the urinary bladder is emptied and contrast medium instilled (50 mL usually is sufficient) to fill the dependent part of the bladder. At this stage, vaginal contrast is instilled, and sometimes intraperitoneal contrast as well (52) (Figure 3.1(ii).8). The patient is seated and a spot film is taken at rest and during straining. The cystographic phase should be performed prior to instillation of rectal contrast, as a contrast-filled rectum may prevent the bladder base from descending. Some authors also have drained the bladder before instillation of contrast medium into the rectum to avoid the descending bladder and preventing visualization of an enterocele or minimizing the detected size of a rectocele (15). We have not found this necessary because

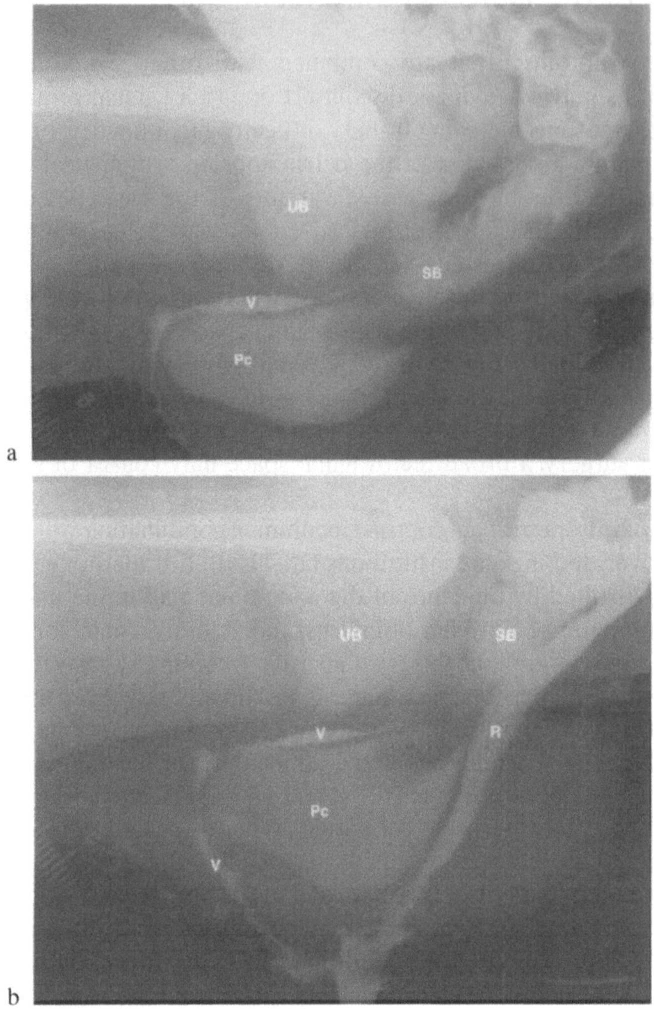

FIGURE 3.1(ii).7. A 72-year-old woman with two years of increasing symptoms of rectal emptying difficulty. Defecography with contrast medium in the urinary bladder, intraperitoneally, in the vagina, rectum, and the small bowel was performed. (a) Contrast medium was administered in the small bowel, urinary bladder, intraperitoneally, and into the vagina. A peritoneocele is seen during straining. (b) Rectal contrast also was administered. A large peritoneocele is demonstrated during straining and evacuation of the rectum. Air-filled bowel is seen descending down into the peritoneocele; namely, this patient has an enterocele. V, vagina; UB, urinary bladder; SB, small bowel; Pc, peritoneocele; R, rectum.

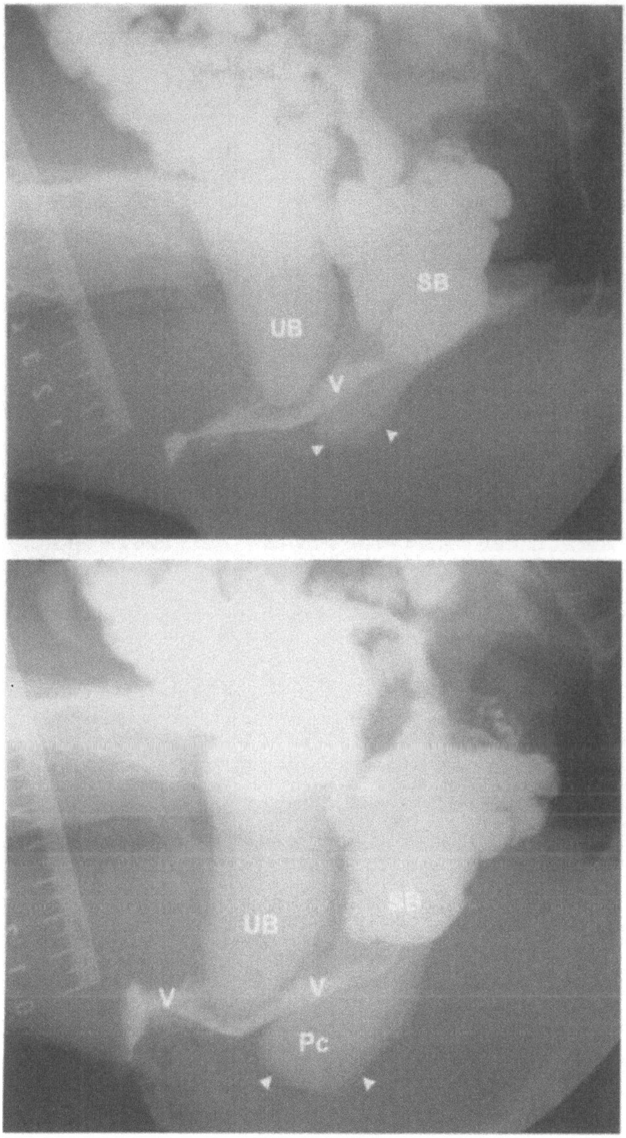

FIGURE 3.1(ii).8. A 62-year-old woman with discomfort due to a vaginal protrusion and rectal emptying difficulty with the need for digitation per vaginam during defecation. Radiological investigation with contrast medium in the urinary bladder, intraperitoneally, in the vagina, rectum, and the small bowel was performed. (a) Contrast medium was administered into the small bowel, urinary bladder, intraperitoneally, and into the vagina. The peritoneal outline was demonstrated and a peritoneocele was easily demonstrated at rest. (b) During straining the peritoneocele enlarges and the bladder base descends.

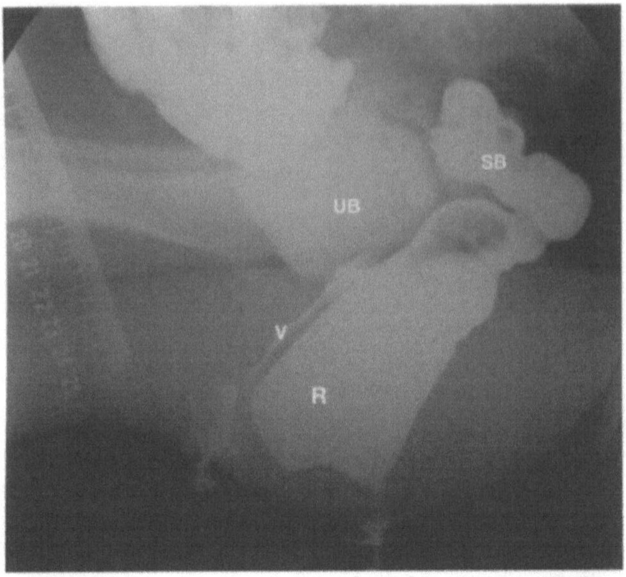

c

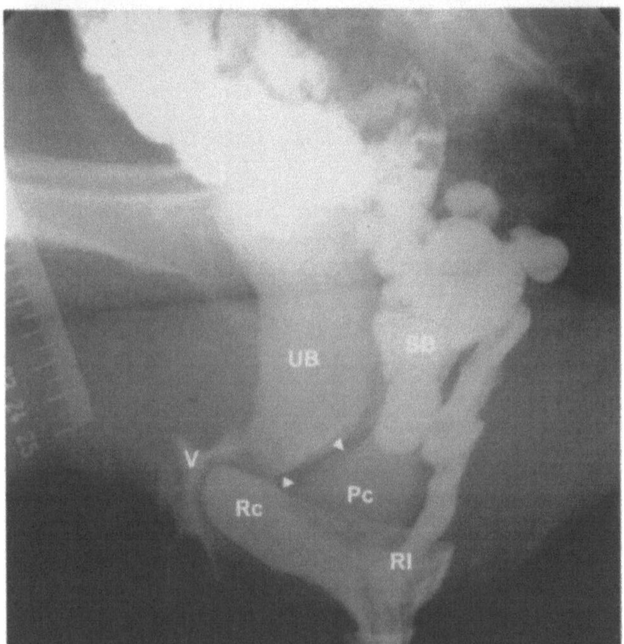

d

FIGURE 3.1(ii).8. (c) Rectal contrast also was administered. At rest, there is a bulge of the anterior rectal wall and the peritoneocele is not seen at this point. (d) During straining and rectal evacuation, a rectocele develops and the peritoneocele is once again demonstrated where the bladder base descends. At the end of evacuation, a rectal intussusception reaching down into the anal canal is also evident. V, vagina; UB, urinary bladder; SB, small bowel; R, rectum; Pc, peritoneocele; Rc, rectocele; RI, rectal intussusception; arrowhead, peritoneal outline.

the volume instilled in the bladder is small and the force from the rectal side is more pronounced.

Defecography and variants of the technique are performed with the patient in the upright position, which is an advantage when studying the alterations in the pelvic peritoneal cavity during rectal emptying. However, it is important to remember that the patient is asked to strain and that a "normal" evacuation initiated by a defecation reflex is not obtained.

Conclusion

We recommend standard use of contrast medium in the rectum, vagina, and small bowel. However, intraperitoneal contrast medium is preferable in the diagnosis of enterocele and peritoneocele, but this method is more invasive. Bladder contrast should be used only in patients with complex pelvic floor disorders and/or previous pelvic floor surgery. It is easy to diagnose an anterior vaginal wall prolapse at clinical examination, and it is very rare that it consists of other abdominal content than the bladder.

References

1. Burhenne HJ. Intestinal evacuation study: a new roentgenologic technique. Radiol Clin. 1964;33:79–84.
2. Brodén B and Snellman B. Procidentia of the rectum studied with cineradiography: a contribution to the discussion of causative mechanism. Dis Colon Rectum. 1968;11:330–47.
3. Kerremans R. Radio-cinematographic examination of the rectum and the anal canal in cases of rectal constipation. Acta Gastroenterol Belg. 1968;31:561–70.
4. Mahieu P, Pringot J, and Bodart P. Defecography: I. Description of a new procedure and results in normal patients. Gastrointest Radiol. 1984;9:247–51.
5. Mahieu P, Pringot J, and Bodart P. Defecography: II. Contribution to the diagnosis of defecation disorders. Gastrointest Radiol. 1984;9:253–61.
6. Ekberg O, Nylander G, and Fork FT. Defecography. Radiology 1985;155:45–8.
7. Mellgren A, Anzén B, Nilsson BY, Johansson C, Dolk A, Gillgren P, et al. Results of rectocele repair, a prospective study. Dis Colon Rectum 1995;38:7–13.
8. Sarles JC, Arnaud A, Selezneff I, and Olivier S. Endo-rectal repair of rectocele. Int J Colorectal Dis. 1989;4:167–71.
9. Kelvin FM, Maglinte DD, and Benson JT. Evacuation proctography (defecography): an aid to the investigation of pelvic floor disorders. Obstet Gynecol. 1994;83:307–14.
10. Hock D, Lombard R, Jehaes C, Markiewicz S, Penders L, Fontaine F, et al. Colpocystodefecography. Dis Colon Rectum. 1993;36:1015–21.
11. Altringer WE, Saclarides TJ, Dominguez JM, Brubaker LT, and Smith CS. Four-contrast defecography: pelvic "floor-oscopy". Dis Colon Rectum. 1995;38:695–9.
12. Gullmo Å. Herniography. The diagnosis of hernia in the groin and incompetence of the pouch of Douglas and pelvic floor. Acta Radiol. 1980;Supplementum 361.

13. Bremmer S, Ahlbäck SO, Udén R, and Mellgren A. Simultaneous defecography and peritoneography in defecation disorders. Dis Colon Rectum. 1995;38: 969–73.
14. Halligan SBC, Hall C, and Wingate J. Enterocele Revealed by Simultaneous Evacuation Proctography and Peritoneography. AJR Am J Roentgenol. 1996; 167:461–6.
15. Kelvin FM and Maglinte DD. Dynamic evaluation of female pelvic organ prolapse by extended proctography. Radiol Clin North Am. 2003;41:395–407.
16. Mellgren A, Bremmer S, Johansson C, Dolk A, Udén R, Ahlbäck S-O, et al. Defecography, results of investigations in 2816 patients. Dis Colon Rectum. 1994;37:1133–41.
17. Skomorowska E, Henrichsen S, Christiansen J, and Hegedüs V. Videodefaecography combined with measurement of the anorectal angle and of perineal descent. Acta Radiol. 1987;28:559–62.
18. Roe AM, Bartolo DCC, and Mortensen NJM. Techniques in evacuation proctography in the diagnosis of intractable constipation and related disorders. J R Soc Med. 1986;79:331–3.
19. Bartolo DCC, Roe AM, Virjee J, Mortensen NJM, and Locke-Edmunds JC. An analysis of rectal morphology in obstructed defaecation. Int J Colorectal Dis. 1988;3:17–22.
20. Freimanis MG, Wald A, Caruana B, and Bauman DH. Evacuation proctography in normal volunteers. Invest Radiol. 1991;26:581–5.
21. Archer BD, Somers S, and Stevenson GW. Contrast medium gel for marking vaginal position during defecography. Radiology. 1992;182:278–9.
22. Ho LM, Low VH, and Freed KS. Vaginal opacification during defecography: utility of placing a folded gauze square at the introitus. Abdom Imaging. 1999;24:562–4.
23. McGee SG and Bartram CI. Intra-anal intussusception: diagnosis by posteroanterior stress proctography. Abdom Imaging. 1993;18:136–40.
24. Shorvon PJ, McHugh S, Diamant NE, Somers S, and Stevenson GW. Defecography in normal volunteers: results and implications. Gut. 1989;30:1737–49.
25. Pescatori M and Quondamcarlo C. A new grading of rectal internal mucosal prolapse and its correlation with diagnosis and treatment. Int J Colorectal Dis. 1999;14:245–9.
26. Stoker J, Halligan S, and Bartram CI. Pelvic floor imaging. Radiology. 2001;218:621–41.
27. Goei R, van Engelshoven J, Schouten H, Baeten C, and Stassen C. Anorectal function: defecographic measurement in asymptomatic subjects. Radiology. 1989;173:137–41.
28. Ferrante SL, Perry RE, Schreiman JS, Cheng SC, and Frick MP. The reproducibility of measuring the anorectal angle in defecography. Dis Colon Rectum. 1991;34:51–5.
29. Beer-Gabel M, Teshler M, Barzilai N, Lurie Y, Malnick S, Bass D, and Zbar AP. Dynamic transperineal ultrasound in the diagnosis of pelvic floor disorders: pilot study. Dis Colon Rectum. 2002;45:239–48.
30. Penninckx F, Debruyne C, Lestar B, and Kerremans R. Observer variation in the radiological measurement of the anorectal angle. Int J Colorectal Dis. 1990;5:94–7.

31. Jorge JMN, Wexner SD, Ger GC, Salanga VD, Nogueras JJ, and Jagelman DG. Cinedefecography and electromyography in the diagnosis of nonrelaxing puborectalis syndrome. Dis Colon Rectum. 1993;36:668–76.
32. Ger GC, Wexner SD, Jorge JM, and Salanga VD. Anorectal manometry in the diagnosis of paradoxical puborectalis syndrome. Dis Colon Rectum. 1993; 36:816–25.
33. Miller R, Duthie GS, Bartolo DCC, Roe AM, Locke-Edmunds J, and Mortensen NJM. Anismus in patients with normal and slow transit constipation. Br J Surg. 1991;78:690–2.
34. Barnes PRH and Lennard-Jones JE. Function of the striated anal sphincter during straining in control subjects and constipated patients with a radiologically normal rectum or idiopathic megacolon. Int J Colorectal Dis. 1988;3:207–9.
35. Bleijenberg G and Kuijpers HC. Biofeedback treatment of constipation: a comparison of two methods. Am J Gastroenterol. 1994;89:1021–6.
36. Christiansen J, Zhu BW, Rasmussen Ø, and Sørensen M. Internal rectal intussusception: results of surgical repair. Dis Colon Rectum. 1992;35: 1026–9.
37. Orrom WJ, Bartolo DCC, Miller R, Mortensen NJM, and Roe AM. Rectopexy is an ineffective treatment for obstructed defecation. Dis Colon Rectum. 1991;34:41–6.
38. Sitzler PJ, Kamm MA, Nicholls RJ, and McKee RF. Long-term clinical outcome of surgery for solitary rectal ulcer syndrome. Br J Surg. 1998;85:1246–50.
39. Ting KH, Mangel E, Eibl-Eibesfeldt B, and Muller-Lissner SA. Is the volume retained after defecation a valuable parameter at defecography. Dis Colon Rectum. 1992;35:762–8.
40. Halligan S and Bartram CI. Is barium trapping in rectoceles significant? Dis Colon Rectum. 1995;38:764–8.
41. Murthy VK, Orkin BA, Smith LE, and Glassman LM. Excellent outcome using selective criteria for rectocele repair. Dis Colon Rectum. 1996;39:374–8.
42. Karlbom U, Graf W, Nilsson S, and Pahlman L. Does surgical repair of a rectocele improve rectal emptying? Dis Colon Rectum. 1996;39:1296–302.
43. Janssen LW and van Dijke CF. Selection criteria for anterior rectal wall repair in symptomatic rectocele and anterior rectal wall prolapse. Dis Colon Rectum. 1994;37:1100–7.
44. van Dam JH, Ginai AZ, Gosselink MJ, Huisman WM, Bonjer HJ, Hop WC, et al. Role of defecography in predicting clinical outcome of rectocele repair. Dis Colon Rectum. 1997;40:201–7.
45. Nichols DH and Randall CL. Enterocele. In: Nichols DH, editor. Vaginal surgery. Baltimore, MD: Williams & Wilkins; 1996. p. 319–20.
46. Lienemann A, Anthuber C, Baron A, and Resier M. Diagnosing enteroceles using dynamic magnetic resonance imaging. Dis Colon Rectum. 2000;43:205–12.
47. Dietz HP and Wilson PD. The influence of bladder volume on the position and mobility of the urethrovesical junction. Int J Urogynecol J Pelvic Floor Dysfunct. 1998;9:365–9.
48. Parks AG, Porter NH, and Hardcastle J. The syndrome of the descending perineum. Proc R Soc Med. 1966;59:477–82.
49. Halligan S and Bartram CI. Evacuation proctography combined with positive contrast peritoneography to demonstrate pelvic floor hernias. Abdom Imaging. 1995;20:442–5.

50. Sentovich SM, Rivela LJ, Thorson AG, Christensen MA, and Blatchford GJ. Simultaneous dynamic proctography and peritoneography for pelvic floor disorders. Dis Colon Rectum. 1995;38:912–15.
51. Bremmer S, Mellgren A, Holmström B, Lopez A, and Udén R. Peritoneocele: Visualization with defecography and peritoneography performed simultaneously. Radiology. 1997;202:373–7.
52. Lopez A, Anzen B, Bremmer S, Kierkegaard J, Mellgren A, Zetterstrom J, et al. Cystodefecoperitoneography in patients with genital prolapse. Int Urogynecol J. 2002;13:22–9.

Chapter 3.2(i) Ultrasound in Coloproctologic Practice: Endorectal/ Endoanal Ultrasound

Ponnandai J. Arumugam, Bharat Patel, and John Beynon

Endorectal and endoanal ultrasound has revolutionized the management of colorectal pathology over the last 20 years. The field of endosonography has seen changes from the primitive four megahertz transducers to the most recent three-dimensional (3D) machines, producing excellent resolution and imaging of complex anorectal disorders. The clinical applications of this technique are expanding, and in this chapter, its present role in various colorectal disorders and the challenges it is facing from other newer techniques will be looked at. The first section covers our unit's approach to the use of rectal ultrasound in rectal cancer and its limitations and results. In the latter part of the chapter, we define our experience with endoanal ultrasound and its value in surgical proctologic practice.

Endorectal Ultrasound

Introduction

Rectal cancer traditionally has been treated by radical en bloc excision of the rectum with its lymphatic drainage, either by a restorative procedure or by an abdominoperineal excision. Recently, preoperative radiotherapy as a short or long course is administered for T3 and T4 tumors, respectively. Some studies also advocate preoperative chemoradiation (1) for such advanced rectal cancer. The recent Dutch adjuvant trial (2) using directed preoperative irradiation has found a favorable reduction in loco-regional recurrence rates in mid- and low rectal cancers where patients have undergone a total mesorectal excision with curative intent; however, this trial failed to show a survival advantage after a two-year follow-up. These adjuvant therapeutic strategies for rectal cancer management are based on an accurate assessment of the depth of tumor invasion and the presence of nodal involvement.

Clinical evaluation of the rectum traditionally has relied on subjective digital examination, proctoscopy, and rigid sigmoidoscopy, which has proven accurate (in experienced coloproctological "hands") only in the delineation of locally advanced cases (3). Various modalities have been tried to improve the accuracy of local staging, including endorectal ultrasound, computed tomography (CT), thin-section high-resolution magnetic resonance imaging (MRI) (4), and endorectal coil MRI (5,6). The most accessible, inexpensive, and accurate of these to date has been that of endorectal sonography (ES).

Endorectal Sonography in Rectal Cancer

Digital examination is inaccurate for the assessment of stage; however, in experienced hands, the accuracy will vary (and be somewhat stage dependent) from 60 to 80% (3,7). Similarly, involvement of pararectal lymph nodes is assessed poorly on clinical examination. Digital examination is also somewhat limited in that only the lower third of the rectum is accessible to the examining digit.

Management decisions regarding surgical or adjuvant treatment would be assisted by more accurate information. The main areas where this sort of information would be of benefit are in:

1. The accurate preoperative staging of both local invasion and pararectal lymph node involvement, thus guiding the choice of individual surgical procedures, whether by radical surgery (with or without neoadjuvant therapy) or by perianal local excision.
2. Identifying patients who have advanced local disease only, which may be suitable for an endoanal resection or transendoscopic microsurgery (TEMS) or in the identification of those who are not candidates for primary surgical treatment and should be considered for primary chemoradiotherapy. In this latter group, re-evaluation using ES following radiotherapy might show that some of these cases would then be amenable to surgical excision, although the accuracy of ES after radiotherapy in stage reduction has been brought into question (8).
3. The detection and evaluation of local recurrence, particularly if that recurrence is arising outside the rectal lumen.

Other potential clinical applications of ES in rectal neoplasms include:

1. The detection of malignant change in villous lesions,
2. The assessment of lesions following downstaging chemo-radiotherapy,
3. Transrectal biopsies of extrarectal (and presacral) or mesenchymal rectal tumors.

The History and Development of ES

Endorectal sonography was first introduced in 1952 by Wild and Reid, with their development of an "echoendo probe" (9–11). The first instrument produced, which resembles those used today, was a hand-held probe with a flexible shaft whose ellipsoidal sound head contained the piezoelectric crystal, drive shaft, and drive motor. A water-filled balloon covered the transducer, which produced a sound beam at right angles to its long axis. A second instrument with a rigid shaft soon followed that allowed introduction into the rectum through a sigmoidoscope. Images then could be taken for each revolution of the sound head within the bowel. The first layered image of the bowel wall was produced using this early equipment, and subsequently the first crude images of a rectal cancer became available with this technology. Technical limitations resulted in being this form of imaging of the gastrointestinal tract were introduced into clinical practice over thirty years later by Dragsted and Gammelgaard (12). Using a Bruel and Kjaer ultrasound scanner Type 8901 and rigid probe equipped with a four and a half megahertz transducer (initially designed for prostatic imaging), thirteen primary rectal cancers were assessed with staging results compared with postoperative histopathology. Invasion was correctly predicted in 11 cases.

Hildebrandt and Fiefel (13,14) successfully staged 23 of 25 patients using the same equipment with a 4.0 megahertz transducer. They found that of the 25 patients examined, eight tumors could not be assessed digitally, but 15 of the others were assessed correctly by the examining finger, with two patients being overstaged. Their suggestion that an ultrasonic variation of the UICC (Union Internationale Contre Le Cancer) system for staging should be adopted for use in ultrasonic staging by the use of the prefix "u", that is, uT1–uT4 has found favor with endosonographers and coloproctologists alike. Initial problems that were encountered in this report were that the distinction between T1 and T2 tumors using the 4 megahertz probe was difficult, as was the examination of stenotic tumors not permitting adequate placement and contact of the probe. As with the previous report by Dragsted and Gammelgaard, no reporting criteria were defined for determining the degree of invasion. Clearly, new systems have to guard against understaging of tumors where, in an age of adjuvant preoperative chemoradiation, such performance characteristics would prove detrimental to cancer-specific outcome. Overstaging is perceived to be less of a concern, although it will likely result in unnecessary preoperative adjuvant radiation therapy.

Technique and Equipment

The plane of scanning is either transverse or longitudinal, and there are some probes capable of scanning in both planes. Images produced by a radial scanner are easier to interpret as they can be related directly to the operative appearance at surgery. These 360-degree images are only produced by mechanically rotating probes requiring the presence of a water-filled balloon to cover the transducer for acoustic contact. Another major advantage of the balloon is that it distends the rectum, preventing distortion by infolding. If the tumor is stenosing it may prevent positioning of the probe to achieve adequate imaging.

Among the authors who have published data related to ES, the majority have used equipment produced by Bruel and Kjaer (Denmark: Probe type 1850) in conjunction with both a five and a half megahertz or seven megahertz transducer, and more recently a ten megahertz probe. In most series, the seven megahertz transducer (focal length 2–5 cm) has been the one of choice. For the best imaging, the rectum should be clear of feces, which can be accomplished using a disposable enema or suppositories. Examinations traditionally have been performed in the left lateral position with the endoprobe either introduced blindly or through a rectoscope. This latter method is an advantage when examining higher or stenotic lesions. Following insertion, the balloon is inflated and the transducer switched on. Then the probe is positioned to scan the area of interest. To obtain optimum images, both the position of the probe and the volume of water in the balloon can be altered.

In recent times, 3D endosonographic imaging (15) with a rigid 3D probe has shown improved accuracy of around 90% for T2 and 84% for T3 tumors, with an accuracy of assessment of nodal involvement of 84%. These authors claim a 10 to 15% improved accuracy rate for this technique when compared with conventional ES; however, their data did not achieve statistical significance. In addition to this technique, flexible endorectal ultrasound (16) also has been tried to improve the staging; however, in one study, it proved to be less accurate in assessing the level of tumor invasion (49%). It also should be recognized that many modalities will have comparatively poor accuracy in the delineation of positive pararectal nodes. This is in keeping with the small size of lymph nodes retrieved by pathologists in the mesorectum using fat clearance techniques (17), many of which lie outside the field of view of the probe, and since up to 20% of resected specimens will have involved nodes that have a maximal diameter of less than three millimeters (18). Moreover, up to two-thirds of metastatic deposits within nodes are themselves less than five millimeters (19). In these circumstances, non-ultrasonographic modalities (such as CT and MRI) are entirely reliant on nodal size as a marker of metastatic involvement, although unique sonographic features of malignant involvement include enlargement with sonolucency and homogeneous acoustic impedance and echogenicity (20,21).

Image Interpretation

Correct identification of the image and its relationship to the histological structure of the rectal wall is imperative for interpretation of endosonographic images and assessment of the extent of local tumor invasion. Five separate layers can be identified clearly in the rectal wall in most endosonographic scans. There are three hyperechoic layers separated by two hypoechoic layers.

The five-layered system of interpretation proposed by Beynon et al. (22) is now recognized as the standard for rectal sonography and has been confirmed by most endosonographers.

These layers are defined as follows (Figure 3.2(i).1):

First Hyperechoic layer—Interface between the water/balloon and the mucosal surface
Second Hypoechoic layer—Combined image produced by the mucosa and muscularis mucosae
Third Hyperechoic layer—Submucosa
Fourth Hypoechoic layer—Muscularis propria
Fifth Hyperechoic layer—Interface between the muscularis propria and perirectal fat or serosa if present.

When an examination is being performed, an additional hyperechoic layer will occasionally be imaged within the fourth hypoechoic layer (the

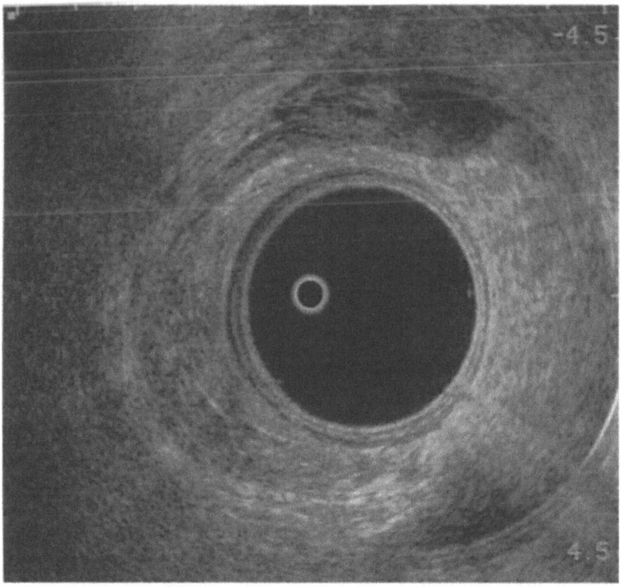

FIGURE 3.2(i).1. Normal rectal wall.

muscularis propria). Although not proven, it is likely that this represents an interface created by the two true muscle layers of the rectum (circular and longitudinal). Thus, the morphological layers of the rectum, with the exception of the muscularis mucosae (which produces a combined image with the mucosa), are represented by the five-layered image. The balloon covering the transducer during patient examinations also produces a hyperechoic image that merges with that of the mucosa—water interface.

The Assessment of Local Invasion in Rectal Cancer

On the whole, carcinomas of the rectum are readily staged by ES, appearing ultrasonically hypoechoic. The Tumor-Node-Metastasis (TNM) classification is used to stage tumors as all anatomical layers can be imaged. A prefix "u" is used to indicate an ultrasonic staging where (23):

uT1 = Tumor confined to the submucosa with an intact bright middle hyperechoic layer (Figure 3.2(i).2).
uT2 = Tumor limited by the hypoechoic layer of the muscularis propria with no disruption of the bright interface between it and the surrounding fat (Figure 3.2(i).3).
uT3 = Tumor penetrating the wall of the rectum to invade the adjacent fat. The tumor edge is usually irregular with saw tooth projections (Figure 3.2(i).4).
uT4 = Tumor invading an adjacent structure (Figure 3.2(i).5).

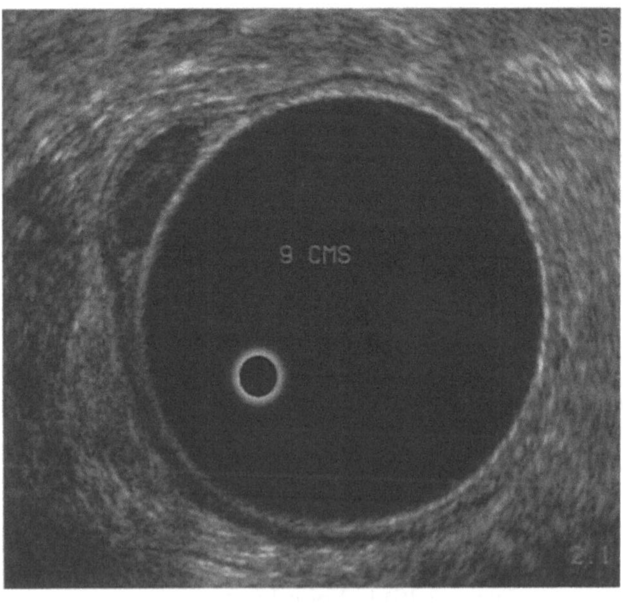

FIGURE 3.2(i).2. uT1 rectal tumor.

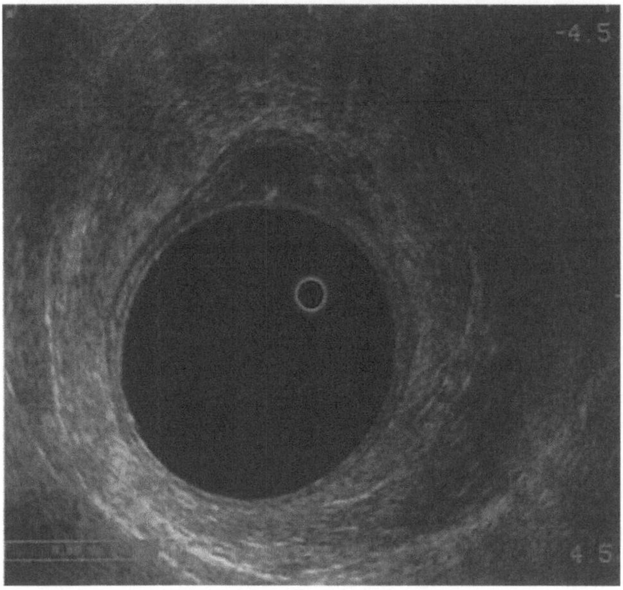

FIGURE 3.2(i).3. uT2 rectal tumor.

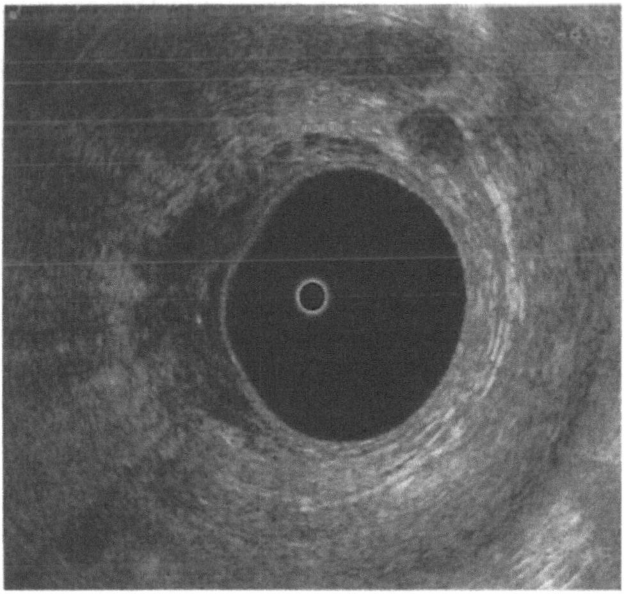

FIGURE 3.2(i).4. uT3 rectal tumor with adjacent lymph node.

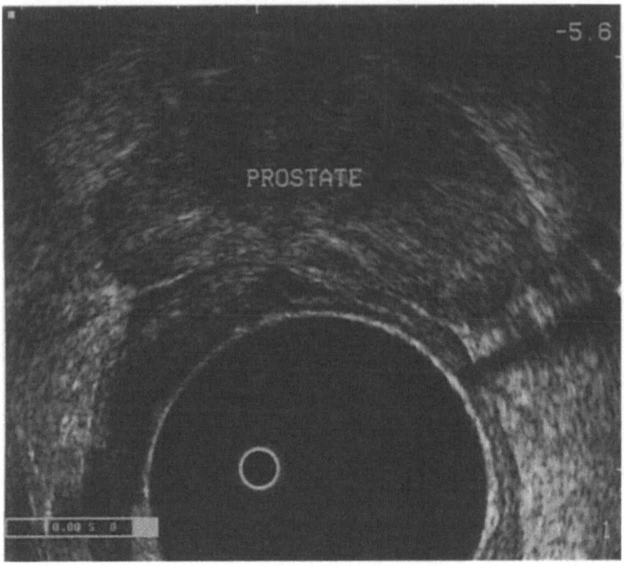

FIGURE 3.2(i).5. uT4 rectal tumor.

Mackay et al. (24) recently have proposed an alternative staging system that splits the uT2 stage into uT2a and uT2b, identifying focal and extensive muscularis propria involvement, respectively. They argue that a uT2b tumor is clinically likely to behave as a uT3 tumor and should be treated as such in the way that this staging will influence management decisions.

Over the last 20 years, various studies on the effectiveness of endosonography in staging rectal cancer have appeared in the literature. Using different scanners, both radial (Bruel and Kjaer 1846 and/or 1849, or Aloka 520) and linear (Toshiba SAL50A, Aloka 280 SL, Kramed, GE RT3000) in type, Rifkin and coworkers (25) identified all seven patients with extension of their tumors into the pararectal fat out of 26 patients with rectal cancers who were examined. They later reported that tumor was identified in 79 of 85 patients with two failures of examination (26). Patients were classified more crudely endosonographically into those either with tumor confined to or extending beyond the rectal wall. Invasion through the muscularis propria was identified in 25 patients, but eight were overstaged. Forty-three patients without invasion were correctly identified, but five patients were understaged. Prediction of extension had a sensitivity in this study of 83%, a specificity of 84%, a positive predictive value (PPV) of 76%, and a negative predictive value (NPV) of 90%. An accuracy for the staging of local invasion in rectal cancer of 85.8% was achieved by Fiefel et al. with their first sixty patients, 42 of whom had been examined by ES prospectively and subsequently subjected to surgery. They later reported the results with a total of 129 cases, using in the more recent examinations a seven megahertz transducer (14). Eighteen patients had no preoperative sonogram and 19 examinations were inadequate because of stenosis. Palliative treatment was offered in fifteen cases. In the remaining 76 cases, both endosonographic and histological assessments were available. In this later series, one tumor was understaged and eight tumors were overstaged.

An early Italian study in which 23 patients with histologically proven rectal cancers were examined provided similarly good results using a CGR probe (SONEL 3000) (27). In 20 cases, tumors were correctly staged ultrasonically according to the UICC TNM system. One tumor was overstaged as T2 and two tumors understaged as T2. Again, no attempt was made to define the ultrasonographically based reporting criteria. Glaser et al. (28) and Holdsworth et al. (29), studying 86 and 36 patients, respectively, found ES was accurate in 88% and 86% of cases, respectively. Invasion through the rectal wall in the latter study was predicted with a sensitivity of 96% and a specificity of 50%, but was limited in that a transducer of only five and a half megahertz was used.

The potential advantage of preoperative ES also resides in the determination of early rectal cancers. In order to define tumors suitable for per anal local excision, ES has been used to image small rectal tumors (30). In discriminating between T1 and T2/3 tumors and between T1/2 and T3 tumors, the positive predictive values were 93% and 100%, respectively, in a study by Detry and Kartheuser, while the NPV were 94% and 93%, respectively, in this series. Katsura et al. have reported an accuracy of 92% for the determination of the level of invasion with 8.3% of cases being overstaged (31), whereas Beynon et al., who studied 100 patients, achieved an ES staging accuracy of 93% in the assessment of the level of tumor invasion (32).

Orrom et al. have attempted to quantify the learning curve in ES by studying three groups of patients during consecutive periods of time (33). Their overall accuracy was 75%, but in the first 27 patients studied, the accuracy was only 60%, with 77% for the next 30 patients assessed and 95% for the final 20 cases examined. In contrast, Garciá-Aguilar et al. (34) from Minnesota have published the largest series of 1184 patients and analyzed 545 patients who did not have preoperative chemoradiation. Their overall accuracy was 69%, with 18% of tumors overstaged and 13% understaged. They concluded that their accuracy was lower than the previous studies reported, being lower more specifically for early tumors, and they believed that the accuracy was largely operator dependent. This study is different from others in that they reported a better accuracy in differentiating benign villous lesions from early cancers, adopting the system advocated by Beynon et al. (22) where lesions that were shown to expand the inner hypoechoic layer and were surrounded by a uniform middle hyperechoic layer are considered villous adenomas, and lesions expanding the inner hypoechoic layer demonstrating distinct defects of the middle hyperechoic layer are considered uT1 invasive tumors.

TABLE 3.2(i)-1. Accuracy of endosonography in staging primary rectal cancer.

	Number of Patients	Accuracy (%)
Dragsted and Gammelgaard (12)	13	85
Hildebrandt and Fiefel (13)	25	92
Romano et al. (27)	23	91
Hildebrandt et al. (21)	76	88
Rifkin and Wechsler (26)	81	84
Beynon (32)	100	93
Holdsworth et al. (29)	36	86
Orrom et al. (33)	77	75
Glaser et al. (28)	86	88
Katsura et al. (31)	120	92
Garciá-Aguilar et al. (34)	545	69
Kim et al. (45)	89	81
Gualdi et al. (44)	26	77
Sailer et al. (36)	162	78
Mackay et al. (24)	356	89

Adams et al. (35) studied 62 consecutive patients with villous lesions and found 12 lesions contained cancer of which only two showed clinical signs of induration. Here, the PPV of endoanal ultrasound in detecting a malignant focus was 66.7%, with a NPV of 88.7%, a sensitivity of only 50%, but a specificity of 94%. They concluded that sensitivity was compromised in large exophytic lesions, particularly if they lay close to the anal verge. At the other extreme of the rectum, Sailer et al. (36), in a study involving 162 patients, concluded that "high" lesions (>12 cm from the anal verge) had an accuracy of T staging of 88% when compared with low lesions (68%); however, they were unable to show any difference in the predictive value of ES with regard to the circumferential position of the rectal tumor. Table 3.2(i)-1 shows some reported series assessing the accuracy of ES in the determination of T stage in rectal cancer.

Post-radiotherapy changes in the rectum are a challenge to endosonographers. Poor resolution of the rectal wall and its post-radiotherapy thickening probably hamper interpretation of the extent of invasion. A recent study by Gavioli et al. (8) claimed that after high-dose preoperative radiotherapy, endorectal ultrasound no longer stages the tumor, but rather the fibrosis that takes place; however, they concluded that a residual tumor will always be inside the fibrosis, but that ES cannot guarantee whether the tumor has been sterilized as a result of the radiotherapy. As a consequence, they advocated downstaging ultrasound as a routine practice.

Lymph Node Assessment

Involvement of lymph nodes is associated with decreasing survival rates and increasing loco-regional recurrence. The success of ES in staging local invasion naturally led into studies on the detection of lymph node metastases, where there are now several reports on the effectiveness of endosonography in the detection of mesorectal nodes (13,15,16,24,26,29,32–34).

Hildebrandt et al., using a seven megahertz transducer, first reported the detection of lymph node metastases (14). In this series, metastatic involvement of pararectal lymph nodes was predicted in 12 of their 27 patients scanned preoperatively; however, these predictions were confirmed in only six cases while the other six patients showed reactive changes only. There was one false-negative case. Ten of 13 patients with positive nodes were identified by Rifkin and Wechsler, with six false positives in the remaining 66 patients (26) resulting in an overall sensitivity of 67%, with a specificity of 91%, a PPV of 63%, and a NPV of 92%. An accuracy of 73.2% for the node positive group has been achieved using an ultrasonic endoscope and similarly a sensitivity of 82.3% for the node negative group (19 false positives and three false negatives), where metastatic and non-metastatic nodes as small as five millimeters could be detected (26). Equally, Hildebrandt et al. found differences in an in vitro study comparing attenuation coefficients between nonspecific inflamed nodes and metastatic nodes (21) where reactive nodes tended to have internal echoes and metastatic nodes had low acoustic impedance and internal echoes. Attempts to differentiate inflammatory nodes from tumor-involved nodes subsequently were made based on their appearance (namely hyperechoic *versus* hypoechoic). Using these criteria, metastatic nodes were predicted with a sensitivity of 72% while inflammatory nodes were predicted with a specificity of 83% and an overall accuracy of 78%. Micrometastases, mixed lymph nodes, and changing echo patterns within inflammatory nodes were thought to explain the lack of improvement using this newer methodology when compared with other studies.

Beynon et al. (37) also have reported 83% accuracy with ES in predicting mesorectal node involvement while, in comparison, CT returned only 57% accuracy. Additionally, involved lymph nodes were of a significantly larger size in their study than inflammatory nodes. Despite this, when hypoechoic nodes are imaged and called positive, the accuracies in the various series lie between 61% and 88%. Katsura et al., using a flexible instrument, have tried to differentiate inflammatory nodes from metastatic nodes based on these differing echo-patterns (31). Here, nodes were divided into two types based on their sonographic appearances. "A" nodes had an ill-defined border and an even and hyperechoic pattern. The incidence of metastases in these nodal types was 18.4%. In type "B" nodes (defined as having a well-defined border and an uneven and markedly hyperechoic intranodal pattern), the incidence of metastases was 72%. These observations do not reflect the experience of other endosonographers who have observed that involved nodes tend to have a generally hypoechoic appearance.

How does endosonography compare with other modalities in predicting nodal involvement? Beynon et al., in a comparative study, found CT to be inferior to ES in predicting the presence of lymph node metastases (38).

Milsom et al. have approached the problem by performing ultrasonically guided biopsy of suspicious nodes to obtain a definitive staging (39), and Lindmark et al. have used Doppler ultrasound in 53 patients to help discriminate between lymph nodes and blood vessels (40). The evaluation of nodal status in this latter study was correct in 43 patients (accuracy 81%). Nine of their patients had one or several metastases, but ES did not identify all involved nodes in each case. Thirty-four patients had no involved nodes, and there were two false positives and eight false negatives in this series. Therefore, endorectal sonography can clearly identify extrarectal manifestations of malignancy as circumscribed echo-poor areas although islands of tumor, due to local invasion, cannot be readily distinguished from involved nodes. The limitation of ES is that false-positive diagnoses occur that are not explained by the architecture of the nodes or by their size, limiting the overall sensitivity of any of these modalities, particularly when there are micrometastases. In the latter circumstances, it may be that positron emission tomography (PET) scanning or radioimmunoscintigraphy will only prove beneficial, particularly following radiation therapy (41–43).

In a comparative study by Gualdi et al. (44), EUS showed a 72% sensitivity and an 80% specificity for nodal assessment whereas endorectal MRI reported an 81% sensitivity and a 66% specificity, respectively. In a study of 89 patiebts, Kim et al. (45) reported 63.5% accuracy for nodal staging using ES compared with 56% with CT and 63% with endorectal MRI. Table 3.2(i)-2 shows a selected series of reported accuracics using ES in the prediction of nodal involvement in rectal cancer. Brown and her group at the Royal Marsden Hospital in London (46) reported improved accuracies for positive nodal detection using high-resolution MRI for preoperative staging, as well as defining great accuracy for the prediction of circumferential margin involvement (see Chapter 3.3).

TABLE 3.2(i)-2. The accuracy of endosonography in predicting nodal involvement.

	Number of Patients	Accuracy (%)
Hildebrandt et al. (14)	27	74
Rifkin and Wechsler (26)	81	88
Beynon et al. (32)	95	83
Holdsworth et al. (29)	36	61
Orrom et al. (33)	77	82
Glaser et al. (28)	73	80
Hildebrandt et al. (21)	113	78
Garciá-Aguilar et al. (34)	238	64
Katsura et al. (31)	98	72
Kim et al. (45)	85	63
Gualdi et al. (44)	26	72
Mackay et al. (24)	263	66

The Detection of Local Recurrence

Despite apparently successful primary radical surgery, local recurrence occurs in five to 10% of cases (2). Local recurrence is more common in tumors that are located in the lower third of the rectum, which are large and locally invasive, and in those with lymphatic metastases. Implantation of viable cells at surgery giving true suture line recurrence readily detectable on sigmoidoscopy is probably a rare event. The more usual so-called anastomotic recurrence more likely results from local recurrence within the pelvis, which breaks through and presents at the anastomosis, a phenomenon that latterly has been thought to occur because of incomplete excision of the mesorectum (47).

Is there any evidence that ES—which is so accurate in the preoperative staging of rectal cancer—is of any use in the assessment and diagnosis of local tumor recurrence? Because it is relatively inexpensive, portable, and the examination is of short duration, it can be included in routine follow-up along with clinical examination and sigmoidoscopy; female patients treated by restorative resection or abdominoperineal excision also can be scanned transvaginally. Assessment of the neorectum is, in essence, no different to preoperative examination in that five layers can still be clearly identified. The presence of a stapled colorectal anastomosis also does not affect the interpretation of the images, where staples are seen as small bright echoes without any attendant acoustic shadowing. The ultrasonic anatomy of the pelvis may alter following surgery, and care in interpretation is required where scanning is ideally performed approximately three months following treatment.

Established locally recurrent cancer, detectable by digital and sigmoidoscopic examination, has endosonographic appearances identical to those of the primary rectal cancer because they are echo poor in nature. The extent of invasion can be assessed as with primary tumors because again there is disruption of the recognizable ultrasonic layers. Extrarectal locally recurrent tumors can be detected at an early stage. Here, tumors appear as a circumscribed echo-poor area within the para-anastomotic tissues, although the presence of tumors cannot always be diagnosed easily using only ES technology. In these situations, one of two policies can be adopted, namely:

a) A repeat ultrasound scan can be performed after a suitable period of a month or six weeks. An increase in size usually will indicate recurrent malignancy or,
b) a percutaneous transperineal biopsy can be performed using the endoprobe as a needle guide.

The effectiveness of ES in the follow-up of patients has been reported from a few centers. Twenty-two recurrences were detected by Hildebrandt et al. using ES, but only six of these were noted with ultrasound alone (14). Three cases also had an elevated carcinoembryonic antigen (CEA) level while ten cases had digital or endoscopic signs with an elevated serum CEA. Eight local recurrences were detected by Romano and colleagues in their follow-up group of 42 patients (27). Two ultrasonically false-positive cases of fibrosis were confirmed by percutaneous ultrasound-guided biopsy. Beynon et al. imaged 22 recurrences in 85 patients, of which only three where solely detected by ES (48). All other recurrences in this study could be palpated digitally or were obvious on sigmoidoscopic examination.

In another study from Italy, 120 patients were followed up by Mascagni et al. (49). Seventeen recurrences were detected in this analysis, of which six were asymptomatic. Twelve recurrences were detected by endorectal ultrasound, whereas five were found using endovaginal sonography, resulting in an accuracy of 97%, with a sensitivity and specificity of 94% and 98%, respectively. In six of their patients, recurrences could be detected by either digital examination or by simple endoscopy. Small extrarectal recurrences can therefore be detected before there is any evidence of luminal recurrence using ES, which may secondarily benefit guided biopsy. The routine use of ES following the surgical treatment of rectal cancer also permits a detailed examination of the pelvis, not previously possible without the use of more expensive techniques such as CT scan or MRI. In this context, when used routinely from three months after surgery, ES would possibly allow the detection of early recurrence in a larger number of patients although prospective cost benefit analyses of its use in the follow-up algorithm are at present unavailable and ES-driven second-look laparotomy in the management of loco-regional recurrence is still unclear.

Pitfalls of ES

1. In assessing polyps, "carpeting" villous lesions can decrease the accuracy of assessment of the depth of invasion, particularly if lesions are near or at the anal verge.
2. Post-radiation assessment of depth of invasion is limited, as it is impossible to differentiate between tumor and fibrosis and to define the standard ultrasonographically described rectal wall layers.
3. Anastomotic recurrence could be over diagnosed with ES where granulomas at the anastomotic site can cause confusion.
4. High stenotic lesions can only be partly assessed by ES, as they do not permit adequate acoustic coupling of the probe and may be limited by the rostral extent of the tumor, which exceeds that of the probe.
5. Care must be taken when assessing lower tumors of the rectum rather than higher ones due to the anatomy of the rectal wall.

Summary

Endorectal sonography has a role in deciding the treatment of benign rectal lesions, primary rectal cancer, and recurrent rectal cancer. It is of particular use in:

1. The identification of those lesions, benign and malignant, suitable for perianal local excision and conversely those that are not.
2. The determination of whether locally advanced tumors are resectable or whether radiotherapy or chemo-radiotherapy should be considered as a primary form of treatment before surgery (either adjuvant or neoadjuvant).
3. The close follow-up of patients after surgical treatment to detect local recurrence.
4. The investigation of pelvic abnormalities.
5. Endorectal sonography complements and serves as a valuable adjunct with CT and MRI in the investigation of specific colorectal disorders (e.g., extrarectal or presacral tumors resulting in evacuatory difficulty) (Figure 3.2(i).6) (50).
6. Endorectal sonography is highly operator dependent and studies have shown the importance of the learning curve.

Endoanal Ultrasound

Anal endosonography (AES) is a minimally invasive, easily accessible technique that provides detailed resolution of the internal and external anal sphincter musculature. It complements anal manometry and proctography and is mandatory in the investigation of fecal incontinence. It has a place in the management of perianal sepsis, obstructed defecation, and other functional bowel disorders. Endoluminal probes initially used for the assessment of prostatic and rectal lesions have been adopted for the anal canal (51,52). The balloon system was replaced by a plastic hard cone to cope with the inherent tone of the anal sphincters.

Endoanal ultrasound has various applications.

1. Assessment of fecal incontinence—pre- and postoperative period.
2. Assessing complex fistula-in-ano.
3. Staging of anal carcinoma.
4. Planning radiotherapy for anal carcinomas.
5. Follow-up of anal carcinoma.
6. Evaluation of functional disorders such as solitary rectal ulcer and obstructed defecation.

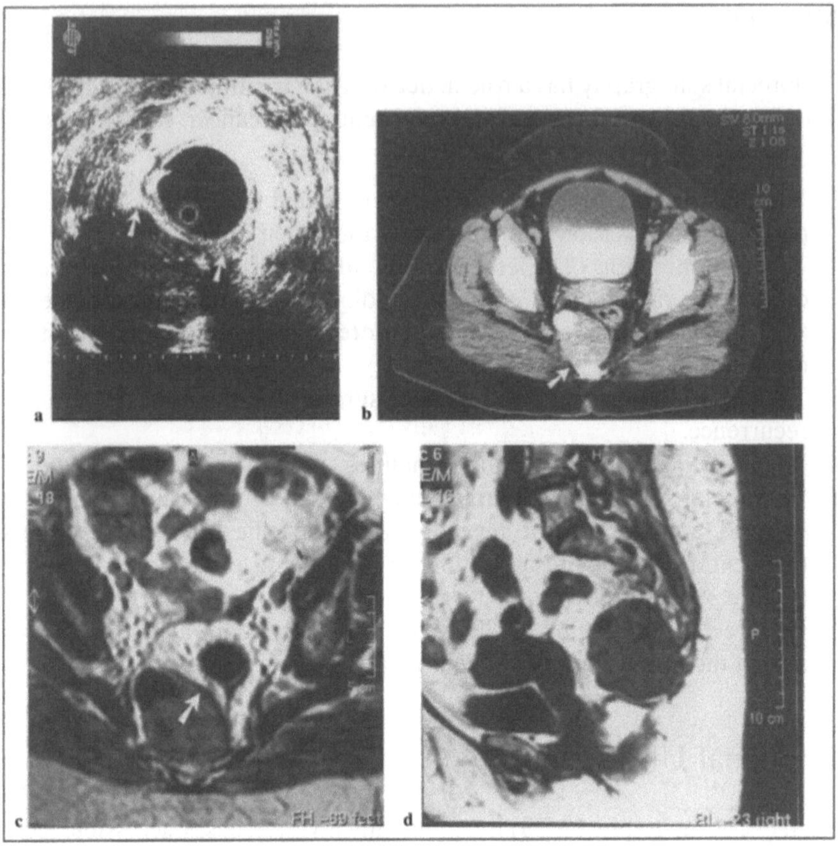

FIGURE 3.2(i).6. Endorectal ultrasound of a presacral mass showing infiltration of the echogenic rectal muscularis (arrows). Figure b is the representative CT scan and figures c and d the axial and mid-sagittal MRI scans respectively of the same tumor. [Reprinted with permission from Wolpert A, Beer-Gabel M, Lifschitz O, and Zbar AP. The management of presacral masses in the adult. Tech Coloproctol. 2002;6:43–9, Springer-Verlag Publishers].

Technique and Instrument

Preliminary studies were performed using a 7 megahertz Bruel and Kjaer endoprobe. A hard plastic cone with an outer diameter of 1.7 centimeters was used. The transducer is rotated mechanically at 1.9 to 2.8 cycles per second and the focal length of the probe is two to four and a half centimeters. The beam is emitted at right angles so that a 360 degree radial-swept image is obtained (53). In recent times, a ten megahertz transducer with a focal range of five to forty-five millimeters and a transverse resolution of less than 0.05 millimeters and a lateral resolution of one-half to one millimeter has been used. The assembly is filled with degassed water for acoustic coupling and covered with a lubricated condom for insertion. Subjects are examined in the prone position to avoid perineal asymmetry, with the image orientated such that the anterior edge is uppermost (54).

The endosonographic anatomy is as follows:

1. First hyperechoic layer = subepithelium
2. Second hypoechoic layer = internal anal sphincter (IAS)
3. Third hyperechoic layer = longitudinal muscle
4. Fourth hyperechoic layer = external anal sphincter (EAS)

The thickness of the IAS shows a positive correlation with age in the high and middle anal canal in female asymptomatic nulliparous women, where there is a gradual thickening of the recognizable hypoechoic IAS with age (55,56). The EAS tends to show a negative correlation with age at high, mid, and low anal levels, and there is no significant correlation between the thickness of longitudinal muscle and the puborectalis. In patients less than 55 years of age, the IAS can be between 2.4 to 2.7 millimeters thick, while in patients above 55 years of age, it can measure anywhere from 2.8 to 3.4 millimeters thick. Excessive thickness of this muscle has been noted by Kamm and colleagues in their description of a polyglucosan inclusion disorder that they have labeled as hereditary internal sphincter myopathy, a condition presenting with familial clustering of severe proctalgia fugax (57). Conversely, the same group has used endosonographic measurements to define the presence of objective IAS atrophy that they have correlated with the presentation of age-related passive fecal incontinence (58).

The conjoint longitudinal muscle coat surrounding the IAS is a continuation of the outer longitudinal muscle coat of the rectum (see Chapter 1). It forms a prominent hyperechoic layer between the internal and external sphincters. This layer is not sonographically uniform, and thin, short hypoechoic areas within it may be due to segments of smooth muscle devoid of connective tissue. The EAS is complex, presenting a trilaminar arrangement that generally is accepted as having deep, superficial, and subcutaneous parts. As the probe is withdrawn, the hyperechoic U-shaped sling of the puborectalis comes into view. The EAS is identified as converging fibers anteriorly as the probe comes down with the formation of a complete annular ring (59). In females, the EAS may be very thin anteriorly, whereas in males it is more symmetrical and annular at all levels, with an outer hypoechoic ring. In women, the echogenicity of all EAS components is identical and the layers are more difficult to delineate (Figure 3.2(i).7). In recent times 3D ultrasonography has been introduced (60). Its clinical use and results are presented in Chapter 3.2(iii). Conventional axial imaging may not give the accurate length of a sphincter tear, but 3D imaging produces a digital volume that may be viewed in any plane (Figure 3.2(i).8).

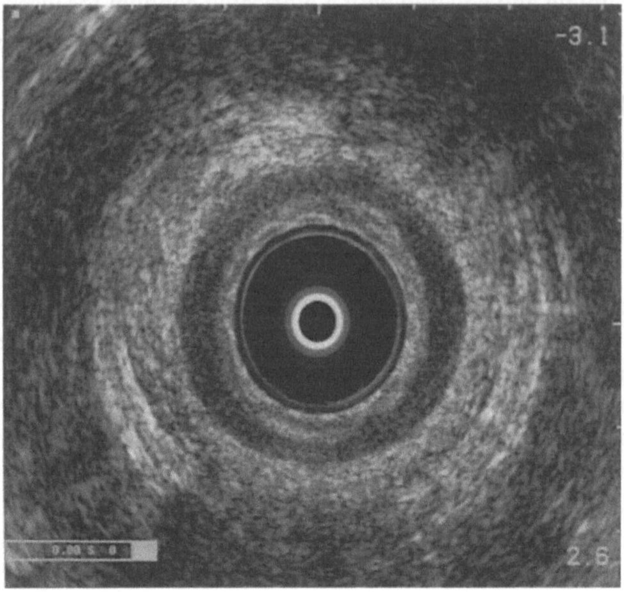

FIGURE 3.2(i).7. Normal anal canal lower third.

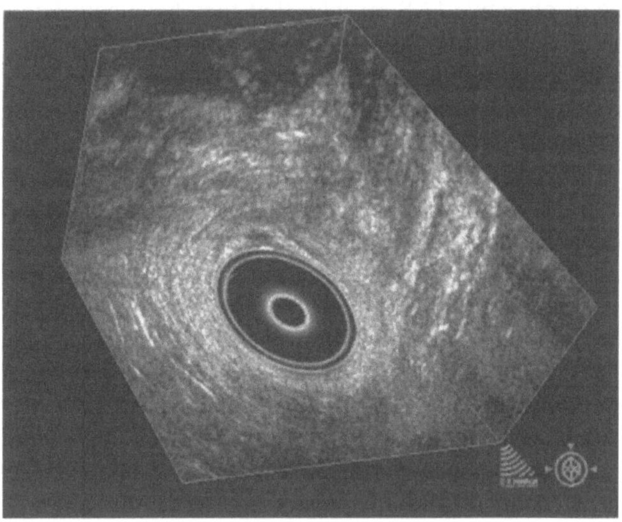

FIGURE 3.2(i).8. Three-dimensional image of anal canal.

Fecal Incontinence

Anal endosonography has been shown in various studies to be a useful tool in mapping sphincter defects. It distinguishes patients with sphincter defects from those with "idiopathic" fecal incontinence and allows the surgeon to manage this complex condition by successful sphincteroplasty. Anal endosonography also has a role in assessing the sphincters after primary or secondary repair of sphincter defects because it has been recognized that inadequate repair (and sometimes primary repairs of obstetric defects performed by non-coloproctologists) may require repeat sphincteroplasty (61). One should be aware of the physiological variation in the thickness of the IAS and the discernable sexual differences. The posterolateral aspect of the EAS should be intact at all levels in both sexes, but tends to be "deficient" anteriorly in females at a high anal canal level, although it presents an intact ring at the mid and low anal canal levels (62) (Figure 3.2(i).9).

Manual dilatation of the anus produces varying degrees of tear at multiple points when compared with deliberate internal anal sphincterotomy, and both can be delineated by AES. Remnants of the sphincter will appear hyperechoic, suggesting fibrotic replacement after manual dilatation; however, lateral internal anal sphincterotomy produces a clean break in the sphincter (62) (Figure 3.2(i).10). Similar changes have been noted after internal anal sphincterotomy using high-resolution endoanal MRI (63),

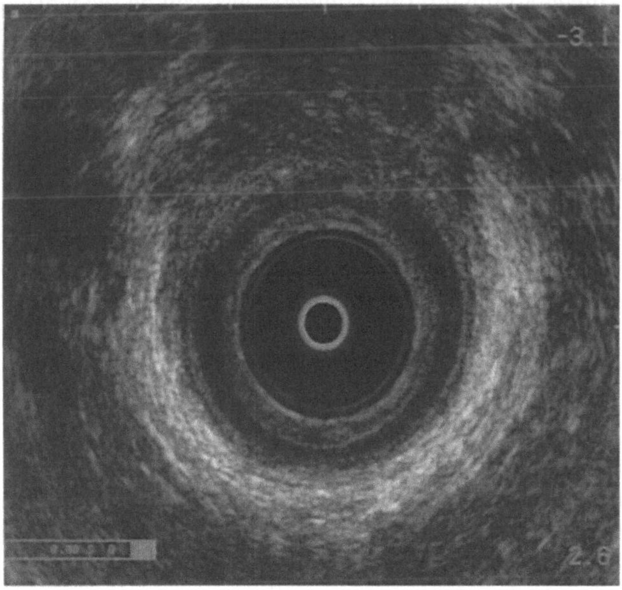

FIGURE 3.2(i).9. Anal canal with deficient EAS anteriorly.

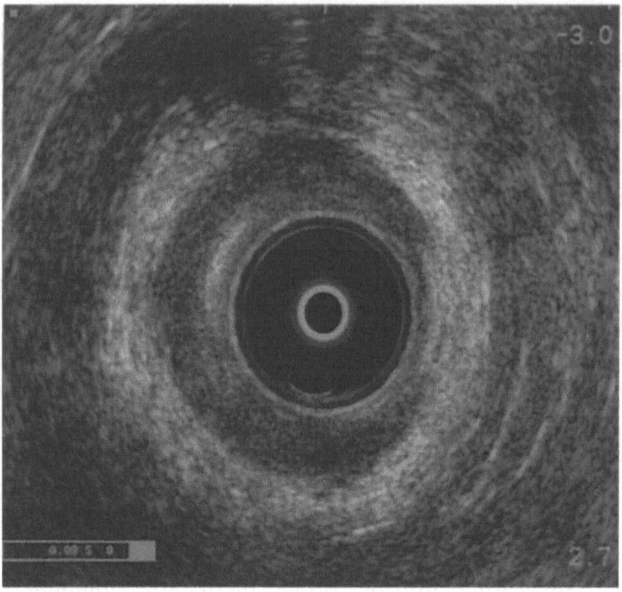

FIGURE 3.2(i).10. Internal anal sphincterotomy.

where with both modalities, the ends are well defined and rounded. External sphincter defects appear hypoechoic relative to the normal sphincter. Surgical damage to the internal sphincter also can be recognized following a fistulotomy for complex perirectal sepsis (Figure 3.2(i).11).

Speakman et al. (62) studied 12 patients with fecal incontinence who had manual dilatation for anal fissure. In this study, endoanal ultrasound showed extensive disruption of IAS in ten patients. In a study by Nielsen et al. (64), 65% of patients undergoing anal dilatation had demonstrable sphincter defects and 12.5% had some degree of fecal incontinence. Bartram et al. (65) have emphasized the role of AES in preventing damage to either the internal and external sphincters because it shows exactly what procedures are associated with sphincter injuries. In this respect, Sultan et al. (66) assessed the effect of internal anal sphincterotomy for anal fissures and showed in women with a shorter anal canal length that a more extensive sphincterotomy than the surgeon intended or anticipated often was performed. In this study, the entire length of the internal sphincter had been divided in nine of ten women.

In a further landmark study that heralded the injurious effects on the anal sphincter of assisted vaginal delivery and the clinical role of AES, the same group showed that 13% of nulliparous women and 23% of multiparous women had anal incontinence six weeks after delivery (67). In this work, 35% of nulliparous women showed sphincter defects, and these defects were still evident at six months. They also showed that sphincter defects were more common after forceps delivery than after vacuum extractions.

Gold et al. (60) assessed the new 3D endoanal ultrasonography and emphasized the role of AES in showing the longitudinal and radial extent of the tear (which appeared to correlate), suggesting that these parameters play a significant role in the success of one's surgical repair of sphincter defects and emphasizing the need for a repair of sufficient sphincter length. Ho et al. (68) also showed the usefulness of AES in delineating sphincter defects iatrogenically caused by stapling instruments in low restorative resection where the functional results have been less than optimal.

Fistula in ano

Complex fistulas have a potential of a high recurrence rate and a high incidence of attendant iatrogenic fecal incontinence due to damage to the anal sphincters as a result of fistulectomy and repeated surgery. Anal endosonography, along with MRI, are valuable tools in the management of complex fistulas.

Deen et al. (69), in a small study of 18 patients, showed that AES is useful in showing horseshoe tracks in 50% of patients and collections in 45% of cases. Here, the surgical findings matched the endosonographic findings in 94%. Hussain et al. (70), in a study comparing AES, endoanal MRI, and

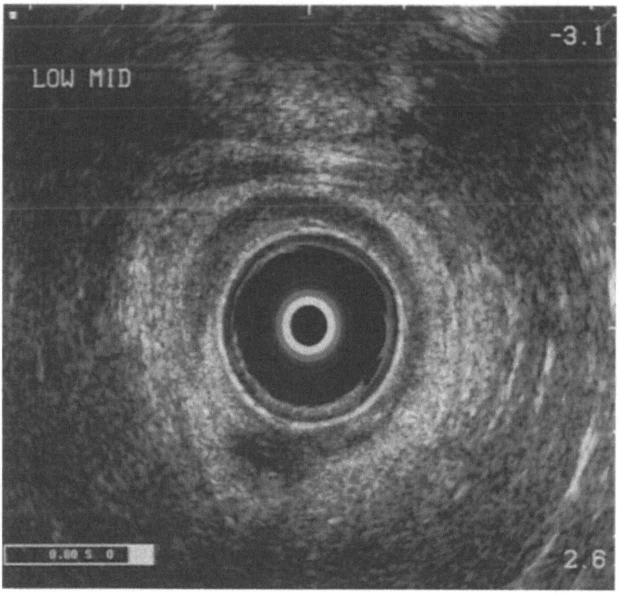

FIGURE 3.2(i).11. Fistula-in-ano with sepsis and sphincterotomy.

surgery, found the accuracy of AES in classifying fistula-in-ano was 69%, with MRI at 89% and surgery at 93%; however, the accuracy of detecting fluid collections by AES and MRI were equivalent. The internal fistula opening, which is a vital component of imaging in the prevention of fistula recurrence, was detected in 43% of cases using AES, in 71% of cases using endoanal MRI, and in 86% with surgery. Laurence et al. (71) studied the role of AES in rectovaginal fistulae and concluded that it may not be as useful a tool in mapping out the fistula, but is useful in management decisions to identify coincidental sphincter defects that have resulted from either surgery or destructive sepsis. Here, the goals of preoperative imaging are not just to define the primary collection (or track), its relationship to the main puborectalis bundle, and the site of the internal fistula opening, although these are all important. The coloproctologist also will benefit from delineation of the secondary effects of uncontrolled and destructive perirectal infection, which may in themselves necessitate staged perineal surgery. Such information will demonstrate the presence of a sphincter defect (EAS and IAS), the integrity of the perineal body, the presence of significant horseshoeing in the retrorectal and anteroanal spaces, and the presence of a rectovaginal or anovaginal fistula.

Kruskal et al. (72) have analyzed the role of peroxide-enhanced AES in perirectal sepsis and found in 60 patients that it was helpful in detecting the number and the internal course of these fistulae.

The issues in preoperative imaging of high and/or recurrent fistula-in-ano are complex (73). By its nature, endoanal probe technology—AES, enhanced AES, 3D AES, and endoanal MRI—will each have limitations in two areas of particular interest to the coloproctologist faced with a complex multiply recurrent fistula-in-ano. The first area pertains to the laterally placed extrasphincteric fistula that lies beyond the focal distance of the probe; the second is in the delineation of a translevator extension where coupling contact of the probe above the puborectalis is not possible. In both of these circumstances, vital information may not be provided by such "newer" endoanal technology, and this is compounded by a lack of information of some cases of primary pelvirectal sepsis that has broken through the levator plate and presented in the ischiorectal fossa. In this latter circumstance, injudicious drainage of sepsis via the ischiorectal space will result in a high extrasphincteric fistula that occasionally requires proctectomy; such suspicious cases need to be assessed preoperatively by surface MRI. Moreover, in recurrent and recrudescent perirectal sepsis, AES is unable to distinguish active sepsis from burnt-out tracks (74), and because of its acoustic shadowing, it may overcall cases of intersphincteric sepsis as trans-sphincteric sepsis. In this circumstance, if the AES is solely relied upon to direct the surgery, it may result in inadvertently excessive sphincter division (75,76).

Anal Canal Carcinoma

Anal endosonography is useful in selecting patients for local resection of anal carcinoma somewhat analogous to the use of transrectal ultrasound in local excision of rectal cancer. It also has a role in the surveillance of these lesions and of the precursor lesion anal intraepithelial neoplasia (77). Tarantino et al. (78), in a small study, showed that AES was accurate in assessing the depth of tumor penetration and is useful in selecting patients suitable for surgery as the primary modality, as well as in assessing the response to chemoradiation.

A new staging system has been proposed for staging anal canal carcinomas (78) based on their AES appearance, where:

uT1 = Confined to submucosa.
uT2a = Lesion invading the internal anal sphincter.
uT2b = Lesion penetrating external anal sphincter.
uT3 = Lesion invading beyond the sphincters into perianal tissues.
uT4 = Lesion invading adjacent structures.

Post-chemoradiation scarring and edema seem to be a challenge in restaging these lesions, but as it appears to diminish after 16 weeks follow-up, reports of longer-term AES changes in this specialized group of patients are required. Giovannini et al. (79), in a study of 146 patients, demonstrated the superiority of an endoanal ultrasound-based staging system in the prediction of outcomes such as local recurrence and patient survival. In this respect, Lohnert et al. (80) used 3D tumor reconstruction based on endoanal ultrasound images utilizing these dimensional geometric assessments for the planning of ultrasound-guided after-loading brachytherapy, showing promising initial results for this new modality of therapy. The radiation target fields were optimized by computer-generated simulation and endosonographically guided implantation of after-loading needles.

Role of Endoanal Ultrasonography in Functional Bowel Disorders

Halligan et al. (81) showed marked thickness of the internal and external anal sphincters in patients with solitary rectal ulcer syndrome (SRUS) when compared with age-matched asymptomatic controls. The precise etiology of this condition is unknown; however, it has been proposed that a combination of mucosal rectal prolapse and increased rectal pressure (due in part to a thickened internal anal sphincter) could be responsible. Marshall et al. (82), in a small study, demonstrated the predictive value of IAS thickness measurement for the diagnosis of rectoanal intussusception in patients with SRUS. They concluded that AES has a 91% PPV in detecting an abnormally thickened IAS in SRUS patients with rectoanal intussusception; however, in this study, the NPV was only 57%. Anal endosonography also may have a role in patients who fail to evacuate during defecating proctography, as well as in pregnant patients presenting with evacuatory difficulty where radiation is an issue and is contraindicated.

Thus, anal endosonography is part of the investigative armamentarium for the assessment of obstructed defecation, as well as to assess the sphincters. In these patients, only the recent technique of dynamic transperineal ultrasound (83) has been shown to correlate well with defecating proctography in detecting rectorectal intussusception, rectoceles, and enteroceles. This subject is addressed in Chapter 3.2(ii).

Summary

Endoanal ultrasound is gaining importance in staging, treatment, and follow-up of anal carcinomas, and with the new 3D reconstructions, it will be interesting to see the impact it will have on neoplastic and functional anorectal disorders. It also shares an important role in assessing complex fistula-in-ano with MRI and is indispensable in the management of fecal incontinence. Its value and its limitations have been discussed in this section of the chapter.

References

1. Barrett MW. Chemoradiation for rectal cancer: current methods. Semin Surg Oncol. 1998;15:114–9.
2. Kapiteijn E, Marijnen CA, Nagtegaal ID, et al. Preoperative radiotherapy combined with total mesorectal excision for resectable rectal cancer. N Engl J Med. 2001;345:638–46.
3. Nicholls RJ, Mason AY, Morson BC, Dixon AK, and Fry IK. The clinical staging of rectal cancer. Br J Surg. 1982;69:404–9.
4. Brown G, Radcliffe AG, Newcombe RG, Dallimore NS, Bourne MW, and Williams GT. Preoperative assessment of prognostic factors in rectal cancer using high-resolution magnetic resonance imaging. Br J Surg. 2003;90:355–64.
5. Zbar AP, deSouza NM, Strickland N, Pignatelli M, and Kmiot WA. Comparison of endoanal magnetic resonance imaging and computed tomography in the preoperative staging of rectal cancer: a pilot study. Tech Coloproctol. 1998;2:61–6.
6. Drew PJ, Farouk R, Turnbull LW, Ward SC, Hartley JE, and Monson JR. Preoperative magnetic resonance staging of rectal cancer with an endorectal coil and dynamic gadolinium enhancement. Br J Surg. 1999;86:250–4.
7. Beynon J, Mortenson NJMcC, Foy DMA, Channer JL, Virjee J, and Goddard P. Endorectal sonography: Laboratory and clinical experience in Bristol. Int J Colorectal Dis. 1986;1:212–5.
8. Gavioli M, Bagni A, Piccagli I, Fundaro S, and Natalini G. Usefulness of endorectal ultrasound after preoperative radiotherapy in rectal cancer: comparison between sonographic and histopathologic changes. Dis Colon Rectum. 2000;43:1075–83.
9. Wild JJ and Reid JM. Diagnostic use of ultrasound. Br J Phys Med. 1956; 19:248–57.

10. Wild JJ and Foderick JW. The feasibility of echometric detection of cancer in the lower gastrointestinal tract. Am J Proct Gastro Col Rectal Surg. 1978; Jan–Feb:16–25.
11. Wild JJ and Foderick JW. The feasibility of echometric detection of cancer of the lower gastrointestinal tract II. Am J Proct Gastro Col Rectal Surg. 1978; Mar–Apr:11–20.
12. Dragsted J and Gamelgaard J. Endoluminal ultrasonic scanning in the evaluation of rectal cancer. Gastrointest Radiol. 1983;8:367–9.
13. Hildebrandt U and Fiefel G. Pre-operative staging of rectal cancer by intrarectal ultrasound. Dis Colon Rectum. 1985;28:42–6.
14. Hildebrandt U, Fiefel G, Schwarz HP, and Scherr O. Endorectal ultrasound: Instrumentation and clinical aspects. Int J Colorectal Dis. 1986;1:203–7.
15. Kim JC, Cho YK, Kim SY, Park SK, and Lee MG. Comparative study of three-dimensional and conventional endorectal ultrasonography used in rectal cancer staging. Surg Endosc. 2002;16(9):1280–5.
16. Steele SR, Martin MJ, and Place RJ. Flexible endorectal ultrasound for predicting pathologic stage of rectal cancers. Am J Surg. 2002;184(2):126–30.
17. Poller DN. Method of specimen fixation and pathological dissection of colorectal cancer influences retrieval of lymph nodes and tumour nodal stage. Eur J Surg Oncol. 2000;26:758–62.
18. Herrera-Ornelas L, Justiniano J, Castillo N, Petrelli NJ, Stule JP, and Nittelman A. Metastases in small lymph nodes from colon cancer. Arch Surg. 1987;122: 1253–6.
19. Dworak O. Number and size of lymph nodes and node metastases in rectal carcinomas. Surg Endosc. 1989;3:96–9.
20. Catalano MF, Sivak MV, Rice T, Gragg LA, and Van Dam J. Endosonographic features predictive of lymph node metastasis. Gastrointest Endosc. 1994;40: 442–6.
21. Hildebrandt U, Klein T, Feifel G, Schwarz HP, Koch B, and Schmitt RM. Endosonography of pararectal lymph nodes. In vitro and in vivo evaluation. Dis Colon Rectum. 1990;33:863–8.
22. Beynon J, Foy DMA, Channer JL, Temple LN, Virjee J, and Mortensen NJM. The endosonic appearances of normal colon and rectum. Dis Colon Rectum. 1986;29:810–3.
23. Hermanek, Hutter RVP, Sobin LH, Wagner G, Wittekind C, and Spiess B. TNM atlas: illustrated guide to the TNM/pTNM classification of malignant tumors. Berlin: Springer-Verlag; 1997.
24. Mackay SG, Pager CK, Joseph D, Stewart PJ, and Solomon MJ. Assessment of the accuracy of transrectal ultrasonography in anorectal neoplasia. Br J Surg. 2003;90:346–50.
25. Rifkin MD and Marks GJ. Transrectal US as an adjunct in the diagnosis of rectal and extrarectal tumours. Radiology. 1985;157:499–502.
26. Rifkin M and Wechsler RJ. A comparison of computed tomography and endorectal ultrasound in staging rectal cancer. Int J Colorectal Dis. 1986;1: 219–23.
27. Romano G, De Rosa P, Vallone G, Rontando A, Grassi R, and Santangelo ML. Intrarectal ultrasound and computed tomography in the pre- and postoperative assessment of patients with rectal carcinoma. Br J Surg. 1985;72(Suppl): S117–19.

28. Glaser F, Schlag P, and Herfarth C. Endorectal ultrasonography for the assessment of invasion of rectal tumours and lymph node involvement. Br J Surg. 1990;77:883–7.
29. Holdsworth PJ, Johnston D, Chalmers AG, Chennels P, Dixon MF, Finan PJ, Primrose JN, and Quirke P. Endoluminal ultrasound and computed tomography in the staging of rectal cancer. Br J Surg. 1988;75:1019–22.
30. Detry R and Kartheuser A. Endorectal ultrasonography in staging small rectal tumours. Br J Surg. 1992;79(Suppl):S30.
31. Katsura Y, Yamada K, Ishizawa T, Yoshinaka H, and Shimazu H. Endorectal ultrasonography for the assessment of wall invasion and lymph node metastasis in rectal cancer. Dis Colon Rectum. 1992;35:362–68.
32. Beynon J. An evaluation of the role of rectal endosonography in rectal cancer. Ann R Coll Surg Engl. 1989;71(2):131–9.
33. Orrom WJ, Wong WD, Rothenberger DA, Jensen LL, and Goldberg SM. Endorectal ultrasound in the preoperative staging of rectal tumours. A learning experience. Dis Colon Rectum. 1990;33:654–9.
34. Garciá-Aguilar J, Pollack J, Lee S, et al. Accuracy of endorectal ultrasound in preoperative staging of rectal tumours. Dis Colon Rectum. 2002;45:10–15.
35. Adams WJ and Wong WD. Endorectal ultrasonic detection of malignancy within rectal villous lesions. Dis Colon Rectum. 1995;38:1093–6.
36. Sailer M, Leppert R, Bussen D, Fuchs KH, and Thiede A. Influence of tumour position on accuracy of endorectal ultrasound staging. Dis Colon Rectum. 1997;40:1180–6.
37. Beynon J, Mortensen NJM, Foy DMA, Channer JL, Rigby H, and Virjee J. Preoperative assessment of meso-rectal lymph node involvement in rectal cancer. Br J Surg. 1989;76:276–9.
38. Beynon J, Mortensen NJM, Foy DMA, Channer JL, Virjee J, and Goddard P. Preoperative assessment of local invasion in rectal cancer: digital examination, endoluminal sonography or computed tomography? Br J Surg. 1986;73:1015–17.
39. Milsom JW, Lavery IC, Stolfi VM, et al. The expanding utility of endoluminal ultrasonography in the management of rectal cancer. Surgery. 1992;112:832–41.
40. Lindmark G, Elvin A, Pahlman L, and Glimelius B. The value of endosonography in preoperative staging of rectal cancer. Int J Colorectal Dis. 1992:7: 162–6.
41. Gupta NC, Falk PM, Frank AL, Thorson AM, Frick MP, and Bowman B. Pre-operative staging of colorectal carcinoma using positron emission tomography. Nebr Med J. 1993;211:30–55.
42. Behr TM, Becker WS, Bair HJ, et al. Comparison of complete versus fragmented technetwin-99m-labeled anti-CEA monoclonal antibodies for immunoscintigraphy in colorectal cancer. J Nucl Med. 1995;36:430–41.
43. Sironi S, Ferrero C, Gainolli L, Landoni C, Del Maschio A, Fazio F, and Zbar AP. The role of imaging in the diagnosis and staging of primary and recurrent rectal cancer. In: Audisio RA, Geraghty JG, and Longo WE, editors. Modern management of cancer of the rectum. London: Springer-Verlag; 2001. p. 33–49.
44. Gualdi GF, Casciani E, Guadalaxara A, d'Orta C, Polettini E, and Pappalardo G. Local staging of rectal cancer with transrectal ultrasound and endorectal magnetic resonance imaging. Dis Colon Rectum. 2000;43:338–45.

45. Kim NK, Kim MJ, Yun SH, Sohn SK, and Min JS. Comparative study of transrectal ultrasound, pelvic computerized tomography, and magnetic resonance imaging in preoperative staging of rectal cancer. Dis Colon Rectum. 1999;42:770–5.
46. Brown G, Radcliffe AG, Newcombe RG, Dallimore NS, Bourne MW, and Williams GT. Preoperative assessment of prognostic factors in rectal cancer using high-resolution magnetic resonance imaging. Br J Surg. 2003;90:355–64.
47. Wood CB, Ratcliffe JG, Burt TW, Malcolm AJH, and Blumgart LH. Local tumour invasion as a prognostic factor in colorectal carcinoma. Br J Surg. 1981;68:326–8.
48. Beynon J, Mortensen NJM, Foy DMA, Rigby HS, Channer JL, and Virjee J. The detection and evaluation of locally recurrent rectal cancer with rectal endosonography. Dis Colon Rectum. 1989;32:509–17.
49. Mascagni D, Corellini L, Urciuoli P, and Di Matteo G. Endoluminal ultrasound for early detection of local recurrence of rectal cancer. Br J Surg. 1989;76:1176–80.
50. Wolpert A, Beer-Gabel M, Lifschitz O, and Zbar AP. The management of presacral masses in the adult. Tech Coloproctol. 2002;6:43–9.
51. Sultan AH, kamm MA, Hudson CN, Nicholas JR, and Bartram CI. Endosonography of the anal sphincters: normal anatomy and comparison with manometry. Clin Radiol. 1994;49:368–74.
52. Schafer A, Erick P, Furst G, Kahn T, Frieling T, and Lubke HJ. Anatomy of the anal sphincter; comparison of anal endosonography to magnetic resonance imaging. Dis Colon Rectum. 1994;137:777–81.
53. Sultan AH, Nicholls RJ, Kamm MA, Hudson CN, Beynon J, and Bartram CI. Anal endosonography and correlation with in vitro and in vivo anatomy. Br J Surg. 1993;80:508–11.
54. Bartram CI and Frudinger A. Handbook of anal endosonography. United Kingdom: Wrightson Biomedical Publishing Ltd; 1997.
55. Burnett SJ and Bartram CI. Endosonographic variations in the normal internal anal sphincter. Int J Colorectal Dis. 1991;6:2–4.
56. Frudinger A, Halligan S, Bartram CI, Price AB, Kamm MA, and Winter R. Female anal sphincter: Age related differences in asymptomatic volunteers with high—frequency endoanal US. Radiology. 2002;224:417–23.
57. Kamm MA, Hoyle CH, Burleigh DE, Law PJ, Swash M, Martin JE, Nicholls RJ, and Northover JM. Hereditary internal anal sphincter myopathy causing proctalgia fugax and constipation. A newly identified condition. Gastroenterology. 1991;100:805–10.
58. Vaizey CJ, Kamm MA, and Bartram CI. Primary degeneration of the internal anal sphincter as a cause of passive faecal incontinence. Lancet. 1997;349(9052):612–15.
59. Bartram CI. Anal endosonography. Alimentary tract radiology. 5th ed. St. Louis: Freeney and Stevenson; 1994.
60. Gold DM, Bartram CI, Halligan S, Humphries KN, Kamm MA, and Kmiot WA. Three dimensional endoanal sonography in assessing anal canal injury. Br J Surg. 1999;86:365–70.
61. Pinedo G, Vaizey CJ, Nicholls RJ, Roach R, Halligan S, and Kamm MA. Result of repeat anal sphincter repair. Br J Surg. 1999;86:66–9.

62. Speakman CTM, Burnett SJD, Kamm MA, and Bartram CI. Sphincter injury after anal dilatation demonstrated by anal endosonography. Br J Surg. 1991;78: 1429–30.
63. Zbar AP and deSouza NM. The anal sphincter. In: deSouza NM, editor. Endocavitary MRI of the pelvis. London: Harwood Academic Publishers; 2001. p. 91–109.
64. Nielsen MB, Rasmussen OO, Pederson JF, and Chritiansen J. Risk of sphincter damage and anal incontinence after anal dilatation for fissure-in-ano. Dis Colon Rectum. 1993;36:677–80.
65. Bartram CI and Sultan AH. Anal endosonography in faecal incontinenece. Gut. 1995;37:4–6.
66. Sultan AH, Kamm MA, Nicholls RJ, and Bartram CI. Prospective study of the extent of lateral anal sphincterotomy division during lateral sphinctertomy. Dis Colon Rectum. 1994;37:1031–3.
67. Sultan AH, Kamm MA, Hudson CN, Thomas J, and Bartram CI. Anal-sphincter disruption during vaginal delivery. N Engl J Med. 1993;329:1905–11.
68. Ho YH, Tsang C, Tang CL, Nyam D, Eu KW, and Seow-Choen F. Anal sphincter injuries from stapling instruments introduced transanally. Dis Colon Rectum. 200;43:169–73.
69. Deen KI, Williams JG, Hutchinson R, Keighley MRB, and Kumar D. Fitulas in ano: endoanal ultrasongraphic assessment assists decision making for surgery. Gut. 1994;35:391–4.
70. Hussain SM, Stoker J, Schouten WR, Hop WC, and Lameris JS. Fistula in ano: Endoanal sonography versus endoanal MR imaging in classification. Radiology. 1996;200:475–81.
71. Laurence FY, Birnbaum EH, Read TE, Kodner IJ, and Fleshman JW. Use of endoanal ultrasound in patients with rectovaginal fistulas. Dis Colon Rectum. 1999;42:1057–64.
72. Kruskal JB, Kane RA, and Morrin MM. Peroxide-enhanced anal endosonography; technique, image interpretation, and clinical applications. Radiographics. 2001;21;S173–89.
73. Lunniss PJ, Kamm MA, and Phillips RKS. Factors affecting continence after surgery for anal fistula. Br J Surg. 1994;81:1382–5.
74. Zbar AP and deSouza NM. Prospective comparison of endosonography, magnetic resonance imaging and surgical findings in anorectal fistula and abscess complicating Crohn's disease. Br J Surg. 1999;86:1093–4.
75. Zbar AP, deSouza NM, Puni R, and Kmiot WA. Comparison of endoanal magnetic resonance imaging with surgical findings in perirectal sepsis. Br J Surg. 1998;85:111–14.
76. Zimmerman DDE. Diagnosis and treatment of transsphincteric perianal fistulas [thesis]. Rotterdam, The Netherlands: Erasmus University; 2003.
77. Zbar AP, Fenger C, Efron C, Beer-Gabel M, and Wexner SD. The pathology and molecular biology of anal intraepithelial neoplasia: comparisons with cervical and vulvar intraepithelial carcinoma. Int J Colorectal Dis. 2002;17:203–15.
78. Tarantino D and Bernstein MA. Endoanal ultrasound in the staging and management of squamous-cell carcinoma of the anal canal. Potential implications of a new ultrasound staging system. Dis Colon Rectum. 2002;45:16–22.

79. Giovannini M, Bardou VJ, Barclay R, et al. Anal carcinoma; prognostic value of endorectal ultrasound (ERUS). Results of a prospective multicenter study. Endoscopy. 2001;33(3):231–6.
80. Lohnert M, Doniec JM, Kovacs G, Schroder J, and Dohrmann P. New method of radiotherapy for anal cancer with three-dimensional tumour reconstruction based on endoanal ultrasound and ultrasound-guided afterloading therapy. Dis Colon Rectum. 1998;41(2):169–76.
81. Halligan S, Sultan AH, Rottenberg G, and Bartram CI. Endosonography of the anal sphincters in solitary rectal ulcer syndrome. Int J Colorectal Dis. 1995; 10:79–82.
82. Marshall M, Halligan S, Fotheringham T, Bartram C, and Nicholls RJ. Predictive value of internal anal sphincter thickness for diagnosis of rectal intussusception in patients with solitary rectal ulcer syndrome. Br J Surg. 2002;89:1281–5.
83. Beer-Gabel M, Teshler M, Barzilai N, Lurie Y, Malnick S, Bass D, and Zbar A. Dynamic transperineal ultrasound in the diagnosis of pelvic floor disorders. Dis Colon Rectum. 2002;45:239–48.

Editorial Commentary

The use of endoluminal ultrasound has revolutionized our understanding of anal sphincter anatomy and the clinical history of postobstetric injury and its relationship to fecal incontinence. It has been used to effect in complex perirectal sepsis although because of its acoustic characteristics, there are limitations in extensive intersphincteric abscesses and it has limitations in trans-sphincteric sepsis (where the proble couples poorly above the puborectalis) and in extrasphincteric fistulae (which tend to lie beyond the focal range of the transducer). In rectal cancer, endoanal ultrasonography is of value in T and N staging although it has been unable to predict the T1/T2 distinction which would define the clear role of local excisional therapies. Moreover, its use after irradiation is limited as is its delineation of involved pararectal lymph nodes some of which lie outside the field of view of the probe and a considerable proportion of which harbor micrometasases.

AZ

Chapter 3.2(ii)
Ultrasound in Coloproctologic Practice: Dynamic Transperineal Ultrasound and Transvaginal Sonography

Marc Beer-Gabel, Andrea Frudinger, and Andrew P. Zbar

A. Dynamic Transperineal Ultrasonography (DTP-US)—A New Aid to Clinical Proctological Practice

Marc Beer-Gabel

Introduction

Dynamic transperineal ultrasonography (DTP-US) is a recently developed and studied novel and simple means for the real-time assessment of component parts of the anterior, middle, and posterior pelvic compartments and their interaction during provocative maneuvers such as straining and simulated defecation. Although it potentially rivals axial endoanal ultrasonography in the quality and resolution of images that it provides statically for the assessment of the integrity of the internal and external anal sphincters, it also may be most useful in dynamic mode for the assessment of patients primarily presenting with evacuatory dysfunction or those with defecation difficulty following pelvic surgery.

There is generally a poor correlation between the symptoms attributed to pelvic floor dysfunction and radiologically demonstrated anatomical findings (1), and studies have shown that the vast majority of patients presenting with evacuatory disorders have a multiplicity of pathology (2). The traditional assessment of these patients often involves a fairly poorly tolerated "extended" defecographic technique requiring opacification of the small bowel, bladder, vagina, and even the peritoneal cavity to determine pathology of the pelvic floor compartments (3) with a presumptive decision-making process to define what represents the dominant pathology in such patients (4). Recently, static DTP-US has been used to assess the morphology and integrity of the anal sphincter components in nullipara (particularly where expensive endoluminal probes are not available), producing images that are as accurate as axial endoanal ultrasonography (5,6).

Dynamic real-time TP-US is a new noninvasive technique simply performed (and learned) that assesses the anterior, middle, and posterior perineal and pelvic compartments, providing clear high-resolution images of the anal canal, anal sphincters, puborectalis sling, bladder base, urethra and urethrovesical angle, vaginal vault, and the rectovaginal (rectogenital) septum, which recently has been reported by our group in an unselected group of patients presenting with a variety of anorectal disorders (7). This first part of the chapter describes the basic technique, advantages, and limitations in specific pelvic floor disorders and accuracy in those select patients presenting to a pelvic floor dysfunction unit with primary disorders of rectal evacuation.

Technical Aspects of DTP-US

No preparation is required for the examination. The procedure is videotaped for orthograde and retrograde scrolling of dynamic images, and static representative images may be used for clinical measurement. Dynamic transperineal ultrasonography is performed with a 7.5 megahertz curvilinear transducer (C 4-7 and C 8-12), as well as a linear-array transducer (L 5-10 ATL: HDI 3000; Advanced Technology Laboratories, Bothell, WA, USA). A latex condom is used for protection of the transducer head, and for best visualization, the patient's rectum is filled with 50 milliliters of ultrasonographic coupling gel (Ultra-Gel: Aquarius 101; Medilab USA) using a standard Luer syringe and a soft-end rubber catheter. A similar volume of acoustic gel is instilled into the vagina (without distending the vaginal vault), and gel is liberally applied to the perineum. For the complete procedure, 50 milliliters of Gastrografin (Schering UK) diluted one to one with tap water is ingested by the patient one hour prior to the procedure to visualize the small bowel.

The perineum of the patient generally is examined in the left lateral position with systematic examination where the probe is placed first in a midsagittal plane on the perineal body to outline a general view of the pelvic floor and viscera and then rotated posteriorly onto the anus to define the posterior perineal structures. The anterior perineum is examined next by placing the probe at (but not in) the vaginal introitus. With this technique, images of the infralevator viscera, soft tissues, and the pelvic floor musculature are obtained at rest, during maximal straining, and with the patient asked to squeeze in order to prevent evacuation. Posterior perineal images show the anus and distal rectum, and the anal sphincters are visualized using coronal images of the anal canal and sphincter musculature, which are identified by holding the transducer head in a transverse plane at the introitus. Sagittal examination of the anterior perineum shows the distal vagina, bladder, and urethra, and it is used to identify contrast-filled enteric loops—if present—between the rectal and vaginal walls in the territory of the rectovaginal septum should the patient have an enterocele. This approach is also desirable in patients who have evacuatory difficulty following a hysterectomy and who may have vaginal vault prolapse consequent upon poor sacrospinous fixation. Towards the end of the procedure, patients are encouraged to evacuate as much of the intrarectal acoustic gel as possible.

Although the measurement of rectal morphologic parameters is of no clinical use, we have assessed this technique for the measurement of anorectal angles (ARAs) and anorectal junction (ARJ) movement in an attempt to compare it with defecography at rest and during maximal straining in an effort to validate the new modality (8). Real-time movement of the anterior and posterior pelvic floor elements during sustained straining and squeezing are clearly seen with DTP-US and provide an opportunity for measurement of several parameters, including the perimeters of the puborectalis muscle, as well as calculation of both the anorectal and posterior urethrovesical angles. These measurements correspond to those normally obtained during defecography and voiding cystourethrography, respectively.

The dynamic function of the puborectalis muscle can be examined and measured by this method during evacuation and straining. In the sagittal view, the distance between the posterior margin of the pubis and the posterior limit of the ARJ defines the perimeters of the puborectalis, with the difference in length between rest and squeeze representing normal shortening of the muscle during contraction. This measurement is shown schematically as D1 in Figure 3.2(ii).1 and is comparable to measurements

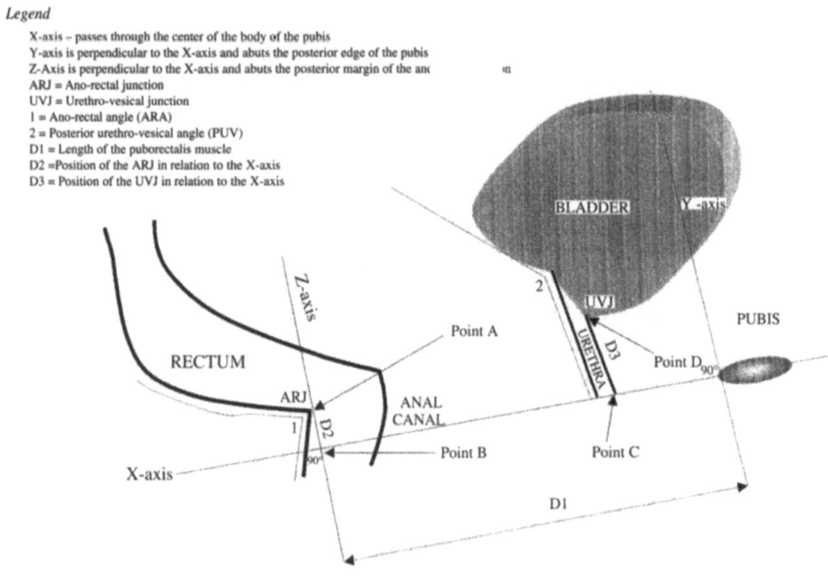

FIGURE 3.2(ii).1. Schematic representation of the pelvic floor at rest using sagittal DTP-US (vagina not shown). (Reprinted with permission from Beer-Gabel M, Teshler M, Barzilai N, Lurie Y, Malnick S, Bass D, and Zbar AP. Dynamic transperineal ultrasound in the diagnosis of pelvic floor disorders. Pilot study. Dis Colon Rectum. 2002;45:239–48.)

obtained with dynamic magnetic resonance imaging (MRI) (9). This measurement directly connects two lines (the *y* and *z* axes) that both lie perpendicular to a line passing through the mid point between the superior and inferior borders of the pubic symphysis. This equatorial line—designated as the *x* axis—is defined more easily by this technique than by conventional defecography because both cortical margins of the symphysis are more frequently readily visible. The *y* axis lies at the posterior limit of the pubis and the *z* axis crosses the posterior aspect of the ARJ. The ARA is measured easily at the confluence of a line forming the longitudinal axis of the anal canal with that of the posterior border of the rectal wall, and the movement of the ARJ is calculated in a coordinate system defined by the axes described above. The point where the *z* axis touches the posterior margin of the ARJ is called Point A and the point where the *z* axis crosses the *x* axis is called Point B. The distance between Points A and B is measured at rest and during sustained squeeze and strain, representing the vertical movement of the ARJ during these maneuvers. This measurement is shown as D2 in Figure 3.2(ii).1. Strict comparisons between these measures at defecography and during DTP-US cannot be made because there is a tendency for the ARJ to lie higher at rest in the left lateral position and for the ARJ to descend more precipitously during straining or attempted gel evacuation in the seated position.

The motion of the soft tissues of the anterior perineum is assessed using a similar coordinate reference system. The position of the urethrovesical junction (UVJ), which is important in the diagnosis of urinary stress incontinence and cystocele, is determined in relation to a perpendicular line drawn from the *x* axis (Point C) to the anterior margin of the bladder base (Point D) with the patient at rest, as described by Schaer et al. (10). Measurements are made and static images taken with a full bladder, although the extent of filling may affect the exact measurement of UVJ movement. The motion of the UVJ during maximal straining (i.e., the distance between Point C and Point D) represents the amount of bladder neck mobility and is shown as measurement D3 in Figure 3.2(ii).1. The posterior urethrovesical angle (PUV), as described by Green et al. (11), also may be measured accurately using DTP-US, where it is defined as the angle created by a line joining the urethral axis to the posterior margin of the bladder base.

When a rectocele is evident, its depth also may be measured accurately using the DTP-US technique; this is schematically shown in Figure 3.2(ii).2. This measurement is made by constructing two axes; the *v* axis (drawn perpendicular to the *x* axis already described and that passes through the anterior aspect of the anal canal) and the *w* axis (which is parallel to the *x* axis and that passes through the most anterior part of the rectocele). Point E is defined then as the point where the *w* axis crosses the most anterior part of the rectocele, and Point F is the point where the *v* and the *w* axes meet. The distance between Point E and Point F (designated as D4 in Figure 3.2(ii).2) is the measurable depth of the rectocele.

Legend:
V-axis passes through the anterior aspect of the anal canal at right angles to the X-axis
W-axis is a line drawn at right angles to the V-axis through the most anterior part of the rectocele
X-axis passes through the center of the body of the pubis
Point E = the most anterior part of the rectocele
Point F = junction of the V and W axes
D4 = the measured depth of the rectocele during maximal straining
RVS = Rectovaginal septum

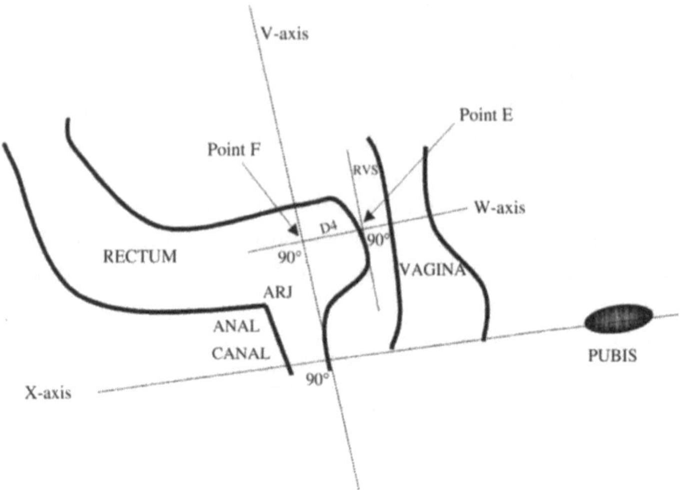

FIGURE 3.2(ii).2. Rectocele depth measurement using DTP-US. Schematic sagittal view of the rectum during maximal strain (bladder and urethra not shown). (Reprinted with permission Beer-Gabel M, Teshler M, Barzilai N, Lurie Y, Malnick S, Bass D, and Zbar AP. Dynamic transperineal ultrasound in the diagnosis of pelvic floor disorders. Pilot study. Dis Colon Rectum. 2002;45:239–48.)

DTP-US in Health and Disease

Axial images with static TP-US rivals those obtained with conventional endoanal probes (Figure 3.2(ii).3). Longitudinal (sagittal) views provide images of the rectoanal junction and an end-on view of the puborectalis bundle (Figure 3.2(ii).4), as well as providing high-resolution images of the perineal structures and the rectovaginal septum. The mucosa in the axial images is well recognized with a hyperechoic uncompressed image, having the potential of diagnosing hemorrhoids and rectal mucosal prolapse. Real-time dynamic imaging corresponds to the movement of the anterior and posterior perineal and infralevator compartments, with variation from the resting position during maximal straining providing evidence of a rectocele (Figure 3.2(ii).5), rectoanal intussusception (Figure 3.2(ii).6), and full-thickness rectal prolapse (Figure 3.2(ii).7). Specialized images may confirm the presence of unusual perirectal mesenchymal masses, which result in evacuatory difficulty (Figure 3.2(ii).8) and assist in the differentiation of a peritoneocele (defined as a widened rectovaginal septum alone) and an

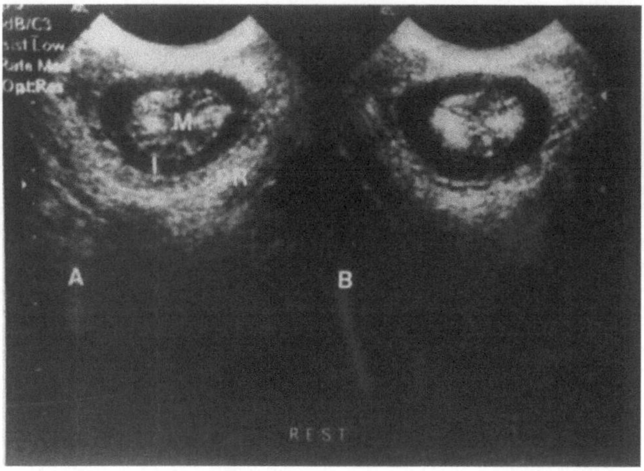

FIGURE 3.2(ii).3. Transverse dynamic transperineal ultrasound of the anal sphincters at the proximal sphincter level. A. The internal anal sphincter (designated as I) is seen as a hypoechoic ring and the puborectalis/external sphincter complex (at the left) appears as an echogenic U-shaped sling posterior to the internal anal sphincter (PR). The mucosa and submucosa (M) is seen as a central echoic luminal structure. B. A similar transverse image through the midsphincter scanned below the puborectalis level. (Reprinted with permission from Beer-Gabel M, Teshler M, Barzilai N, Lurie Y, Malnick S, Bass D, and Zbar AP. Dynamic transperineal ultrasound in the diagnosis of pelvic floor disorders. Pilot study. Dis Colon Rectum. 2002;45:239–48.)

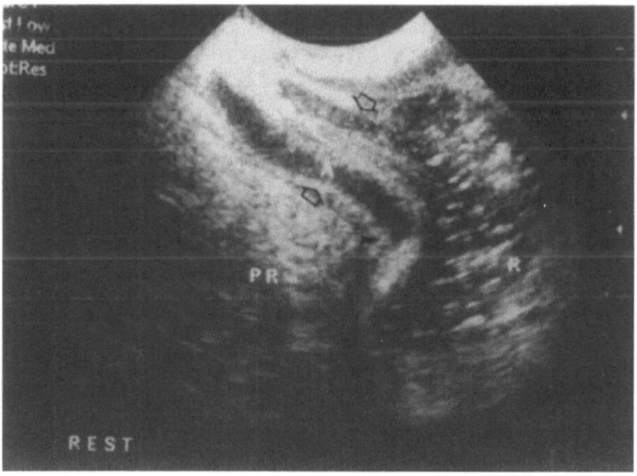

FIGURE 3.2(ii).4. Sagittal dynamic transperineal ultrasound of the anal canal and distal rectum. The internal anal sphincter (A) is seen as two longitudinal hypoechoic parallel layers (open arrows) lying on both sides of the lumen against the hyperechoic mucosa and submucosa. The puborectalis muscle (PR) is seen as a hyperechoic bundle posterior to the anorectal angle (arrowhead). The rectum (R) is filled with echogenic acoustic gel. (Reprinted with permission from Beer-Gabel M, Teshler M, Barzilai N, Lurie Y, Malnick S, Bass D, and Zbar AP. Dynamic transperineal ultrasound in the diagnosis of pelvic floor disorders. Pilot study. Dis Colon Rectum. 2002;45:239–48.)

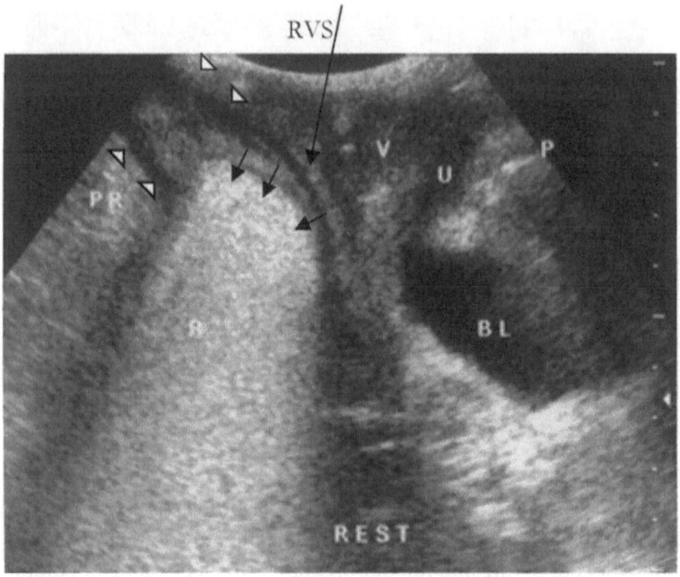

FIGURE 3.2(ii).5. Rectocele on DTP-US (short arrows). PR, puborectalis; R, rectum; BL, bladder; U, urethra; P, pubis; V, vagina; RVS, rectovaginal septum. Arrowheads point to the internal anal sphincter seen in mid-sagittal plane. (Reprinted with permission from Zbar AP, Lienemann A, Fritsch H, Beer-Gabel M, and Pescatgori M. Rectocele: pathogenesis and surgical management. Int J Colorectal Dis. 2003;18:369–84.)

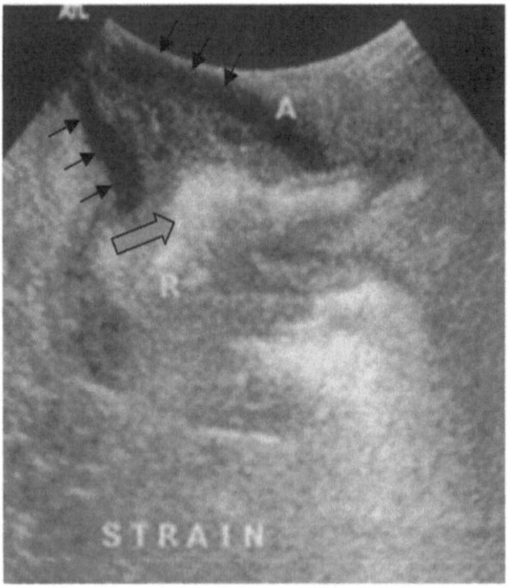

FIGURE 3.2(ii).6. Dynamic transperineal ultrasonography of rectoanal untussusception. The contrast-filled rectum can be seen to contain an intussuscepting leading edge (intussusceptum; black arrow) infolding into the apex of the anal canal. The hypoechoic IAS is marked by white arrows.

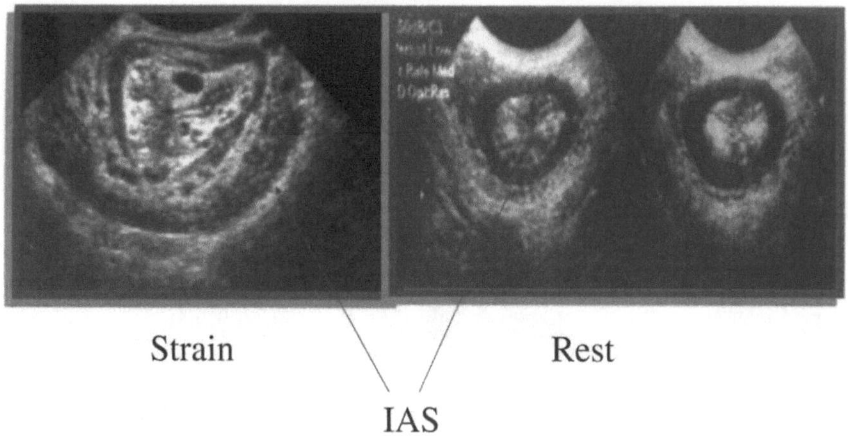

FIGURE 3.2(ii).7. Axial DTP-US image of a rectal prolapse showing edema of the rectal mucosa with vascular congestion.

enterocele (Figure 3.2(ii).9). The anterior compartment may be assessed for abnormal widening of the urethrovesical angle (somewhat dependent upon the filling status of the bladder during dynamic imaging), as well as in the diagnosis of a cystocele (Figure 3.2(ii).10).

In a recently published study from our group, we assessed 33 women who presented with long-standing difficulty in evacuation, comparing blinded assessment of defecography with DTP-US (8) where evacuation difficulty exceeded six months in duration, where there was less than one bowel movement every four days (or longer), or if 25% or greater of bowel

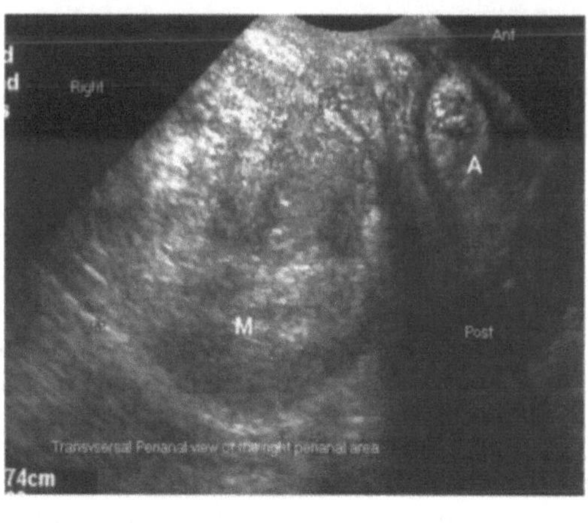

FIGURE 3.2(ii)8. Sagittal view of a perirectal mesenchymal mass (M) causing defacation difficulty. The anal canal is labeled as A.

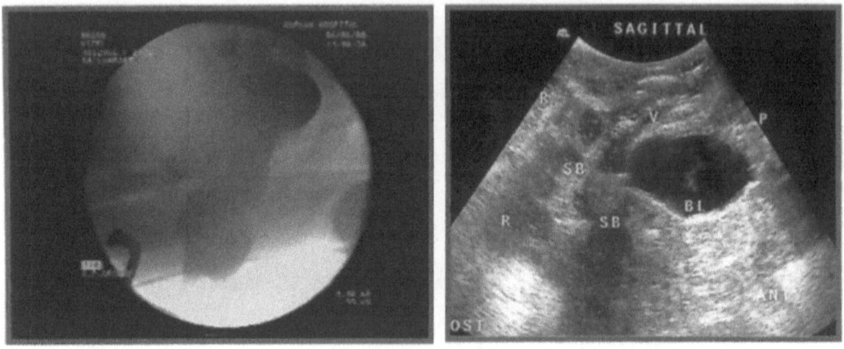

FIGURE 3.2(ii).9. The left-hand figure shows a defecating proctogram with an enterocele. This is also evident on the DTP-US (right-hand figure) where small bowel loops (SB) are seen distending the rectovaginal septum. BL, bladder; R, rectum; V, vagina; P, pubis.

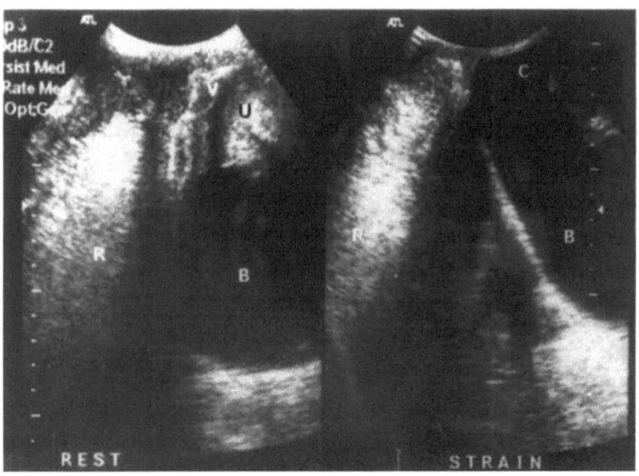

FIGURE 3.2(ii).10. Sagittal dynamic transperineal ultrasound at rest and during straining showing a cystocele. The rectum (R), vagina (V), urethra (U), and the bladder (B) are well seen. At rest, the bladder is seen as an anechoic structure distended with urine with the urethra appearing as a hypoechoic channel. Posteriorly, the vagina is outlined by contrast and is seen as a hypoechoic line. The rectum is filled with echogenic contrast. During straining, the anterior part of the rectum moves anteriorly to form a small rectocele. The anechoic bladder prolapses downward to form a large cystocele (C). (Reprinted with permission from Beer-Gabel M, Teshler M, Barzilai N, Lurie Y, Malnick S, Bass D, and Zbar AP. Dynamic transperineal ultrasound in the diagnosis of pelvic floor disorders. Pilot study. Dis Colon Rectum. 2002;45:239–48.

movements were accompanied by excessive straining as previously reported and defined (12,13). Comparisons were made with a standard proctographic technique where comparative measurements were recorded of the ARA (at rest and during straining) and of displacement of the ARJ during maximal straining from a position of rest.

The overall diagnostic categorization with both techniques showed good agreement for the main diagnoses of rectocele, enterocele, rectoanal intussusception, and rectal prolapse. In general, more enteroceles are diagnosed with DTP-US, particularly when there is a coincident rectocele and in the post-hysterectomy patient—a point of considerable import when the surgeon is contemplating operating on the patient presenting with evacuation difficulty and where the dominant finding is that of a sizeable rectocele. Dynamic transperineal ultrasonography also tends to show a greater multiplicity of pelvic pathologies when compared with defecography in this unselected patient group. Our group has demonstrated a high correlation between resting and straining ARA and measured displacement of the ARJ on maximal straining, validating this technique (Table 3.2(ii)-1).

What is clear is that the technique is simple, easily trained, inexpensive, and well tolerated. It dynamically provides useful information concerning the anterior, as well as the posterior, pelvic floor and perineal structures where there is frequent coincident pathology of note, and it appears to provide more information than transintroital US, which has been used in

TABLE 3.2(ii)-1. Measurements of the anorectal angle (ARA) at rest and during maximal straining and the position at rest and movement during maximal straining of the anorectal junction (ARJ) as calculated using defecography and DTP-US (mean difference value obtained by DTP-US subtracted from the value measured at defecography, CI 95% confidence interval).*

	Mean ± SEM	Mean difference	95% CI	*P*
ARA at rest				0.92
Defecography	102.9 ± 3.75	−0.39	−8.29 to +7.5	
DTP-US	103.3 ± 2.86		—	
ARA during straining				0.09
Defecography	123.3 ± 4.32	+6.91	−0.75 to +14.57	
DTP-US	116.4 ± 3.32		—	
ARJ position at rest (mm)				0.72
Defecography	14.17 ± 4.9	1.23	−5.89 to +8.35	
DTP-US	12.94 ± 3.4		—	
ARJ movement during straining (mm)				0.49
Defecography	34.73 ± 10.6	2.78	−5.63 to +1.19	
DTP-US	31.94 ± 5.14		—	

* Reprinted with permission from Beer-Gabel M, Teshler M, Schechtman E, and Zbar AP. Dynamic transperineal ultrasound vs. defecography in patients with evacuatory difficulty a pilot study. Int J Colorectal Dis. 2003. e-pub DOI 10.1007/s00384-003-0508-x.

urinary stress incontinence, transvaginal delineation of the anal sphincter (vide infra), and transintroital balloon sonography (14–16). In this regard, DTP-US appears to result in less perineal distortion than any of these other described techniques. At present, the full potential of this technique is unclear. Sagittal views afforded by DTP-US may assist in the definition of the rostral extent of sphincteric defects and transsphincteric fistula-in-ano without requiring the complex software necessary for three-dimensional (3D) endoanal sonography or of its comparatively difficult image interpretation. Moreover, the images provided of the undistorted mucosa and submucosal space may assist in the delineation of the course of fistulae and their internal openings so necessary for successful mucosal advancement anoplasty.

It should be recognized, however, that there are some inherent problems with this new technique. It has a significant learning curve and requires considerable dedication. In some patients, there is reticence to carry out either provocative maneuvers of full straining (perhaps because of the proximity of the probe or the position of the operator's hand to the perineum), resulting in the risk of under diagnosis. The position of these patients in left lateral is certainly not physiological, and straining of gel can only represent, at best, a simulated attempt at defecation, which may fail to diagnose conditions where maximal straining is a physiological posture at the end of "defecation" is important. These conditions notably include full-thickness rectal prolapse and rectoanal intussusception, which cluster in such patients. The newer techniques discussed in this book, such as dynamic MRI, are more expensive and are not as readily allocated or available for functional anorectal disorders (17), and they too do not represent true physiological simulation of defecation unless open architecture units are available (18).

Summary

The wide availability of such technology and its ease of use, patient tolerance, and low cost make this an attractive imaging modality in patients presenting with specialized and complex complaints presenting to a pelvic floor unit. Dynamic transperineal ultrasonography necessitates further prospective evaluation in specific subgroups of patients and in the prospective assessment of the effects hysterectomy imposes on the pelvic floor and perineal structures. The avoidance of complex software programs and computerized algorithms (as part of 3D endoanal ultrasonography or dynamic MRI) or of radiation exposure (particularly in extended defecographic procedures) are significant advantages of this modality (19).

References

1. Maglinte DD, Kelvin FM, Fitzgerald K, Hale DS, and Benson T. Association of compartment defects in pelvic floor dysfunction. AJR Am J Roentgenol. 1999;172:439–44.

2. Kenton K, Shott S, and Brubaker L. The anatomic and functional variability of rectocele in women. Int Urogynecol J Pelvic Floor Dysfunct. 1999;10:96–9.
3. Kelvin FM, Hale DS, Maglinte DD, Patten BJ, and Benson JT. Female pelvic organ prolapse: diagnostic contribution of dynamic cystoproctography and comparison with physical examination. AJR Am J Roentgenol. 1999;173:31–7.
4. Siproudhis L, Robert A, Vilotte J, Bretagne JF, Heresbach D, Raoul JL, and Gosselin M. How accurate is clinical examination in diagnosing and quantifying pelvirectal disorders? A prospective study in a group of 50 patients complaining of defecatory difficulties. Dis Colon Rectum. 1993;36:430–8.
5. Kleinübing H Jr, Janini JF, Malafaia O, Brenner S, and Pinho M. Transperineal ultrasonography: new method to image the anorectal region. Dis Colon Rectum. 2000;43:1572–4.
6. Piloni V. Dynamic imaging of the pelvic floor with transperineal sonography. Tech Coloproctol. 2001;5:103–5.
7. Beer-Gabel M, Teshler M, Barzilai N, Lurie Y, Malnick S, Bass D, and Zbar AP. Dynamic transperineal ultrasound in the diagnosis of pelvic floor disorders. Pilot study. Dis Colon Rectum. 2002;45:239–48.
8. Beer-Gabel M, Teshler M, Schechtman E, and Zbar AP. Dynamic transperineal ultrasound versus defecography in patients with evacuatory difficulty: a pilot study. Int J Colorect Dis. 2004;19:60–7.
9. Healy JC, Halligan S, Reznek RH, Watson S, Phillips RK, and Armstrong P. Patterns of prolapse in women and symptoms of pelvic floor weakness: assessment of MR imaging. Radiology. 1997;203:77–81.
10. Schaer GN, Koechli OR, Schuessler B, and Haller U. Perineal ultrasound for evaluating the bladder neck in urinary stress incontinence. Obstet Gynecol. 1995;85:220–4.
11. Green TH. Urinary stress incontinence: differential diagnosis, pathophysiology and management. Am J Obstet Gynecol. 1975;122:368–400.
12. Favetta U, Amato A, Interisano A, and Pescatori M. Clinical, manometri and sonographic assessment of the anal sphincters: a comparative prospective study. Int J Colorectal Dis. 1996;11:163–6.
13. Zbar AP, Aslam M, Gold DM, Gatzen C, Gosling A, and Kmiot WA. Parameters of the rectoanal inhibitory reflex in patients with idiopathic fecal incontinence and chronic constipation. Dis Colon Rectum. 1998;41:200–8.
14. Koebl H, Bernaschek G, and Dentinger J. Assessment of female urinary incontinence by introital sonography. J Clin Ultrasound. 1990;18:370–4.
15. Quinn MJ, Beynon J, Mortensen NJ, and Smith PJ. Transvaginal endosonography: a new method to study the anatomy of the lower urinary tract in urinary stress incontinence. Br J Urol. 1988;62:414–18.
16. Poen AC, Felt-Bersma RJ, Cuesta MA, and Meuwissen GM. Vaginal endosonography of the anal sphincter complex is important in the assessment of faecal incontinence and perianal sepsis. Br J Surg. 1998;85:359–63.
17. Lienemann A, Anthuber C, Baron A, Kohr P, and Reiser M. Dynamic MR colpocystorectography assessing pelvic floor descent. Eur Radiol. 1997; 7:1309–17.
18. Schoenenberger AW, Debatin JF, Guldenschuh I, Hany TF, Steiner P, and Krestin GP. Dynamic MR defecography with a superconducting open-configuration MR system. Radiology. 1998;206:641–6.
19. Beer-Gabel M and Zbar AP. Dynamic transperineal ultrasonography (DTP-US) in patients presenting with obstructed defecation. Tech Coloproctol. 2002;6:141.

B. Transvaginal Endosonography in the Assessment of the Anorectal Sphincter

Andrea Frudinger and Andrew P. Zbar

Introduction

There are comparatively few reports in the literature concerning this technique, and it has not gained an established place in coloproctology because of relatively poor resolution of the anterior external anal sphincter, the perineal body, or rectovaginal fistulae (1,2). Many pelvic floor units combine the use of endoanal and transvaginal ultrasonography in the assessment of their patients, and it is unclear how much (if anything) the transvaginal examination either demonstrates or contributes to the anorectal assessment or to specific decision making. The technique has largely not been adopted by the colorectal fraternity because it has been considered relatively inaccurate in the assessment of the anterior EAS, as there are anatomical limitations imposed on the axial images (3), although it may be used in units where there is the requirement for post-obstetric assessment of the anal sphincters when there is no available endoanal probe. Here, only the grossest anterior EAS defects will be visualized. Moreover, the hoped-for delineation by transvaginal ultrasound of the sonographic appearances of the perineal body structure (and definition of what may represent a perineocele) has been disappointing (4,5).

Technical Details

Standard probes as used either for endoanal or prostatic scanning may be employed for this technique (6), or one may use dedicated endovaginal probes as typically used by gynecologists for the assessment of ovarian pathology (7), latterly with 3D transvaginal reconstruction (8) or recently by our group in the diagnosis of acute pelvic appendicitis (9). The probe needs to be inserted at least three centimeters into the vagina; therefore, the procedure is different from transintroital ultrasonography (10). Moderate balloon distension is required for adequate acoustic coupling and reasonable resolution of the anal sphincter on probe withdrawal. Examinations may be made either in the left lateral or the supine (dorsal) position. Adequate probe movement with the probe tip directed posteriorly beyond the hymenal ring will define the cross-sectional appearance of the anal canal, the perineal body, and the puborectalis sling. Inherent differences exist between the transvaginal and endoanal ultrasonographic approaches. With transvaginal sonography, there is no closed EAS ring in the most proximal part of the anal canal. Here, the fibers of the sphincter move forwards and downwards to form a ring only in the lower part of the anal canal so that

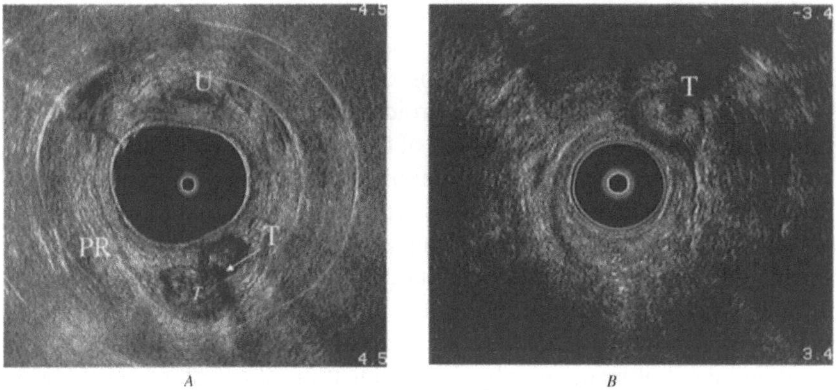

FIGURE 3.2(ii).1. A. Sixty-seven year old female with a palpable benign expression (T) in the rectovaginal septum seen on transvaginal ultrasound using a B&K 360 degree rotating 10 megahertz probe. Orientation: U, urethra; PR, puborectalis sling. B. The same, well-delineated expansion (T) on endoanal ultrasound, compressing the external anal sphincter.

this effect cannot be visualized with the transvaginal technique, making the interpretation of EAS defects unreliable.

Figures 3.2(ii).1 and 3.2(ii).2 show the value of the transvaginal technique in the delineation of the extent of infiltration of masses invading the rectovaginal space.

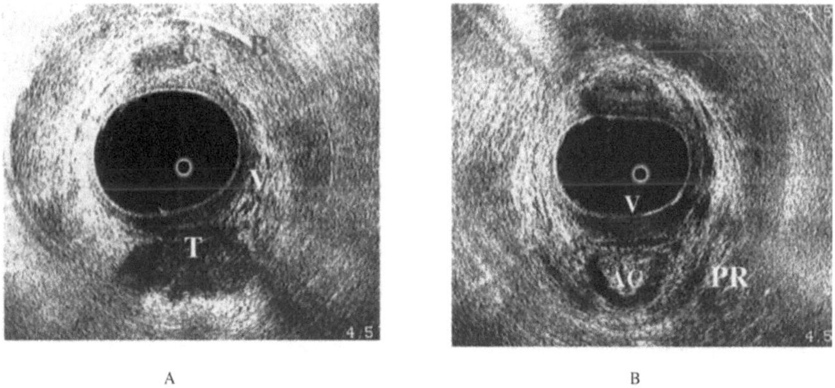

FIGURE 3.2(ii).2. A. A 75-year old female with an ill-defined malignant expansion (T) involving the posterolateral vaginal wall and infiltrating the rectovaginal septum. The image was taken above the anorectal verge using a B&K 360 degree rotating 10 megahertz probe. Orientation: U, urethra; B, bladder; V, vaginal wall. B. The same 75-year old female. The transvaginal image was taken at the anorectal verge (PR) using a B&K 360 degree rotating 10 megahertz probe. Orientation: U, urethra; V, vaginal wall; AC, anal canal; PR, puborectalis sling.

Published Results

In this technique, the rectum is collapsed with visualization of the mucosal folds and submucosa and the hemorroidal plexus/cushions as is seen with transperineal ultrasound. Withdrawal of the probe after identification of the puborectalis sling shows the anorectal junction as a change in diameter of the hyperechoic shadow as it moves from a larger flattened rectum to a well-defined annular anal canal. Transvaginal endosonography does not provide adequate separation of the puborectalis from the deep component of the EAS (11). The appearance of the EAS as a complete or incomplete ring (defining anterior EAS defects) is akin to that obtained with conventional endoanal ultrasonography. The delineation of an inferomedial slope of the anterior EAS in women needs to be defined using this modality, and the appearance can be difficult to appreciate, limiting the use of the technique in subtle and incomplete EAS tears (12).

The diagnosis and calibration of hemorrhoids with transvaginal ultrasound has not been reported adequately, although it is possible because of the lack of mucosal distortion with directional color Doppler (13). In their original study, Sultan and colleagues assessed 10 healthy females and 10 patients presenting with fecal incontinence using transvaginal endosonography (1) and were able to define sphincter defects in all cases, each of which was confirmed at surgery. The limited value of this small study was confirmed by Alexander et al. (2), where 28 women were assessed with a side-fire transrectal probe modified for transvaginal use. These authors also reported accurate diagnosis of low rectovaginal fistulae and anovaginal fistulae, particularly in patients presenting with fecal leakage after unsuccessful primary repairs of fourth degree obstetric-related perineal lacerations. For the diagnosis of rectovaginal fistula, supplementation of the image may be provided by the ultrasonic identification of water flow following transrectal instillation into the vaginal vault using a 10 Fr. catheter positioned at the anorectal junction. In a publication by Frudinger et al. (3), comparison of transvaginal and endoanal ultrasound in 47 patients presenting with fecal incontinence proved comparatively disappointing, showing sphincter defects in only one-half of the cases examined, where multiple attempts at transvaginal scanning were required in some cases because single-shot scanning proved too limited.

However, this view was refuted in a study by Stewart and Wilson (5) with 50 patients in all examined with the two techniques (32 presenting with fecal incontinence), where although both types of ultrasound were in agreement in 40 of 44 cases; there were four patients who had normal endoanal ultrasounds with an anterior defect of the EAS demonstrated by transvaginal endosonography and who subsequently had operative confirmation of a sphincter defect. This study calls into the question some of the image interpretation. In general, the measured IAS thickness using endoanal ultrasound appears to be less than that obtained with transvaginal endosonography, which may have to do with the luminal distortion exerted on the anal canal by the endoanal probe.

Summary

In theory, transvaginal ultrasonic imaging of the anal sphincters has several advantages. The anus lays undisturbed, providing accurate determination of IAS damage and thickness, definition of the subepithelial space for determination of the internal opening of fistulae, and potential categorization of hemorrhoids and what could constitute the normal perineal body. It would appear that defects of either the IAS or the EAS, which are of critical importance in operative decision making for patients presenting with fecal incontinence, are not readily demonstrated using this technique where transvaginal imaging is particularly limited in showing the proximal anal canal and in definition of the perineal soft tissues (and their integrity) below the introital level. This may arise as the vaginal axis diverges from that of the anal canal because the latter cannot be adequately scanned in a plane parallel to its longitudinal axis. Moreover, although oblique views of the puborectalis sling are accurately defined with the transvaginal probe, the posterior wall of the anal canal and the distal anterior anal canal are incompletely viewed because of poor acoustic contact. Any attempt to assist in contact appears to distort the perineum, creating reverberation artifact, and resulting in a non-anatomical alignment of the rectovaginal space and its soft-tissues.

As a result in practice, extensive distal IAS and EAS defects will tend to be missed using this technique. This view, as experienced by Frudinger and colleagues (3), may be partly obviated by a more dedicated transvaginal biplane probe and by gentle pressure on the perineal body with the patient supine as the probe is withdrawn. For these reasons, the technology has not advanced over the years and it is hardly used in colopropctologic practice except to confirm the findings noted either on endoanal or transperineal sonography. In theory, it may have a place in the delineation of a high anterior EAS defect in a patient with an attendant anal canal stenosis that does not permit the placement of a standard endoanal probe and in the occasional patient with complex perianal Crohn's disease and an anovaginal fistula where it may complement transperineal sonography in documentation of the course of the fistulous track. It is certainly a valuable tool for the visualization of the rectovaginal space and expansions involving this part of the pelvic structures.

References

1. Sultan AH, Loder PB, Bartram CI, Kamm MA, and Hudson CN. Vaginal endosonography: new approach to image the undisturbed anal sphincter. Dis Colon Rectum. 1994;37:1296–9.

2. Alexander AR, Liu J, Menton DA, and Nagle DA. Fecal incontinence: transvaginal ultrasound evaluation of anatomic causes. Radiology. 1996;199:529–32.
3. Frudinger A, Bartram CI, and Kamm MA. Transvaginal versus anal endosonography for detecting damage to the anal sphincter. AJR Am J Roentgenol. 1997;168:1435–8.
4. Sultan AH, Kamm MA, Hudson CN, Thomas JM, and Bartram CI. Anal sphincter disruption during vaginal delivery. N Engl J Med. 1993;321:1905–11.
5. Stewart L and Wilson SR. Transvaginal sonography of the anal sphincter: reliable or not? AJR Am J Roentgenol. 1999;173:179–85.
6. Frentzel-Beyne B, Schwartz J, and Aurich B. Die transrektale prostatosonographie (TPS). CT-Sonographie. 1982;2:68–75.
7. Alcazar JL, Galan MJ, Ceamanos C, and Garcia-Manero M. Transvaginal grayscale and color Doppler sonography in primary ovarian cancer and metastatic tumors to the ovary. J Ultrasound Med. 2003;22:243–7.
8. Kurjak A, Kupesic S, Sparac V, Prka M, and Bekavac I. The detection of stage I ovarian cancer by three-dimensional sonography and power Doppler. Gynecol Oncol. 2003;90:258–64.
9. Caspi B, Zbar AP, Mavor E, Hagay Z, and Appelman Z. The contribution of transvaginal ultrasound in the diagnosis of acute appendicitis: an observational study. Ultrasound Obstet Gynecol. 2003;21:273–6.
10. Koebl H, Bernaschek G, and Dentinger J. Assessment of fgemale urinary incontinence by introital sonography. J Clin Ultrasound. 1990;18:370–4.
11. Fucini C, Elbetti C, and Messerini L. Anatomic plane of separation between external anal sphincter and puborectalis muscle: clinical implications. Dis Colon Rectum. 1999;42:374–9.
12. Sandridge DA and Thorp JM Jr. Vaginal endosonography in the assessment of the anorectum. Obstet Gynecol. 1995;86:1007–9.
13. Jaspersen G, Koerner T, Schorr W, and Hammar CH. Proctoscopic Doppler ultrasound in diagnostics and treatment of bleeding haemorrhoids. Dis Colon Rectum. 1993;36:942–5.

Chapter 3.2(iii) Three-Dimensional Endoanal Ultrasound in Proctological Practice

Andrew P. Zbar and Andrea Frudinger

Introduction

Conventional axial endoanal ultrasonography is somewhat limited in its utility to adequately appreciate the longitudinal extent of normal anal structures and that of perianal pathology (1). The linear extent of disease is of considerable importance in perirectal sepsis where it may adequately define the relationship of some complex fistulous tracks to the main sphincter muscle mass. In fecal incontinence, there is some evidence that less than satisfactory functional results following overlapping external anal sphincteroplasty can result from an incomplete repair of the full extent of the external anal sphincter (EAS) muscle defect itself (2,3). Here, there is a fine balance between excessive mobilization of the EAS for adequate repair and devascularization/denervation of the muscle that results in a less-than-optimal outcome, providing some potential advantages in a preoperative imaging modality that accurately defines the rostral extent of the EAS defect. This view would be reinforced by the available results of techniques that provide high-resolution coronal images of the anal canal [most notably, endoanal magnetic resonance imaging (MRI)] and that appear to correlate anatomically with conventional endoanal ultrasonographic images and with operative findings at sphincteroplasty (4–10).

Three-dimensional (3D) endoanal ultrasound represents a novel method of reconstruction from close-stepped axial endosonographic images of the anal canal using computerized software with data interpolation to create 3D images of the anal canal (11). Although not widely available and still somewhat experimental, the potential advantages of this modality will be to define constitutive gender and age differences in the normal anal canal and to validate this technique for clinical preoperative use in decision making of complex and recurrent high trans- and suprasphincteric fistula-in-ano where there tends to be poor coupling of conventional endoanal probes against the puborectalis, and consequently a relative inability with traditional technology in adequate definition of the translevator extent of disease. In theory, 3D endoanal reconstructed images also may assist in defining the morphological reasons for poor functional outcome due to incomplete overlapping EAS sphincteroplasty (12,13).

This chapter presents a personal view of the potential benefits of 3D reconstructed ultrasonographic technology in clinical coloproctological practice.

Technical Aspects

The basic technique of 3D endoanal ultrasound utilizes a standard endoanal 7.5–10 megahertz probe (Hawk 2102 B-K Sandhofen, Copenhagen, Denmark) with 360-degree rotation (focal range; 2.0–45 mm) where axial images are stored at 0.2-millimeter step intervals using a special colorectal pullback mover as a mechanical rig. The B&K Medical pullback mover can be operated at different levels of resolution. Data is captured on a PC-video card system for 3D-interpolated reconstruction over the length of the internal anal sphincter (IAS)/external anal sphincter (EAS) complex. Each volume dataset is seeded in the axial plane for slicing in coronal and sagittal orientations and multiplanar volume set identification utilizing Voxblast ® Windows software (Version 1.3.1., VayTek Inc., Fairfield, Iowa). This reconstruction begins at the commencement of the recognizable puborectalis muscle and is extended to the most distal part of the subcutaneous EAS muscle for analysis. The most distal component for analysis is recognized as the last caudal reverberation echoes detectable. Anteriorly, the EAS generally is measured in the mid sagittal plane from the proximal formation of a complete muscular ring (given the standard differences between the genders), and as with conventional endoanal axial ultrasound images, the extent and morphology of the IAS is more readily identified for coronal and sagittal reconstructions. Mediolateral markers are made for the EAS, transverse perinii, puboanalis, and bulbospongiosis muscles. Anteroposterior muscle lengths are assessed in mid sagittal reconstructions, with the IAS length measured mid coronally. Sphincter symmetry is detected by sequential slicing of the coronal dataset.

The data volume obtained is outlined at precise points on the clock face, as well as with mediolateral muscle markings that can be fixed within data points for recognition in any plane and for identification and measurement using the Scion computer package (Scion Image; Frederick, MD) for determination of the anal canal length (anteroposterior/sagittal), puborectalis dimensions (end sagittal/reconstructed), and IAS calculation (mid-coronal).

3D Endoanal Ultrasound Use in Health and Disease

Normal Anatomical Variations

Figure 3.2(iii).1 shows a normal EAS complex using 3D reconstruction. Using this technique, EAS subdivisions, as demonstrated using endoanal magnetic resonance imaging (MRI), are not visible (8). In keeping with standard axial imaging reports and those of endoanal MRI (8), Gold and colleagues have confirmed a generally longer EAS and anal canal length in males when compared with females (11). These have been reported as a mean anal canal length in males of 32.6 millimeters (±5.3 mm) compared with 25.1 millimeters (±3.4 mm) in females ($p < 0.001$; 95% CI, 3.4–11.8 mm). The differences in the IAS between males and females were found to be 25.6 millimeters (±6.3 mm) versus 19.8 millimeters (±4.2 mm), respectively ($p < 0.02$; 95% CI, 0.9–10.9 mm). This finding is complicated, however, because the mean proportion of the IAS/total anal canal length appears to be roughly equivalent in both sexes at around 78% of the total anal canal. The overall mean EAS length in the male has been reported by this group as 32.6 millimeters (±5.3 mm) compared with the female at 15.3 millimeters (±2.8 mm) ($p < 0.001$; 95% CI, 13.4–21.4 mm). Figure 3.2(iii).2 shows the standard two-dimensional (2D) endoanal ultrasound images at different anal canal levels juxtaposed with the 3D reconstructed image of

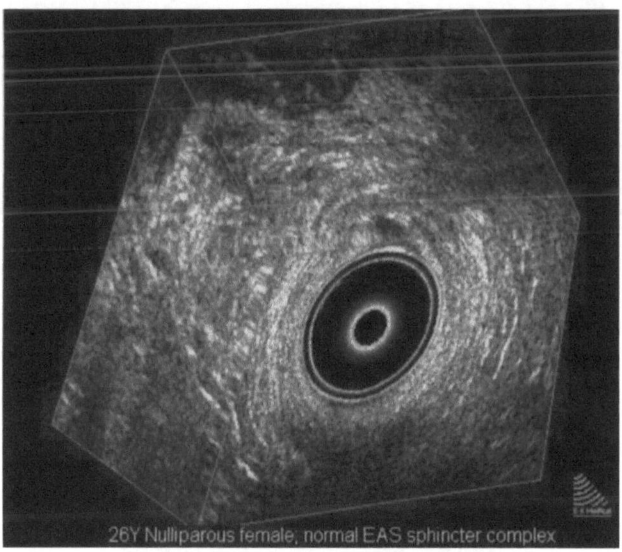

FIGURE 3.2(iii).1. Three-dimensional reconstruction of a normal female nulliparous anal sphincter.

the entire anal canal in a nulliparous woman. Figure 3.2(iii).3 shows the comparative 3D image in a normal male.

Attempts have been made by this group of authors to allocate station-specific tonic motor activity to anatomically defined correlative images (14), although these studies should be viewed with caution (15). In this respect, it should be recognized that these approaches are strictly constructs because only about 60% of the resting anal tone is attributed solely to IAS tonic contraction (16–18). The designation of manometric zones to functional parts of morphological reconstructions has been equated with the recognizable limits of the puborectalis muscle, the puborectalis/EAS overlap, the EAS/IAS overlap, and the distal EAS. Whereas these studies have shown that the anal canal length in males is longer than that of females as a direct result of a longer EAS (without any recognizable difference in puborectalis length or in anteroposterior IAS/EAS orientation), it appears that the anterior EAS occupies less of the anal canal in the female when compared with the male (38% vs 58%, respectively; $p < 0.001$). If this data is true, it would appear that the puborectalis muscle occupies a significantly larger proportion of the anal canal in women (61% vs 41%, respectively; $p = 0.02$), and because it has been shown that there is a clear anatomical separation between the puborectalis and the deep component of the EAS, these find-

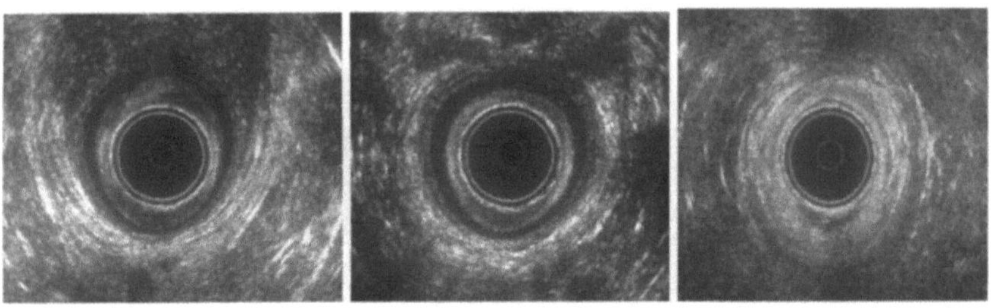

2-D AES, Nullipara, high anal canal (puborectalis sling)

2-D AES. Nullipara, mid anal canal (transverse perineii level)

2-D AES. Low anal canal, subcutaneous external anal sphincter

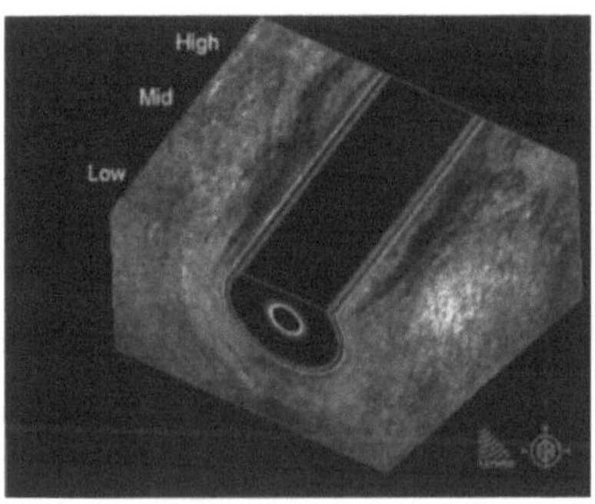

3-D reconstruction. Nulliparous female. Levels of the anal canal and corresponding musculature (in comparison with the 2-D images above).

FIGURE 3.2(iii).2. Two-dimensional endoanal ultrasonographic images of the different levels of the anal sphincter with a 3D total anal canal reconstruction (female).

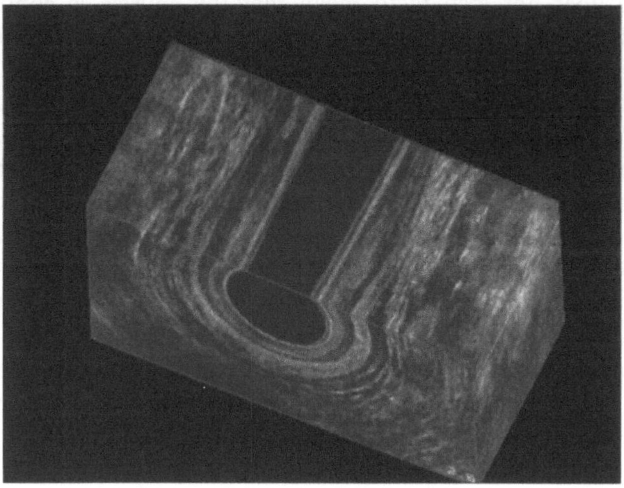

FIGURE 3.2(iii).3. Three-dimensional reconstruction of a normal male anal sphincter.

ings would suggest that this area should be revisited in the dissecting room (19). No detectable differences in IAS length have been shown utilizing this technique (as confirmed by our group using endoanal magnetic resonance imaging) or in its overall relationship to total anal canal length.

In fact, these findings are of considerable importance, where our group has shown previously that constitutive IAS/EAS overlap is limited in some patients presenting with EAS atrophy and fecal incontinence, as well as in some patients with chronic anal fissure. Here, inadvertent internal anal sphincterotomy is likely to be a major contributor to postoperative fecal soiling by rendering the distal anal canal relatively unsupported where there is this preexistent anatomical configuration (20). Moreover, these studies utilizing 3D endoanal ultrasound to attribute functional muscle disposition have proved somewhat contradictory to manometric findings where the high-pressure zone (HPZ) length at rest has been shown to extend caudally beyond the IAS termination and where the mean resting anal pressure in both genders has been suggested as being located at the IAS termination. In these studies, the suggestion that the upper extent of the HPZ is located caudal to the most recognizable parts of the IAS is at variance with vectorvolume data provided by our group, which has shown that there are no differences in HPZ length at rest following lateral internal anal sphincterotomy for topically resistant chronic anal fissure between patients who have continent or incontinent outcomes (21,22).

However, care must be taken in the interpretation of the study by Williams and colleagues (14), where functional activity is attributed to the morphological recognition of a muscle group because the mere presence of a muscle does not ipso facto mean that this muscle is contributing to recorded pressure. Moreover, there appears to be a moderate difficulty with the 3D endoanal ultrasound technique in the definition of the EAS/puborectalis orientation, providing conflict between the results serially reported by the same group at St. Mark's hospital (11,14,23). Squeeze pressures using this technology have been shown to be maximally located at the EAS/puborectalis overlap point (although located somewhat more distally in women), with a longer overall demonstrable subcutaneous EAS in men that appears to be associated with a higher percentage of the maximal squeeze pressure contribution in women. These results also would appear at variance with observed manometry, although given the enhanced role of the puborectalis muscle in squeeze pressure generation proposed by these workers, this finding provides an explanation why some patients remain relatively continent even when large sections of the EAS are divided as in high transsphincteric fistula surgery.

The 3D technique also provides unique views of the puboanalis muscle—a striated muscle derived from the puborectalis that enters the longitudinal muscle of the anal canal and that provides an ultrasonographically recognizable landmark. This muscle is recognized as a low reflective structure located medial to the puborectalis sling high in the anal canal (see Chapter 1).

3D Endoanal Ultrasound in Fecal Incontinence

As outlined above, gender variations in IAS/EAS morphology and disposition have been suggested as primary causes of continence differences when inadvertent or deliberate sphincter injury is undertaken. The story of postoperative incontinence is much more complicated than this, but what is clear from these and other modality studies of the sphincter mass and orientation in incontinence is that the traditional view as advanced by axial anal endosonography by Sultan et al. (24) is overly simplistic. It would seem more realistic to recognize that there are segmental constitutive differences in individuals of both sexes that may lead to predictable functional disturbance in some patients even after minimal surgeries (22,25). Three-dimensional endoanal ultrasound has shown that the visible length of EAS tears correlates with the destruction angle of the EAS defect—in effect, how far apart the sphincter ends are separated. This phenomenon is perhaps reflective of the fibroelastic tone of the sphincter and confirmed in the study by Gold and colleagues for both IAS and EAS defects (11). Such wide defects are important to define preoperatively as they alert the surgeon to the fact that these tears are of proportionate length—information that may lead to a broader EAS sphincteroplasty and a better potential long-term postsphincteroplasty outcome, although this needs to be tempered with overzealous EAS mobilization. This also may explain the relatively poor long-term outcomes already reported by experts in the field using conventional technology to guide repair (26) because sphincteroplasty failures tend to correlate with persistent EAS defects even when the angle of the recognizable defect has been reduced (27). These reconstructed images are also more likely to define cases of IAS atrophy in patients presenting with passive fecal incontinence where standardized measurements tend to be made and where the IAS thickness appears most symmetrical—about four to five millimeters rostral to its termination (28,29).

3D Endoanal Ultrasound in Perirectal Sepsis and Fistula in ano

Conventional endoanal ultrasonography has difficulty in defining lateral extrasphincteric fistulae (by virtue of the focal distance of the probe), trans- or supralevator disease (because of poor coupling of the endoanal probe with the rectal luminal surface above the puborectalis), and in the distinction of burnt-out fistula tracks from areas of recurrent or residual recrudescent disease. The literature on the use of 3D endoanal ultrasonography in complex perirectal sepsis is at present limited; however, since this modality is reconstructed from endoluminal images, the same limitations would be expected to apply (30). This technique currently is not sufficiently real time to permit extended dynamic hydrogen peroxide enhancement (31). The advantages of this technique are unclear and somewhat specialized, perhaps defining echogenic breaches in the submucosa as internal openings in multiple-operated patients where clinical examination is unreliable. In this, the only prospective randomized study in perirectal sepsis compares endoanal MRI with hydrogen peroxide-enhanced 3D reconstructed endoanal ultrasonography (32). Circuitous secondary tracks appear if anything to be better defined using MRI, although there was no operative correlation of fistula anatomy in this small study, and there was a considerable time delay between the two individual investigative examinations (median 66 days; IQR = 21–160 days).

At this time, the use of this new modality for the assessment of complex perirectal infection must be regarded as experimental, and it is unclear what advantages the technique offers over surface MRI, which now appears to be the gold standard of investigation (33). We also has some reservations concerning the acoustic impedance inherent in the use of conventional endoanal probes, where acoustic shadowing of intersphincteric collections may "overcall" these as transsphincteric, potentially placing more sphincter muscle at risk if this imaging is solely relied upon for operative decision making (34). Figure 3.2(iii).4 shows a reconstructed image in association with a standard endosonographic image of perirectal intersphincteric sepsis. The 3D image assisted in the delineation and location of a translevator abscess extension. Figure 3.2(iii).5 shows the 2D and 3D comparative

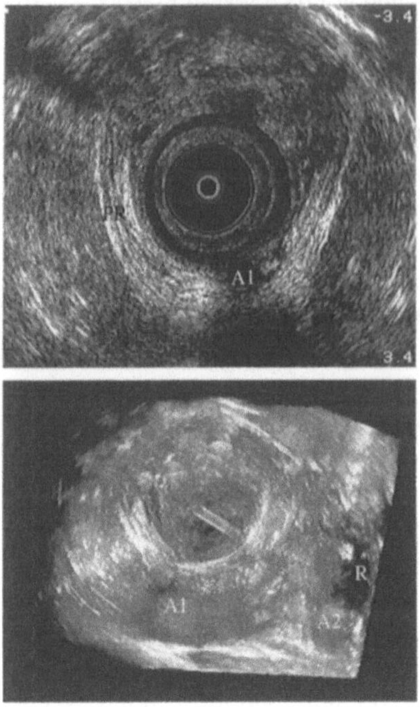

2D AES of a 39 year old female patient with severe pain due to anal and perirectal sepsis. No internal opening was evident but there was a clinical impression of induration at the level of the puborectalis-sling.
Orientation: 12 o'clock anterior,
PR (puborectalis), A 1(abscess 1)

3-D-reconstruction of the same patient showing a second, isolated, perirectal abscess above the levator muscle.
Orientation: 12 o'clock anterior,
A1 (abscess 1), A2 (abscess 2), R (rectum)

FIGURE 3.2(iii).4. Two-dimensional and 3D images of perirectal sepsis. The 3D image shows an additional unrecognized translevator abscess collection.

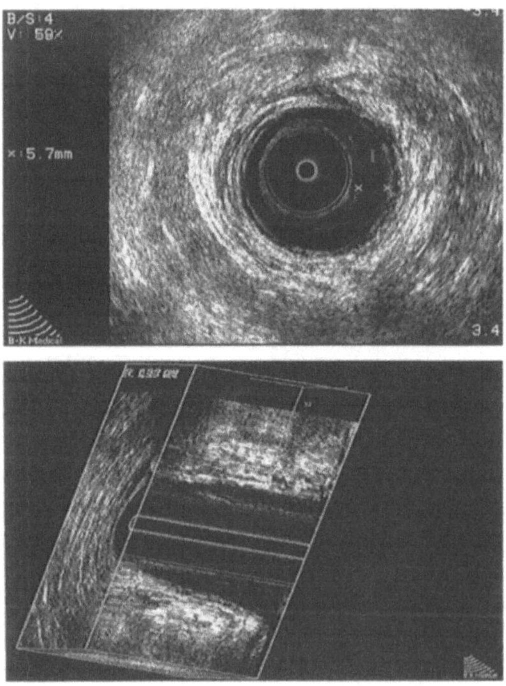

2D AES-image of a 35 year male patient with proctalgia fugax due to a myohyperplastic internal anal sphincter muscle (I, 5.7 mm). A 10 MHz B&K 360 ° rotating transducer was used..
Orientation: 12 o'clock anterior,
E (external anal sphincter)

3-D reconstruction of the same patient, lateral view.
I (IAS), E (EAS)

FIGURE 3.2(iii).5. Two-dimensional and 3D images of a male patient presenting with severe proctalgia fugax showing internal anal sphincter myohypertrophy.

images of a patient with hereditary internal anal sphincter hypertrophy—a rare cause of hereditary proctalgia (35).

Summary

Three-dimensional endoanal ultrasonography is still an experimental procedure. It is not widely available (being used in only a few European centers) and requires specialized software for interpretation. It attempts to reconstruct coronal and sagittal images from axial scans with multi-acquisition of data between registered points using data interpolation. Initial results showing gender differences of IAS/EAS orientation have been conflicting, and comparisons with station point physiological measurements and sphincter configurations have contrasted with manometric data. The theoretical advantages of such technology would lie in new orientations for delineation of complex perirectal sepsis close to the anal canal when surface Gadolinium-enhanced MRI is not available, although limitations of any endorectal/endoanal technology in some of the complicated cases must be recognized. Despite these forms of image alignment, there still will be cases where specific surface technology is required to define a pelvirectal origin of sepsis where pus breaks through the levator plate and presents as an ischiorectal abscess. Failure to adequately show these cases will result in a high extrasphincteric fistula if sepsis is drained through the ischiorectal space without diagnosis of its primary origin (36). It may be that prospective 3D data might also preoperatively define some patients where combined EAS overlapping sphincteroplasty and levatorplasty for the treatment of fecal incontinence is advised or where a more proximal EAS sphincteroplasty is needed after failed primary sphincter repair. At present, this information regarding these technical points is simply not available.

This technology is not yet standardized, where data acquisition seems to be very much operator dependent, varying with the equipment used. Another problem is the current lack of integration of harmonic gray-scale imaging, so there is some sacrifice of image quality with 3D reconstruction. Volume acquisition takes time, and in the future, faster volume acquisition is likely to make this a more standardized and usable technology.

References

1. Law PJ and Bartram CI. Anal endosonography: technique and normal anatomy. Gastrointestinal Radiol. 1989;14:349–53.
2. Nielsen MB, Dammegaard L, and Pedersen JT. Endosonographic assessment of the anal sphincter after surgical reconstruction. Dis Colon Rectum. 1994;37: 434–8.

3. Londono-Schimmer EE, Garcia-Duperly R, Nicholls RJ, Ritchie JK, Hanley PR, and Thompson JP. Overlapping anal sphincter repair for faecal incontinence due to sphincter trauma: 5-year follow-up functional results. Int J Colorectal Dis. 1994;9:110–3.
4. Deen KI, Kumar D, Williams JG, Oluff J, and Keighley MR. Anal sphincter defects: correlation between endoanal; ultrasound and surgery. Ann Surg. 1993;218:201–5.
5. Sultan AH, Kamm MA, Talbot IC, Nicholls RJ, and Bartram CI. Anal endosonography for identifying external sphincter defects confirmed histologically. Br J Surg. 1994;81:463–5.
6. Schafer A, Enck P, Furst G, Kahn T, Freiling T, and Lubke HJ. Anatomy of the anal sphincters: comparison of endosonography to magnetic resonance imaging. Dis Colon Rectum. 1994;37:777–81.
7. Hussain SM, Stoker J, and Lameris JS. Anal sphincter complex: endoanal magnetic resonance imaging of normal anatomy. Radiology. 1995;197:671–7.
8. deSouza NM, Puni R, Zbar A, Gilderdale DJ, Coutts GA, and Krausz T. MR imaging of the anal sphincter in multiparous women using an endoanal coil: correlation with in vitro anatomy and appearances in fecal incontinence. AJR Am J Roentgenol. 1996;167:1465–71.
9. Rociu E, Stoker J, Zwamborn AW, and Lameris JS. Endoanal MR imaging of the anal sphincter in fecal incontinence. Radiographics. 1999;Suppl:S171–7.
10. Briel JW, Zimmerman DD, Stoker J, Rociu E, Lameris JS, Mooi WJ, and Schouten WR. Relationship between sphincter morphology on endoanal MRI and histopathological aspects of the external anal sphincter. Int J Colorectal Dis. 2000;15:87–90.
11. Gold DM, Bartram CI, Halligan S, Humphries KN, Kamm MA, and Kmiot WA. 3-D endoanal sonography in assessing anal canal injury. Br J Surg. 1999; 86:365–70.
12. Engel AF, Kamm MA, Sultan AH, Bartram CI, and Nicholls RJ. Anterior anal sphincter repair in patients with obstetric trauma. Br J Surg. 1994;81:1231–4.
13. Pinedo G, Vaizey CJ, Nicholls RJ, Roach R, Halligan S, and Kamm MA. Results of repeat anal sphincter repair. Br J Surg. 1999;86:66–9.
14. Williams AB, Cheetham MJ, Bartram CI, Halligan S, Kamm MA, Nicholls RJ, and Kmiot WA. Gender differences in the longitudinal pressure profile of the anal canal related to anatomical structure as demonstrated on three-dimensional anal endosonography. Br J Surg. 2000;87:1674–9.
15. Zbar AP and Beer-Gabel M. Gender differences in the longitudinal pressure profiule of the anal canal related to anatomical structure as demonstrated on three-dimensional anal endosonography. Br J Surg. 2001;88:1016.
16. Frenckner B and Euler CVR. Influence of pudendal block on the function of the anal sphincters. Gut. 1975;16:482–9.
17. Lestar B, Penninckx F, and Kerremans R. The composition of anal basal pressure: an in vitro study in man. Int J Colorectal Dis. 1989;4:118–22.
18. Zbar AP, Jayne DG, Mathur D, Ambrose NS, and Guillou PJ. The importance of the internal anal; sphincter (IAS) in maintaining continence: anatomical, physiological and pharmacological considerations. Colorectal Dis. 2000;2:193–202.

19. Fucini C, Elbetti C, and Messerini L. Anatomic plane of separation between external anal sphincter and puborectalis muscle: clinical implications. Dis Colon Rectum. 1999;42:374–9.
20. Zbar AP, Kmiot WA, Aslam M, Williams A, Hider A, Audisio RA, Chiappa AC, and deSouza NM. Use of vector volume manometry and endoanal magnetic resonance imaging in the adult female for assessment of anal sphincter dysfunction. Dis Colon Rectum. 1999;42:1411–8.
21. Zbar AP, Aslam M, and Allgar V. Faecal incontinence after internal sphincterotomy for anal fissure. Tech Coloproctol. 2000;4:25–8.
22. Zbar AP, Beer-Gabel M, Chiappa AC, and Aslam M. Fecal incontinence after minor anorectal surgery. Dis Colon Rectum. 2001;44:1610–23.
23. Williams AB, Bartram CI, Halligan S, Marshall MM, Nicholls RJ, and Kmiot WA. Multiplanar anal endosonography—normal canal anatomy. Colorectal Dis. 2001;3:169–74.
24. Sultan AH, Kamm MA, Hudson CN, Nicholls RJ, and Bartram CI. Endosonography of the anal sphincters: Normal anatomy and comparison with manometry. Clin Radiol. 1994;49:368–74.
25. Hussain SM, Stoker J, Zwamborn AW, et al. Endoanal MRI of the anal sphincter complex: correlation with cross-sectional anatomy and histology. J Anat. 1996;189:677–82.
26. Halverson AL and Hull TL. Long-term outcome of overlapping anal sphincter repair. Dis Colon Rectum. 2002;45:345–8.
27. Engel AF, Kamm MA, Sultan AH, Bartram CI, and Nicholls RJ. Anterior anal sphincter repair in patients with obstetric trauma. Br J Surg. 1994;81:1231–4.
28. Enck P, Heyert T, Gantke B, et al. How reproducible are measures of the anal sphincter muscle diameter by endoanal ultrasound? Am J Gastroenterol. 1997;92:293–6.
29. Vaizey CJ, Kamm MA, and Bartram CI. Primary degeneration of the internal anal sphincter as a cause of passive faecal incontinence. Lancet. 1997;349:612–5.
30. Zimmerman DDE. Diagnostik en bahnadlung van transsfincterische perianale fistels [Diagnosis and treatment of trans-sphincteric perianal fistulas] [thesis]. Rotterdam, The Netherlands: Erasmus University; 2003.
31. West RI, Zimmerman DDE, Dwarkasing S, Hop WCJ, Hussaain SM, Schouten WR, Kuipers EJ, and Felt-Bersma RJ. Prospective comparison of hydrogen peroxide-enhanced 3-D endoanal ultrasonography and endoanal MR imaging of perianal fistulas. In: Zimmerman DDE, editor. Diagnostik en bahnadlung van transsfincterische perianale fistels [Diagnosis and treatment of trans-sphincteric perianal fistulas] [thesis]. Rotterdam, The Netherlands: Erasmus University; 2003. p. 45–64.
32. Halligan S. Imaging fistula-in-ano [review]. Clin Radiol. 1998;53:85–95.
33. Orsoni P, Barthet M, Portier F, Panninck M, Desjeux A, and Grimaud JC. Prospective comparison of endosonography, MR imaging and surgical findings in anorectal fistula and abscesses complicating Crohn's disease. Br J Surg. 1999;86:360–4. Comment: Zbar AP, deSouza NM. Br J Surg. 1999;86:1093–4.
34. Zbar AP, deSouza NM, Puni R, and Kmiot WA. Comparison of endoanal magnetic resonance imaging with surgical findings in perirectal sepsis. Br J Surg. 1998;85:111–4.

35. Kamm MA, Hoyle CH, Burleigh DE, Law PJ, Swash M, Martin JE, Nicholls RJ, and Northover JM. Hereditary internal anal sphincter myopathy causing proctalgia fugax and constipation. A newly defined condition. Gastroenterology. 1991;100:805–10.
36. Zbar AP. Magnetic resonance imaging and the coloproctologist. Tech Coloproctol. 2001;5:1–7.

Chapter 3.3(i)
MRI in Colorectal Surgery: Surface Magnetic Resonance Imaging in Anorectal Practice

Gina Brown and Andrew P. Zbar

Introduction

The advent of endoanal ultrasonography has effectively clarified the age-old arguments concerning the component morphology of the anal sphincter (see Chapter 1) and redefined the clinical significance of external anal sphincter (EAS) injury in the pathogenesis of fecal incontinence. More recently surface magnetic resonance imaging (MRI) has become the modality of choice in the preoperative locale staging of rectal and anal cancers, defining those patients likely to benefit from preoperative neoadjuvant therapies (1). In the anal canal, there is considerable evidence for its selected use in recurrent and clinically complex perirectal fistulous disease, where it has been hailed as the gold standard for the delineation of the primary track and its extensions and their relationship to the main puborectalis musculature (2).

This chapter outlines the indications and pitfalls in the use of MRI in proctological practice, with specific reference to its use in complex peri rectal infection and in low rectal, anal, and pararectal tumors.

The MRI Definition of Normal Anatomy

The recent introduction of high-resolution surface and endoanal MRI has contributed substantially to the clarification of the anatomy of the internal anal sphincter (IAS), the EAS, and the longitudinal muscle, as well as their intrinsic relationships (3–5). This has effectively confirmed the EAS a tri-layered structure including the subcutaneous, superficial, and deep components as was suggested many years ago (6,7) with a recently clarified relationship between the distal EAS and its overlap of the termination of the IAS (8). Endoanal and surface MRI may not be strictly comparable, however, because they define the intersphincteric space slightly differently and there are differences that may rely on the amount of fibroelastic muscular content for adequate definition of the outer margins of the EAS and puborectalis complex. Magnetic resonance imaging has a myriad of uses in specialized coloproctology, with applications in the definition of congenital anorectal anomalies (9,10) and their surgical functional aftermath (11), the definition of the rostral extent of presacral tumors (12), and in the evaluation of neurologic and myopathic disorders secondarily affecting the anorectum (13).

Surface MRI and Complex Perirectal Sepsis

The vast majority of perirectal sepsis is simple and does not require specialized preoperative imaging (14). The basic surgical requirements in perirectal infection are a knowledge of the site of the primary track (along with associated collections), the presence of secondary extensions, horseshoeing of the track in the retrorectal or anteroanal spaces, the site of the internal fistula opening, and the relationship of collections and tracks to the main puborectalis sling. Recurrences of fistulae are related to a failure to appreciate one, some, or all of these requirements (15). The coloproctologist, however, is likely to be referred complex and recurrent cases, including patients with difficult and atypical infections, perianal Crohn's disease, Behcet's disease, post-irradiation sepsis, HIV-related infection, and rarely malignant transformation of an anal gland presenting as sepsis where clinical examination may be misleading or even relatively impossible, and in these specialist cases, there may be considerable reliance on accurate and specialized preoperative imaging that will require sophisticated interpretation. A more specialized knowledge of the secondary effects of destructive perirectal sepsis seeks to assess the status of the sphincters (internal and external), the destructive effects on the perineal body (which may require secondary reconstruction), and the presence of an ano- or rectovaginal fistula. For these latter pieces of information, it may be necessary to combine surface MRI with endoluminal technology (16). Here, examinations usually are conducted with T1-weighted spin-echo imaging in the coronal plane using supplemental short TI inversion recovery (STIR) sequencing along with spin-echo T2-weighted axial imaging. Gadolinium is employed at 10, 30, and 50 second intervals after intravenous (IV) bolus injection (0.1 mmol/Kg body weight) with out-of-phase gradient-echo sequencing using fast low-angle shot software to render short time to echo (TE) in contiguous slices.

In this respect, there have been many recent reports of the accuracy in the delineation of inter-, trans-, and extrasphincteric tracks and collections using surface MRI with or without Gadolinium enhancement (17–20), where it has been shown to function effectively as a gold standard in blinded comparison with surgery when concerned with the diagnosis of primary track locale and horseshoeing of abscess collections (17). The distinct advantage in some cases includes the ability of pelvic-phased array MRI to define some rare cases of extrasphincteric fistulae, where the origin of the sepsis is abdominopelvic (i.e., pelvirectal). Here, injudicious drainage of an ischiorectal collection through the perineum will result inevitably in a high extrasphincteric fistula that will occasionally necessitate proctectomy (16). This type of problem needs to be distinguished from a translevator extension of a trans-sphincteric fistula-related ischiorectal abscess, where drainage via the ischiorectal fossa (and drainage of the levator) results in cure.

Surface MRI is not perfect, however, and it should be remembered that its soft tissue resolution is such that the subepithelial space is poorly defined (in comparison with endoluminal probe technology), so that in some cases the exact site of the internal opening can only essentially be inferred. This is important to remember for several reasons. Firstly, in those patients undergoing a mucosal (or cutaneous) advancement anoplasty for recalcitrant sepsis, the exact site of the internal opening must be defined. Moreover, recent suggestions that the angulation of the track as it enters the EAS (where more obtuse angles are associated with higher internal openings) imply that the preoperative definition of track angle may spare sphincter where it traditionally has been supposed that the fistula enters the anal canal more transversely (21). Here, it may be equally important to ascertain what the angulation of the track is to the IAS, as it recently has been suggested that IAS preservation in complex fistula surgery may be as (if not more) important than low EAS preservation in the maintenance of continence, particularly in the multiply operated patient (22). Nevertheless, the advantage here with MRI is its multiplanar capacity for coronal demonstration of extension around of tracks and collections around the front or the back of the anal canal, particularly when the tissue is relatively woody to the touch because of previous surgery.

To some extent, the advantages of one technique are the disadvantages of another. In comparison with endoanal ultrasound, the added advantage of MRI is that Gadolinium enhancement can by and large distinguish residual or recrudescent sepsis from "burnt-out" tracks (23,24). Any endoluminal technology (ultrasound or MR) will have serious limitations in two uncommon (but important) circumstances precisely where the coloproctologist seeks specific information—namely in lateral extrasphincteric fistulae and in delineating the presence of supralevator extensions. In the former case, the fistula may simply lie beyond the field of view of the endoluminal probe, necessitating surface imaging, whereas in the latter scenario, poor coupling of the probe above the puborectalis sling will prevent diagnosis of significant trans- or supralevator collections.

Although MRI-directed fistula-in-ano classification systems have been devised (19), it is unclear at this time whether MRI in these selected cases represents a cost-beneficial investigation (24) and whether long-term fistula-related outcome (namely the incidence of recurrence) is improved with the more ready use of MRI. In addition to this, prospective data is required regarding the impact that the more routine use of MRI may have

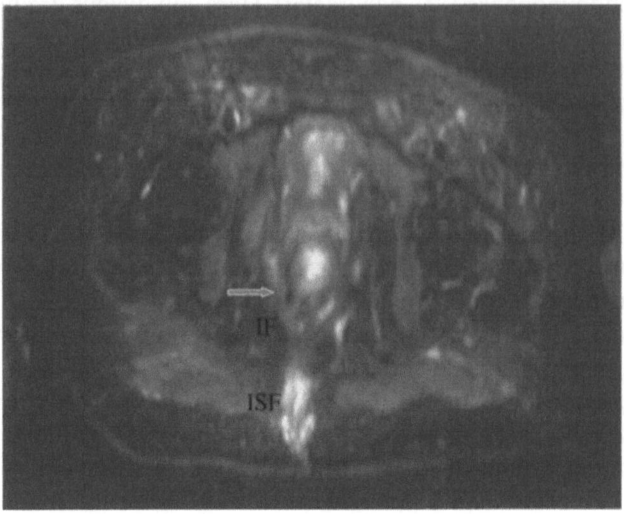

FIGURE 3.3(i).1. Gadolinium-enhancing intersphinteric fistula (ISF). Levator plate, block arrow; ischiorectal fossa (IF).

on fistula-specific quality-of-life parameters (25). At the present time, we would advocate the use of contrast-enhanced MRI for perirectal sepsis (where available) that is unexpectedly recurrent, in complex perianal Crohn's disease, HIV- or radiation-related fistulae, perianal lymphoma or leukemic infiltration, and in perirectal sepsis in neutropenia or pancytopenia. These indications are likely to expand with time as expertise in this technique and MRI availability increase. An example of a Gadolinium-enhanced intersphincteric fistula is shown in Figure 3.3(i).1. Figure 3.3(i).2 shows a high trans-sphincteric fistula. Figure 3.3(i).3 is an example of a pelvirectal abscess originating above the levator plate. In this circumstance, MR imaging preoperatively protects against transischiorectal fossa drainage, which would result in an extrasphincteric fistula.

MRI in the Preoperative Assessment of Rectal, Anal, and Presacral Tumors

In rectal cancer, the availability of a range of operative approaches and preoperative therapeutic options has raised the importance of accurate preoperative staging where it has been shown in some series that preoperative adjuvant radiation has been associated with reduced loco-regional recurrence and even enhanced cancer-specific survival (26). High spatial resolution MRI is being used increasingly as a method for accurately staging not

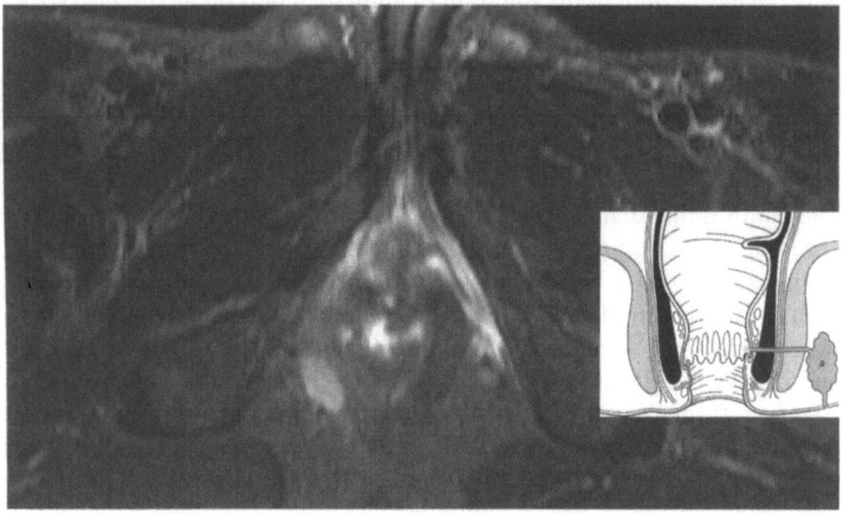

FIGURE 3.3(i).2. Trans-sphincteric fistula (STIR sequencing) with attached schematic.

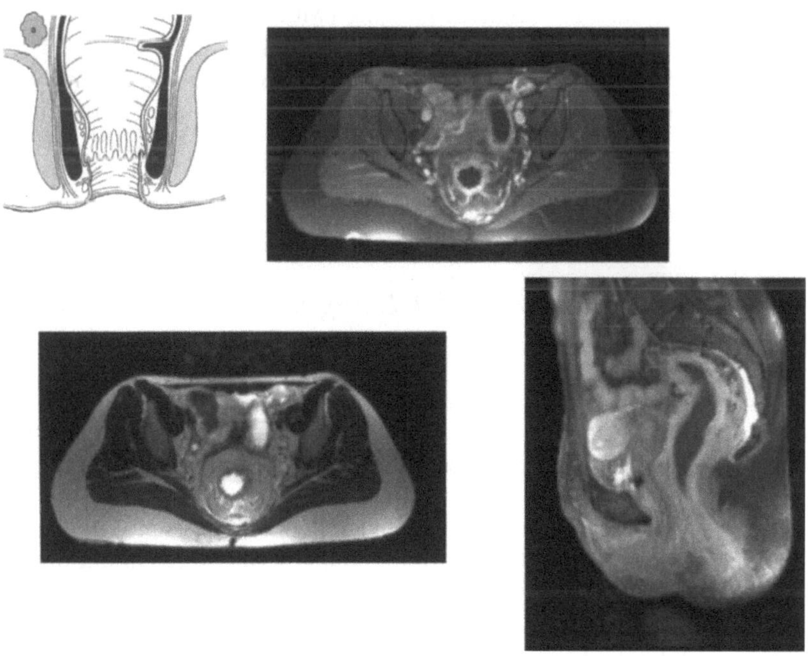

FIGURE 3.3(i).3. Axial and coronal MR images of a pelvirectal abscess originating above the levator plate (see text).

only the local extent of the tumor in relation to important anatomical structures, but also in identifying these important prognostic factors that influence the use of preoperative therapies.

Technical Considerations of MRI Technique

The features that define MR image quality are the signal-to-noise ratio, the speed of acquisition of images, and the image resolution. Improvements in image quality have been achieved through technological developments such as stronger gradients (enhancing greater signaling), advances in software for imaging sequences, and improvements in the coils that transmit and receive the signal from the scanned area. In particular, coil design has advanced from using the body coil of the magnetic gantry at some distance from the area being examined (with a relatively poor signal-to-noise ratio) to dedicated coils designed to maximize the signal detected. An early advance in coil design was the endorectal coil, which received a signal at a point of direct contact with the bowel wall; however, in recent years more sophisticated multiple-element coil arrays have been constructed, designed to maximize signal-to-noise ratios over the region examined without having to position the coil within the endoluminal cavity.

T2-weighted imaging is the best method for demonstrating the primary tumor, and additional sequences such as STIR (short tau inversion recovery sequencing) and T1-weighted imaging (with or without fat saturation or contrast enhancement) have been used. It would appear that the latter sequences add little additional useful staging information and generally are not used in our unit, where they provide no clear distinction between the tumor and surrounding normal anatomic structures. In the past, this has accounted for reports using T1-weighted sequences that have overstaged low rectal tumors (27).

Patient Preparation for MRI Using the Pelvic Phased Array Surface Coil

No specific patient preparation is required for this examination; however, image degradation can be problematic with motion artifact. This can be improved if the following technical points are taken in to consideration:

- By far the most common cause of image degradation is motion artifact caused by movement of the lower abdominal wall during patient breathing, which can be overcome by applying firm compression to the lower abdomen by means of foam padding between the pelvic surface coil and anterior abdominal wall. A distended bladder should be avoided, as this also worsens image quality and prevents adequate lower abdominal compression.

- Air insufflation worsens the image quality by introducing further bowel motion related to expulsion of insufflated air and consequent collapse of the bowel wall.
- The introduction of intraluminal contrast agents may cause discomfort and may result in excessive bowel wall motion while not providing any additional staging information because tumor staging does not require delineation of the luminal component of the tumor, but relies on the mural and extramural spread of tumour—a feature unaided by intraluminal contrast.
- It is critical that the patient is comfortable during the MR examination, taking steps that ensure the patient has emptied their bladder prior to the examination, explaining the likely duration of scans (up to 10 minutes per sequence), and ensuring that the patient is pain free during the examination.
- In the author's experience, small bowel motion only very rarely results in any significant image degradation. On occasion, however, patients who have undergone previous hysterectomy may have low-lying loops of small bowel that can cause image degradation of the mid- and upper rectum and that may justify the use of antispasmodics in selected cases.

Recommended Imaging Parameters for Obtaining High Spatial Resolution Images

Magnetic resonance imaging is performed with a 1.5 Tesla whole body system using a quadruple element surface coil. Axial and sagittal T2-weighted fast-spin echo acquisitions of the anatomical pelvis are conducted using a 24-centimeter field of view, 5-millimter contiguous slice thickness, TR 4000 ms, TE 85 ms, 512 × 256 matrix, and an echo train length of 8, with no fat saturation and a bandwidth of 32 kilohertz with two acquisitions. These scans then are used to plan high-resolution axial scans (perpendicular to the long axis of the tumour) through the rectal tumor and adjacent pararectal tissues.

Although current generation MRI scanners can employ a 512 matrix to produce high-resolution images, these images have a poor signal-to-noise ratio and generally produce poor overall image quality. The highest resolution achievable on most 1.5 T machines with an acceptable signal-to-noise ratio is obtained by using a 256 × 256 image matrix with three-millimeter slice thickness, a 16-centimeter field of view, and four excitations.

Surgical Considerations and Relevance to MRI Reporting

The widespread adoption of total mesorectal excision (TME) surgery resulting in removal of the mesorectal lymphovascular package with its intact enveloping mesorectal fascia (the fascia propria) has been one of the single most important factors in reducing loco-regional recurrence in rectal cancer. The technique has been promulgated by Heald, who has demonstrated local recurrence rates of only 6% compared with more than 40% in centers not using this technique in non-randomized studies (28–30). The principal rationale for this method of surgery is:

- Total removal of rectum and its draining lymph nodes en bloc (Figure 3.3(i).4)
- Anal sphincter preservation
- Autonomic nerve preservation

Despite the widespread use of this form of surgery, the wide variation in local recurrence rates amongst surgeons has been attributed, at least in part, to the quality of the surgical technique (31), an operation that can effectively be taught by special workshop (32). Here, attention has focused on judging the quality of the resected specimen as an indicator of the quality of surgery itself. Despite the success of optimized TME surgery in substantially reducing local recurrence rates, there remain a number of important surgical issues preventing a successful curative resection in a significant number of patients, and both preoperative imaging and multidisciplinary discussion of the imaging is an essential part of enabling appropriate tailored surgical planning. In MRI, it is important to specifically assess certain tumor-related aspects; namely:

- If the tumor is clear of adjacent structures; namely, the prostate, seminal vesicles, bladder, and pelvic sidewalls. Invasion of the pelvic sidewalls and prostate indicates that primary surgery is highly unlikely to achieve a curative (R0) resection and necessitates neoadjuvant downstaging therapy, which may be monitored on MRI (33).
- If the tumor is clear of the mesorectal fascia (>1 mm from the fascia). Tumor extending to the mesorectal fascia or breaching the fascia can result in resection margin violation during standard TME surgery.
- If the tumor is not invading through the rectal wall below the level of the levator ani origin or extending into the main sphincter complex. The preservation of a clear circumferential resection margin in these cases is more challenging, particularly when abdominoperineal excision is performed.
- Assessment of all sites of disease within the pelvis, including tumor deposits lateral to the mesorectal fascia, and thus, lateral to the conventional surgical resection plane, necessitating an R1 resection with extended lymphadenectomy in some cases (34).

Failure to resolve these important issues preoperatively can result in non-curative resection and the lost opportunity to provide intensive preoperative therapy aimed at downstaging the tumor and rendering disease

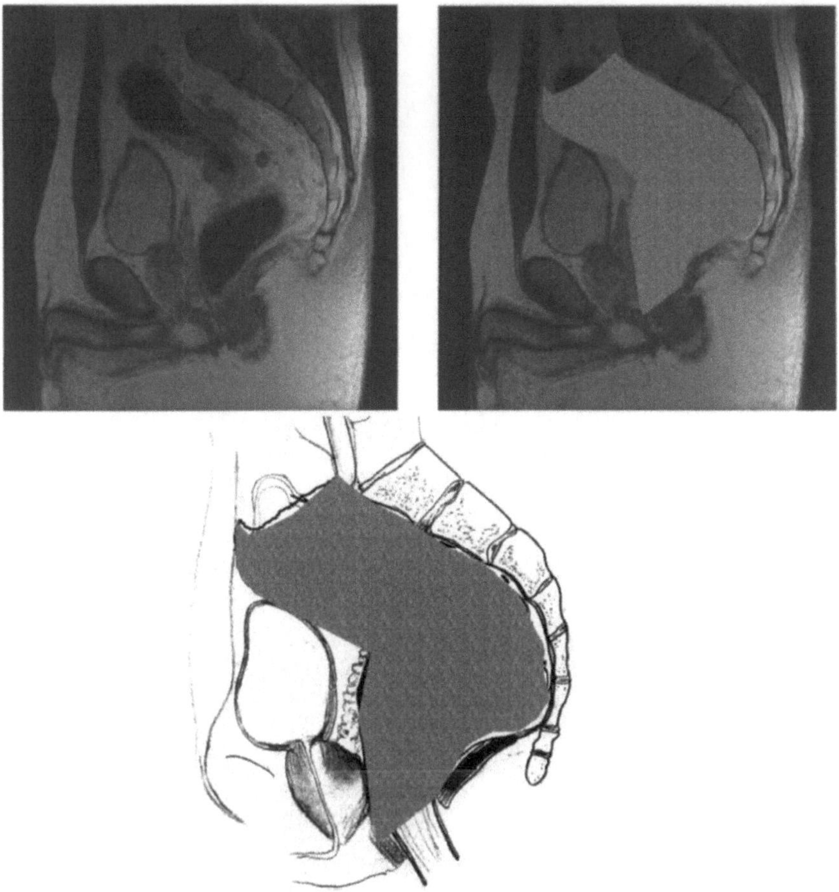

FIGURE 3.3(i).4. Surgical excision plane in TME surgery. The colored shaded area represents the tissue comprising the rectum and mesorectum removed during TME surgery. In TME surgery, the whole mesorectum is removed and a low anastomosis between proximal rectum, rectosigmoid, and the anal canal is performed. The precise height of the anastomosis from the sphincter is determined by the distance of the lowermost edge of tumor from the sphincter. In patients with tumors of the upper third of the rectum, the mesorectum often is transected five centimeters below the distal edge of the tumor.

resectable and locally curative. Conversely, overstaging by inaccurate preoperative and operative assessment may result in classifying potentially operable patients as inoperable for cure or result in the use of inappropriate adjuvant treatments (35). Figure 3.3(i).5(a, b) shows the normal mesorectum on T2-weighted MRI, along with a tumor infiltrating the mesorectum near adjacent normal vessels.

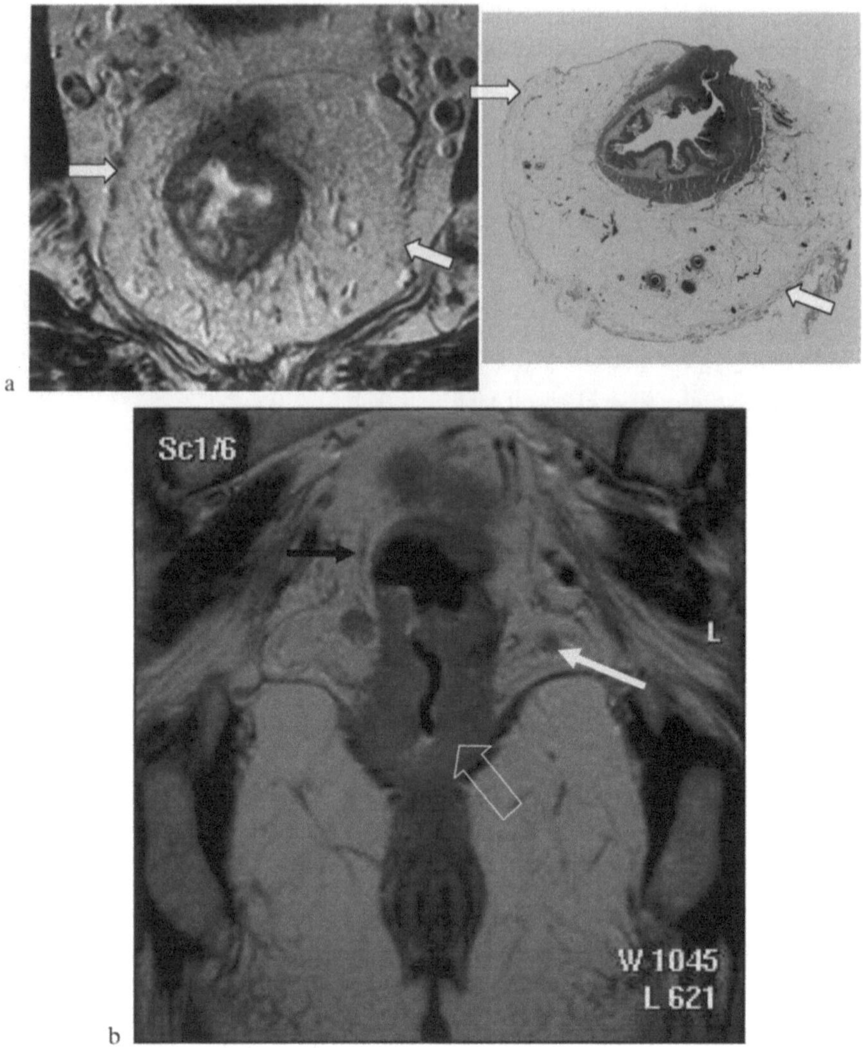

FIGURE 3.3(i).5. (a) The mesorectal fascia (MRI) and the whole mount section showing mesorectal fascia. The mesorectal fascia (arrows) demonstrated on an axial T2-weighted MR image as a low signal layer surrounding the mesorectum. (b) Coronal T2-weighted fast spin-echo image of a low rectal tumor. The intermediate signal intensity tumor (open arrow) is demonstrated within the bowel wall and small vessels (black arrow) and lymph nodes (white arrow) are clearly resolved within the mesorectum.

MRI Anatomy Relevant to TME Surgery

An understanding of the detailed anatomy of the mesorectal fascia is of importance in relation to staging and TME surgery. Bissett et al. (36) dissected the mesorectal fascia (fascia propria of the rectum), showing that the fascia was a continuous structure that encircles the rectum and mesorectum, fusing with the peritoneum as it is reflected off the rectal wall. At the level of the anorectal junction, the mesorectum thins out as a recognizable structure. The mesorectal fascia is demonstrated clearly on MRI, permitting an assessment of the distance of tumor from the potential radial circumferential margin—a factor of importance in the prevention of loco-regional pelvic recurrence (37).

MRI Appearance of the Mesorectal Fascia

The mesorectal fascia is best appreciated on axial section and is seen as a low signal linear structure surrounding the mesorectum. It is depicted consistently on thin-slice MRI. The mesorectum is demonstrated as a high signal intensity (fat signal) envelope surrounding the rectum, containing vessels that are depicted as low signal components due to signal void produced by blood flow. Lymph nodes are shown as high signal ovoid structures within the mesorectum due to a high fluid content. Small nerves are not visualized within the mesorectum, but interlacing connective tissue is recognized as low signal intensity strands.

Pathologic Considerations and High Spatial MRI Correlation

Microscopic and Macroscopic Appearances

On high spatial resolution MRI, rectal tumors are most commonly demonstrated as an elevated plaque of intermediate signal that projects into the lumen forming a U-shaped thickened disc corresponding to an annular or semiannular plaque of tumor on histologic sections. Figures 3.3(i).6, 3.3(i).7, and 3.3(i).8 depict T2-weighted axial MR images of semiannular plaque, annular plaque, and polypoidal rectal cancers with corresponding histological whole-mount specimens for comparison. In some patients, plaques may show a central depression forming a mass with a central crater that corresponds to tumor with central ulceration and raised rolled edges on histology sections (Figure 3.3(i).6). Central ulceration of the tumor may produce focal thinning or erosion of the rectal wall. In these cases, thinning of the rectal wall is also associated with loss of distinction of individual bowel wall layers and is associated with a marked desmoplastic reaction (Figure 3.3(i).9).

Exophytic or polypoidal tumors typically have a pronounced protuberant appearance with the tumor mass projecting into the lumen. A number

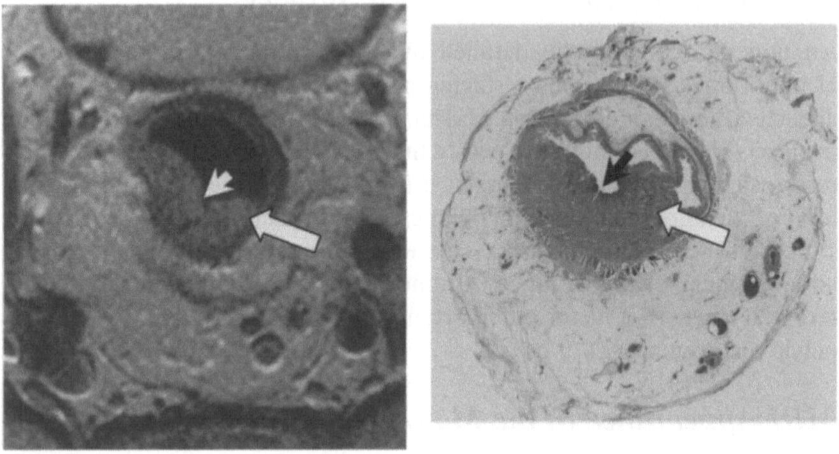

FIGURE 3.3(i).6. Axial T2-weighted fast spin-echo MR image and corresponding histological (H&E stained) whole mount section demonstrating a semiannular plaque of tumor with central ulceration (arrowhead) and raised rolled edges (arrows).

of studies have observed that such polypoidal lesions are often of a relatively low-grade malignancy (38). On high spatial resolution MRI, these polypoidal tumors are shown as intermediate signal intensity, rounded, protuberant mass lesions that project into the lumen (Figure 3.3(i).8). The surface of these polypoidal tumor mass lesions often shows high signal intensity clefts corresponding to mucinous fluid on the tumor surface. These mucinous tumors form a distinct morphological subgroup of rectal cancers characterized by their gelatinous appearance with a propensity for more extensive intramural spread. On MRI, they show very high signal intensity

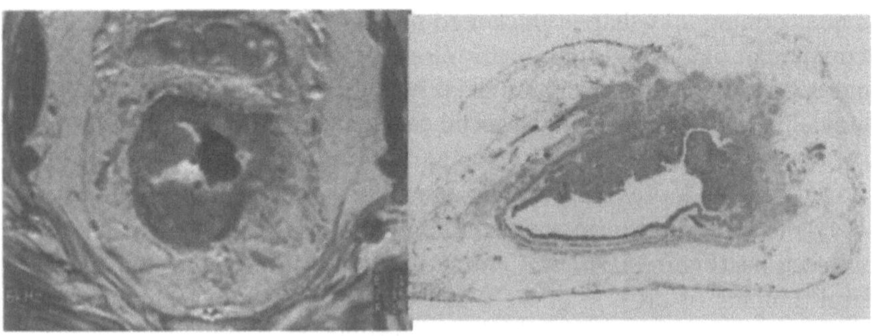

FIGURE 3.3(i).7. Axial T2-weighted fast spin-echo image and corresponding histological (H&E stained) whole mount section demonstrating an annular plaque of tumor. This is the most common pattern forming a disc-like protrusion of tumor into the bowel lumen.

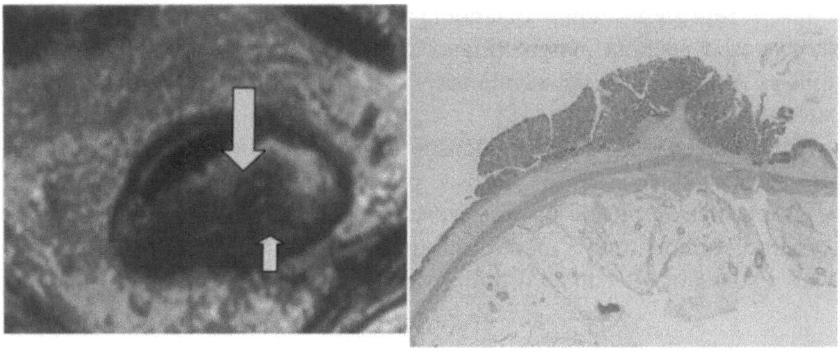

FIGURE 3.3(i).8. High-resolution T2-weighted image and corresponding histological (H&E stained) whole mount section demonstrating a T1 polypoid carcinoma (arrow). There is partial preservation of the submucosal layer (short arrow) seen as a thin rim of high signal intensity deep into the tumor. The tumor does not extend into the muscularis propria layer.

that is isointense to fluid within the layers of the rectal wall, and the layers typically show high signal intensity expansion (Figure 3.3(i).10).

Patterns of Spread

When rectal tumors invade through the bowel wall into the perirectal fat, they commonly do so with a fairly well-circumscribed margin. In 25% of cases, however, the pattern of spread is widely infiltrative with ill-defined borders. This pattern of spread has been shown to worsen prognosis, whereas conversely, the presence of an inflammatory response at the advancing margin of the tumor represents a favorable prognostic feature (39,40). Regardless of differentiation, colorectal tumors—unlike upper gastrointestinal tumors—rarely show submucosal or intramural spread beyond their macroscopic borders. This characteristic is important in the surgical planning of distal resection margins, and current evidence based on data examining intramural spread suggests that a one-centimeter distal clearance is sufficient to ensure curative resection of the tumor (41).

The Extent of Local Spread

Dukes highlighted the importance of the extent of extramural spread in the prediction of local recurrence, as well as in cancer-specific survival. Here, the measurement of extramural spread is taken from the outer edge of the longitudinal muscle layer, and it has been shown that once spread occurs beyond the bowel wall, the incidence of lymph node invasion increases, rising from 14.2% in tumors confined to the bowel wall to 43.2% in those tumors extending beyond the bowel wall. On MRI, intermediate signal intensity represents tumor extending into the perirectal fat either with a broad-based pushing margin (Figure 3.3(i).11) or with finger-like projections of intermediate signal intensity forming nodular extensions into the perirectal fat (Figure 3.3(i).12).

Fine spicules of low signal intensity often are seen in the perirectal fat corresponding to areas of fibrosis, perivascular cuffing, or peritumoral desmoplastic response. This appearance is seen most commonly in cases of "eroding" tumors and is most pronounced in the perirectal tissues immediately adjacent to the rectal wall at the level of the tumor itself.

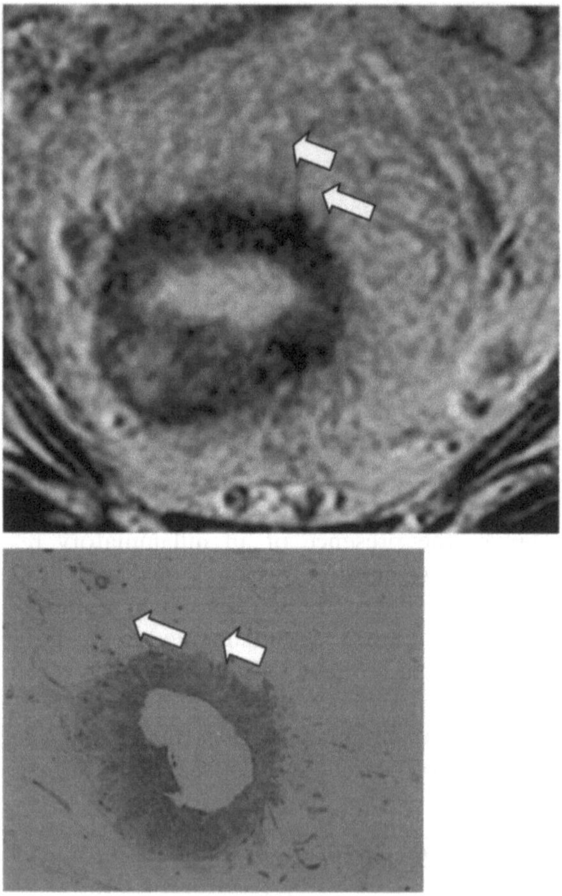

FIGURE 3.3(i).9. Axial T2-weighted fast spin-echo image and corresponding histological (H&E stained) whole mount section demonstrating an eroding tumor. This is characterized by the focal thinning of the rectal wall due to erosion of the tumor into the bowel wall layers preventing the MR demonstration of discrete layers. Marked spiculation (arrows) is shown corresponding histologically with a desmoplastic response.

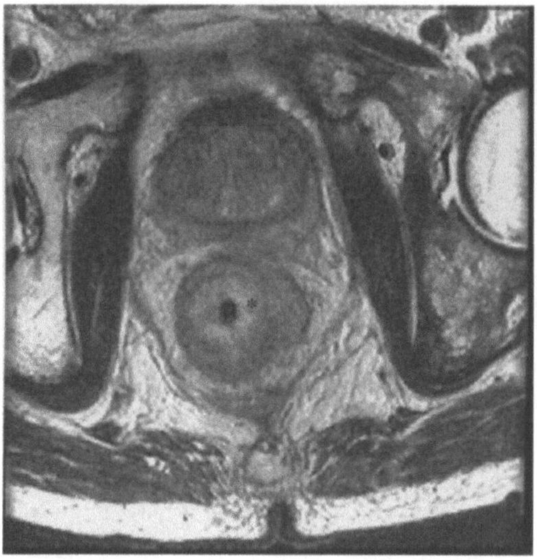

FIGURE 3.3(i).10. Axial T2-weighted fast spin-echo MR image demonstrating a mucinous tumor characterized by a very high signal intensity (high water content). The tumor (asterisk) infiltrates the bowel wall without destroying the boundaries between the individual layers, resulting in accentuation (thickening) of the bowel wall.

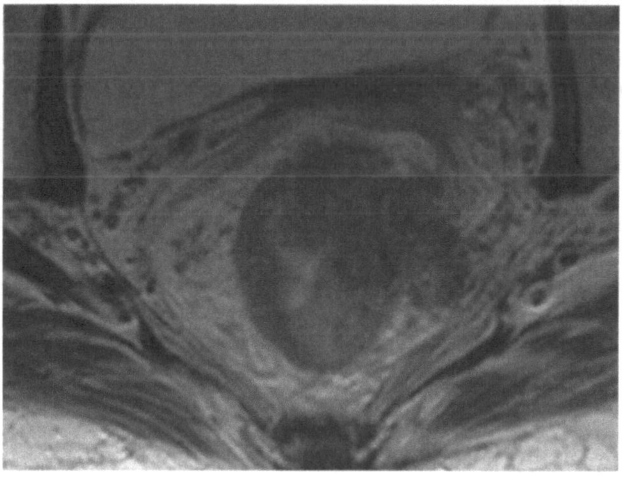

FIGURE 3.3(i).11. Axial high-resolution T2-weighted image showing a tumor with a pushing edge. The advancing edge of the tumor has a well-circumscribed margin with a sharp border between the advancing edge of the tumor and the perirectal fat. This is the most common pattern of tumor spread.

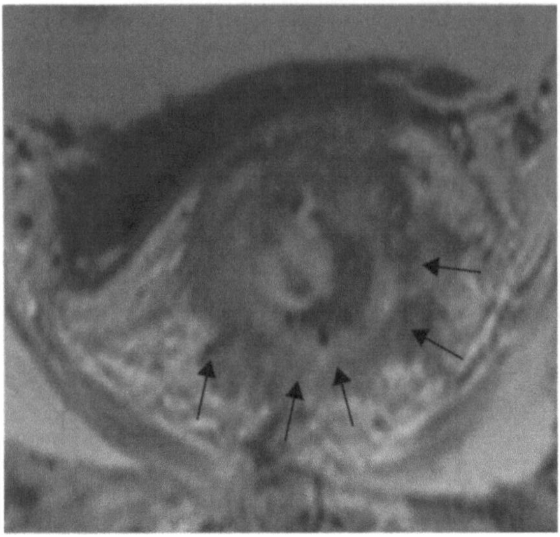

FIGURE 3.3(i).12. Axial T2-weighted FSE image showing nodular extension with ill-defined margins. The tumor is spreading into the perirectal fat at its leading edge.

Venous Spread

It has been shown that the presence of invasion of large extramural veins by tumor is independently associated with a low five-year survival rate in rectal cancer (42) and that microscopic venous invasion correlates with hepatic metastatic disease as a manifestation of treatment failure, even in patients with node-negative tumors (43). Thus, venous invasion is not only a predictor of poor survival, but is also the third most powerful independent predictor of metastasis, after lymph node involvement and the local extent of local tumor infiltration (44). On MRI, the formation of discrete tubular projections of tumor extending into the perirectal fat that appear to follow the course of a perirectal vessel is thought to correspond to extramural venous invasion (Figure 3.3(i).13) and, when detected, is highly predictive of venous invasion on subsequent histopathological assessment (45).

Spread Beyond the Peritoneal Membrane

Perforation of the peritoneal membrane by tumor and the consequent spillage of tumor cells results in both local recurrence and widespread intra-abdominal peritoneal dissemination. Local peritoneal involvement is detected in 25% (54 of 209) of cases depending on the technique used (cytological vs molecular biological) (46) and is also an independent prognostic factor for local recurrence after rectal resectional surgery (47). On MRI, tumor may be demonstrated extending through the anterior rectum at the point of attachment of the peritoneal reflection corresponding on histology to peritoneal perforation (pT4 tumor).

The Circumferential (Radial) Resection Margin (CRM)

When the surgically excised specimen is sectioned transversely, the lateral border of the specimen is termed the circumferential (or radial) resection margin (CRM). The importance of the circumferential margin involvement by tumor and its relation to local recurrence has been demonstrated by Quirke et al. and is one of the principal factors governing loco-regional tumor relapse (37). Here, the risk of local recurrence in CRM-positive patients are significantly higher than that of CRM-negative patients, and when compared with CRM-negative cases, the risk of death with CRM-positivity is three times higher (48). In their initial study, each tumor was embedded in its entirety with preparation of multiple whole-mount tissue blocks. Quirke and colleagues later showed that visual inspection of the macroscopic slices was sufficient to select sections with suspected CRM involvement (49). This proved to be robust in practice and reproducible in other institutions (50).

On high spatial resolution MRI, involvement of the mesorectal fascia (the potential circumferential margin) with tumor is defined as an image where the primary tumor, a tumor deposit, or a positive lymph node abuts or extends through the mesorectal fascia or extends to within one millimeter of the mesorectal edge. There is generally good agreement for close mesorectal margin assessment by preoperative MRI in dedicated units (51).

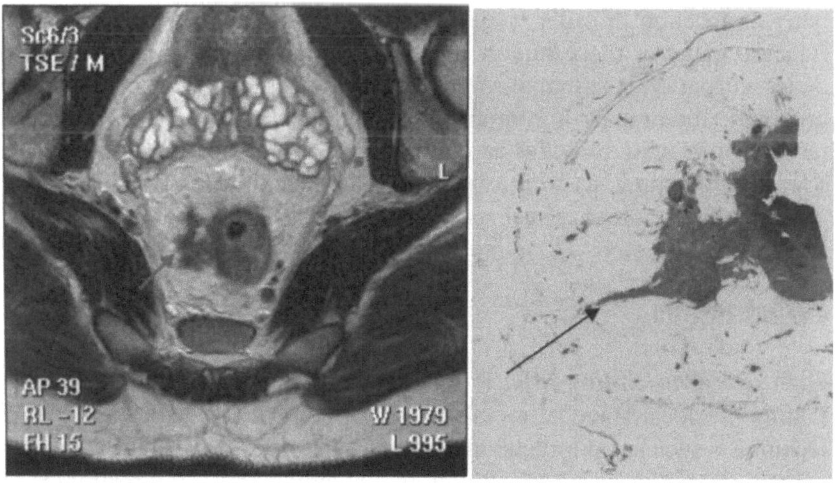

FIGURE 3.3(i).13. Nodular projection of tumor corresponding to extramural venous invasion. There is serpiginous extension of the tumor into the perirectal fat (arrow) following a presumed vessel that was shown histologically to be thick-walled extramural venous invasion.

MRI in Recurrent Rectal Cancer

Up to 40% of patients with rectal cancer resected for cure will develop recurrence, and up to one-third of these patients may die without evidence of systemic metastatic disease (52). This disease, if untreated, is associated with less than a 5% five-year survival, with an average life expectancy of seven months (53). Postoperative changes (with or without radiotherapy) will obscure the diagnosis of recurrence using computed tomography (CT) scan or MRI, and it has been advocated to obtain a baseline MRI scan after rectal resection (particularly when abdominoperineal resection has been performed) to assess for serial changes during follow-up. This strategy, however, is not practical in many units (54). Here, masses of soft tissue density may be due to tumor recurrence, granulation tissue, organized (ing) hematoma, or fibrosis (55,56). Most recurrences have intermediate to high signal intensity on T2-weighted images when compared with fibrous tissue. There is recent evidence that computerized semi-quantitative assessments of Gadolinium enhancement in recalled sequences has a moderately high sensitivity for the diagnosis of pelvic recurrence (57), particularly if this involved the pelvic side walls (58).

The Use of MRI in Presacral Tumors

Presacral (retrorectal) tumors are uncommon in both children and adults. In children, left untreated, many will become malignant, whereas in adults they often are found on incidental rectal examination and are usually benign (12). The coloproctologist needs to define the upper limit of these lesions and the presence or absence of presacral infiltration and/or sacral bony destruction in order to decide about the optimal surgical approach. Because many of these tumors are cystic (either wholly or in part), complete extirpation is essential to prevent recurrence, with a choice between presacral, abdominal, or combined abdominosacral approaches. Magnetic resonance imaging provides an optimal mid sagittal view for accurate preoperative planning, as well as providing information in some cases concerning other anomalies such as spinal dysraphism (59).

Conclusions

High spatial resolution MRI is gaining acceptance as a method of determining the local stage of rectal cancer. In comparison with endoluminal techniques such as endorectal ultrasound, MRI offers inherent advantages, namely, the ability to assess all tumors (extending above the rostral extent of the endoluminal probe) and bulky obstructing or stenosing cancers that limit probe placement. Moreover, the larger field of view permits assessment of the entire mesorectum, as well as the relationship of the tumor to the mesorectal fascia—a factor that crucially corresponds to the radial margin in TME rectal resection. The accuracy of the assessment of tumor depth (T status) is high, although there is variable reporting regarding its nodal (N) status sensitivity. This is partly because, with new fat clearance histopathological technology, pathologists are dissecting more nodes in TME specimens that harbor micrometastatic disease (60). Here, border contour and signal intensity are more important than nodal size in the MR definition of possible malignant involvement (61). The sensitivity for high caliber extramural venous involvement and peritoneal infiltration is also high with high resolution MRI (62).

Its high contrast resolution using T2-weighted fast spin-echo sequences enables perirectal fibrosis to be distinguished from tumor by virtue of signal intensity characteristics, and its ability to depict the outer muscle coat as a distinct layer on MR images permits accurate assessment of the depth of extramural spread from the outer muscle coat. The introduction of the pelvic phased-array coil has enabled a major improvement in the detail and reproducibility of rectal cancer imaging. It has been shown to be of high accuracy in staging the depth of extramural spread and in predicting the relationship of the tumor close to the mesorectal fascia. The recent advances in MRI technology have provided a much more accurate way of defining the group of patients in whom the specialist rectal surgeon is unlikely to be able to perform an R0 resection. It remains to be seen whether this is beneficial for cancer-specific survival where MRI-directed prospective studies guide the use of preoperative adjuvant and neoadjuvant therapy.

References

1. Martling A, Holm T, Bremmer S, Lindholm J, Cedermark B, and Blomqvist L. Prognostic value of preoperative magnetic resonance imaging of the pelvis in rectal cancer. Br J Surg. 2003;90:1422–8.
2. Schaefer O, Lohrmann C, and Langer M. Assessment of anal fistulas with high-resolution subtraction MR-fistulography. Comparison with surgical findings. J Magn Reson Imaging. 2004;19:91–8.
3. Lunniss PJ and Phillips RK. Anatomy and function of the anal longitudinal muscle. Br J Surg. 1992;79:882–4.
4. deSouza NM, Puni R, Zbar A, Gilderdale DJ, Couttts GA, and Krausz T. MR imaging of the anal sphincter in multiparous women using an endoanal coil: correlation with in vitro anatomy and appearances in fecal incontinence. AJR Am J Roentgenol. 1996;167:1465–71.
5. Fucini C, Elbetti C, and Messerini L. Anatomic plane of separation between external anal sphincter and puborectalis muscle. Clinical implications. Dis Colon Rectum. 1999;42:374–9.
6. Milligan ETC and Morgan CN. Surgical anatomy of the anal canal with special reference to ano-rectal fistulae. Lancet. 1934;2:150(6);1213–27.

7. Fowler R. Landmarks and legends of the anal canal. Aust N Z J Surg. 1957;27: 1–8.
8. Zbar AP, Kmiot WA, Aslam M, Williams A, Hider A, Audisio RA, Chiappa AC, and deSouza NM. Vectorvolume manometry and endoanal magnetic resonance imaging in the adult female for assessment of anal sphincter dysfunction. Dis Colon Rectum. 1999;42:1411–8.
9. Aslam A, Grier DJ, Duncan AW, and Spicer RD. The role of magnetic resonance imaging in the preoperative assessment of anorectal anomalies. Pediatr Surg Int. 1998;14:71–3.
10. McHugh K. The role of radiology in children with anorectal anomalies: with particular emphasis on MRI. Eur J Radiol. 1998;26:194–9.
11. Husberg B, Rosenborg M, and Frenckner B. Magnetic resonance imaging of anal sphincters after reconstruction of high or intermediate anorectal anomalies with posterior sagittal anorectoplasty and fistula-preserving technique. J Pediatr Surg. 1997;32:1436–42.
12. Wolpert A, Beer-Gabel M, Lifschitz O, and Zbar AP. The management of presacral masses in the adult. Tech Coloproctol. 2002;6:43–9.
13. deSouza NM, Williams AD, Wilson HJ, Gilderdale DJ, Coutts GA, and Black CM. Fecal incontinence in scleroderma: assessment of the anal sphincter with thin-section endoanal MR imaging. Radiology. 1998;208:529–35.
14. Sangwan YP, Rosen L, Riether RD, Stasik JJ, Sheets JA, and Khubchandani IT. Is simple fistula-in-ano simple? Dis Colon Rectum. 1994;37:885–9.
15. Garcia-Aguilar J, Belmonte C, Wong WD, Goldberg SM, and Madoff RD. Anal fistula surgery. Factors associated with recurrence and incontinence. Dis Colon Rectum. 1996;39:723–9.
16. Zbar AP. Magnetic resonance imaging and the coloproctologist. Tech Coloproctol. 2001;5:1–7.
17. Barker PG, Lunniss PJ, Armstrong P, Reznek RH, Cottam K, and Phillips RK. Magnetic resonance imaging of fistula-in-ano:technique, interpretation and accuracy. Clin Radiol. 1994;49:7–13.
18. Spencer JA, Ward J, Beckingham IJ, Adams C, and Ambrose NS. Dynamic contrast-enhanced MR imaging of perianal fistulas. AJR Am J Roentgenol. 1996;167:735–41.
19. Spencer J, Chapple K, Wilson D, Ward J, Windsoe ACJ, and Ambrose NS. Outcome after surgery for perianal fistula: predictive value of MR imaging. AJR Am J Roentgenol. 1998;171:403–6.
20. Maruyama R, Noguchi T, Takano M, Takagi K, Morita N, Kikuchi R, and Uchida Y. Usefulness of magnetic resonance imaging for diagnosing deep anorectal abscess. Dis Colon Rectum. 2000;43 (Suppl):S2–S5.
21. Buchanan GN, Williams AB, Bartram CI, Halligan S, Nicholls RJ, and Cohen CRG. Potential clinical implications of direction of a trans-sphincteric anal fistula track. Br J Surg. 2003;90:1250–5.
22. Zbar AP, Ramesh J, BeerGabel M, Salazar R, and Pescatori M. Conventional cutting versus internal anal sphincter-preserving seton for high trans-sphincteric fistula: a prospective randomized manometric and clinical trial. Tech Coloproctol. 2003;7:89–94.
23. Zbar AP, deSouza NM, Puni R, and Kmiot WA. Comparison of endoanal magnetic resonance imaging with surgical findings in perirectal sepsis. Br J Surg. 1998;85:111–4.

24. Chapple KS, Spencer JA, Windsor ACJ, Wilson D, Ward J, and Ambrose NS. Prognostic value of magnetic resonance imaging in the management of fistula-in-ano. Dis Colon Rectum. 2000;43:511–6.
25. Cavanaugh M, Hyman N, and Osler T. Fecal incontinence severity index after fistulotomy: a predictor of quality of life. Dis Colon Rectum. 2002;45: 349–53.
26. Dahlberg M, Stenborg A, Pahlman L, Glimelius B; Swedish Rectal Cancer Trial. Cost-effectiveness of preoperative radiotherapy in rectal cancer: Results for the Swedish Rectal Cancer Trial. Int J Radiat Oncol Biol Phys. 2002;54:654–60.
27. Kim MJ, Park JS, Park SI, Kim NK, Kim JH, Moon HJ, Park YM, and Kim WH. Accuracy in differentiation of mucinous and non-mucinous rectal carcinoma on MR imaging. J Comput Assist Tomogr. 2003;27:48–55.
28. Heald RJ and Ryall RD. Recurrence and survival after total mesorectal excision for rectal cancer. Lancet. 1986;I:1479–82.
29. Heald RJ, Moran BJ, Ryall RD, Sexton R, and MacFarlance JK. Rectal cancer: the Basingstoke experience of total mesorectal excision, 1978–1997. Arch Surg. 1998;133:894–9.
30. Dahlberg M, Glimelius B, and Pahlman L. Changing strategy for rectal cancer is associated with improved outcome. Br J Surg. 1999;86:379–84.
31. Hermanek P. Impact of surgeon's technique on outcome after treatment of rectal carcinoma. Dis Colon Rectum. 1999;42:559–62.
32. Kapiteijn E, Putter H, van de Velde CJ; Cooperative Investigators of the Dutch ColoRectal Cancer Group. Impact of the introduction and training of total mesorectal excision on recurrence and survival in rectal cancer in the Netherlands. Br J Surg. 2002;89:1142–9.
33. Kremser C, Judmaier W, Hein P, Griebel J, Lukas P, and de Vries A. Preliminary results on the influence of chemoradiation on apparent diffusion coefficients of primary rectal carcinoma measured by magnetic resonance imaging. Strahlenther Onkol. 2003;179:641–9.
34. Watanabe T, Tsurita G, Muto T, Sawada T, Sunouchi K, Higuchi Y, Komuro Y, Kanazawa T, Iijima T, Miyaki M, and Nagawa H. Extended lymphadenectomy and preoperative radiotherapy for lower rectal cancers. Surgery. 2002;132:27–33.
35. Durdey P and Williams NS. The effect of malignant and inflammatory fixation of rectal carcinoma on prognosis after rectal excision. Br J Surg. 1984;71:787–90.
36. Bissett IP, Fernando CC, Hough DM, Cowan BR, Chau KY, Young AA, Parry BR, and Hill GL. Identification of the fascia propria by magnetic resonance imaging and its relevance to preoperative assessment of rectal cancer. Dis Colon Rectum. 2001;44:259–65.
37. Quirke P, Durdey P, Dixon MF, and Williams NS. Local recurrence of rectal adenocarcinoma due to inadequate surgical resection: histopathological study of lateral tumour spread and surgical excision. Lancet. 1986;ii:996–9.
38. Bjerkeset T, Morild I, Mork S, and Soreide O. Tumor characteristics in colorectal cancer and their relationship to treatment and prognosis. Dis Colon Rectum. 1987;30:934–8.
39. Halvorsen TB and Seim E. Association between invasiveness, inflammatory reaction, desmoplasia and survival in colorectal cancer. J Clin Pathol. 1989; 42:162–6.
40. Murphy J, O'Sullivan GC, Lee G, Madden M, Shanahan F, Collins JK, and Talbot IC. The inflammatory response within Dukes' B colorectal cancers: implications

for progression of micrometastases and patient survival. Am J Gastroenterol. 2000;95:3607–14.

41. Moore HG, Reidel E, Minsky BD, Saltz L, Paty P, Wong D, Cohen AM, and Guillem JG. Adequacy of 1-cm distal margin after restorative rectal cancer resection with sharp mesorectal excision and preoperative combined-modality therapy. Ann Surg Oncol. 2003;10:80–5.
42. Talbot IC, Ritchie S, Leighton MH, Hughes AO, Bussey HJ, and Morson BC. The clinical significance of invasion of veins by rectal cancer. Br J Surg. 1980;67:439–42.
43. Ouchi K, Sugawara T, Ono H, Fujiya T, Kamiyama Y, Kakugawa Y, Mikuni J, and Tateno H. Histologic features and clinical significance of venous invasion in colorectal carcinoma with hepatic metastasis. Cancer. 1996;78:2313–7.
44. Harrison JC, Dean PJ, el-Zeky F, and Vander Zwaag R. From Dukes through Jass: pathological prognostic indicators in rectal cancer. Hum Pathol. 1994;25:498–505.
45. Brown G, Radcliffe AG, Newcombe RG, Dallimore NS, Bourne MW, and Williams GT. Preoperative assessment of prognostic factors in rectal cancer using high-resolution magnetic resonance imaging. Br J Surg. 2003;90:355–64.
46. Shepherd NA, Baxter KJ, and Love SB. Influence of local peritoneal involvement on pelvic recurrence and prognosis in rectal cancer. J Clin Pathol. 1995;48:849–55.
47. Solomon MJ, Egan M, Roberts RA, Philips J, and Russell P. Incidence of free colorectal cancer cells on the peritoneal surface. Dis Colon Rectum. 1997; 40:1294–8.
48. Beets-Tan RG and Beets GL. Rectal cancer: how accurate can imaging predict the T stage and the circumferential resection margin? Int J Colorectal Dis. 2003;18:385–91.
49. Quirke P and Dixon MF. The prediction of local recurrence in rectal adenocarcinoma by histopathological examination. Int J Colorect Dis. 1988;3:127–31.
50. de Has-Kock DF, Baeten CG, Jager JJ, Langendijk JA, Schouten LJ, Volovics A, and Arends JW. Prognostic significance of radial margins of clearance in rectal cancer. Br J Surg. 1996;83:781–5.
51. Beets-Tan RG, Beets GL, Vliegen RF, Kessels AG, van Boven H, De Bruine A, von Meyenfeldt MF, Baeten CG, and van Engelshoven JM. Accuracy of magnetic resonance imaging in prediction of tumour-free resection margin resection margin in rectal cancer surgery. Lancet. 2001;357(9255):497–504.
52. Abulafi AM and Williams NS. Local recurrence of colorectal cancer: the problem, mechanisms, management and adjuvant therapy. Br J Surg. 1994; 81:7–19.
53. Gunderson LL and Sosin H. Areas of failure found at reoperation (second or symptomatic look) following “curative surgery” for adenocarcinoma of the rectum. Clinicopathologic correlation and implications for adjuvant therapy. Cancer. 1974;34:1278–92.
54. Sagar P. Reoperative surgery for recurrent rectal cancer. In: Longo WE and Northover J, editors. Reoperative colon and rectal surgery. London: Martin Dunitz; 2003. pp. 221–51.
55. Ebner F, Kressel HY, Mintz MC, et al. Tumor recurrence versus fibrosis in the female pelvis: differentiation with MR imaging at 1.5T. Radiology. 1988; 166:333–40.

56. Rafto SE, Amendola MA, and Gefter WB. MR imaging of recurrent colorectal carcinoma versus fibrosis. J Comput Assist Tomogr. 1988;12:307–11.
57. Torricelli P, Pecchi A, Luppi G, and Romagnoli R. Gadolinium-enhanced MRI with dynamic evaluation in diagnosing the local recurrence of rectal cancer. Abdom Imaging. 2003;28:19–27.
58. Robinson P, Carrington BM, Swindell R, Shanks JH, and O'Dwyer ST. Recurrent or residual pelvic bowel cancer: accuracy of MRI local extent before salvage surgery. Clin Radiol. 2002;57:514–22.
59. Moulopoulos LA, Karvouni E, Kehagias D, Dimopoulos MA, Gouliamos A, and Vlahos L. MR imaging of complex tailgut cysts. Clin Radiol. 1999;54:118–22.
60. Dworak O. Number and size of lymph nodes and node metastases in rectal carcinomas. Surg Endosc. 1989;3:96–9.
61. Brown G, Richards CJ, Bourne NW, Newcombe RG, Radcliffe AG, Dallimore NS, and Williams GT. Morphologic predictors of lymph node status in rectal cancer with use of high-spatial-resolution MR imaging with histopathologic comparison. Radiology. 2003;227:371–7.
62. Brown G, Radcliffe AG, Newcombe RG, Dallimore NS, Bourne MW, and Williams GT. Pre-operative assessment of prognostic factors in rectal cancer using high-resolution magnetic resonance imaging. Br J Surg. 2003;90:355–64.

Chapter 3.3(ii)
MRI in Colorectal Surgery: Endoluminal MR Imaging of Anorectal Diseases

Jaap Stoker

Introduction

Several common anorectal diseases—fecal incontinence, complex and recurrent perianal fistulas, and rectal tumors—require imaging for proper management. Magnetic resonance imaging (MRI) has become a valuable alternative to endosonography, with superiority in several aspects of diagnosis and management. Initially, MRI with the use of a body coil and surface coil MRI were introduced. Although the potential of the technique was demonstrated, both MRI methods had drawbacks, as the spatial resolution of body coil MRI was too limited and the effective volume of external surface coils too small (1). Further developments included the introduction of endoluminal coils and phased array coils, which have given a boost to the use and diagnostic accuracy of MRI (2–6). Both types of coils give a higher signal-to-noise ratio, which can be used to increase spatial resolution. The use of endoluminal coils results in the highest signal-to-noise for a limited field of view, whereas phased array coils have the advantage of larger fields of view.

In this chapter, the merits and limitations of endoluminal MRI of anorectal diseases are discussed. The role of endoluminal MRI in anorectal diseases has been studied primarily in fecal incontinence and in perianal fistulas, with more limited study in certain anorectal tumors.

Endoanal MRI Technique

Endoluminal coils can be used at any field strength, but mainly will be used at field strengths of 1 Tesla and higher. For endoluminal MRI of the rectum, a coil with a balloon or a cylindrical rigid coil can be used, while a cylindrical rigid coil is the most optimal for endoanal MRI (7). T2-weighted sequences (turbo spin-echo) are commonly used, as these give optimal tissue contrast in this area. T1-weighted sequences after intravenous (IV) contrast medium are not routine, but may be valuable in inflammatory and neoplastic disease. The axial plane is the most informative plane, and one or more additional longitudinal planes should be used to fully evaluate the anal anatomy and anal sphincter pathology (7). The imaging planes should be parallel or orthogonal to the coil and anorectum to reduce partial volume effects. As the angle of the anus is different to the angle of the rectum, one oblique axial sequence will not suffice for axial evaluation in patients with diseases involving both the anus and rectum. In these cases, at least one additional axial sequence with different angulation should be used.

Patient discomfort is limited with endoanal MRI, except in some patients with perianal fistulas. In our experience, approximately 10% of the patients with perianal fistulas experience discomfort, whereas the examination will not be possible in 2% (8). Bowel relaxants can be given to reduce artifacts caused by bowel motion. The total examination time (room time) will depend on the imaging protocol used and therefore will vary between 20 and 60 minutes. For more details on the technique of endoluminal MRI, the reader is referred to the literature and textbooks on this subject (6–9).

There are no absolute values for tissue contrast [as there are, for example, in computed tomography (CT)], and therefore contrast of a tissue or structure on MRI is compared with surrounding tissues and described as a relative difference in signal intensity, where references at T2-weighted sequences (fat or fluid) are used. These are generally very hyperintense (white), whereas very hypointense (black) structures such as fibrous tissue (e.g., tendon or aponeurosis) and cortical structures are used as references at the other end of the MR signal spectrum.

Normal Anorectal Anatomy on Endoluminal MRI

The layered anatomy of the rectum comprises the mucosa and submucosa, the muscularis propria (the inner circular layer and the outer longitudinal layer), and the surrounding perirectal fat. With endoluminal MRI, using T2-weighted images, the muscularis propria can be identified as a relatively low-intensity structure, distinct from the relatively hyperintense inner (sub)mucosal layers and the relatively hyperintense outer perirectal fat.

The anal sphincter is composed of several cylindrical layers identifiable on MRI (Figures 3.3(ii).1 and 3.3(ii).2) (2,6,10). The innermost layer is evident on T2-weighted turbo spin-echo sequences as a relatively hyperintense subepithelium/submucosa that effectively seals off the anal canal (so-called anal cushions). The next layer is the relatively hyperintense cylindrical smooth muscle of the internal anal sphincter (IAS) (more hyperintense than the subepithelium), the continuation of the circular muscular layer of the muscularis propria of the rectum. Outside the IAS is the relatively hypointense longitudinal muscle layer, a continuation of the longitudinal layer of the muscularis propria. The longitudinal layer courses through the relatively hyperintense fat-containing layer that represents the surgical intersphincteric space. The outermost layer is the relatively hypointense striated muscle of the external anal sphincter (EAS) and the puborectalis (PR) muscle. The EAS forms the lower outer ring of the sphincter complex (Figure 3.3(ii).2), while the sling-like PR (pubovisceralis) forms the upper part.

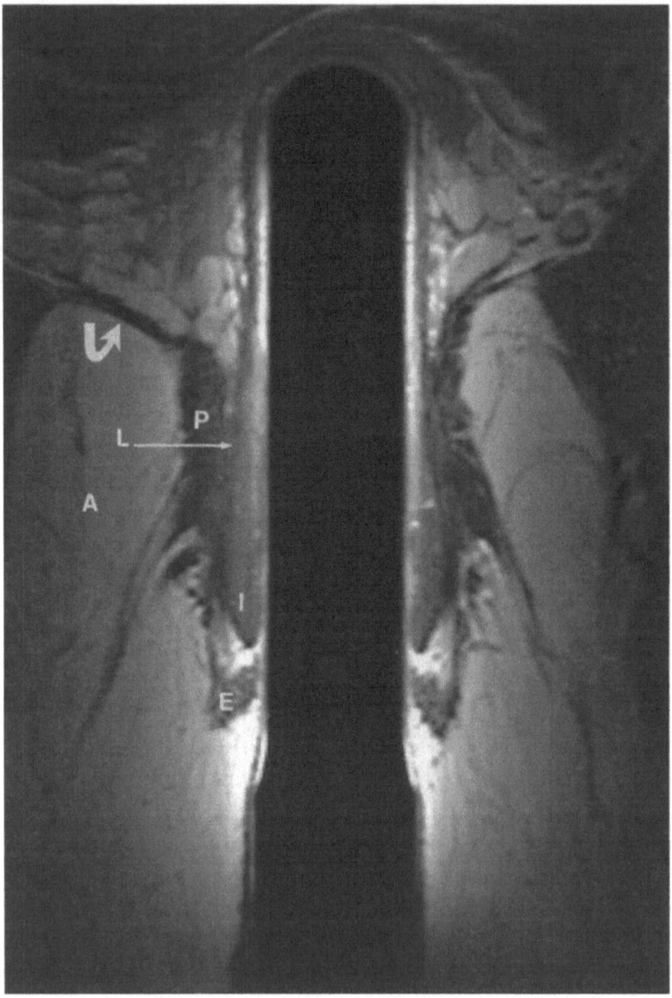

FIGURE 3.3(ii).1. Coronal T2-weighted MRI demonstrates the multilayer morphology of the anal sphincter. Innermost are the mucosa/submucosa and consecutively, the relatively hyperintense internal anal sphincter (I), the relatively hypointense longitudinal muscle (L) in the intersphincteric space, the external anal sphincter (E), and puborectalis (pubovisceral) muscle (P). The levator ani muscle (curved arrow) and ischioanal fossa (A) also are shown.

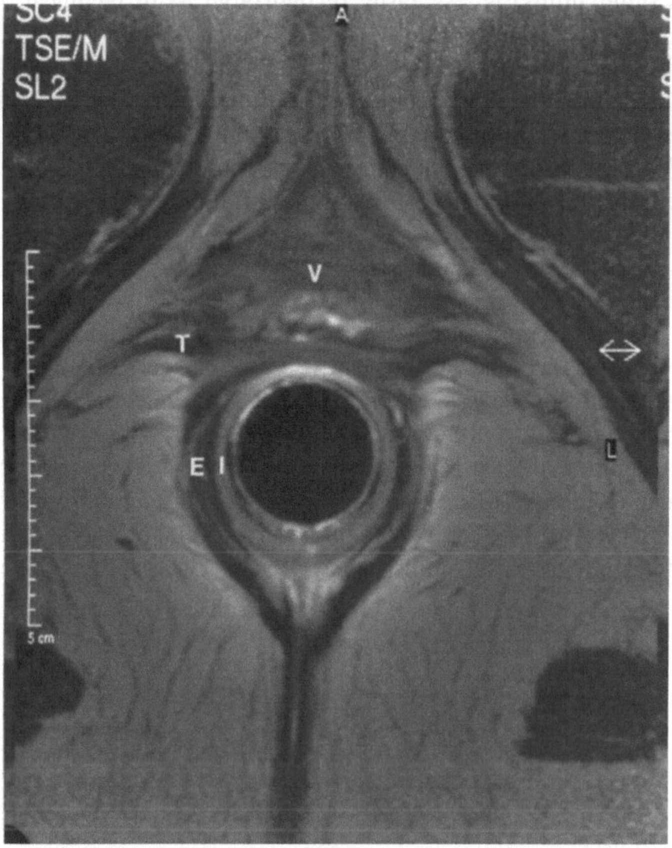

FIGURE 3.3.(ii).2. Axial T2-weighted MRI showing the relatively hyperintense internal anal sphincter (I) signal, the relatively hypointense external anal sphincter (E) signal, Vaginal introitus (V), and transverse perineal muscle (T).

Endoanal MRI and Fecal Incontinence

Anal sphincter defects are an important cause of fecal incontinence. Initially, digital examination, anal manometry, and electromyography were used for identifying anal sphincter defects; however, these techniques have limitations (limited accuracy and relative invasiveness) and have been surpassed by endoluminal imaging with respect to detection of sphincter defects.

Endosonography was the first endoluminal technique introduced in the work up of patients with fecal incontinence, and this methodology has become an important integral part of the diagnostic work up in anorectal units. The IAS and PR muscles are readily visualized, although the EAS (and its outer limits) is less easily recognizable. With technical developments and greater awareness of the sonographic features of the EAS, there has been improvement in the visualization of the boundaries of the muscle and in the delineation of EAS defects. This limited visualization of the EAS at endosonography prompted the introduction of endoanal MRI in the mid 1990s. With this technique, all components of the sphincter can be visualized accurately in the axial, coronal, and sagittal planes, providing the possibility not only of evaluating the sphincter boundaries, but also showing the internal structure of the muscle, which appears to be a prerequisite for the detection of external sphincter atrophy.

Initial studies using endoanal MRI have disclosed that anal sphincter anatomy is visualized accurately with this technique (2). Several studies have evaluated the accuracy of endoanal MRI in detecting lesions of the anal sphincter. Lesions of both the IAS and EAS are visualized accurately, with an accuracy of 95% for EAS lesions (11). Several types of sphincter lesions can be identified, including defects, scar tissue, and atrophy (Figures 3.3(ii).3–3.3(ii).6). The overall inter-observer agreement for the assessment of sphincter integrity using endoanal MRI is strongest if the sphincters are

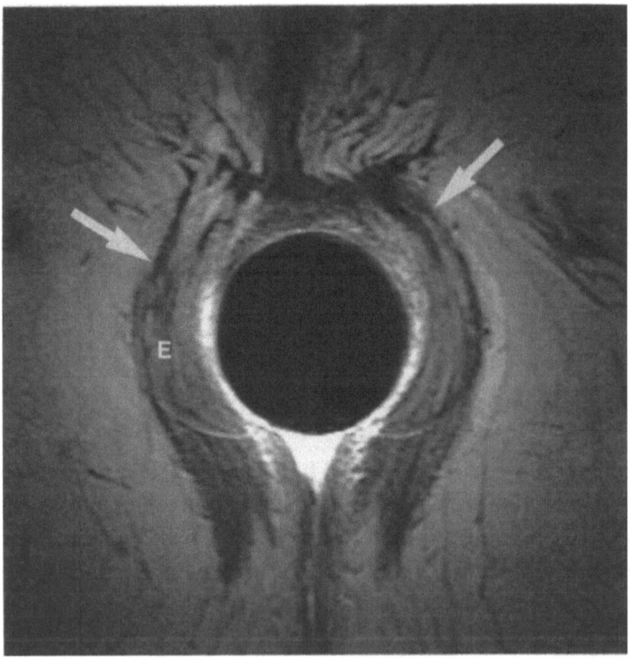

FIGURE 3.3(ii).3. Axial T2-weighted MRI demonstrating hypointense scar tissue (arrows) at the anterior EAS. Compare the distorted architecture anteriorly with Figure 3.3(ii).2 and the remaining normal external anal sphincter (E).

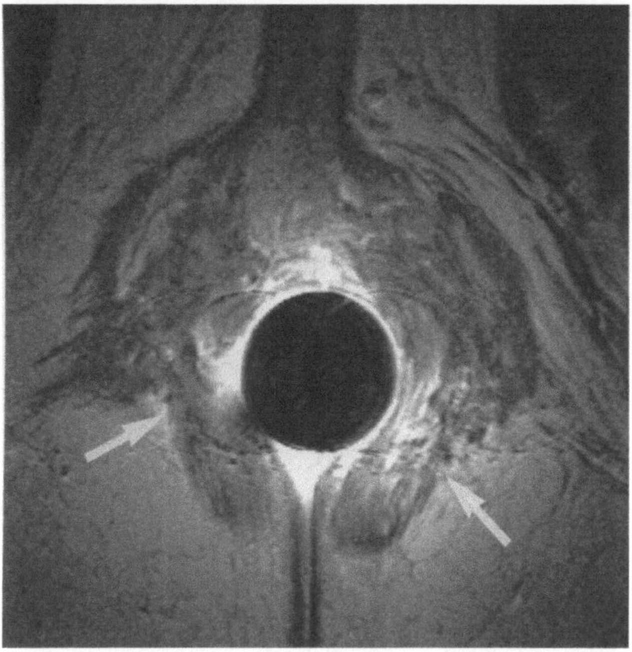

FIGURE 3.3(ii).4. On axial T2-weighted MRI there is complete distortion of the anterior external anal sphincter (compare with Figure 3.3(ii).2). Only the posterior part has remained intact (arrows).

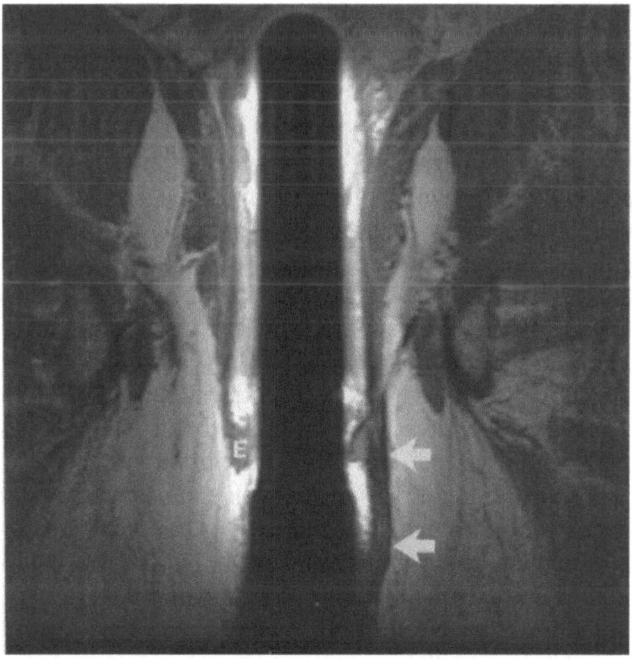

FIGURE 3.3(ii).5. Coronal T2-weighted MRI reveals longitudinal scarring after fistula. Scarring inferior of the sphincter and at the left external sphincter (arrows). Compare to normal external sphincter (E) at the right.

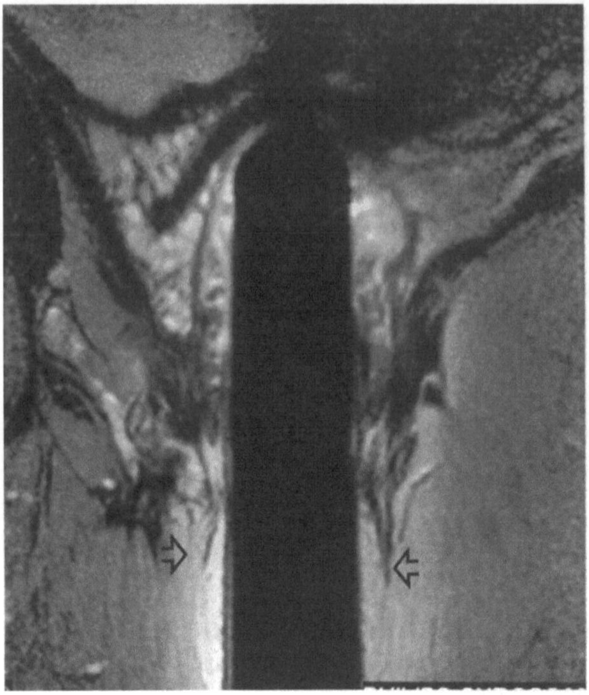

FIGURE 3.3(ii).6. Coronal T2-weighted MRI shows atrophy of the external sphincter (open arrows). Compare to Figure 3.3(ii).1.

either both intact or both disrupted (12) where the full extent of the damage is best appreciated in a combined evaluation of the axial and longitudinal plane sequences. Secondary changes to the architecture of adjacent structures (longitudinal muscle and perianal fat) provide supportive evidence of a tear, and although the opposite side may be atrophic, if it remains relatively normal, it still may be compared with the "torn" side.

Studies on the role of endoanal MRI in the work up as compared with anorectal functional tests have not been performed as yet. Until now, two comparative studies of endosonography and endoanal MRI in fecal incontinence have been published, with partly discordant findings. A retrospective study by Rociu et al. of 22 patients with sphincter defects compared anal endosonography and endoanal MRI with surgery. In this series, MRI was found to be the most accurate technique (11). External anal sphincter defects were detected with sonography and endoanal MRI in 16 (73%) and 20 (91%) patients, respectively, and IAS defects in 15 (68%) and 17 (77%) cases, respectively. In a similar prospective study by Malouf et al. in 52 consecutive patients presenting with fecal incontinence, it was suggested that endosonography and endoanal MRI are comparable for the delineation of EAS defects and that endosonography is superior in defining IAS defects (13). This may be partly expected given the endosonographic features of the IAS and the MR features of the EAS. In this study, comparisons of imaging findings were made by consensus of a gastroenterologist and a surgeon. The differences between the results of both studies are at least partly related to differences in patient populations, study design, and experience with either technique. Most likely, endosonography and endoanal MRI are comparable in detecting IAS and EAS defects. There may be some differences in sensitivity, but the level of experience of the radiologist is probably of greater importance than the technique used.

Apart from focal lesions, there may be generalized sphincter muscle changes of the internal or external anal sphincters. This primarily concerns the definition of muscle thinning (atrophy). Atrophy of the IAS in idiopathic degeneration can present as passive incontinence (14). Atrophy of the IAS also may be found in patients with scleroderma (15), and the diagnosis of IAS atrophy is made on endoluminal MRI when the IAS thickness is less than two millimeters. As the IAS is accurately demonstrated using both endosonography and endoanal MRI, this diagnosis can be established with either technique.

Recent publications on endoanal MRI have reemphasized the importance of EAS atrophy. This entity had become somewhat neglected following the widespread introduction of endosonography and subsequent removal of electromyography from the work up in many institutions. Until the introduction of endoanal MRI, no endosonographic study addressed the issue of EAS atrophy. The problem with an endosonographic diagnosis of atrophy is that although the outer border of the external sphincter is visible in normals, this is no longer possible with fat replacement in patients with significant atrophy. The accurate visualization of the EAS boundaries and internal structure on endoanal MRI provided the possibility of evaluating both the presence of sphincter lesions, as well as EAS atrophy in one examination (Figure 3.3(ii).1). On endoanal MRI, EAS atrophy is characterized by generalized sphincter thinning and fatty replacement (Figure 3.3(ii).6). Endoanal MRI has been demonstrated to be accurate in this evaluation, which has been validated both surgically and histologically (16,17). In a study with histological confirmation, endoanal MRI has been demonstrated to be accurate in evaluating EAS atrophy in 93% (14 of 15) cases (17). A recent study delineated the EAS with endoanal MRI and found that there is a relationship between function (e.g., squeeze pressure) and EAS bulk, although no functional relationship was found with the fat content of the anal sphincter (18).

External anal sphincter atrophy on endoanal MRI is also a negative predictor of the outcome of sphincter repair. In a comparative study of 20 female patients, no EAS was detected with endosonography, while the presence of EAS atrophy with endoanal MRI (as defined) correlated ($p = 0.004$) with a poor functional outcome following anal sphincter repair ($P = 0.004$) (16).

Alternative MRI Techniques

The role of external phased array coil MRI in the work up of fecal incontinence has not yet been evaluated. Potential advantages include a simpler examination without the need to introduce an endoluminal coil, as well as cheaper cost. Although the anatomy of the pelvic floor anatomy can be demonstrated accurately (19), it remains to be demonstrated whether phased array coil MRI does allow enough delineation of pelvic muscles for accurate detection of sphincter defects and atrophy. Endovaginal MRI can be used for evaluation of the anal sphincter without distension by an endoanal coil; however, the increased distance between the sphincter and the coil is a significant disadvantage, and distension of the anal sphincter does not have to be considered an obvious disadvantage. The torn ends of a ruptured sphincter may be identified more clearly when there is less overlay of the torn sphincter parts.

Although recently three-dimensional (3D) endosonography of the anal canal has shown a direct correlation between the angle of the EAS defect and its length (20), it is unclear whether endoanal distraction is a real disadvantage as such, and comparisons with transvaginal MRI have not been made in patients presenting with fecal incontinence and known EAS defects.

Present Work Up

In the work up of patients with fecal incontinence, endoanal MRI can be used as a primary imaging technique, as a problem-solving technique, or as additional technique after endosonography. In most institutions, endosonography will be the primary imaging modality, as this is more widely available and most likely less costly than endoanal MRI. With the present knowledge, this strategy can be used with, however, one important caveat. When disruption of the EAS has been diagnosed, MRI is strongly recommended prior to EAS repair to exclude significant sphincter atrophy. When endoanal MRI is used as the primary imaging technique, this will give an accurate, complete evaluation concerning lesions or generalized atrophy of the sphincter in one procedure. Whether the benefits of this approach outweigh the costs needs to be studied and will, amongst other things, depend on the prevalence of EAS atrophy presenting to any given institution and the presence of reliable MR image interpretation.

Complex Perirectal Sepsis

The presence of an active perianal fistula is often obvious on clinical grounds. In these patients, imaging may be performed for classification or follow-up after treatment. In others, imaging is performed for the detection of fistulas where symptoms may be nonspecific or where previous disease with fibrous scarring prevents an accurate evaluation on physical examination. Such examples may occur in multiply operated patients with perianal Crohn's disease, where the determination of significant horseshoeing (anteroanal or retrorectal) may be difficult (8,21). Magnetic resonance imaging and endosonography have surpassed fistulography, which has been demonstrated to be an inaccurate (and occasionally complicated) technique (22).

In initial reports using MRI, the value of the body coil MRI in the identification and classification of perianal fistulas has been demonstrated; however, the spatial resolution was somewhat limited. Later studies with the use of higher spatial resolution techniques (endoluminal MRI, external phased array coil MRI) have demonstrated the advantage of these techniques over body coil MRI in perianal fistulas (1,23). Successful surgery for complex perirectal sepsis is reliant on delineation of the primary track, secondary tracks and collections, the internal fistula opening, and their relationship to the main sphincter muscle mass.

Primary Track

Initial studies with a body coil or external surface coil showed accuracy for primary track identification and for definitive classification in up to 92% of cases studied, but later studies have reported conflicting lower accuracies. A major advance has been the introduction of high spatial resolution MRI with the use of endoluminal or external phased array coils. Magnetic resonance imaging with an endoluminal coil has been demonstrated to be superior to external surface coil MRI in cryptoglandular fistulas (accuracy 86% vs. 43%, respectively) (5) (Figures 3.3(ii).7 and 3.3(ii).8), with different results reflecting differences in imaging sequences for both coils along with variations in the initial use of more sensitive sequences (such as the fat-suppression technique) utilized with the body coil MRI. In one of these early studies (5), patients with perianal Crohn's disease were included although it is most likely that endoluminal MRI is not optimal in Crohn's disease. Here, tracks may extend outside the limited field of view of an endoluminal coil, and where there is an expected extrasphincteric fistula, the site and course of the primary track will lie beyond the field of any endoluminal probe, whether that be MRI or ultrasound (24).

In a comparative study of endosonography and endoluminal MRI in 26 patients with cryptoglandular fistulas treated by surgery, our group

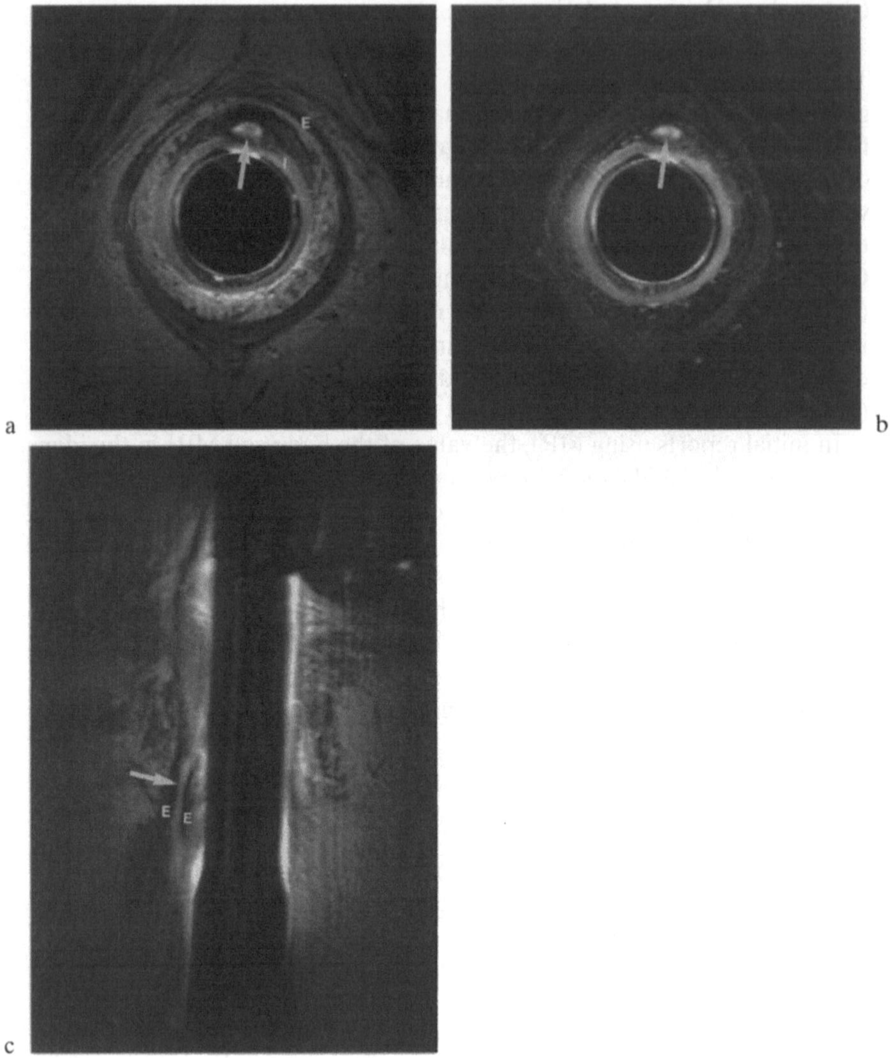

Figure 3.3(ii).7. At axial T2-weighted (a) and axial fat saturated T2-weighted (b) T2-weighted MRI an anterior fistula is visible in the intersphincteric space between external sphincter (E) and lower edge of the internal sphincter (I). The track has an inferior trans-sphincteric course through the anterior external sphincter as visible at a sagittal sequence (c). With fat saturation (b), the fluid within the track is more conspicuous and therefore track identification is facilitated, but the anatomy less clearly identified (b).

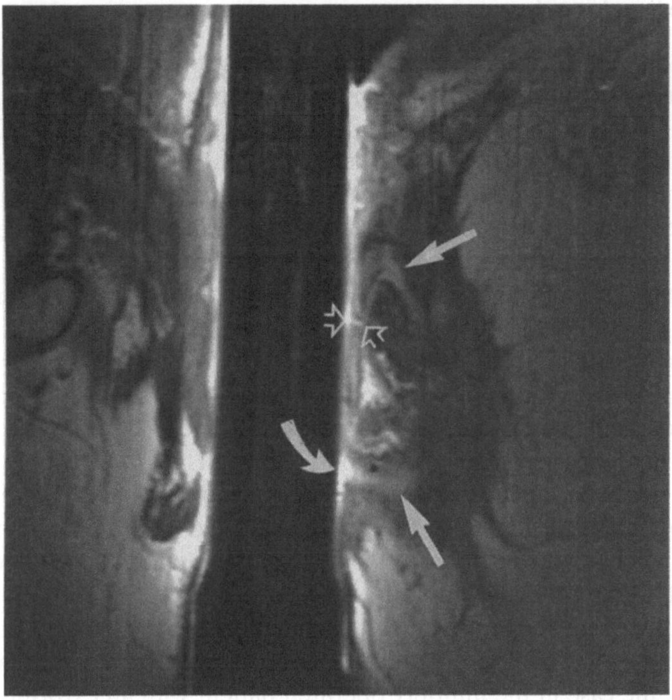

FIGURE 3.3(ii).8. Sagittal oblique T2-weighted MRI shows a trans-sphincteric fistula surrounded by scar tissue. The track (arrows; track partly visualized in this slice) courses through both external sphincter and puborectal (pubovisceral) muscle. Both openings are within the anal canal. The internal opening and the track to the internal opening are subtle (open arrows) and very likely not visualized at external coil MRI. The inferior opening is less subtle (curved arrow).

previously has shown that endoluminal MRI was more accurate in delineation of the primary track (61% vs. 89%, respectively) (3). At endosonography, major difficulties were encountered in the differentiation between scar tissue and an active (or recrudescent) track. The use of hydrogen peroxide has been shown in anal endosonography to facilitate this differentiation (25), and, to date, only one study has assessed this effect, comparing endoluminal MRI with phased array coil MRI or hydrogen peroxide-enhanced endosonography (26). In Crohn's disease, as tracks may be present or extend outside the sensitive region of the endoluminal techniques, external phased array MRI may be preferred in selected cases (Figure 3.3(ii).8).

Complex Fistulas

The coloproctologist also needs to ascertain whether there is any suprasphincteric or translevator component in some complicated cases, where again all forms of endoluminal technology (MRI or ultrasound) will couple poorly above the main PR sling. In such cases, the selective use of combined endoluminal and phased array MRI techniques will be needed. This approach is also of relevance in circumstances where the primary etiology of the sepsis is pelvirectal and where infection breaks through the levator plate. In this circumstance, injudicious drainage of the abscess presenting in the ischioanal fossa will invariably result in a high extrasphincteric fistula, which may occasion proctectomy.

Complex fistulas may have secondary tracks, interconnecting ramifications, horseshoe configurations, or abscesses. Endosonography has limitations in detecting secondary extensions, but results improve with hydrogen peroxide-enhanced endosonography. Data on endoluminal MRI are sparse, and most papers using MRI have only evaluated external coils. In these studies, MRI has been demonstrated to be more accurate than either digital examination or surgical exploration in secondary track identification when the results of a preoperative MR examination are revealed to the coloproctologist after clinical operative decisions have been made. This is particularly the case in the multiply operated patient with an extrasphincteric fistula (27). A study assessing eight patients with complex fistulas compared endoluminal MRI and phased array coil MRI with surgery. Endoluminal MRI was superior to phased array MRI in delineating secondary tracks and their site (92% vs. 54%, respectively) (4).

Internal Opening

Identification of the internal opening often is difficult with endosonography, although the use of hydrogen peroxide has led to improved results. This part of the examination is of vital concern for the prevention of recurrence (28), and particularly where mucosal advancement anoplasty is contemplated for fistula cure (29). Endoluminal MRI has been demonstrated to be superior to non-hydrogen peroxide-enhanced endosonography (71% vs. 43%) and phased array MRI (72% vs. 61%) (3), and the combination of high spatial resolution and high intrinsic contrast resolution leads to identification of even very small internal openings (Figure 3.3(ii).8).

Fluid Collections

Endoluminal MRI has been reported to be superior to phased array MRI in sphincteric abscess identification and location in both patients with simple tracks (100% vs. 50%) and complex tracks (93% vs. 79%) (1,3). However, in daily clinical practice, the superiority of endoluminal MRI for these abscesses is unclear (30). Many sphincteric abscesses will be detected with external phased array coil MRI, although endoluminal MRI may be superior in small abscesses. In a comparative study of endosonography and endoluminal MRI in 28 patients with cryptoglandular fistulas, all abscesses were detected using both techniques (3). In patients with Crohn's disease, tracks or fluid collections may extend outside the sensitive region of the endoluminal coil, as well as endosonography transducer as stated above, necessitating the use of surface imaging technology. It also should be remembered that endoanal ultrasound, because of its acoustic impedance, may overcall sizeable intersphincteric abscesses as trans-sphincteric collections, placing sphincter musculature at risk if this modality alone is relied upon for operative decision making (8,24).

Outcome

With MRI, tracks can be identified in areas not explored at surgery. Several studies using external coils have demonstrated that tracks that were detected at MRI and not identified at surgery proved to be present at follow-up or upon reevaluation at surgery after disclosure of the imaging results. Until now, one series has reported superiority of examination under general anesthesia over endosonography and external phased array coil MRI (31). No study has evaluated outcome for patients studied with endoluminal MRI. With the use of external coils, the beneficial effect of preoperative MRI on clinical outcome in patients presenting with a primary perianal fistula, as well as in patients with recurrent fistulas, has been demonstrated (32,33).

Anovaginal and Rectovaginal Fistulas

Anovaginal and rectovaginal fistulas often are caused by obstetric trauma, inflammation (e.g., Crohn's disease, Behçet's disease), or have an iatrogenic cause (surgery, radiotherapy). These fistulas are uncommon and data on imaging are sparse. Contrast studies of the vagina or rectum have been surpassed by cross-sectional imaging techniques, as the track is often not demonstrated well and the relation of the track to the sphincter is poorly visualized.

Endosonography and endoluminal MRI can demonstrate the track and its relationship to the anal sphincter. The optimal technique has not yet been established, but high-resolution techniques can be expected to be preferable, as the tracks tend to be short, thin walled, and often collapsed (Figure 3.3(ii).9). Until now, one comparative study of endoanal/endorectal sonography and endoanal/endorectal MRI has been published. In this study, endosonography and endoluminal MRI had comparable results with a specificity and positive predictive value for fistula detection of 100% and

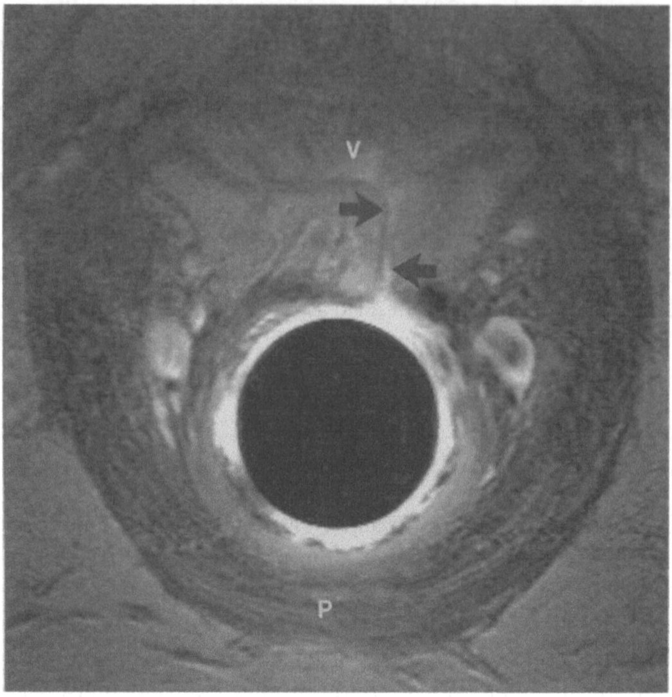

FIGURE 3.3(ii).9. Axial T2-weighted MRI shows an anovaginal fistula (arrows). Vagina (V), puborectal (pubovisceral) muscle (P).

92%, respectively (34). No data are available at the current time concerning the accuracy of external phased array MRI in anovaginal and rectovaginal fistulas.

Recommended Current Work Up

Magnetic resonance imaging is an accurate technique for the work up of some patients with perianal fistula. This is the case for perianal Crohn's disease, especially complex reoperated patients, specialist disorders such as Behçet's disease, perianal inflammation where the anatomy is expected to be complicated (post-irradiation, carcinoma of the anal canal presenting as primary perirectal sepsis, HIV-related fistulas), as well as for unexpected recurrent fistula, presumed extra- or suprasphincteric disease, or where pelvirectal sepsis is suspected. Such imaging also will be advantageous in cases where mucosal or anocutaneous advancement anoplasty is contemplated in which endoanal MRI gives accurate information on both fistula visualization and sphincter integrity (ultrasonography may be used as an alternative). For cryptoglandular tracks, endoluminal MRI is the preferred option for the optimal identification of the track, and especially for the internal opening, because the subepithelial space is relatively poorly demonstrated using surface technology. In Crohn's disease, external phased array MRI is believed to be superior to endoluminal imaging for some of the reasons mentioned above, particularly where disease lies beyond the effective volume of the endoluminal coil or where there is expected supra- or translevator disease. Endoluminal imaging has been demonstrated to be valuable in the preoperative assessment of anovaginal and rectovaginal fistulas where primary repair, interposition grafting, and perineoplasty are contemplated.

Anorectal Tumors

The treatment of rectal tumors has changed substantially over the last few decades, and this has led to a substantial role for preoperative imaging in the staging and management of this disease. Initial work primarily focused on the presence of invasion in or through the wall (T-staging), as well as lymph node (N) staging. More recent studies have emphasized the importance of determining the distance between the tumor and the mesorectal fascia in T3-tumors for the performance of total mesorectal excision with the assessment of radial resection margins. Until now, the number of studies on endoluminal imaging of rectal cancer has been relatively limited, and most studies on MRI of rectal cancer have used external coils [see Chapter 3.3(i)]. Endoluminal MRI is intrinsically limited to local staging, as is endosonography.

Local Staging

Endoluminal MRI can visualize the anorectal wall and small tumors in detail. In general, T2-weighted sequences are used for local staging. As in endosonography, only the lower part of the tumor will be visualized in larger tumors, proximal tumors, and stenotic tumors (Fig. 3.3(ii).10). The accuracy of T-staging of rectal tumor is approximately 75 to 85% (Fig. 3.3(ii).11) (35–37). Comparative studies with other imaging techniques are sparse and do not demonstrate superiority of endoanal MRI over endosonography or external phased array coil MRI (38). In a study comparing endoluminal MRI and external phased array MRI, the use of an endoluminal coil resulted in a more detailed demonstration of the rectal wall, but this did not result in an improved staging accuracy (39). With each technique (endosonography, endoluminal MRI, external phased array MRI), limitations in accuracy are subject to understaging caused by microscopic invasion and overstaging caused by desmoplastic reaction (40).

a 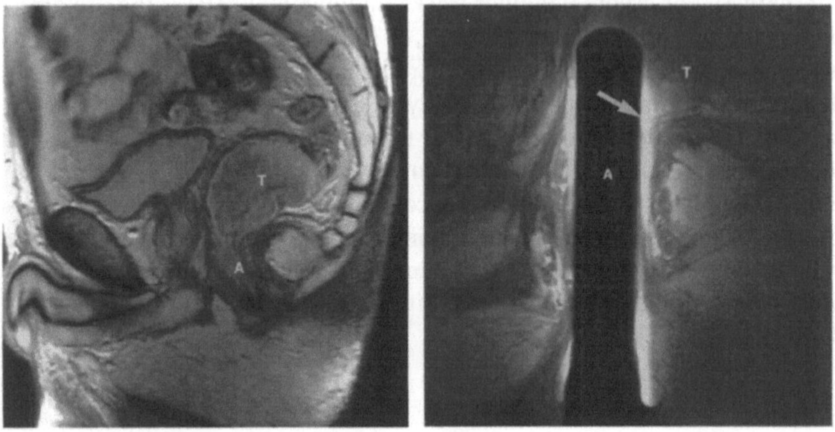 b

Figure 3.3(ii).10. Sagittal T2-weighted MRI with external phased array coil (a) demonstrates a villous adenoma posterior in the distal rectum. The complete tumor (T) can be evaluated for extension through the wall. With endoluminal MRI in identical plane (b), the relation of the tumor (T) to the anal sphincter and anorectal junction (arrow) is more easily appreciated. Only the inferior part of the tumor (T) is visualized. Anus (A).

a 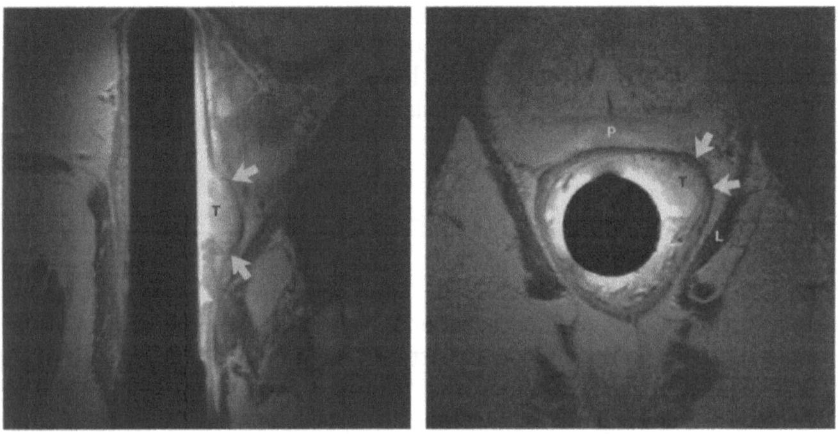 b

Figure 3.3(ii).11. Sagittal oblique T2-weighted MRI (a) shows a distal rectal tumor (T) without extension through the relatively hypointense muscular wall (arrows). Levator ani muscle (L), anorectal junction (large arrow). Axial plane (b) confirms the findings. The tumor (T) does not extend through the relatively hypointense wall (arrows). Levator ani muscle (L), prostate (P).

The more routine use of fat-clearance technology has expanded the lymph node yield after total mesorectal excision, whether that is performed open or laparoscopic assisted (41). In these lymph node retrievals, up to one-quarter of the glands are less than five millimeters in maximal diameter (42), with at least one-third of metastases being less than two millimeters in size (43). In this regard, present standard imaging techniques (surface or endoluminal) will not prove sufficiently accurate in the preoperative delineation of such micrometastatic disease. However, a new development is the use of a lymph node specific contrast medium [ultra small paramagnetic iron oxide (USPIO)] (44). This facilitates identification of metastatic involvement in lymph nodes considered benign with standard imaging (see section on local lymph node staging).

Transanal endoscopic microsurgery (TEMS) can be performed for T1 tumors where detailed preoperative information provided by high soft tissue resolution imaging on tumor depth might be valuable. For the work up of these patients, endosonography has the theoretical advantage over endoluminal MRI that the rectal wall is more detailed in its visualization. On endoluminal MRI, only one superficial layer is readily identified, reflecting both the mucosa and the submucosa, which is bordered by muscularis propria (Figures 3.3(ii).10 and 3.3(ii).11), and the hope that endoluminal MRI would successfully differentiate T1 from T2 tumors (and define the role of local excision) has not been realized (40). The mucosa and submucosa also have multiple reflective interfaces on endosonography. Until now, no study has compared both endoluminal imaging techniques in a substantial number of patients with early rectal cancer. The introduction of clinical higher field MR systems (3 Tesla) might lead to improved visualization of the rectal wall at endoluminal MRI.

The sensitive region of an endoluminal coil is often too limited for an adequate visualization of the mesorectal fascia, especially as the tumor will increase the distance between the coil and the mesorectum. Endosonography also has this limitation, effectively precluding evaluation of tumor extension to the mesorectal fascia—a finding normally accurately demonstrated with external phased array MRI (45). Several studies using external phased array coils have shown limitations of MRI in T-staging, but a high accuracy in determining the spread to the mesorectal fascia (45,46). Limitations in T-staging are an important drawback for predicting those patients likely to benefit from preoperative neoadjuvant therapies. Endoluminal MRI has not been shown to be more accurate than external phased array MRI in this respect, although the data are sparse. Multimodality assessment may be of value where the tumors are deemed to be either bulky or where their rostral extent exceeds the linear dimensions of the endoanal MR probe. The mesorectal fascia also is visualized with multi-slice spiral-CT. Computed tomography has the advantage of simultaneous evaluation of lymph nodes, liver, and lungs. Present research is evaluating the role of multi-slice CT in the staging of rectal cancer.

Theoretically, endorectal MRI might be superior to phased array MRI in determining infiltration of the anal sphincter and in anal cancer; however, sufficient data to support this view are currently lacking. Other units have reported more promising results than those alluded to above by Hadfield and colleagues. A recent study of 61 patients using an external phased array MRI evaluated the sensitivity and specificity of this technique in determining anal sphincter infiltration in distal rectal cancer (47), where values were 98% and 100%, respectively.

Local Lymph Node Staging

The data on lymph node staging of rectal tumors with endoluminal MRI are limited. One study has reported an accuracy of 80% (48), while in another series, a sensitivity of only 80% was reported (36). In this latter series by Hünerbein et al., there was not a significant difference between endosonography, 3D endosonography, and endorectal MRI. The specificity has been reported to be between 50 and 70%. With endoluminal techniques, small perirectal lymph nodes are detected more easily than with external coil MRI, but parailiac and paraaortic lymph nodes are not detectable. The reservations regarding positive lymph node detection in rectal cancer afforded by endoluminal probes is discussed above. In a study by Blomqvist and colleagues comparing phased array coil MRI alone to phased array coil MRI combined with an endoluminal coil, the accuracy for local lymph nodes was essentially the same, indicating some preference for phased array coil MRI alone (39). There are limitations with either technique, primarily as the size criterion used is not accurate. Lymph node-specific contrast agents have been developed to address this problem. Ultra small paramagnetic iron oxide is injected intravenously and taken up by non-metastatic lymph nodes (macrophages). With this contrast agent, the signal intensity of normal lymph nodes reduces on T2-weighted gradient echo sequences, while metastases do not show reduced signal intensity. This technique has been demonstrated to be promising in prostate cancer, and preliminary results in rectal cancer are promising (44,49,50). With the use of external phased array coils, all relevant lymph node stations can be evaluated.

Suggested Present Role for Endorectal MRI in Rectal Cancer

The role of endorectal MRI in rectal cancer is limited. At present, no clear evidence exists favoring the use of this technique over external phased array coil MRI or endosonography. Imaging strategies for patients with rectal cancer will depend on local expertise and preference, but may encompass endosonography for early cancer and MRI with external phased array coils in more advanced cases. The role of multi-slice spiral-CT is also yet to be determined.

Conclusions

Endoluminal MRI is in many aspects superior to body coil MRI and in some aspects superior to external phased array MRI and endosonography. The latter primarily concerns the evaluation of EAS atrophy in fecal incontinence. When an EAS defect diagnosed at endosonography is considered for surgical repair, then an endoluminal MRI should be performed (where available) to exclude substantial external sphincter atrophy. Until now, no data are available on external phased array MRI in fecal incontinence. In perianal fistulas, endoanal MRI is preferable in cryptoglandular fistulas, while in Crohn's disease, preliminary evidence suggests a benefit in external phased array coil MRI. The limitations in endoanal probe technology for some important questions in complex perirectal sepsis still apply and have been outlined in this chapter; however, Gadolinium or saline enhancement will readily distinguish residual or recrudescent sepsis from burnt-out scar tissue. In rectal cancer, endorectal MRI has not been demonstrated to be superior to endosonography or external phased array MRI, and its role appears limited. Unfortunately, it has not proven useful in the differentiation between T1 and T2 tumors despite high resolution of the soft tissues, and therefore it cannot enhance surgical decision making regarding curative TEMS. The use of endoluminal MRI might be advantageous in anal tumors for determining depth of infiltration; however, until now, no study has sufficiently evaluated endoluminal MRI in this condition.

References

1. Stoker J, Hussain SM, van Kempen D, Elevelt AJ, and Laméris JS. Endoanal coil in MR imaging of anal fistulas. AJR Am J Roentgenol. 1996;166:360–2.
2. Hussain SM, Stoker J, and Laméris JS. Anal sphincter complex: endoanal MR imaging of normal anatomy. Radiology. 1995;197:671–7.
3. Hussain SM, Stoker J, Schouten WR, Hop WCJ, and Laméris JS. Fistulo-in-ano: endoanal sonography vs endoanal MR imaging in classification. Radiology. 1996;200:475–81.
4. deSouza NM, Gilderdale DJ, Coutts GA, Puni R, and Steiner RE. MRI of fistulo-in-ano: a comparison of endoanal coil with external phased array coil techniques. J Comput Assist Tomogr. 1998;22:357–63.
5. Beets-Tan RG, Beets GL, van der Hoop AG, et al. Preoperative MR imaging of anal fistulas: Does it really help the surgeon? Radiology. 2001;218:75–84.
6. Zbar AP and deSouza NM. The anal sphincter. In: de Souza NM, editor. Endocavitary MRI of the pelvis. London: Harwood Academic Publishers; 2001. pp. 91–109.

7. Stoker J, Rociu E, Zwamborn AW, Schouten WR, and Laméris JS. Endoluminal MR imaging of the rectum and anus: Technique, applications, and pitfalls. Radiographics. 1999;19:383–98.
8. Zbar AP, deSouza NM, Puni R, and Kmiot WA. Comparison of endoanal magnetic resonance imaging with surgical findings in perirectal sepsis. Br J Surg. 1998;85:111–4.
9. Rociu E and Stoker J. Endoanal magnetic resonance imaging. In: Bartram CI and DeLancey JOL, editors. Imaging pelvic floor disorders. Berlin: Springer Verlag; 2003 in press.
10. Rociu E, Stoker J, Eijkemans MJ, and Laméris JS. Normal anal sphincter anatomy and age- and sex-related variations at high-spatial-resolution endoanal MR imaging. Radiology. 2000;217:395–401.
11. Rociu E, Stoker J, Eijkemans MJC, Schouten WR, and Laméris JS. Fecal incontinence: endoanal US versus endoanal MR imaging. Radiology. 1999; 212:453–8.
12. Malouf AJ, Halligan S, Williams AB, Bartram CI, Dhillon S, and Kamm MA. Prospective assessment of interobserver agreement for endoanal MRI in fecal incontinence. Abdom Imaging. 2001;26:76–8.
13. Malouf AJ, Williams AB, Halligan S, Bartram CI, Dhillon S, and Kamm MA. Prospective assessment of accuracy of endoanal MR imaging and endosonography in patients with fecal incontinence. AJR Am J Roentgenol. 2000; 175:741–5.
14. Vaizey CJ, Kamm MA, and Bartram CI. Primary degeneration of the internal anal sphincter as a cause of passive faecal incontinence. Lancet. 1997;349 (9052):612–5.
15. deSouza NM, Williams AD, Wilson HJ, Gilderdale DJ, Coutts GA, and Black CM. Fecal incontinence in systemic sclerosis: assessment of the anal sphincter using high resolution endoanal MR imaging. Radiology. 1998;208:529–35.
16. Briel JW, Stoker J, Rociu E, Laméris JS, Hop WCJ, and Schouten WR. External anal sphincter atrophy on endoanal magnetic resonance imaging adversely affects continence after sphincteroplasty. Br J Surg. 1999;86:1322–7.
17. Briel JW, Zimmerman D, Stoker J, Rociu E, Laméris JS, Mooi WJ, and Schouten WR. Relationship between sphincter morphology on endoanal MRI and histopathological aspects of the external sphincter. Int J Colorectal Dis. 2000;15:87–90.
18. Williams AB, Malouf AJ, Bartram CI, Halligan S, Kamm MA, and Kmiot WA. Assessment of external anal sphincter morphology in idiopathic fecal incontinence with endocoil magnetic resonance imaging. Dig Dis Sci. 2001;46:1466–71.
19. Beets-Tan RG, Morren GL, Beets GL, et al. Measurement of anal sphincter muscles: endoanal US, endoanal MR imaging, or phased-array MR imaging? A study with healthy volunteers. Radiology. 2001;220:81–9.
20. Gold DM, Bartram CI, Halligan S, Humphries KN, Kamm MA, and Kmiot WA. 3-D endoanal sonography in assessing anal canal injury. Br J Surg. 1999;86: 365–70.
21. Tio TL, Mulder CJJ, Wijers OB, Sars PRA, and Tytgat GNJ. Endosonography of peri-anal and peri-colorectal fistula and/or abscess in Crohn's disease. Gastrointest Endosc. 1990;36:331–6.
22. Weisman RI, Orsay CP, Pearl RK, and Abcarian H. The role of fistulography in fistula-in-ano. Dis Colon Rectum. 1991;34:181–4.

23. Spencer JA, Ward J, Beckingham IJ, Adams C, and Ambrose NS. Dynamic contrast-enhanced MR imaging of perianal fistulas. AJR Am J Roentgenol. 1996;191:545–9.
24. Zbar AP and deSouza NM. Prospective comparison of endosonography, magnetic resonance imaging and surgical findings in anorectal fistula and abscess complicating Crohn's disease. Br J Surg. 1999;86:1093–4.
25. Cheong DMO, Nogueras JJ, Wexner SD, and Jagelman DG. Anal endonography for recurrent anal fistulas: image enhancement with hydrogen peroxide. Dis Colon Rectum. 1993;36:1158–60.
26. West RL, Zimmerman DDE, Dwarkasing S, Hop WCJ, Hussain SM, Schouten WR, Kuipers EJ, and Felt-Bersma RJ. Prospective comparison of hydrogen peroxide-enhanced 3-dimensional endoanal ultrasonography and endoanal MR-imaging of perianal fistulas. In: Zimmerman DDE, editor. Diagnosis and treatment of trans-sphincteric perianal fistulas [thesis]. Rotterdam, The Netherlands: Erasmus University; 2003. pp. 45–64.
27. Barker PG, Lunniss PJ, Armstrong P, Reznek RH, Cottam K, and Phillips RK. Magnetic resonance imaging of fistula in ano: technique, interpretation and accuracy. Clin Radiol. 1994;49:7–13.
28. Garcia-Aguilar J, Belmonte C, Wong WD, Goldberg SM, and Madoff RD. Anal fistula surgery: factors associated with recurrence and incontinence. Dis Colon Rectum. 1996;39:723–9.
29. Shemesh EI, Kodner IJ, Fry RD, and Neufeld DM. Endorectal sliding flap repair of complicated anterior anoperineal fistulas. Dis Colon Rectum. 1988;31:22–4.
30. Shouler PJ, Grimley RP, Keighley MRB, and Alexander-Williams J. Fistula in ano is usually simple to manage surgically. Int J Colorectal Dis. 1986;1:113–5.
31. Schwartz DA, Wiersema MJ, Dudiak KM, et al. A comparison of endoscopic ultrasound, magnetic resonance imaging, and exam under anesthesia for evaluation of Crohn's perianal fistulas. Gastroenterology. 2001;121:1064–72.
32. Buchanan GN, Halligan S, Williams AB, Cohen RCG, Tarroni D, Phillips RKS, and Bartram CI. Magnetic resonance imaging for primary fistula in ano. Br J Surg. 2003;90:877–81.
33. Buchanan G, Halligan S, Williams A, Cohen CR, Tarroni D, Phillips RK, and Bartram CI. Effect of MRI on clinical outcome of recurrent fistula-in-ano. Lancet. 2002;360:1661–2.
34. Stoker J, Rociu E, Schouten WR, and Laméris JS. Anovaginal and rectovaginal fistulas: endoluminal sonography versus endoluminal MR imaging. AJR Am J Roentgenol. 2002;178:737–41.
35. Zagoria RJ, Schlarb CA, Ott DJ, et al. Assessment of rectal tumor infiltration utilizing endorectal MR imaging and comparison with endoscopic rectal sonography. J Surg Oncol. 1997;64:312–7.
36. Hünerbein M, Pegios W, Rau B, Vogl TJ, Felix R, and Schlag PM. Prospective comparison of endorectal ultrasound, three-dimensional endorectal ultrasound, and endorectal MRI in the preoperative evaluation of rectal tumors. Surg Endosc. 2000;14:1005–9.
37. Gualdi GF, Casciani E, Guadalaxara A, d'Orta C, Polletini E, and Pappalardo G. Local staging of rectal cancer with transrectal ultrasound and endorectal magnetic resonance imaging: comparison with histologic findings. Dis Colon Rectum. 2000;43:338–45.

38. Bipat S, Glas AS, Slors FJ, Zwinderman AH, Bossuyt PM, and Stoker J. Rectal cancer: local staging and assessment of lymph node involvement with endoluminal US, CT, and MR imaging—a metal-analysis. Radiology. 2004;232:773–83.
39. Blomqvist L, Holm T, Rubio C, and Hindmarsh T. Rectal tumours. MR imaging with endorectal and/or phased array coils, and histopathological staging on giant sections. Acta Radiol. 1997;38:437–44.
40. Zbar AP, deSouza NM, Strickland N, Pignatelli M, and Kmiot WA. Comparison of endoanal magnetic resonance imaging and computerized tomography in the preoperative staging of rectal cancer: a pilot study. Tech Coloproctol. 1998;2:61–6.
41. Jass JR, Miller K, and Northover JM. Fat clearance method versus manual dissection of lymph nodes in specimens of rectal cancer. Int J Colorectal Dis. 1986;1:155–6.
42. Herrera-Ornelas L, Justiniano J, Castillo N, Petrelli NJ, Stulc JP, and Mittelman A. Metastases in small lymph nodes from colon cancer. Arch Surg. 1987; 122:1253–6.
44. Dworak O. Number and size of lymph nodes and node metastases in rectal carcinomas. Surg Endosc. 1989;3:96–9.
45. Koh D, Brown G, Temple L, Raja A, Toomey P, and Husband JE. MR imaging of pelvic lymph nodes in rectal cancer using USPIO: preliminary observations. Radiology. 2002;225:244.
46. Beets-Tan RG, Beets GL, Vliegen RF, et al. Accuracy of magnetic resonance imaging in prediction of tumour-free resection margin in rectal cancer surgery. Lancet. 2001;357:497–504.
47. Hadfield MB, Nicholson AA, MacDonald AW, Farouk R, Lee PWR, Duthie GS, and Monson JRT. Preoperative staging of rectal carcinoma by magnetic resonance imaging with a pelvic phased-array coil. Br J Surg. 1997;84:529–31.
48. Urban M, Rosen HR, Hölbling N, et al. MR imaging for the preoperative planning of sphincter-saving surgery for tumors of the lower third of the rectum: use of intravenous and endorectal contrast materials. Radiology. 2000;214: 503–8.
49. Indinnimeo M, Grasso RF, Cicchini C, et al. Endorectal magnetic resonance imaging in the preoperative staging of rectal tumors. Int Surg. 1996;81:419–22.
50. Harisinghani MG, Barentsz J, Hahn PF, Deserno WM, Tabatabaei S, van de Kaa CH, de la Rosette J, and Weissleder R. Noninvasive detection of clinically occult lymph-node metastases in prostate cancer. N Engl J Med. 2003;348:2491–9.

Editorial Commentary

This technology represents another endoluminal imaging method which has confirmed the basic anatomical configuration of the sphincter musculature but which although providing better soft-tissue resolution images than endoanal ultrasound, suffers from the same limitations in the investigation of anal and rectal pathology as any other endoluminal method. The delineation of the internal opening and course of intersphincteric and transsphincteric fistulae appears to be an advance over ultrasonography and Gadolinium-enhancement distinguishes burnt-out tracks from active recrudescent sepsis. The staging of rectal cancer has been a little disappointing although it affords reasonable T status prediction without an ability to make the important T1/T2 distinction. This methodology is still being validated and may require supplemented pelvic phased-array support in selected cases. It is currently providing very high-resolution images of clinical value in congenital anorectal malformations and in their postoperative assessment.

AZ

Chapter 3.3(iii)
MRI in Colorectal Surgery: Dynamic Magnetic Resonance Imaging

Andreas Lienemann and Tanja Fischer

Introduction

For years, the understanding of pelvic floor anatomy has been obtained by dissection of the human cadaver. This information, although extremely valuable, has produced artifacts that have been written into the anatomic folklore, some secondary to the embalming process itself. As a result, the clinician has, in part, been faced with a wrong (or at least distorted) image of the anatomy and histomorphology of the region. Magnetic resonance imaging (MRI) is a well-established radiological imaging technique that, as a noninvasive modality, allows for the depiction of relevant anatomy in the living subject. Because of its superb soft tissue contrast, multiplanar imaging capability, and lack of ionizing radiation, MRI is now the tool of choice in the diagnosis and research of pelvic floor disorders.

This chapter will briefly review one of the main radiological methods for the dynamic evaluation of the pelvic floor—namely, Functional Cine-MRI, which has developed as a specialized dynamic imaging technique for the "real-time" assessment of the pelvic floor structures (supra- and infralevator), as well as the perineal soft tissues. Following a general outline of the method and details of the technique, there is a description of the available literature on the use of dynamic MRI for patients presenting with evacuatory difficulty and its recommended role in the coloproctologist's armamentarium, as well as its limitations.

General Considerations Concerning the Dynamic Approach

Functional cine-MRI of the pelvic floor can be explained as the conjunction of an imaging modality (MRI with its distinct features) and an adequate method of examination (freezing of motion). It should not be confused with dynamic MRI using intravenous (IV) or arterial contrast media. At present, the imaging sequences utilized do not permit a sufficient depiction of motion using true three-dimensional (3D) techniques. To overcome this limitation and to record motion, two different approaches have been used, including multiple single slices at the same slice position or one stack of slices covering a whole anatomical region. The first approach allows for a higher temporal resolution and can analyze intrinsic (bowel motility) or extrinsic (straining) motion continuously in more detail at any given anatomical position. The duration of one single measurement has to be less than the expected frequency of the motion itself. One disadvantage of this sequencing is the limited overview given by the field of view and the thickness of a single slice. In order to overcome this problem, a stack of slices can be used as an alternative to describe a region of interest. Here, however, due to the increased acquisition time, the temporal resolution is limited and the specified load (e.g., pelvic floor contraction or straining) should not, where possible, vary over the whole duration of the measurement. In this event, it is difficult for the patient to maintain a continuous "posture of strain" over a period of more then 8 seconds without producing blurring artifacts on the images. Moreover, only one snapshot might conceal clinically relevant findings or the further development of existing significant pathologies.

History of Dynamic MRI Development

In the 1991 February issue of *The Lancet*, Hugosson et al. commented in a letter on the important role of the muscles of the abdominal wall (1). They indicated that they had also examined one single female volunteer using MRI to document the changes of the levator ani muscle during rest, contraction, and a Valsalva's maneuver. A few months after this report, Yang and colleagues (2) and Kruyt et al. (3) independently introduced functional cine-MRI of the pelvic floor where both reported on the movement of the bladder, vagina, and rectum in relation to the pubococcygeal and symphysiosacral reference line. Goodrich et al. (4) recommended the technique for the pre- and postoperative evaluation of the pelvic floor in women following vaginal suspension procedures in contrast to the results published by Dellemare and colleagues (5), where the technique appeared to lack adequate clinical application in the examination of the anorectum.

Subsequently, a plethora of publications have focused on different aspects and modifications of the basic method, each stressing the usefulness of functional cine-MRI in the evaluation of the pelvic floor (6–10). These varying techniques have led to a mixed standardization of technique as reflected in the complexity of reporting (Table 3.3(iii)-1).

TABLE 3.3(iii)-1. Functional cine MRI of the pelvic floor: Survey of the literature.

First author	Tesla	Positioning	Type of sequence dynamic	Single slice or slab?	Slice orientation	Patient instruction	Reference line	Opacification
Constantinou	1.5	supine	TSE	slab	ax, sag	r,c	Subtract Ima	B full
Bertschinger	1.5	supine	SSFSE; SP-GRE	slice	sag	r,c,s	PCL3 per; grading	B emptied, R (potato mash +Gd)
	0.5	sitting	SP-GRE	slice	sag	r,c,s,d	PCL3 per; grading	B emptied, R (potato mash +Gd)
Roos	0.5	sitting	SP-GRE	slice	sag, (cor)	r,c,s,d	PCL3 per; grading	B emptied, R (potato mash +Gd)
Fielding	?	supine	SSFSE	slice	sag	r,s	HMO	—
Singh	1.5	supine	FSE	slab	ax, sag, cor	r,s	—	—
Hodroff	1.5	supine	?	slab	sag	r,c,s	PCL1 per	B (NaCl + Gd), VR (Gel + Gd), U (5FKath)
Stoker	?	?	?	?	?	?	?	?
Rentsch	1.5	supine	TrueFISP	slice	sag	r,s,d	PCL1 per	R (Gel + Gd)
Singh	1.5	supine	FSE	slab	ax, sag, cor	r,s	MPL per; grading	—
Unterweger	1.5	supine	SSFSE	slice	sag	r,s	PCL 3 obl	B emptied
Hoyte	1.5	supine	?	slice	sag	r,s	PCL ?	—
Lienemann	1.5	supine	TrueFISP	slice	sag, obl	r,c,s,d	PCL 3 per	B emptied; V + R (Gel)
Bo	0.5	sitting	GE	slice	sag	c,s	PCL 1 per	—
Gousse	1.5	supine	SSFSE	slice	sag	r,s	PSL; grading	—
Pannu	1.5	supine	SSFSE	slice	ax, sag, cor	r,s	?	R?
Goh	1.0	supine	FFE	slab	ax, sag, cor	r,s	PCL 3 per; grading	—
Sprenger	1.5	supine	TrueFISP	slice	ax, sag, (cor)	r,c,s,d	PCL 3 per; HL per	B emptied; V + R (Gel)

Kelvin	1.5	supine	TrueFISP	slice	sag	r,c,s,d	PCL 1 per; grading	B emptied; V + R (Gel)
Comiter	1.5	supine	HASTE; SSFSE	slice	sag	r,s	HMO; grading	—
Vanbeckevoort	1.5	supine	HASTE	slab	sag	r,s	PCL 1 per	R (Gel)
Gufler	1	supine	HASTE	slice	sag	r,c,s	PCL 2	—
Lienemann	1.5	supine	TrueFISP	slice	sag, ax, (obl)	r,c,s,d	PCL 3 per; HL per	B (emptied or NaCl), U (none or Thread + NaCl), V + R (Gel)
Fielding	0.5	sitting/supine	FSE	slice	sag	r,s	PCL 3	B full; Rectal ballon for pressure meas
Schoenenberger	0.5	sitting	GE	slice	sag	r,s	—	R (potato mash +Gd)
Mikuma	1.5	supine	FSE	slab	sag, cor	r,c	—	—
Hilfiker	0.5	sitting	GE	slice	sag	r,c,s,d	—	R (potato mash + Gd)
Hjartardottir	1.0	supine	GE, TSE	slab	ax, sag, cor	r,c,s	PCL 1 per	B full
Healy	1.5	supine	GRASS	slab	sag	r,s	PCL 3 per	V + R (Rubber tube)
Lienemann	1.5	supine	True FISP; HASTE	slice	sag	r,c,s	PCL 1 per	B (NaCl), U (Thread + NaCl), V + R (Gel)
Healy	1.5	supine	GRASS	slab	ax, sag, cor	r,s	PCL 1 per	V + R (Rubber tube)
Lienemann	1.5	supine	True FISP; HASTE	slice	sag	r,c,s	PCL 1 per	B (NaCl), U (Thread + NaCl), V + R (Gel)
Christensen	1.5	supine	FSE	slab	sag, cor	r,s	Subtract Ima	—
Delemarre	1.5	prone	GE	slice	sag	r,s	SSL per	B emptied
Goddrich	1.5	supine	GRASS	?	sag, cor	r,s	PSL; grading	—
Yang	1.5	supine	GRASS	slice	sag, (cor)	r,c,s	PCL 3 obl	—
Kruyt	0.5/1.5	prone	GE	slice; ?	sag	r,c,p	SSL	B emptied; R (normal air)

r, rest; c, contract; S, strain; d, defecate; per, perpendicular; obl, oblique; PCL, pubococcygeal line; MPL, mid pubic line; SSL, symphysiosacral line; PSL, pubosacral line; 1, sym-sacrococcygeal; 2, sym-lev insertion coccygeus; 3, sym-last intervert.

B = Bladder

R = Rectum

V = Vagina

Technique

Taking the literature on functional cine-MRI into consideration, the smallest common denominators for the procedure itself include the following points: the use of a high-field system, the supine or sitting position of the patient using surface array coils, and the utilization of a non-echo-planar imaging sequence to produce a mid sagittal image with the patient either at rest or during straining.

MR System and Patient Positioning

Due to lack of a dedicated MR system for the examination of the pelvic floor, most authors use an all-purpose high-field system of 1.5 Tesla with the possibility of sub-second scans and a 512 matrix in combination with an acceptable signal-to-noise ratio (4,6,8,9,11). In other reports, a mid field system of 0.5 Tesla with an open magnet configuration has been used (3,9,12,13). The latter offers the advantage of evaluating the patient in either a sitting or a standing position, which is a more physiological position for simulated defecation where, at the end of this simulation, certain pathologies (notably full-thickness rectal prolapse and rectoanal intussusception) will become evident. With respect to positioning, however, the supine position proved to be steadier in imaging and was reported as preferable by the patients and more comfortable than the decubitus or prone positions (3,5). The relative disadvantages of the open configuration system include a restricted signal-to-noise ratio due to an occasionally unfavorable design of the surface coils with these open magnets, along with a limited spatial and temporal resolution resulting in generally poorer image quality.

Sequence Protocol

The sequence protocol preferred by most authors includes a set of either T1- or T2-weighted Turbo Spin-Echo sequences with acquisition of a stack of images in two or all three orientations. This type of sequence has been approved in various settings of diseases of the pelvis and provides a high spatial resolution of the selected anatomic region of interest (14,15). This approach facilitates the assessment of the urethral and anal sphincter complexes, as well as the perivaginal spaces (16,17). In addition, the course of an organ such as the sigmoid colon over several slices or of incidental findings such as an intra-abdominal desmoid can be traced (18).

To create the necessary freezing of motion and in accordance with the type of machine and manufacturers instructions, a variety of fast non-echo-planar sequence techniques for image acquisition have been described. Our group first introduced a gradient-echo technique with fully refocused transverse magnetization [true Fast Imaging with Steady Precession (trueFISP)].

This gradient-echo sequence combines both speed (high bandwidth and very short TR) with contrast (mixed T1/T2* contrast), but it is very sensitive to susceptibility gradients. With this sequence, we have achieved an in-plane resolution of one millimeter with a temporal resolution of 1.3 images/second using a 256 matrix and a field of view of 270 millimeters (6). This sequencing has proved superior to gradient-echo techniques with partially refocused transverse magnetization [Fast Field Echo (FFE)] (3,5,19), Gradient Recalled Acquisition in the Steady State (GRASS) (2,20), the multi-echo spin-echo techniques of Rapid Acquisition with Relaxation Enhancement (RARE) (21,22), single snapshot GRASS technology (4), and Half Fourier.

Single-Shot Turbo Spin Echo sequencing (HASTE) (7,23,24). New methods of *k*-space acquisition (11) and recent advances in faster imaging that are not sequence related (so-called "parallel imaging") allow for ultra fast achievement of images that tend to exhibit a lower signal-to-noise ratio.

Slice Orientation

The mid sagittal cut through the pelvis is the most preferred slice orientation throughout the literature (2,3,6,8,9,11,13,20,23). It was first independently introduced by Yang et al. (2) and Kruyt et al. (3), providing an excellent overview of all relevant organs within the different compartments and the bony framework. In addition, radiologists are familiar with this kind of view since the days of conventional cystography or evacuation proctography; however, the complexity of the pelvic floor requires at least two different slice orientations, each perpendicular to the other. As opposed to this in the literature, coronal and axial slices are only occasionally used to acquire additional information (4,9,19,25).

As a result, our own protocol routinely includes a single axial slice, as well as a stack of coronal slices. The axial slice at the level of the inferior border of the symphysis bone and the ischial tuberosities, respectively, nicely depicts the urogenital hiatus with its contents and the puborectalis portion of the levator ani muscle. Changes in the signal intensity of the femoral vein allow for the estimation of the straining effort by the patient, although it is recognized that this slice orientation is subject to changes in the "normal" tilt disposition of the pelvis. Due to the lack of whole coverage of the pelvic floor, coronal images are necessary to evaluate the entire anatomic region (19,25–27). Those images depict the levator ani muscle in more detail and facilitate the detection of lateral rectoceles, levator ani hernias, and rectoanal intussusception. In addition, the uterosacral ligaments are best visualized using this slice orientation.

If some findings on these images remain unclear, an oblique or double-oblique slice orientation adjoining the structure of interest is highly recommended. This presupposes an online survey of the images during the examination assessing specific abnormalities such as asymmetric ballooning of the urogenital hiatus and anticipation of some of the more unusual pelvic floor findings, including a lateral rectocele. We have used this approach in two-thirds of our patients and gained additional information of this type (25).

Organ Opacification

On T2-weighted sequences, fluid-filled structures like the bladder or small bowel loops exhibit high signal intensity. Other organs like the vagina, rectum, anal canal, or muscles normally show an intermediate to low signal intensity, making their evaluation more difficult. This is especially true for T1-weighted sequences. To avoid these difficulties, we introduced a stringent algorithm of opacification of the bladder, urethra, vagina, and rectum (6,25).

Here, the bladder is filled with 60 milliliters of sterile isotonic saline solution using a 26 Fr Foley catheter and the urethra is delineated using a twisted cotton thread soaked with isotonic saline solution and gadopentetate dimeglumine (Magnevist®, Schering, Berlin, Germany) (6). Due to its invasive nature and the potential risk of cystitis or even the loss of the thread in the bladder, we omitted this method of urethral contrast in later studies with no apparent drawback in diagnosis (18). Similar to our group, Hodroff and colleagues (28) have used a 5 Fr catheter to outline the urethra and to fill the bladder with saline solution and gadopentetate dimeglumine. It should be remembered that the presence of the catheter itself might impede the movement of the urethra during dynamic maneuvers. In the available literature, most authors do not administer urethral contrast medium and merely instruct the patients to empty their bladder prior to the examination (8,9,11,22). The latter is necessary to prevent masking of a rectocele or enterocele when there is a full bladder and a concomitant cystocele.

Opacification of the vagina in the literature is also controversial. Ultrasound gel is an easy to handle, well-tolerated, and cheap contrast medium. Delineation of the entire vagina, and especially of the posterior fornix and posterior wall, is always achieved with this technique (6,8). In addition, during the Valsalva maneuver, the gel in the vagina is emptied passively, and thus the movement of the organ itself is not impeded. A similar approach has been employed using intravaginal gel during dynamic transperineal sonography for the investigation and categorization of pelvic floor disorders (29) [see Chapter 3.2(ii)]. With regard to the rectum, a variety of contrast media have again been employed. In those studies where simulated defecation has been attempted, either gel (6,8,25), potato mash (6,12,22), or rubber tubes (20) have been proposed.

Patient Procedural Instruction

In order to achieve satisfactory results, adequate patient instruction prior to the examination is mandatory. According to the literature, most authors examine the patient while at rest and during straining (2,4,6,11,17,20,22,24). To assess the function of the levator ani muscle in patients presenting with primary evacuatory difficulty, it is necessary to contract the pelvic floor at least once during the entire procedure, where Vanbeckevoort et al. (24) have shown the success of this technique when compared with colpocystodefecography. As a result, we advise the following sequence of specified loads; namely, rest → contract → relax → strain → defecate → relax (6,8,12,25). It is necessary for this kind of cycle to be repeated until complete defecation has been documented, where, in our experience, between two and four cycles are needed. If the situation is either too embarrassing for the patient, or he/she cannot empty their rectum at all while lying supine, a triphasic approach as recommended by Kelvin et al. (8) may be suitable. Other specific loads, including coughing or micturition, are possible, but are not commonly used. The overall duration of such an examination normally ranges between 9 and 30 minutes (8,10). Overall, this appears to be a well-tolerated sequence load for most patients where there is a more private atmosphere within the bore of the magnet during the entire examination.

Image Analysis

At the end of the entire examination, the single slices have to be rearranged anatomically according to their slice position and viewed in a cine-loop. Although the visual impression of organ movements is decisive, certain aids have been developed to quantify the extent of the observed pathologies. Unfortunately, no general agreement on categorization and measurement of these pathologies has been reached to date, and this is the current objective of a European Working Party. A guide line for image analysis should include the following points—namely, the bony pelvis, the muscles of the pelvic floor, the recognizable named ligaments, and the degree of movement of organs or reference structures under specified loads.

Functional cine-MRI should not be confused with MR-Pelvimetry, although looking at bony structures sometimes can be helpful in these patients. The lesser pelvis is part of the intra-abdominal cavity and the pelvic floor is exposed to the changing forces within this compartment. The superstructure that surrounds, protects, and supports the soft tissues and pelvic viscera is comprised of the pelvic ring (30). Here, Retzky et al. have described a perpendicular relationship of the abdominal and pelvic cavity in a properly orientated bony pelvis (30), where, in their opinion, this directs pressure towards the pubic symphysis and away from the pelvic floor. In this respect, Lazarevski (31) has compared 340 women with pelvic organ prolapse with a control group of 136 females without any evidence of organ descent. Pelvimetry on conventional X-ray pictures revealed significant changes of bony parameters between the groups, where he showed a more horizontal orientation or tilting of the pelvis with an upward (ventrocranial) movement of the pubic bone amongst the prolapse patient group. In addition, a significant increase in the distance between the posteroinferior border of the pubic symphysis and either the S5 level or the tip of the coccygeal bone was evident. He concluded that this anatomical variation ultimately might lead to an increased pressure load on the pelvic floor.

In our own experience, more than half of the female patients tend to tilt the pelvis as previously described in order to promote the defecation process. In addition, most female patients demonstrate an outward bulging of the ventral abdominal wall due to relaxation of possibly weakened musculature. Moreover, the shape of the sacral and coccygeal bone varies considerably, as can be seen on mid sagittal MR images. A simple computer model of the abdomino-pelvic cavity can make these interrelations apparent where there appears to be an increase in demonstrable relaxation of the abdominal wall and/or a deep sacrococcygeal cavity resulting in diminished force transmission to the pelvic floor. One could postulate that these bony and soft tissue anomalies demonstrable using MRI technology might alter the voluntary triggering of the defecation or voiding processes themselves. Further to this hypothesis, Tarlov (perineural) cysts frequently can be seen at the lumbosacral transition or sacral segments of the spine. The normal prevalence of these cysts is reported to be 4.6% of the general population, but we have noted their presence in up to 12% of our symptomatic patients. These Tarlov cysts can be symptomatic, putting pressure on the nerve roots (32,33); however, the possibility of causing secondary muscular pelvic floor weakness has yet to be proven.

One of the other benefits of dynamic MRI is the demonstration of coincident but significant other pathology where incidental pathologies have included occult stress fractures of the sacral bone and coccydynia. In the latter condition, there is demonstrable bony edema, as well as surrounding small rim periosseous fluid along with altered configuration, and mobility of the coccygeal bone. Here, Bo et al. (34) found a ventrocranial movement of 8.1 millimeters of the pelvic floor during contraction and a caudodorsal movement of 3.7 millimeters during straining, although there were no statistical differences between the continent and incontinent women. This group also has applied the same technology in the assessment of women with primary urinary incontinence (35).

The pelvic floor muscles at large do not represent a simple linear plate or swinging hammock that is interconnected between the bony structures, but rather a complex 3D structure (36); therefore, linear measurements on 2D MR images can vary considerably. In their study, Hoyte et al. (37) measured the anteroposterior dimension of the levator hiatus using slightly rotated images, where calculated and measured values differed with up to 15% variation. There are several reasons for these reported variabilities in pelvic floor movement using dynamic MRI technology. These include:

1. Most cuts through the muscles on MR images are not perpendicular to the muscle itself; therefore, measurements of the diameter are falsified and slightly increased.
2. The position of the subject within the MR scanner can vary. It is highly recommended to position the patient properly during the examination. On the coronal localizer, both acetabular bones should be at the same level. Tilting of the pelvis in the vertical axis during contraction and straining should be eliminated. In our experience. changes of more then five millimeters or 10 degrees already account for visual asymmetry of muscular structures (38).
3. Inter-observer accuracy also has to be taken into account.
4. On most workstations, accuracy of measurements is limited to about one millimeter.

Nevertheless, in the literature a variety of parameters concerning the pelvic floor muscles have been used on functional images, including the width of the levator hiatus on axial imaging (8,13,19,21,25,37,38), coronal (4,36) and sagittal images (23,27), the thickness of the iliococcygeal portion of the levator ani muscle on coronal and axial images (27), the range of movement of the levator ani (iliococcygeal part) on coronal images (36), and the cross-sectional area of the urogenital hiatus on axial images (9,19,38,39), as well as the surface of the levator ani calculated on coronal images (39). In addition, three different angles have been proposed for measurement, including the levator plate (4,19,38,39) and the levator vaginal (4,9) and the iliococcygeal angle (27).

The levator plate angle (LPA) is the angle between the posterior part of the levator ani muscle (the iliococcygeal portion), as seen on the mid sagittal image, and the pubococcygeal reference line (PCL) (vide infra). Similarly, the levator vaginal angle is calculated by measuring the angle between the posterior levator ani and a line drawn through the horizontal axis of the upper third of the vagina, as recommended by Singh et al. (9). Still another parameter to access the orientation and slope of the iliococcygeal muscle is the angle between this muscle and the transverse plane of the pelvis on coronal images (27). To understand better the meaning of such muscular parameters, we can, for example, consider the LPA in more detail. This parameter was introduced by Goodrich et al. (4), who measured it at 16.8 degrees at rest and 1.0 degrees during straining in nulliparous volunteers. Differences from these norms were most evident in multiparous volunteers (18.8 and –2.2 degrees at rest and during straining, respectively), where the range of values could become increasingly negative (–3.0 to –24.6 degrees). In contrast, Healy et al. (39) found statistically significant changes of the LPA between asymptomatic and constipated patients at rest and during straining (12 and 22 degrees vs 0 and 45 degrees, respectively). Asymptomatic women and men did not exhibit any significant changes of the LPA in the study published by Goh et al. (19), where men had a measured LPA of 11 degrees at rest and 20 degrees during straining and women were found to have an LPA of 13 degrees at rest and 17 degrees during straining. In yet another study by Hoyte et al. (38), the range of the LPA differed between asymptomatic and symptomatic patients presenting with either stress incontinence or organ prolapse. The respective data for rest and strain reported in this study were 9.5 degrees and –4.3 degrees in the asymptomatic group compared with 13.2 degrees and –11.5 degrees in the incontinent group and 6.9 degrees and –30.0 degrees in those with prolapse.

These differing results document the dilemmas encountered when making dynamic measurements of the pelvic floor. Even the calculated standard deviations provided above and quoted in other studies are relatively high, indicating either small sample populations or considerable intra-/inter-observer variation. Despite these reservations, assessment of the shape of the various parts of the levator ani muscle reveals useful additional information. Muscle defects with or without hernias are seen best on coronal images where a steep angle of the coccygeal portion of the levator ani muscle on mid sagittal images together with a ballooning of the puborectalis portion on axial images are indicative of pelvic floor weakness. Asymmetry, or even complete loss of the right puborectalis portion of the levator ani, is a frequent finding in multiparous women following episiotomy, whereas we have recognized intramuscular hematomas secondary to excessive straining and a relatively thickened coccygeal portion of the muscle in patients with levator ani syndrome. Many more muscular pathologies are visible on static MR images (40,41).

The ligaments play an important role in supporting the organs of the pelvic floor, and tears within these ligaments have been reported to be relevant in the pathogenesis of rectoceles and of uterine/vaginal descent (42), although their anatomic existence and importance has remained controversial (43–47). With the exception of three ligamentous structures visualized on functional MRI, no other corresponding ligamentous structures are readily discernable. These three structures are the rectovaginal interface, the anococcygeal ligament, and the uterosacral ligament. The first two structures are best seen on mid sagittal images, whereas the uterosacral ligaments are well delineated on coronal images. Using functional MRI, the rectovaginal interface consists of the close relationship between the posterior wall of the vagina and the anterior wall of the rectum, where both structures are of intermediate to low signal intensity. Separation of these two structures by a small rim of high signal intensity on T2-weighted images may just indicate a deep pouch of Douglas, and more correlative anatomical/imaging work in this region is required.

To evaluate the range of movement of the organs of the pelvic floor, a variety of reference lines have been established. The most commonly used reference line is the so-called PCL. This line originally has been used for many years for the evaluation of organ descent on cystography and evacuation proctography (48). This line was first introduced for functional MRI by Yang et al. (2), where it best represents the level of the levator ani muscle and is unaffected by tilting of the pelvis. In this respect, there are three different kinds of PCL mentioned in the literature, with an additional two different methods of measuring the distance between the reference organ and the PCL itself. All PCL reference lines (and points) are drawn on mid sagittal images and start at the posteroinferior rim of the pubic symphysis. The second bony landmark may be variably the first sacrococcygeal joint (8,34,36,39), the last visible coccygeal intervertebral space (2,6,10,11,13,19,20,25,38), or the point of insertion of the coccygeal portion of the levator ani (7). While most authors measure the distance of the organ in respect to the PCL by drawing a perpendicular line, some prefer to use a vertical line (2,11). Other reference lines proposed include a horizontal line on mid sagittal images at the level of the inferior border of the pubic symphysis (18,25), a symphysiosacral line on mid sagittal images between the superior border of the pubic bone and the distal sacral bone (5), and the mid pubic line through the longitudinal axis of the pubic bone (9). The diversity of all these reference lines makes it nearly impossible to compare the results published.

In order to establish definitive pelvic diagnoses, several reference structures have been introduced together with their attendant reference lines. Within the anterior compartment, the bladder base or the most caudal dorsal part of the bladder wall are defined. The cervix or the posterior fornix of the vagina serve as reference structures within the middle compartment, and the anorectal junction is the only relevant reference point of the posterior compartment. By definition, descent of a relevant organ is diagnosed if one or all of the aforementioned reference structures descend below the suitable reference line, where several authors propose a grading system of organ prolapse using steps of two or three centimeters (4,9,10,19,23). The diagnosis of an enterocele is more difficult and is intimately related to the definition of the pouch of Douglas, where the normal depth of the rectouterine space is approximately five centimeters. Depending on the demonstrated depth and/or the visible content of the pouch, a variety of definitions of an enterocele may be used (see Table 3.3(iii)-2) (49). The most widely accepted definition of an rectocele was proposed by Yoshioka et al. (50), where the depth of the rectocele is calculated by measuring the distance between a line drawn parallel to the anal canal and the most ventrocaudal part of the bulging of the anterior rectal wall (Figure 3.3(iii).1B). If the depth of the rectocele exceeds three centimeters, it traditionally has been labeled as pathological, although this does not necessarily mean it is responsible for evacuatory difficulty. Here, a considerable overlap exists

TABLE 3.3(iii)-2. Definition of an enterocele.

Author	Year	Definition
Kuhn	1982	Depth of pouch of Douglas in multiparous women: 5.4 cm
Ekberg	1985	Distance between vagina and rectum dilated
Kelvin	1992, 1994	Distance between upper third of vagina and rectum >2 cm during straining
Mellgren	1994	Small bowel loops within the pouch
Jorge	1994	Sigmoid colon below the PC line
Bremmer	1995	Rectouterine pouch extends below the lower third of vagina
Sentovich	1995	Intraperitoneal contrast media between vagina and rectum
Halligan	1996	Pouch deeper then vaginal apex on lat. Projection
Kelvin	1997	Small bowel loops more then 2 cm within the pouch
Maglinte	1997	Small bowel loops more then 2–4 cm, 4–6 cm, or >6 cm below vaginal apex
Lienemann	1999	Pouch of Douglas below PC line

A

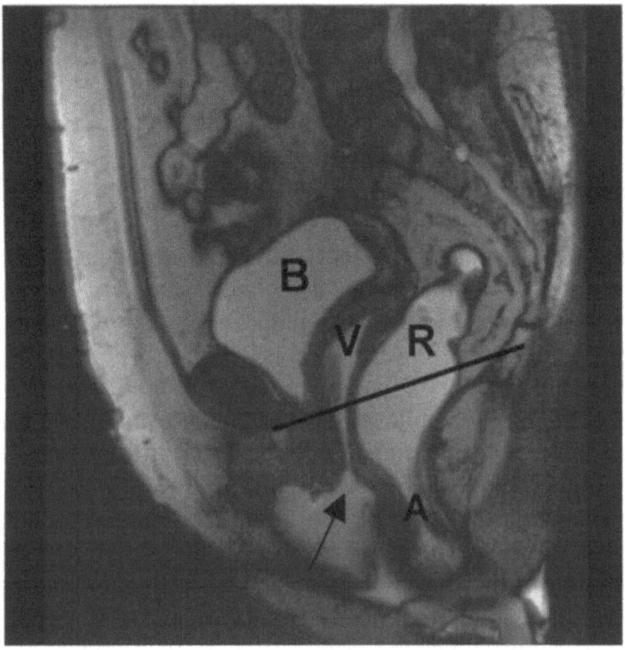

FIGURE 3.3(iii).1. (A–D) Dominant hernial orifice with rectocele and cystocele in a 65-year-old woman. Mid sagittal T2-weighted functional MR images of the pelvis obtained with the patient at rest (A) and during straining (B–D). (A) Normal position of the bladder (B) and vagina (V) above the pubococcygeal reference line. The rectum (R) shows no anterior bulging. A, anal canal, arrow introital level.

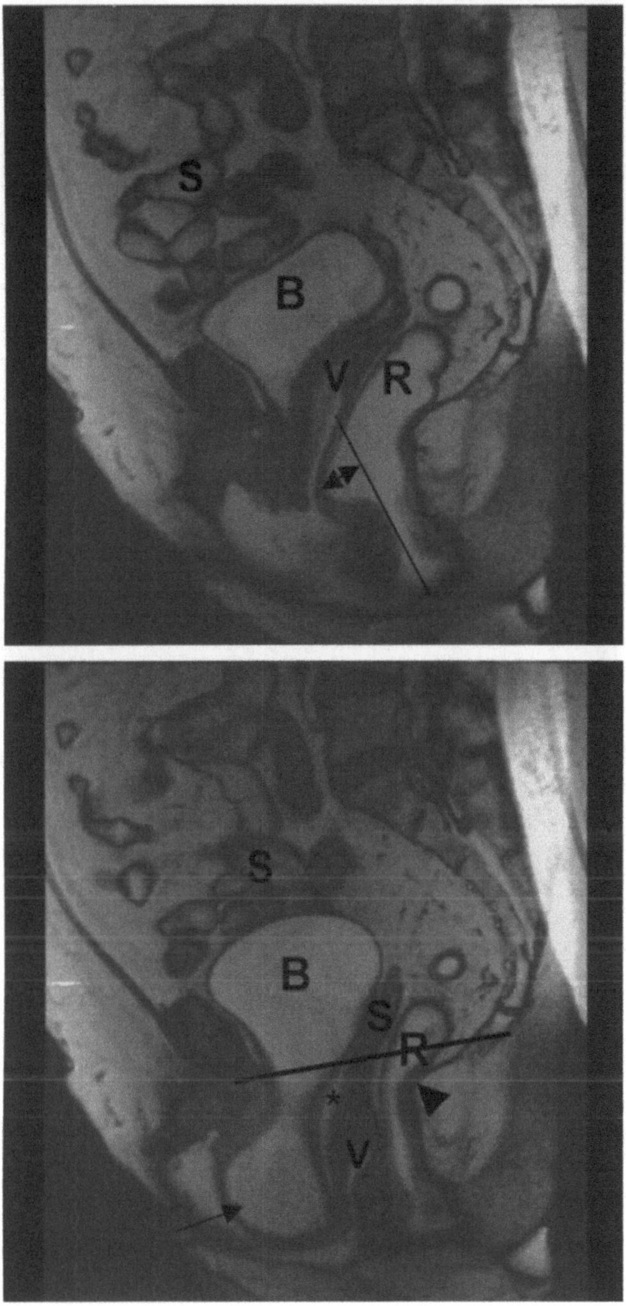

B

C

FIGURE 3.3(iii).1. (B) During the first episode of straining, a bulging of the anterior rectal wall occurs in an anterior direction. As illustrated in the image, the depth of the rectocele can be defined as the distance between the tip of the rectocele and a parallel line along the anal canal. The bladder (B) and the vagina (V) remain in its normal position. (C) After two more episodes of straining and defecation, the rectum (R) has been emptied. Now a large cystocele (arrow), as well as a vaginal descent (V), can be seen. Most of the bladder (B) and the entire vagina are now below the pubococcygeal reference line. The pouch of Douglas is deeper (asterisk) and would allow for an enterocele (S, small bowel loop) to develop if the bladder had been emptied. In addition, the puborectal sling has not completely relaxed (arrowhead).

D

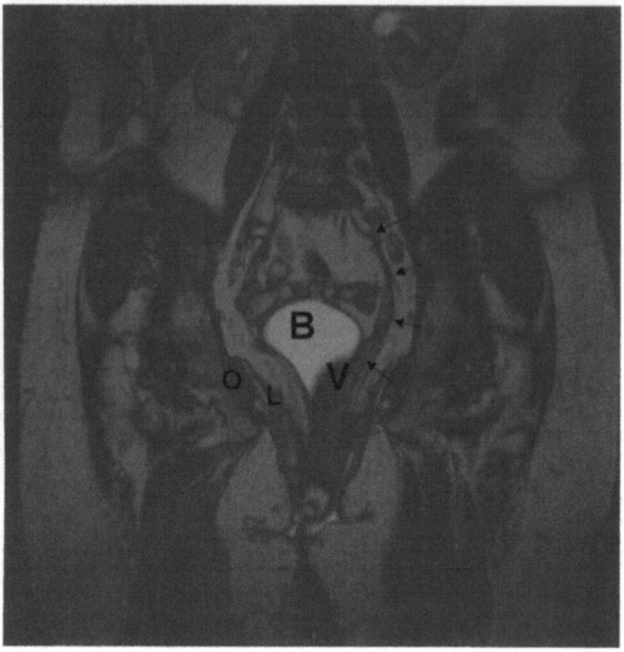

FIGURE 3.3(iii).1. (D) This coronal image at the level of the vesicovaginal pouch nicely demonstrates the course of the sacrouterine ligaments (small arrows), as well as the relationship between the internal obturator muscle (o) and the levator ani muscle (L).

between the findings in normal age-matched volunteers and symptomatic patients (51).

Findings

The Anterior Compartment

The bladder is a fluid-filled, hyperintense structure on T2-weighted images that, at rest, is situated posterosuperiorly to the pubic symphysis and the space of Retzius (Figure 3.3(iii).1A). The urethra is normally not well visualized on the mid sagittal images, although its target-like appearance on axial images is easily noted. Depending on the degree of its filling, the shape of the bladder can vary considerably, ranging from a more triangular to a rounder profile (Figures 3.3(iii).1B and 3.3(iii).2B). Surrounding structures such as small bowel loops can be displaced, but adhesions between the dome of the bladder and bowel loops that occur should be noted. On mid sagittal images, an area of fat-equivalent signal intensity is seen between the pubic bone and the bladder representing the retropubic space—space of Retzius—adding to the impression of bladder displacement (Figures 3.3(iii).2A and 3.3(iii).3A). This area can be enlarged in patients with incontinence (15). The supporting muscular and connective tissue structures surrounding the urethra are still debated and are not readily discerned on functional MRI.

Both the urethra and the bladder are exposed to changes in the intra-abdominal pressure during straining. A cystocele is deemed present when the bladder neck or any part of the posterior wall of the bladder descends

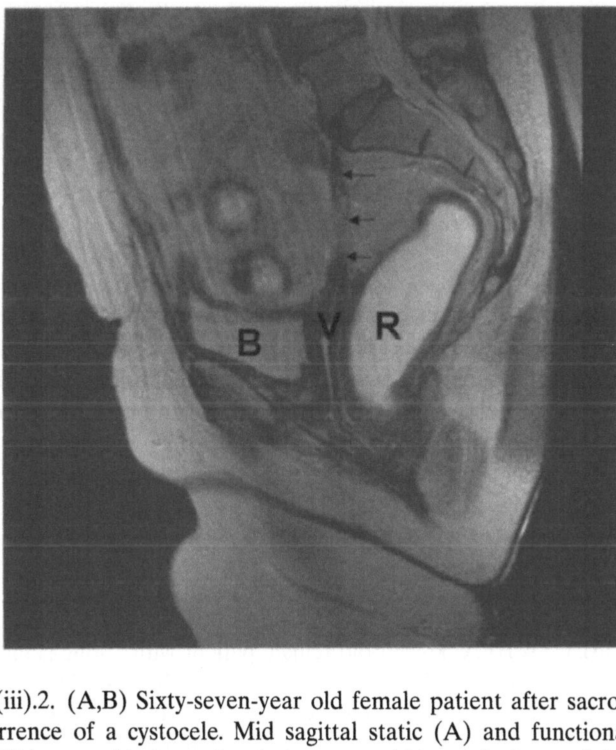

A

FIGURE 3.3(iii).2. (A,B) Sixty-seven-year old female patient after sacrocolpopexy with reocurrence of a cystocele. Mid sagittal static (A) and functional (B) T2-weighted MR image with the patient being at rest (A) and during straining (B). (A) Static MR images nicely demonstrate the foreign material extending from the vaginal apex (V) to the promontory (small arrows). B, bladder; R, rectum. (B) Typical findings in this patient show the normal position of the bladder neck (asterisk) in contrast to the descent of the posterior wall of the bladder (arrow) below the PC line. The vagina (V) is kept in place by the intact foreign material. R, rectum; S, small bowel.

B

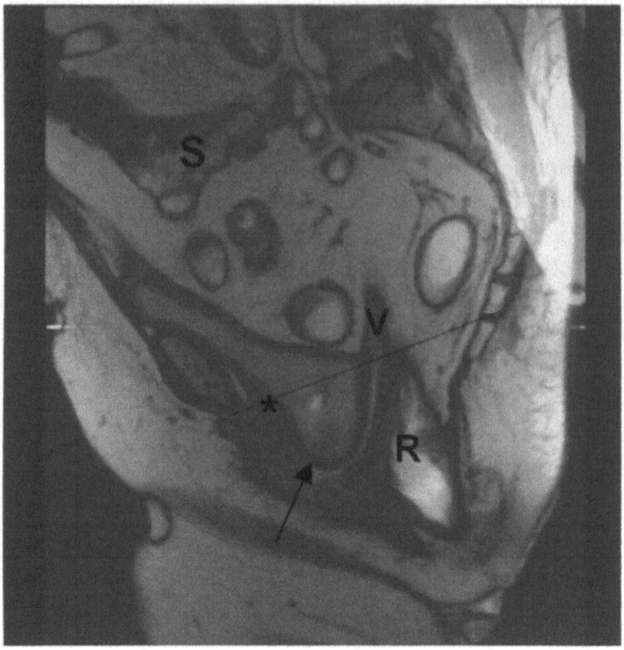

FIGURE 3.3(iii).2. *Continued*

below the PC line. (Figures 3.3(iii).1C and 3.3(iii).4B). Both the proximal urethra and the bladder neck descend and rotate around the pubic bone, initially moving posteroinferiorly. A nonspecific finding in patients with involuntary loss of urine is relative funneling of the proximal urethra, and an additional kinking of the urethra at the urethrovesical junction can be seen in large cystoceles. Furthermore, due to the limited space provided by the urogenital hiatus, a large cystocele can be seen actually masking a rectocele (Figures 3.3(iii).1B and 3.3(iii).1C). Reoccurrence of a cystocele after

FIGURE 3.3(iii).3. (A,B) A 60-year-old female patient with a long-standing history of stool outlet obstruction. Mid sagittal (A) and axial (B) T2-weighted MR images after several unsuccessful efforts to defecate. (A) The anal sphincter complex (A) does not open to allow for emptying of the rectal ampulla. Instead, a large rectocele (R) evolves and a kinking of the rectum (arrow) occurs. The large rectocele (R) resembles a sack (small arrows) and is situated well below the PC line. There is a marked descent of the anorectal junction with a steep, almost vertical, configuration of the dorsal levator ani muscle. These findings are accompanied by a small cystocele and a vaginal vault descent. (B) This axial image at the level of the symphysis pubis shows a ballooning of the levator ani muscle (small arrows) caused by organ descent and muscular weakness. The descending bladder (B), vagina (V), and rectum are noted. *, ischiatic tubera.

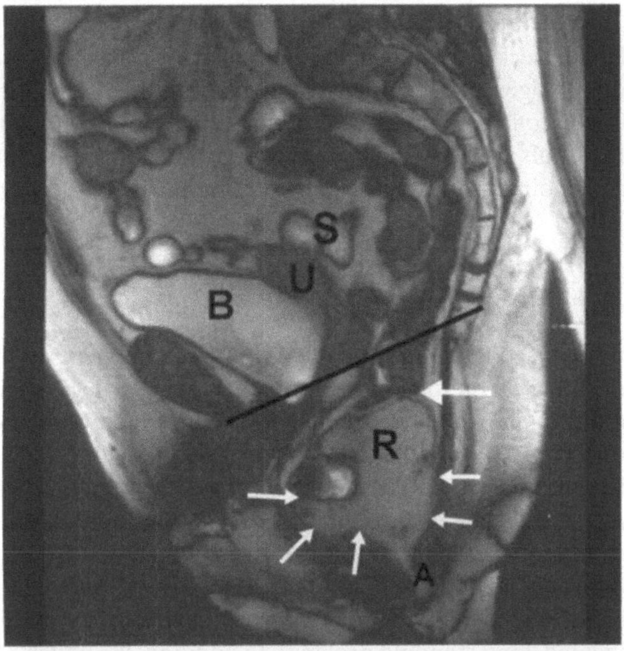

A

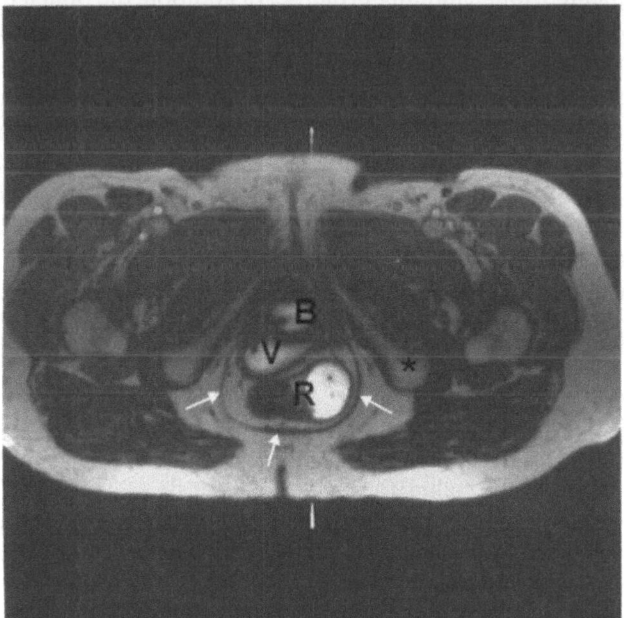

B

retropubic or vaginal procedures performed for stress incontinence can be nicely revealed by functional MRI. In these patients, the proximal urethra/bladder neck maintains its normal position, but the posterior wall of the bladder bulges into the anterior vaginal wall (Figures 3.3(iii).2A and 3.3(iii).2B), and following injections of bulk-enhancing agents, collagen, or the mesh materials used in sling procedures, these operative agents are discernable as hypointense regions readily visible in the periurethral tissues on MRI (52).

The Middle Compartment

The normal vagina, the rectum, and the posterior components of the levator ani muscle tend to lie on top of one another (Figure 3.3(iii).1A), where the position of the vagina and uterus depend to some extent upon the amount of filling of the rectal ampulla. In the presence of significant vaginal (or uterine) descent and only after the rectum has been emptied, both structures move ventrocaudally beyond the PC line (Figures 3.3(iii).4A and 3.3(iii).4B), where the PC line itself can overestimate the extent of organ descent within the middle compartment (8,20). Here, the vagina is foreshortened and the vaginal wall may appear thickened or even everted in cases of repeated, long-standing prolapse. In addition, the pouch of Douglas appears widened, facilitating the development (and diagnosis) of a peritoneocele or enterocele (Figure 3.3(iii).1C). Fascial defects (e.g., paravaginal defects or tears within the rectovaginal septum) cannot be readily appreciated on functional cine-MRI alone, although elongated uterosacral ligaments may be discerned on coronal MR images (Figure 3.3(iii).1D). These diagnoses are of major value in patients presenting with significant symptoms of pelvic fullness and evacuatory difficulty after hysterectomy or colpoperineorrhaphy (53–55).

The pouch of Douglas normally represents the deepest point within the intra-abdominal cavity and predisposes to an internal hernia. This posterior

FIGURE 3.3(iii).4. (A,B) Combined organ descent with uterovaginal prolapse, cystocele, and rectocele in a multiparous 42-year-old female. Mid sagittal T2-weighted MR images of the pelvis obtained with the patient straining. (A) The vagina and rectum (R) are filled with sonography gel. Thus, the anterior and posterior vaginal vault and the cervix are well delineated. The same is true for the rectum, which shows an extensive bulging of the anterior rectal wall in an anterior, perineal, and posterior direction. The rectocele effectuates the position of both the bladder and the uterus, which stay above the PC line. U, uterus. (B) After straining and defecation the uterus (U) and bladder (B) have descended well below the pubococcygeal line. Both organs lie upon the rectum (R) anteriorly and ultimately promote an internal rectal prolapse (asterisk). The sonography gel in the vagina has been evacuated passively. The rectocele shows an incomplete emptying and now contains air (arrow). A, anal canal.

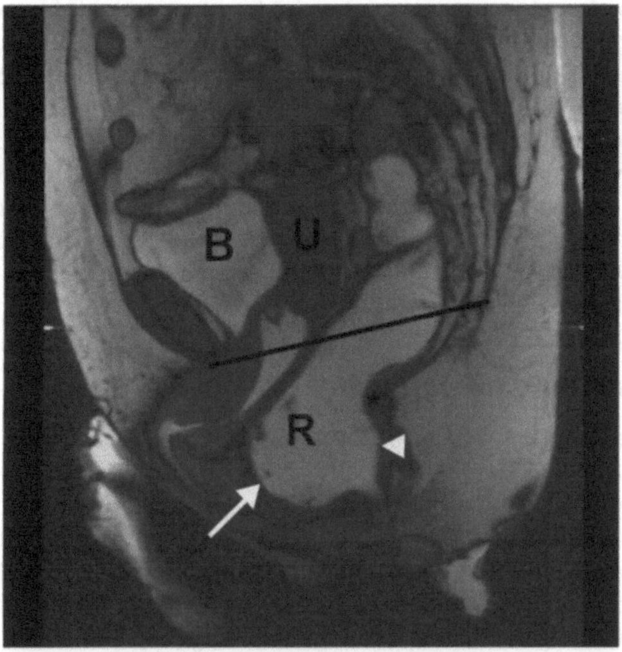

A

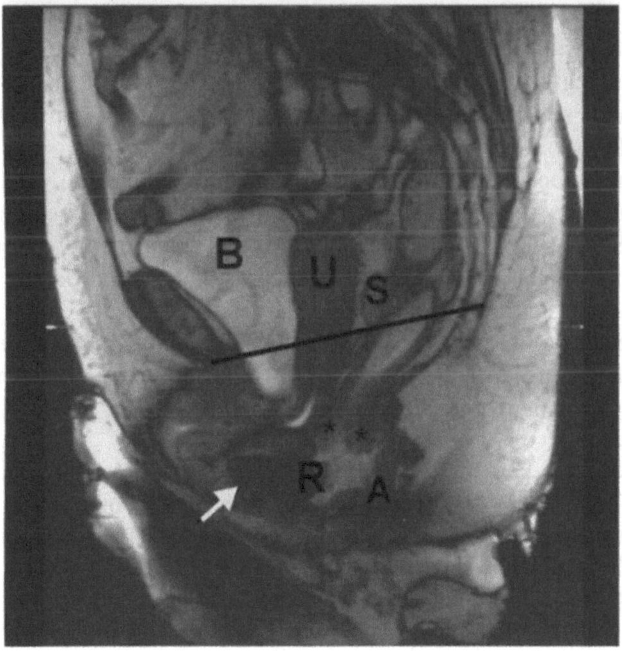

B

herniation of peritoneum may contain fat (peritoneocele) (56), small bowel loops (enterocele), or sigmoid colon (sigmoidocele) (57). The criteria for making the diagnosis of an enterocele is the descent of bowel loops below the PC line (8,49). The hernial sac generally follows the course of the vagina and the rectovaginal septum, where a large enterocele again can mask either a cystocele or a rectocele (25,49). Occasionally, herniation can be lateral or anterior, where, if the mesenteric root is short, an enterocele is unlikely to occur. Following sacrocolpopexy or uteropexy, functional MRI is able to depict the foreign material utilized and to demonstrate its intact function (Figures 3.3(iii).2A and 3.3(iii).2B) (58).

The Posterior Compartment

To some extent, the rectum behaves like a flexible and expansible tube where it can fold in on itself with a lateral or anterior displacement or kinking. Most often a bulging of the anterior rectal wall is noted (26), and these anterior rectoceles can be normal findings with even large rectoceles being clinically asymptomatic (Figures 3.3(iii).1B, 3.3(iii).3A, and 3.3(iii).4A). In the literature, a rectocele with a depth of more than three centimeters is regarded as a pathological finding (51); however, this is controversial (42). The direction of an anterior rectocele is either anteriorly through the distal segment of the posterior vaginal wall or dorsally in association with significant perineal descent (59). The latter tends to occur in patients with severe stool outlet obstruction (Figure 3.3(iii).3A), which occasionally occurs in men (60).

A circumscribed thickening of the rectal mucosa and the wall, together with a caudal movement of this rectal segment, marks the beginning of an internal rectal prolapse (Figures 3.3(iii).4B and 3.3(iii).5A). A more prominent internal rectal prolapse is often seen as a V-shaped or double rectal wall on the mid sagittal image (Figure 3.3(iii).5A), where the internal rectal prolapse eventually may protrude through the anal canal and become an external rectal prolapse (61). Often, an organ descent in the anterior or middle compartment typically leads to a depression of the ventral rectal

FIGURE 3.3(iii).5. (A,B) A 49-year-old women with a feeling of incomplete evacuation and a history of previous surgery for incontinence and organ descent. Mid sagittal (A) and axial (B) T2-weighted MR images taken at rest (B) and during straining and defecation (A). (A) The bladder neck is situated below the PC line. A funneling of the proximal urethra at the urethrovesical junction (small arrow) is seen. The vaginal vault (V) stays above the PC line. The rectum has been emptied, but no physiological rectocele occurred. Instead, the perineal body seems to be enlarged (asterisk). Next to it, an additional thickening of the rectal mucosa is depicted as a kinky structure of slightly elevated signal intensity. B, bladder. (B) Axial image at the level of the introitus shows a marked asymmetry of the perineal body (arrows) due to scaring. F, ischiorectal fossa; Glu, gluteal muscle.

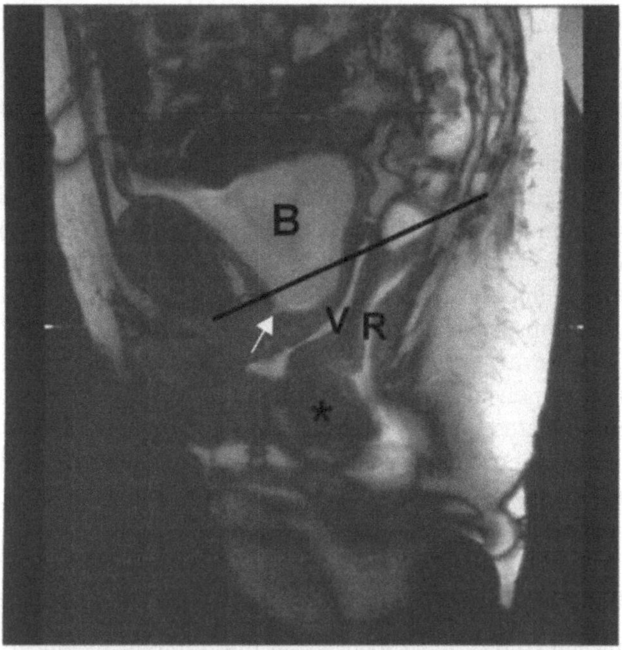

A

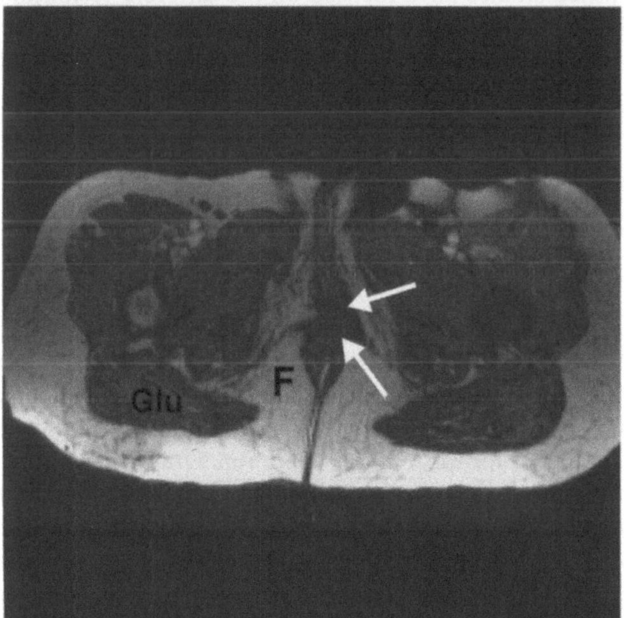

B

wall. This finding can promote an internal rectal prolapse and might account for stool entrapment (Figure 3.3(iii).4B).

Levator Ani Muscle

On the mid sagittal images, the posterior aspects of the levator ani muscle can be delineated. An adequate relaxation of the puborectalis sling during defecation should be noted (Figures 3.3(iii).1C and 3.3(iii).5A), and displacement of the anorectal junction in relation to the PC line is used as a parameter to define rectal descent, as it does in conventional defecography and dynamic transperineal ultrasonography (DTP-US) (3,9,19,20). A ballooning of the levator muscle on axial images is obvious in patients with weakness of the pelvic floor muscles (Figure 3.3(iii).3B). Here, the width of the urogenital hiatus should not exceed five centimeters (38), and on axial images, an asymmetric appearance of the puborectalis part of the levator muscle can occasionally be seen in some patients following episiotomy and grade IV perineal tears.

The Rating of Functional MRI in Clinical Practice

Most published studies have focused on the different technical aspects of the cine-MRI method and confirmed the usefulness of this technique in depicting significant differences between asymptomatic age-matched volunteers and those with significant symptomatic pelvic floor disorders (2–4,11–13,18,23,27,34,36).

Functional MRI versus Fluoroscopy/ Colpocystorectography

Approximately 10 studies have compared functional cine-MRI with conventional defecography. In this respect, Delemarre et al. (5) examined 14 out of 33 patients with functional cine-MRI and evaluated qualitative grading and quantitative measurements of anterior rectoceles with a finding of limited potential for MRI in this condition. Drawbacks of this study are the use of the prone position for patient assessment and failure to opacify the rectum. Our own results in two separate studies tend to favor the use of functional cine-MRI (6,18). In one study, we examined five asymptomatic volunteers and 44 symptomatic female patients. In terms of diagnosis, MRI was either identical with (21 cases) or superior to (18 cases) dynamic fluoroscopy. Functional MRI was especially helpful in the depiction of pathologies within the middle compartment such as descent of the uterus and enteroceles and in revealing changes in the dominant type of prolapse. Healy et al. (20) have found a significant correlation of standard measurements of anorectal configuration using functional MRI and evacuation proctography in ten women with constipation. In addition, functional MRI was able to show significant changes of muscular parameters in 11 women with otherwise normal proctograms (39). Schoenenberger et al. (62) examined 15 patients with defecation disorders using an open-configuration MR system. Magnetic resonance images showed all pathologic findings except for one case of intussusception in a patient with spastic pelvic floor syndrome, whereas defecography missed four pathologic conditions. Measurements of the anorectal angle, as well as a receiver operating characteristic (ROC) analysis showed similarity between the two modalities. In the study performed by Gufler et al. (7), 32 women with urinary incontinence (and/or organ prolapse) were examined using bead-chain cystourethrography or colpocystorectography and functional MRI.

Magnetic resonance imaging correctly diagnosed the condition and the degree of bladder descent with a coefficient of determination of 0.81 and 0.85, respectively, whereas cystourethrography alone missed all rectoceles. The combination of MRI together with colpocystorectography correctly depicted these pathologic findings, and enteroceles in particular could only be diagnosed using cine-MRI. A shortcoming of this study is the different X-ray methods used. Although colpocystorectography is certainly superior to cystourethrography alone, when used without opacification of small bowel, enteroceles are still likely to be missed. Another study comparing conventional X-ray methods with functional MRI was published by Vanbeckevoort (24), where functional MRI was compared to colpocystodefecography with maximum straining and during voiding and defecation in 35 women with pelvic floor descent. When compared with the X-ray method, MRI exhibited a specificity of 100% in all compartments, but the sensitivity of MRI tended to be inferior (being as low as 13%) for the detection of vaginal vault descent and only 56% sensitive for the diagnosis of a rectocele. The authors stated that MRI is unreliable as a result in the anterior and middle compartments. This study demonstrates the impact of the defecation process on diagnosis because functional MRI without defecation was compared with colpocystodefecography with simulated defecation.

In their study, Kelvin et al. (8) compared an extended cystocolpoproctographic technique with opacification of all relevant organs to functional MRI in the supine position with opacification of the bladder, vagina, and rectum. In addition to our own protocol, they added a post-toilet phase. Both examinations were in complete agreement on the presence of both rectoceles and cystoceles. One enterocele was missed using functional MRI due to incomplete emptying of the bladder, and a vaginal vault prolapse on MRI was obscured in another patient with metal clip artifacts. In contrast, the fluoroscopic examination missed a sigmoidocele in one case. The authors concluded that MRI and cystocolpoproctography showed similar detection rates for prolapse of pelvic organs.

Functional MRI in Asymptomatic Subjects

Although most studies include asymptomatic volunteers as a control study group, there are only two reports in the literature that exclusively define the normal range of findings in asymptomatic individuals. Goh et al. (19) examined 25 men and 25 women on a 1.0 Tesla system in the supine position with the volunteers assessed at rest and during straining. They measured the descent of the bladder base and the cervix and anorectal junction in relation to the PC line and calculated the pelvic floor hiatus area and perimeter, as well as the anorectal and levator plate angles. Our own study included 20 female volunteers who all had no pathologic findings on clinical examination or on urodynamics (37). Functional MRI was performed in the supine position using a 1.5 Tesla system and the vagina and rectum were opacified with sonography gel. Among others, we calculated the position of the bladder base, posterior vaginal fornix, and the anorectal junction in relation to the PC line and the horizontal line. The width and area of the levator hiatus, as well as several bony parameters, also were defined, measured, and calculated.

Functional MRI vs Pelvic Organ Prolapse Quantification Staging System

In 1996, the International Continence Society (ICS) introduced the ICS score to standardize the measurement of pelvic organ descent and prolapse. To date, such a widely accepted pelvic organ prolapse quantification staging system (POPQ) has not been developed for imaging of the pelvic floor. In this regard, two questions are of considerable interest—namely, whether functional MRI is able to detect relevant morphological changes in patients with only minor or no clinical findings (POPQ stages I or O) and whether the reference line system adopted by radiologists correlates with the clinical POPQ system. So far, there are only two relevant studies available in the literature that address the above problems. The study by Hodroff et al. (28) showed that functional MRI was able to detect significant anatomic changes in POP stage O patients, whereas the study by Singh et al. (9) tried to define a grading system using functional MRI, where the reference points were the same landmarks as those employed in clinical grading. By using the mid pubic reference line, they found a good correlation between the two reference systems.

Recommended Indications and Perspectives for Functional MRI

Taking the above into account, the indications for functional cine-MRI still remain controversial. The method itself is not yet standardized, and so far only a 2D approach for functional imaging of the pelvic floor exists. With the advent of fast "parallel imaging" a stack of two to three slices within the same time seems possible in the near future. In patients with disorders of support, functional MRI is an alternative to conventional X-ray procedures like urethrocystography, colpocystorectography, or evacuation proctography. Functional MRI has proven to be at least equivalent and sometimes clearly superior to some of these conventional methods due to its multiplanar capability, superb soft tissue contrast, and lack of superimposition, where additional important findings include definition of muscular and ligamentous defects that can be of clinical significance. Functional cine-MRI has proven to be especially helpful in patients with equivocal clinical findings delineating hernial orifices and outlining enteroceles, particularly in the postoperative patient often missed by extended defecographic techniques. It is suggested that functional cine-MRI will be the modality of choice (depending upon availability, allocation, and training) in patients with pelvic floor dysfunction; however, further studies will be needed to determine, among other matters, the cost effectiveness and cost benefit of this relatively new methodology.

References

1. Hugosson C, Joruf H, Lingman G, and Jacobson B. Morphology of the pelvic floor. Lancet. 1991;337:367.
2. Yang A, Mostwin JL, Rosenshein NB, and Zerhouni EA. Pelvic floor descent in women: dynamic evaluation with fast MR imaging and cinematic display. Radiology. 1991;179:25–33.
3. Kruyt RH, Delemarre JVBM, Doornbos J, and Vogel HJ. Normal anorectum: dynamic MR imaging anatomy. Radiology. 1991;179:159–63.
4. Goodrich MA, Webb MJ, King BF, Bampton AEH, Campeau NG, and Riederer SJ. Magnetic resonance imaging of pelvic floor relaxation: dynamic analysis and evaluation of patients before and after surgical repair. Obstet Gynecol. 1993;82: 883–91.
5. Delemarre JVBM, Kruyt RH, Doornbos J, Buyze-Westerweel M, Trimbos JB, Hermans J, and Gooszen HG. Anterior rectocele: assessment with radiographic defecography, dynamic magnetic resonance imaging and physical examination. Dis Colon Rectum. 1994;37:249–59.
6. Lienemann A, Anthuber C, Baron A, Kohz P, and Reiser M. Dynamic MR colpocystorectography assessing pelvic-floor descent. Eur Radiol. 1997;7:1309–17.
7. Gufler H, Laubenberger J, DeGregorio G, Dohnicht S, and Langer M. Pelvic floor descent: dynamic MR imaging using a falf-Fourier RARE sequence. J Magn Reson Imaging. 1999;9:378–83.
8. Kelvin FM, Maglinte DDT, Hale DS, and Benson JT. Female pelvic organ prolapse: a comparison of triphasic dynamic MR imaging and triphasic fluoroscopic cystocolpoproctography. AJR Am J Roentgenol. 2000;174:81–8.
9. Singh K, Reid WMN, and Berger LA. Assessment and grading of pelvic organ prolapse by use of dynamic magnetic resonance imaging. Am J Obstet Gynecol. 2001;185:71–7.
10. Bertschinger KM, Hetzer FH, Roos JE, Treiber K, Marincek B, and Hilfiker PR. Dynamic MR imaging of the pelvic floor performed with patient sitting in an open-magnet unit versus with patient supine in a closed-magnet unit. Radiology. 2002;223:501–8.
11. Unterweger M, Marincek B, Gottstein-Aalame N, Debatin JF, Seifert B, Ochsenkühn-Imhof N, Perucchini D, and Kubik-Huch RA. Ultrafast MR imaging of the pelvic floor. AJR Am J Roentgenol. 2001;176:959–63.

12. Hilfiker PR, Debatin JF, Schwizer W, Schoenenberger AW, Fried M, and Marincek B. MR-defecography: depiction of anorectal anatomy and pathology. J Comput Assist Tomogr. 1998;22:749–55.
13. Fielding JR, Griffiths DJ, Versi E, Mulkern RV, Lee MLT, and Jolesz FA. MR imaging of pelvic floor continence mechanisms in the supine and sitting positions. AJR Am J Roentgenol. 1998;171:1607–1610.
14. Strohbehn K, Ellis JH, Strohbehn JA, and DeLancey JOL. Magnetic resonance imaging of the levator ani with anatomic correlation. Obstet Gynecol. 1996;87: 277–85.
15. Tan IL, Stoker J, Zwamborn AW, Entius KAC, Calame JJ, and Lameris JS. Female pelvic floor: endovaginal MR imaging of normal anatomy. Radiology. 1998;206:777–83.
16. Huddleston HT, Dunnihoo DR, Huddleston III PM, and Meyers PC. Magnetic resonance imaging of defects in DeLancey's vaginal support levels I, II and III. Am J Obstet Gynecol. 1995;172:1778–84.
17. Fielding JR, Hoyte L, and Schierlitz L. Magnetic Resonance imaging of pelvic floor relaxation. J Womens Imaging. 2000;2:82–7.
18. Lienemann A. An easy approach to functional magnetic resonance imaging of pelvic floor disorders. Tech Coloproctol. 1998;2:131–4.
19. Goh V, Halligan S, Kaplan G, Healy JC, and Bartram CI. Dynamic MR imaging of the pelvic floor in asymptomatic subjects. AJR Am J Reontgenol. 2000;174: 661–6.
20. Healy JC, Halligan S, Reznek RH, Watson S, Bartram C, Phillips R, and Armstrong P. Dynamic MR imaging compared with evacuation proctography when evaluating anorectal configuration and pelvic floor movement. AJR Am J Roentgenol. 1997;169:775–9.
21. Fielding J. Practical MR imaging of female pelvic floor weakness. Radiographics. 2002;22:295–304.
22. Roos JE, Weishaupt D, Wildermuth S, Willmann JK, Marincek B, and Hilfiker PR. Experience of 4 years with open MR defecography: pictorial review of anorectal anatomy and disease. Radiographics. 2002;22:817–32.
23. Comiter CV, Vasavada SP, Barbaric ZL, Gousse AE, and Raz S. Grading pelvic prolapse and pelvic floor relaxation using dynamic magnetic resonance imaging. Urology. 1999;54:454–7.
24. Vanbeckevoort D, Van Hoe L, Oyen R, Ponette E, De Ridder D, and Deprest J. Pelvic floor descent in females: comparative study of colpocystorectography and dynamic fast MR imaging. J Magn Reson Imaging. 1999;9:373–7.
25. Sprenger D, Lienemann A, Anthuber C, and Reiser M. Funktionelle MRT des beckenbodens: Normale anatomie und pathologische befunde. Radiologe. 2000;40:451–7.
26. Pannu HK, Kaufman HS, Cundiff GW, Genadry R, Bluemke DA, and Fishman EK. Dynamic MR imaging of pelvic organ prolapse: spectrum of abnormalities. Radiographics. 2000;20:1567–82.
27. Singh K, Reid WMN, and Berger LA. Magnetic resonance imaging of normal levator ani anatomy and function. Obstet Gynecol. 2002;99:433–8.
28. Hodroff MA, Stolpen AH, Denson MA, Bollinger L, and Kreder KJ. Dynamic magnetic resonance imaging of the female pelvis: the relationship with the pelvic organ prolapse quantification system. J Urol. 2002;167:1353–5.
29. Beer-Gabel M, Teshler M, Barzilai N, Lurie Y, Malnick S, Bass D, and Zbar AP. Dynamic transperineal ultrasound in the diagnosis of pelvic floor disorders. Pilot study. Dis Colon Rectum. 2002;45:239–48.

30. Retzky SS, Rogers RM Jr, and Richardson AC. Anatomy of female pelvic support. In: Brubaker LT and Saclarides TJ, editors. The female pelvic floor disorders of function and support. Philadelphia (PA): F.A. Davis Company; 1996.
31. Lazarevski M. Morphotopographic, static and dynamic changes in small pelvis with genital prolapse and urinary stress incontinence [thesis]. Medical Faculty Skopje, Macedonia: 1974.
32. Paulsen RD, Call GA, and Murtagh FR. Prevalence and percutaneous drainage of cysts of the sacral nerve root sheath (Tarlov cysts). Am J Neuroradiol. 1994;15:293–7.
33. Voyadzis JM, Bhargava P, and Henderson FC. Tarlov cysts: a study of 10 cases with review of the literature. J Neurosurg. 2001;95(1 Suppl):25–32.
34. Bo K, Lilleas F, Talseth T, and Hedland H. Dynamic MRI of the pelvic floor muscles in an upright sitting position. Neurourol Urodyn. 2001;20:167–74.
35. Hedlund H, Bo K, Lilleas F, Talseth T, and Tillung T. The clinical value of dynamic magnetic resonance imaging in normal and incontinent women—a preliminary study on micturition. Scand J Urol Nephrol Suppl. 2001;207:87–91.
36. Hjartardottir S, Nilsson J, Petersen C, and Lingman G. The female pelvic floor: A dome—not a basin. Acta Obstet Gynecol Scand. 1997;76:567–71.
37. Hoyte L and Ratiu P. Linear measurements in 2-dimensional pelvic floor imaging: The impact of slice tilt angles on measurement reproducibility. Am J Obstet Gynecol. 2001;185:537–44.
38. Lienemann A, Sprenger D, Janssen U, Anthuber C, and Reiser M. Functional MRI of the pelvic floor. Method and reference values. Radiologe. 2000;40:458–64.
39. Healy JC, Halligan S, Reznek RH, Watson S, Bartram CI, Kamm MA, Phillips RKS, and Armstrong P. Magnetic resonance imaging of the pelvic floor in patients with obstructed defecation. Br J Surg. 1997;84:1555–58.
40. Tunn R, Paris S, Fischer W, Hamm B, and Kuchinke J. Static magnetic resonance imaging of the pelvic floor muscles morphology in women with stress urinary incontinence and pelvic prolapse. Neurourol Urodyn. 1998;17:579–89.
41. Tunn R, DeLancey JO, Howard D, Thorp JM, Ashton-Miller JA, and Quint LE. MR imaging of the levator ani muscle recovery following vaginal delivery. Int Urogynecol J Pelvic Floor Dysfunct. 1999;10:300–7.
42. Zbar AP, Lienemann A, Fritsch H, Beer-Gabel M, and Pescatori M. Rectocele: pathogenesis and surgical management. Int J Colorectal Dis. 2003;18:369–84.
43. Uhlenluth E and Nolley GW. Vaginal fascia, a myth? Obstet Gynecol. 1957;10: 349–58.
44. Milley PS and Nichols DH. A correlative investigation of the human recto-vaginal septum. Anat Rec. 1969;163:443–51.
45. Fritsch H. Topography and subdivision of the pelvic connective tissue in human fetuses and in adult. Surg Radiol Anat. 1994;16:259–65.
46. Fröhlich B, Hötzinger H, and Fritsch H. Tomographical anatomy of the pelvis, pelvic floor and related structures. Clin Anat. 1997;10:223–30.
47. Aigner F, Zbar AP, Ludwikowski B, Kreczy A, Kovacs P, and Fritsch H. The rectogenital septum: morphology, function and clinical relevance. Dis Colon Rectum. 2003 in press.
48. Shorvon PJ, McHugh S, Diamant NE, and Somers Stevenson GW. Defecography in normal volunteers: results and implications. Gut. 1989;30:1737–49.
49. Lienemann A, Anthuber C, Baron A, and Resier M. Diagnosing enteroceles using dynamic magnetic resonance imaging. Dis Colon Rectum. 2000;43:205–13.
50. Yoshioka K, Matsui Y, Yamada Y, et al. Physiologic and anatomic assessment of patients with rectoceles. Dis Colon Rectum. 1991;34:704–8.

51. Shorvon PJ, McHugh S, Diamant NE, Somers S, and Stevenson W. Defecography in normal volunteers: results and implications. Gut. 1989;30:1737–49.
52. Carr LK, Herschorn S, and Leonhardt C. Magnetic resonance imaging after intraurethral collagen injected for stress incontinence. J Urol. 1996;155;1253–5.
53. Jeffcoate TN. Posterior colpoperineorrhaphy. Am J Obstet Gynecol. 1959;77: 490–502.
54. Ross JW. Techniques of laparoscopic repair of total vault eversion after hysterectomy. J Am Assoc Gynecol Laparosc. 1997;4:173–83.
55. Tunn R, Paris S, Taupitz M, Hamm B, and Fischer W. MR imaging in posthysterectomy vaginal prolapse. Int Urogynecol J Pelvic Floor Dysfunct. 2000;11:87–92.
56. Bremmer S, Mellgren A, Holmstrom B, and Uden R. Peritoneocele and enterocele: formation and transformation during rectal evacuation studied by means of defaeco-peritoneography. Acta Radiol. 1998;39:167–75.
57. Fenner DE. Diagnosis and assessment of sigmoidoceles. Am J Obstet Gynecol. 1996;175:1438–42.
58. Lienemann A, Sprenger D, Anthuber C, Baron A, and Resier M. Functional cine magnetic resonance imaging in women after abdominal sacrocolpopexy. Obstet Gynecol. 2001;97:81–5.
59. Shafik AA. Study involving patients with posterior rectocele. Tech Coloproctol. 2002;6:127.
60. Chen HH, Iroatulam A, Alabaz O, Weiss EG, Nogueras JJ, and Wexner SD. Associations of defecography and physiologic findings in male patients with rectocele. Tech Coloproctol. 2001;5:157–61.
61. Pescatori M and Quondamcarlo C. A new grading of rectal internal mucosal prolapse and its correlation with diagnosis and treatment. Int J Colorect Dis. 1999;14:245–9.
62. Schoenenberger AW, Debatin JF, Guldenschuh I, Hany TF, Steiner P, and Krestin GP. Dynamic MR defecography with a superconducting open-configuration MR system. Radiology. 1998;206:641–6.

Editorial Commentary

Dynamic MRI appears to be the way of the future in the assessment of patients with functional pelvic disorders either de novo or following gynecologic surgery. Sequencing (and its modifications) have not yet been firmly worked out or evaluated but the technique in mid-sagittal mode offers a fairly comprehensive view of the anterior, middle and posterior compartments simultaneously with validated data in the diagnosis of rectocele, enterocele and peritoneocele which is superior to the views obtained by extended defecography. The role of the open magnet in more physiological 'defecation' is unclear at the present time but it may assist in the objections to conventional dynamic MRI positioning during simulated defecation for disorders such as rectal prolapse, rectoanal intussusception and descending perineum syndrome where the diagnoses are typically made at the end of straining.

AZ

Chapter 4
Sphincter Pharmacology and Pharmacotherapy

THANESAN RAMALINGAM and NEIL J. MCC MORTENSEN

Introduction

There is little doubt that using the anal sphincter as a pharmacological target has contributed to our understanding of anorectal physiology. The ability to pharmacologically modulate anal sphincter function has led to significant changes in our approach to the management of certain benign anorectal diseases.

In this chapter, we will describe current knowledge of the pharmacology and pharmacotherapy of the anal sphincter, as well as the physiological aspects of the sphincter complex, in particular, its innervation. The discussion includes the current state of knowledge of the neurotransmitters involved in the control of the anal sphincter and suggested mechanisms for their manipulation principally designed to manage patients with anal fissure disease and fecal incontinence.

The anal sphincter consists of an inner ring of smooth muscle, the internal anal sphincter (IAS), surrounded by an outer ring of striated muscle, the external anal sphincter (EAS). The IAS is an involuntary muscle that is in a continuous state of contraction as a result of its intrinsic myogenic properties and extrinsic innervation by the autonomic nerves (1). The EAS, being a voluntary muscle, is innervated by the pudendal (somatic) nerve. Together they play a central role in the maintenance of continence. The IAS contributes up to 85% of the overall resting anal pressure, while the EAS is thought to contribute up to 50% of the anal pressure, particularly during periods of rectal distension (2). When required, the voluntary component can be called upon to momentarily raise the anal pressure in order to defer defecation. The functioning anal sphincter therefore relies on the autonomic and myogenic innervation of the IAS, as well as the somatic innervation of the EAS.

Autonomic Control of the Anal Sphincter

The autonomic nervous system (ANS) consists of the craniosacral parasympathetic and the thoracolumbar sympathetic components (3). They originally were classified by Dale (4) on the basis of the neurotransmitter type released by the nerves, i.e., "cholinergic" nerves released acetylcholine and "adrenergic"nerves released noradrenaline. Cholinergic nerves included almost all preganglionic nerves, all parasympathetic postganglionic nerves, and some sympathetic postganglionic sympathetic nerves. The two main cholinergic receptor types were called "muscarinic" and "nicotinic" based on the alkaloids muscarine and nicotine used to identify them. They differ in that the cholinergic actions of muscarine are mediated via receptors on the effector tissues while nicotine stimulates autonomic ganglia. There are at least two subtypes of nicotinic and muscarinic receptors: N1, N2 and M1, M2. The stimulation of M1 and N1 result in acetylcholine release from myenteric nerves whereas stimulation of M2 and N2 appears to inhibit acetylcholine release from the neurons located in smooth muscle-mediated contraction (5).

Adrenergic nerves include most postganglionic sympathetic nerves. There are also two principal subtypes of adrenergic receptors, namely, α and β. In most smooth muscles, α effects are excitatory and β effects are inhibitory. These receptors can be subclassified further into α_1, α_2 and β_1, β_2, according to their preferential response to archetypal agonists and antagonists. The α_1 receptors are located post junctionally on smooth muscle cells and intrinsic nerves, whereas α_2 receptors may be present at both pre- and post-synaptic sites. Although the β_1 and β_2 adrenergic receptors are found mainly on smooth muscle cells, β_1 receptors also can also be located on some myenteric neurons (6).

For its motor function, the IAS receives its sympathetic input from the hypogastric plexus and its parasympathetic supply from the first to third sacral segments via the pelvic plexus (7). Although the autonomic nerves help regulate sphincter function, Langley (4) recognized that gastrointestinal motility was independent of the extrinsic autonomic nerve supply. This gave rise to the concept of an intramural, intrinsic pathway known as the enteric nervous system.

The Enteric Nervous System and Sphincter Function

The enteric nervous system (ENS) has been described as the third component of the ANS, mainly controlling the gastrointestinal motility. It receives inputs from both the sympathetic and parasympathetic arms of the ANS. In addition, it contains complex reflex pathways that function in afferent, efferent, and interneuronal connections. The ENS consists of two major plexuses of interconnecting ganglia, namely, the submucous (Meissner's) plexus and the myenteric (Auerbach's) plexus (8). These reflex pathways involve numerous neurotransmitters, some of which we are only now beginning to identify, although they not only seem to exert control on gastrointestinal motility, but also to coordinate reflexes such as the rectoanal inhibitory reflex (see Chapter 2.2).

The Rectoanal Inhibitory Reflex (RAIR)

The rectoanal inhibitory reflex (RAIR) was first described by Gowers (9) in 1877. It is characterized by the transient reduction in anal pressure in response to rectal distension, permitting rectal contents to come into contact with the epithelium of the upper anal canal containing sensory receptors. This process, called "anorectal sampling," has been postulated for the discrimination of solid, liquid, and gaseous matter (10).

It seemed that peristalsis was not involved in the reflex as the sphincter relaxes before peristalsis reaches it—a finding that led Denny-Brown and Robertson to suggest that the reflex was intramural (11). Their view was supported by the absence of the RAIR following circumferential myotomy (12) and bowel anastamosis (13), but its presence after sectioning of the hypogastric nerves (14).

This reflex is definitively absent in patients with Hirschsprung's disease, which is characterized by a lack of myenteric ganglia along variable lengths of the colon and rectum (15), and our group has suggested that nitric oxide (NO) is the principal mediator in RAIR. The mechanoreceptors for RAIR are thought to be located in the rectal mucosa because RAIR can be blocked by the installation of topical anesthetic gel into the rectum (12) or by the use of ganglion blocking agents (16). Hirst and colleagues have suggested that rectal distension activates action potentials in ganglion cells, transmitting intramural inhibitory impulses distally (17), and it is thought that the presence of shunt fascicles (bundles of nerve fibers related to the myenteric plexus) also may facilitate this rapid neuronal communication (18).

Physiological Considerations of the Anal Sphincter: The Role of a Nonadrenergic, Noncholinergic (NANC) Neurotransmitter

The ANS and the ENS, together with augmentation from somatic nerve input, regulate the function of the anal sphincter. In order to appreciate the pharmacology of the sphincter, we need to consider the chemical mediators/transmitters involved in its physiology.

Using in vivo experiments, investigators have shown that reduction in IAS tone can be achieved following sympathetic blockade by either high spinal (T6-T12) anesthesia or by infusion of phentolamine, an α-adrenoceptor antagonist. These findings suggest a tonic excitatory sympathetic discharge to the IAS (19). Presacral nerve stimulation at surgery, on the other hand, has been shown to both increase (20) and decrease (12) the IAS tone, where conflicting results are probably explained by the differences in the stimulation parameters to the IAS in different studies.

There does not appear to be a tonic parasympathetic input to the IAS in vivo (1). In addition, superimposed on the tonic state of the IAS, there are two intermittent waveform activities, namely slow and ultraslow variants, according to their respective frequencies (21). The relevance of these waveforms is not yet clear, but it has been suggested that they may either act to oppose rectal pressure waves (22) or to keep the anal canal closed to prevent desensitization of the anoderm (23). However, there do not appear to be characteristic variations in their frequency and pattern in conditions such as full-thickness rectal prolapse, although it has been suggested that this may in part be a factor governing persistent incontinence following mucosal proctectomy (Délorme's operation) or when the mucosa is restored to its normal locale.

Much of our understanding of the physiology of the IAS has been derived from in vitro experiments using the superfusion organ bath (24), where the effects of different mediators on the spontaneous tone generated by strips of IAS have been studied. Unlike rectal smooth muscle, the IAS smooth muscle strips develop a tone that is resistant to tetrodotoxin, a neurotoxin (25). Moreover, this tone also has been shown to be dependant on extracellular calcium and its entry into the smooth muscle cells via L-type calcium channels (26). It seems here that agonist-induced contractions are dependent on calcium release from intracellular stores while relaxation is effected by mechanisms that cause a reduction of cytosolic calcium. Relaxation of the strips also can be brought about by the addition of carbachol (an acetylcholine analogue), and this effect can be blocked by pretreatment with atropine (a muscarinic antagonist) and by nitric oxide synthase inhibitors (27). Noradrenaline, on the other hand, causes a dose-dependent contraction that has been shown to be mediated via β adrenoceptors (where IAS strips have been pretreated with phentolamine, an α receptor antagonist). Furthermore, work using isoprenaline, a β agonist, has been shown to cause relaxation in the strips in vitro (28), suggesting a very specific IAS receptor profile.

Burleigh and colleagues have shown that electric field stimulation of the IAS causes a relaxation that is blocked by tetrodoxin, but not by atropine or guanethidine (25), implying that IAS relaxation is nerve mediated. This effect is not controlled by cholinergic or adrenergic pathways, paving the way for a possible nonadrenergic, noncholinergic (so-called NANC) mediator.

Various transmitters have been suggested as the potential principal NANC mediator in the IAS acting via the intramural ENS to cause relaxation of the muscle. The main contenders include adenosine triphosphate

(ATP), vasoactive intestinal peptide (VIP), and NO. Although ATP is known to be an ENS neurotransmitter, there does not appear to be a reliable histochemical stain to localize it. In this respect, it is known that purinoceptor antagonists such as Suramin (29) can block the pharmacological actions of ATP, but despite its inhibitory actions in other parts of the gastrointestinal tract, the evidence for a similar role for ATP in the IAS is not convincing (25).

In this regard, VIP has been shown to be an inhibitory neurotransmitter causing relaxation in the lower esophageal sphincter (30), where it has been shown to be present in the IAS (31) and where VIP antagonists have been demonstrated to cause IAS relaxation. However, it has been suggested that VIP may be acting via the NO pathway in the opossum IAS (32). Whether this can adequately be translated to the human IAS requires further study.

Working on isolated opossum IAS strips, Rattan and Chakder showed that NO caused tetrodoxin-resistant relaxation and that L-N-9-nitroarginine (an inhibitor of the enzyme responsible for the production of NO) suppressed the fall in IAS tension in electric field-stimulated strips (33). Later, using chemiluminescence, they showed that NO was released in response to NANC stimulation. O'Kelly and colleagues made similar observations in their experiments using isolated human IAS strips where they showed that the concentration-dependent effect of L-N-9-nitroarginine was countered by the addition of the NO precursor, L-arginine (27). This group went on to suggest that muscarinic receptors were present on NO neurons because inhibitors of NO synthase attenuated the response to carbachol (34).

Because the inherent automaticity of the IAS confers the sphincter complex with a resting tone, which in turn helps maintain our subconscious control of continence, there has been a greater emphasis on research looking into the physiology and pharmacology of the IAS compared to the EAS. As far as the EAS is concerned, it has a somatic nerve supply with acetylcholine as the excitatory neurotransmitter at the neuromuscular junction working via nicotinic receptors. The EAS derives its nerve supply from nerves whose cell bodies lie in the ventral horn of the second and third sacral segments of the spinal cord (35).

Recently, we have assessed the nature of the RAIR in NO-knockout mice (36). Here, the issues of rectoanal inhibition appear quite complex where there is only partial attenuation of the RAIR and where field stimulation of potentially inhibitory nerves in the KO mice was still associated with inhibitory activity. In addition, pretreatment with NO synthase, VIP, ATP, and heme oxygenase antagonists variably affected the inhibitory response, implying a role for other inhibitory neurotransmitters in IAS relaxation, at least in this complex model.

Finally, we are aware that there are sensory receptors in the anal canal for touch, pain, and temperature modalities. The high concentration of these in the anal transition zone-ATZ (37) suggests that they have an important role in the anorectal sampling reflex (10).

Putative Therapeutic Agents in Sphincter Function

Much of clinical research to do with sphincter pharmacology has been targeted at agents that reduce IAS tone, where in particular they have been used in the management of patients with chronic anal fissure. This is because it is a relatively common condition that can account for 10% of new outpatient cases (38). Additionally, it is recognized that operative management for fissure disease such as lateral sphincterotomy and manual dilatation of the anus have the significant potential risk of permanent damage to the sphincter complex, leading to incontinence (39–41).

We know that the majority of anal fissures have an idiopathic etiology (42) and that the condition has long been associated with IAS spasm (43). Anal fissures tend to be located posteriorly in the midline of the anal verge and, as work from Klosterhalfen and colleagues (44) have shown, impair the blood circulation to the fissure. Others also have shown that the increased anal pressures in these patients (45) compounds this relatively poor blood flow, inevitably delaying healing and promoting chronicity of the disorder.

Although other derangements, such as increased frequency of ultraslow waves (46) and an abnormal RAIR (47,48), have been noted in fissure patients, the clinical significance of these findings is unknown. Here, it has been postulated that a rapid return to baseline after RAIR induction to a normal pressure may be important in patients whose continence is already compromised (48)—a finding recently confirmed in other studies (49).

The pharmacological agents that have been shown to cause the relaxation of the IAS include NO donors, botulinum toxin, calcium antagonists, muscarinic receptor agonists, α-adrenoceptor inhibitors, and β-adrenoceptor agonists. These agents have been under extensive trial for chronic anal fissure, and prospective randomized controlled comparative trials are awaited.

Nitric Oxide Donors

O'Kelly and colleagues have shown NO to be the predominant neurotransmitter effecting IAS relaxation in their in vitro study (27). This followed earlier work, which showed that using glyceryl trinitrate (GTN), a NO donor, resulted in reduced anal canal pressures (50). This was supported by reports of successful treatment of anal fissures using topical GTN (51,52). A summary of several recent randomized, prospective, controlled studies using topical GTN for chronic anal fissure is provided in Table 4.1.

The study from Lund and colleagues (53) showed significant reduction in anal resting pressure along with an increase in anodermal blood flow (as measured by laser Doppler flowmetry) in the treated group. In their study, Bacher (54) and colleagues included patients with acute fissures in their

TABLE 4-1. Summary of recent prospective, randomized, controlled studies using topical GTN in the treatment of anal fissures.

Study	Patient numbers	Agents used	Duration of therapy (weeks)	Fissure healing rate (Placebo)	Rate of relapse
Lund et al., 1997 (53)	80	0.2% GTN Placebo	8	68% (8%)	3/38 at 4 months
Bacher et al., 1997 (54)	35	0.2% GTN 2% Lignocaine	4	80% (40%)	N/A
Carapeti et al., 1999 (55)	70	0.2% GTN, Rising dose GTN, Placebo	8	65%, 70%, (32%)	9/31 at 9 months (median)
Kennedy et al., 1999 (56)	43	0.2% GTN Placebo	4	46% (16%)	5/8 at 29 months (mean)
Beck et al., 2000 (57)	304	0.1% GTN 0.2% GTN 0.4% GTN Placebo	8	50% (50%)	N/A
Altomare et al., 2000 (58)	119	0.2% GTN Placebo	4	49% (52%)	5/26 at 12 months (median)

treated population, and their definition of a healed fissure was determined not only by clinical examination (the end-point in the other studies on Table 4-1), but also by improvement in patients' symptoms. In so far as whether an increased dose of GTN conferred a better response, Carapeti (55) and colleagues showed that enhanced GTN therapy did not improve results where they found similar healing rates between patients using 0.2% three times a day (65%) and those treated with an initial dose of 0.2% but increased on a weekly basis by 0.1% to a maximum of 0.6% (70%).

The initial successful results of using GTN were countered by separate studies by Beck (57) and Altomare (58), which failed to demonstrate any significant effect of GTN on fissure healing. In the study by Altomare et al. (58), the placebo group actually had a better fissure healing rate of 52% compared with 49% in the treatment group. Beck and colleagues showed that using increased concentrations of GTN (and different regimens, i.e., twice daily compared with three times daily) failed to show any difference between the treatment and placebo groups. It has been argued that the less impressive healing rates in the former study may be due to the short treatment period of four weeks. Assessment of fissure healing at the same time interval in Lund and colleagues' (53) suggested that less than 20% of patients had healed long-term—a finding confirmed by McLeod et al. in a large Canadian cooperative trial comparing medical with surgical therapy, where the recidivism rate in topically treated chronic anal fissure was 73% (59). There are, however, other possible factors diminishing the efficacy of GTN in some reports, including poor patient compliance caused by the high incidence of headache (72%) (55) as a side-effect and the phenomenon of tachyphlaxis (60). Tachyphlaxis is defined as the diminishing therapeutic effects of a drug caused by the increased tolerance of the target tissue to the drug.

The results of studies such as that from Evans and colleagues also seemed to undermine the efficacy of GTN (61), where they compared the outcomes of sphincterotomy and treatment with GTN paste in a prospective, randomized study, showing that the healing rate was worse in the GTN-treated group and that there were negligible rates of incontinence in the surgical group. It could be argued, however, that incontinence may take several years to manifest. Other NO donors are currently being evaluated, including isosorbide dinitrate (ISDN) (62) and L-arginine, a NO precursor, although there is little evidence to show that ISDN is superior to GTN in its efficacy. The use of L-arginine has been shown to reduce mean anal resting pressure by around 40% in volunteers (63).

Botulinum Toxin

Botulinum toxin type A is one of several toxins produced by the bacterium *Clostridium botulinum*. Scott (64) first clinically used it to treat patients with strabismus in 1977, but it was not until 1993 that Jost and colleagues advocated its use for the treatment of patients with anal fissures (65). They injected five units of botulinum toxin into the EAS of 12 patients, and after a period of three months they showed healing in ten of these patients. Later, in a series of 100 patients treated with botulinum toxin, 78% were shown to be pain free after one week, with healing rates of 82% and 79% at three and six months, respectively (66).

Botulinum toxin acts by blocking the presynaptic release of acetylcholine at the neuromuscular junction, and this mode of action would explain its effect on the EAS; however, Gui and colleagues have shown that three injections of botulinum toxin (15 units in total) into the IAS of fissure patients resulted in a 60% healing rate at two months, with one patient developing a transient incontinence of flatus (67).

These results added some sign as to the mechanism of action of botulinum toxin where Jones and colleagues suggested that it causes a reduction in the myogenic tone, blocking the sympathetic nerves in the IAS (68). There are also uncertainties regarding the optimum dose necessary, as well as the optimum site for its administration. This is compounded by the discovery that doses in different commercial preparations are not equivalent even though the measured units of botulinum toxin are related to the median lethal dose in mice (66). As a result, a range of doses between two and a half units (69) to 40 units (70) have been used to treat fissure patients although better healing rates have been observed using 20 units compared with 15 units (71) and 21 units when compared with 10 units or 15 units in several trials (72).

In trying to ascertain the optimum site for injection, work by Maria and colleagues appears to show that injection into the IAS at a site in the posterior midline is most effective in treating posterior fissures (73). It has been suggested that botulinum toxin is more effective than topical GTN, and therefore its use should be considered as first line treatment for fissures (74). In a randomized controlled study where 50 patients were given either 20 units of botulinum toxin injected into the IAS or 0.2% GTN paste for 6 weeks, the healing rate was greater in the botulinum toxin group (96%) compared with the GTN group (60%). In this respect, others also have used botulinum toxin to treat patients with refractory fissures (75). Its apparent superiority can perhaps be attributed to the fact that there are potentially no compliance problems or tachyphylaxis with its use.

Calcium Channel Antagonists

Chrysos and colleagues first showed that a reduction in anal canal pressure could be achieved in volunteers following the administration of sublingual nifedipine, a calcium antagonist (76). In another study involving 15 patients with chronic fissures treated with oral doses of nifedipine retard 20 milligrams twice a day, there was a reduction in mean anal resting pressure of 36%, and after 8 weeks of treatment, fissure healing was observed in nine (60%) patients while a further three patients (20%) were asymptomatic.

Antropoli and colleagues (77) compared the topical use of 0.2% nifedipine gel with a mixture of 1% lignocaine/1% hydrocortisone gel in the treatment of 283 patients with acute anal fissures in a randomized double-blinded study. All patients were treated for 21 days and received a laxative and an anal dilator as part of their treatment protocol. The mean resting and squeeze pressures were found to be reduced in the nifedipine group by 30% and 17%, respectively, whereas there were no significant corresponding changes in the control group. The healing rates were 95% in the nifedipine group and 50% in the control group.

Using topical diltiazem (another calcium channel antagonist), Knight and colleagues (78) showed that the 2% ointment, when used in 71 patients with fissures for a median of 9 weeks, resulted in an 88% healing rate (79). However, at longer term follow-up (median 32 weeks), approximately one-third of these patients had recurrent symptoms. A recent study using 2% topical diltiazem gel showed that it might have a role in treating GTN-resistant fissures (80). In this study involving 39 fissure patients who had previously been treated with GTN, 19 (49%) patients' fissures healed with the use of 2% diltiazem, and the mean anal resting pressure was also reduced by 20%. The advantage that the use of calcium channel antagonists has over that of GTN is that it has fewer side effects, particularly resulting in fewer headaches. When compared with the use of botulinum toxin in fissure patients, calcium channel antagonists are less expensive and less uncomfortable to administer.

Muscarinic Agonists

The use of topical 0.1% bethanecol has been shown to reduce maximum anal resting pressure and to heal fissures (81). In 10 healthy volunteers, the maximum resting pressure was reduced by a mean of 24% (76) where 10 out of 15 patients with chronic fissures healed after an 8-week course of treatment. However, there does not appear to be much momentum at present in research into the use of these agents.

Sympathetic Neuromodulators

Both oral indoramin (an α_1 antagonist) and salbutamol (a β_2 agonist) have been shown to reduce mean anal resting pressure (82,83); however, a randomized controlled study using indoramin was abandoned because of its clinical ineffectiveness (84). There is both in vivo (84) and in vitro (83) evidence to support the notion that β adrenoceptors are upregulated in fissure patients when compared with controls. Inhaled salbutamol has been shown to shorten the duration of severe pain attacks in patients with proctalgia fugax (84). Further studies are awaited to clarify whether β agonists will be effective in the treatment of fissures.

Phosphodiesterase Inhibitors

There has been recent interest in this group of agents, which have been shown to cause IAS relaxation in vitro (85). They act by preventing the breakdown of intracellular cyclic adenosine monophosphate (cAMP) and cyclic guanyl monophosphate (cGMP), both of which cause relaxation of the IAS (86). So far, 11 families of phosphodiesterases (PDE) have been identified, many of these with specific inhibitors (87). An example of this is the drug sildenafil, a PDE-5 inhibitor that has current prominence from its use for the treatment of impotence. Other agents such as trimebutine cause the release and modulation of peptides, which in turn are thought to act via opiate receptors to bring about relaxation of the IAS. Ho and colleagues have investigated the role of trimebutine to see whether it reduced anal sphincter spasm and might contribute to the relief of post-hemorrhoidectomy pain, and they showed in their study of 80 patients (using trimebutine as a suppository) that it reduced the mean anal resting pressure by 35% (88).

Incontinence

Damage to the anal sphincter muscles can lead to fecal incontinence, and although disruption of the EAS may be surgically repaired with a good outcome, the same cannot be said about the IAS. It is possible, given the range of newer more limited therapies for symptomatic hemorrhoids (e.g., Ligasure hemorrhoidectomy, Doppler-guided hemorrhoid artery ligation, and stapled hemorrhoidectomy), that there may be a potential increase in inadvertent IAS injury (and the clinical presentation of passive fecal incontinence) because each of these techniques makes no attempt to display the plane of cleavage between the IAS and the hemorrhoid, particularly when there is substantial preoperative hemorroidal prolapse (89). Furthermore, in many patients presenting with fecal incontinence, the IAS may be structurally intact. Here, the causes of incontinence may be multifactorial where inadvertent IAS damage is only one consideration (41). Other factors may include inadvertent inherent IAS behavior during rectoanal distension and RAIR elicitation (48) intrinsic variations in IAS neuropeptide expression and the distal IAS/EAS anatomical overlap where deliberate IAS sphincterotomy leaves the distal anal canal relatively unsupported when there is a "constitutive" absence of the subcutaneous portion of the EAS (90). These patients often have low anal resting pressures on manometry. Incontinent patients also can have derangement of the slow and ultra slow waveforms (91) and an abnormal anorectal sampling reflex (10). Since the result of surgery to the IAS (plication) has been unrewarding (92), attempts to increase its tone by pharmacotherapy is gaining momentum.

Phenylephrine

The use of topical phenylephrine has been shown to increase the anal sphincter resting pressure (92). In their study of 12 healthy volunteers, Carapeti et al. observed an 8% rise in the maximum resting pressure using 5% phenylephrine gel while application of 10% phenylephrine gel produced a significant 33% increase. A subsequent small randomized controlled blind study using 10% phenylephrine gel to treat 12 patients with incontinence after ileoanal pouch surgery was carried out by the same investigators (93), where 6 of the patients who received the phenylephrine gel improved subjectively compared with only one using placebo, and 4 patients reported complete continence using phenylephrine treatment. Incontinence scores and maximum anal resting pressures were both significantly higher in the treatment group, however, when 10% phenylephrine was used in incontinent patients with a normal sphincter; on ultrasound imaging, the results were not as impressive (94). Here, there was no significant improvement in the incontinence scores, maximum anal resting pressures, or in the anodermal blood flow. Of the 36 patients in this study, 8 (6 on phenylephrine and 2 receiving placebo) reported a 75% subjective improvement in continence.

In this study, the therapeutic effectiveness of concentrations of 0%, 10%, 20%, 30%, and 40% phenylephrine gel was investigated, and although the different concentrations increased the maximum anal resting pressures relative to placebo, there was only a significant difference when using the two highest concentrations of phenylephrine gel. This study, however, omitted to report any symptomatic effects on incontinence (94).

The potential drawbacks of the use of phenylephrine include its cardiovascular side effects and the problem of local dermatitis, particularly when using higher topical concentrations. It has led to the trial of other pharmacologically related agents such as methoxamine, another α-adrenergic agonist. One of its stereoisomers, L-erythromethoxamine, is four times as potent as phenylephrine or the racemate (a mixture containing an equal amount of stereoisomers/enantiomers) at inducing IAS contraction (95). Further in vitro and in vivo studies are awaited using this agent.

Loperamide

Loperamide has long been used in the management of patients with diarrhea (96) and in patients with fecal incontinence (97). It inhibits the binding of naloxone, thus acting as an opiate agonist. Apart from decreasing colonic motility, it causes reduction of net intestinal fluid secretion acting via opiate receptors (98). In the normal anorectum, it increases the volumes needed to elicit the RAIR, but does not appear to significantly affect the anal resting or maximum squeeze pressures (99), although it has been shown to increase anal sphincter tone in animal models (100). Subsequently, loperamide has been used to improve sphincter function and continence in patients after restorative proctocolectomy (101). The effects of loperamide are complex in incontinence, reducing stool weight, and increasing whole gut (but not oral to cecal) transit, along with a direct effect on resting IAS tone (102,103).

Conclusion

The complex pharmacology of the anal sphincter is still in its infancy and is relatively poorly understood. By using the anal sphincter, and in particular the IAS, as a pharmacological target, we have been able to discern more of its normal physiology although we still seem some way away from understanding the neurophysiology of defecation, especially in relation to the afferent pathways and the potential transmitters involved in regulating this process (23). Much of the pharmacotherapy relating to the anal sphincter has been directed at the treatment of anal fissures, which in itself serves as an ideal model of study that has revolutionized the management of this relatively common anorectal condition. Other potential applications of agents to relax the IAS include use in reducing post-hemorrhoidectomy pain (104) and, anecdotally, its use prior to the insertion of the stapling gun head during anterior resections or pouch surgery in order to prevent inadvertent injury to the sphincter. In contrast, the use of pharmacological agents to manage patients with fecal incontinence has not met with as much success perhaps because the subject of continence is complex, with a multitude of factors governing its development primarily or following surgery. No doubt further studies of the anal sphincter complex using techniques such as dynamic magnetic resonance imaging, sacral nerve stimulators, and superfusion organ bath experiments will help unfold further pharmacological secrets and potential therapies for the management of these important anorectal disorders.

References

1. Frenckner B and Ihre T. Influence of autonomic nerves on the internal anal sphincter in man. Gut. 1976;17:306–12.
2. Frenckner B and Euler CV. Influence of pudendal nerve blockade on the function of the anal sphincters. Gut. 1975;16:482–9.
3. Langley JN. The autonomic nervous system. Part 1. Cambridge: Heffer and sons Ltd; 1921.
4. Dale HH. Nomenclature of fibres in the autonomic nervous system and their effects. J Physiol. 1933;80:10–1.
5. Goyal RK and Rattan S. Neurohumoral, hormonal and drug receptors for the lower oesophageal sphincter. Gastroenterology. 1978;74:598–619.
6. De Ponti F, Giaroni C, Cosentino M, Lechini S, and Frigo G. Adrenergic mechanism in the control of gastrointestinal motility: from basic science to clinical applications. Pharmacol Ther. 1996;69:59–78.
7. Schuster MM. Motor action of the rectum and anal sphincters in continence and defecation. Handbook of physiology, alimentary canal. Physiol Soc. 1968;4(6):2121–39.
8. Furness JB and Costa M. The enteric nervous system. New York: Churchill Livingstone; 1987.
9. Gowers WR. The automatic action of the sphincter ani. Proc R Soc Lond B Biol Sci. 1877;26:77–84.
10. Miller R, Bartolo DC, Cervero F, and Mortensen NJ. Anorectal sampling: a comparison of normal and incontinent patients. Br J Surg. 1988;75:44–7.
11. Denny-Brown D and Robertson EG. An investigation of the nervous control of defecation. Brain. 1935;58:256–310.
12. Lubowski DZ, Nicholls RJ, Swash M, and Jordan MJ. Neural control of internal anal sphincter function. Br J Surg. 1987;74:668–70.
13. Gaton EA. The physiology of faecal incontinence. Surg Gynecol Obstet. 1948;87:280–90.
14. Schuster MM, Hendrix TR, and Mendeloff AI. The internal anal sphincter response: manometric studies on its normal physiology, neural pathways and alteration in bowel disorders. J Clin Invest. 1963;42:196–207.
15. O'Kelly TJ, Davies JR, Tam PK, Brading AF, and Mortensen NJM. Abnormalities of nitric oxide producing neurons in Hirschsprung's disease: morphology and implications. J Paediatr Surg. 1994;29:294–300.

16. Meunier P and Mollard P. Control of the internal anal sphincter (manometric study of human subjects). Pflugers Arch. 1977;370:233–9.
17. Hirst GD, Holman ME, and McKirdy HC. Two descending nerve pathways activated by distension of guinea-pig small intestine. J Physiol Lond. 1975;244: 113–27.
18. Kumar D and Phillips SF. Human myenteric plexus: confirmation of unfamiliar structures in adults and neonates. Gastroenterology. 1989;9:1021–8.
19. Gutierrez JG and Shah AN. Autonomic control of the internal anal sphincter in man. In: von Trappen, editor. Vth international symposium on gastrointestinal motility. Leuven: Typoff Press. 1975; p. 63–73.
20. Carlstedt A, Nordgren S, Fasth S, Applegren L, and Hulten L. Sympathetic nervous influence on the internal anal sphincter and rectum in man. Int J Colorectal Dis. 1988;3:90–5.
21. Sun WM, Read NW, Miner PB, Kerrigan DD, and Donnelly TC. The role of transient internal sphincter relaxation in faecal incontinence. Int J Colorectal Dis. 1990;5:31–6.
22. Sorensen SM, Gregersen H, Djurhuus JC. Spontaneous anorectal pressure activity: evidence of internal anal sphincter contractions in response to rectal pressure waves. Scand J Gastroenterol. 1989;2:115–200.
23. Zbar AP, Jayne DG, Mathur D, Ambrose NS, and Guillou PJ. The importance of the internal anal sphincter (IAS) in maintaining continence: anatomical, physiological and pharmacological considerations. Colorectal Dis. 2000;2:193–202.
24. Brading AF and Sibley GN. A superfusion apparatus to study field stimulation of smooth muscle from mammalian urinary bladder. J Physiol (Lond). 1983;334:11–12P.
25. Burleigh DE, D'Mello A, and Parks AG. Responses of isolated human internal anal sphincter to drugs and electrical field stimulation. Gastroenterology. 1979;77:484–90.
26. Cook TA, Brading AF, and Mortensen NJM. Differences in contractile properties of anorectal smooth muscle and the effects of calcium channel blockade. Br J Surg. 1999;86:70–5.
27. O'Kelly TJ, Brading AF, and Mortensen NJM. Nerve mediated relaxation of the human internal anal sphincter: the role of nitric oxide. Gut. 1993;34:689–93.
28. O'Kelly TJ, Brading AF, and Mortensen NJM. In vitro response of the human anal canal longitudinal muscle layer to cholinergic and adrenergic stimulation: evidence of sphincter specialization. Br J Surg. 1993;80:1337–41.
29. Hoyle CHV. Purinergic cotransmission: parasympathetic and enteric nerves. Neurosciences. 1996;8:207–15.
30. Biancani P, Walsh JH, and Behar J. Vasoactive intestinal polypeptide. A neurotransmitter for lower esophageal sphincter relaxation. J Clin Invest. 1984;73:963–7.
31. Alumets J, Hakanson R, Sundler F, and Uddman R. VIP innervation of sphincters. Scand J Gastroenterol. 1978;13(49):6.
32. Chakder S and Rattan S. Evidence for VIP-induced increase in NO production in myenteric neurons of opossum internal anal sphincter. Am J Physiol. 1996;270:G492–7.

33. Chakder S and Rattan S. Release of nitric oxide by activation of nonadrenergic noncholinergic neurons of internal anal sphincter. Am J Physiol. 1993;264: G7–12.
34. O'Kelly TJ, Brading AF, and Mortensen NJM. Nitric oxide mediates cholinergic relaxation of human internal anal sphincter muscle in vitro. Gut. 1992;33: A48.
35. Schroder HD. Onuf's nucleus X: a morphological study of a human spinal nucleus. Anat Embryol (Berl). 1981;162:443–53.
36. Jones AM, Brading AF, and Mortensen NJ. Role of nitric oxide in anorectal function of normal and neuronal nitric oxide synthase knockout mice: a novel approach to anorectal disease. Dis Colon Rectum. 2003;46:963–70.
37. Duthie HL and Gairns FW. Sensory nerve endings and sensation in the anal region in man. Br J Surg. 1990;47:585–95.
38. Pescatori M and Interisano A. Annual report of the Italian coloproctology units. Tech Coloproctol. 1995;3:29–30.
39. Snooks S, Henry MM, and Swash M. Faecal incontinence after anal dilatation. Br J Surg. 1984;71:617–8.
40. Khubchandani IT and Reed JF. Sequelae of internal sphincterotomy for chronic fissure-in-ano. Br J Surg. 1989;76:431–4.
41. Zbar AP, BeerGabel M, Chiappa AC, and Aslam M. Fecal incontinence after minor anorectal surgery. Dis Colon Rectum. 2002;44:1610–23.
42. Lund JN and Scholefield JH. Aetiology and treatment of anal fissure. Br J Surg. 1996;83:1335–44.
43. Brodie BC. Lectures on diseases of the rectum; lecture III; preternatural contraction of the sphincter ani. Lond Med Gaz. 1835;16:26–31.
44. Klosterhalfen B, Vogel P, Rixen H, and Mittermayer C. Topography of the inferior rectal artery: a possible cause of chronic primary anal fissure. Dis Colon Rectum. 1989;2:43–52.
45. Gibbons CP and Read NW. Anal hypertonia in fissures: cause or effect? Br J Surg. 1986;73:443–5.
46. Keck JO, Staniunas RJ, Coller JA, Barrett RC, and Oster ME. Computer-generated profiles of the anal canal in patients with anal fissure. Dis Colon Rectum. 1995;38:72–9.
47. Northmann BJ and Schuster MM. Internal anal sphincter derangement with anal fissures. Gastroenterology. 1974;67:216–20.
48. Zbar AP, Aslam M, Gold DM, Gatzen C, Gosling A, and Kmiot WA. Parameters of the rectoanal inhibitory reflex in patients with idiopathic fecal incontinence and chronic constipation. Dis Colon Rectum. 1998;41:200–8.
49. Kaur G, Gardiner A, and Duthie GS. Rectoanal reflex parameters in incontinence and constipation. Dis Colon Rectum. 2002;45:928–33.
50. Guillemot F, Lone YC, Leroi H, Lamblin MD, and Cortot A. Nitroglycerin in situ reduces upper anal canal pressure. Dig Dis Sci. 1992;37:155.
51. Kennedy ML, Lubowski DZ, and King DW. Chemical sphincterotomy for anal fissure. Tripartite Meeting, Sydney 1993 as quoted by Watson SJ, Kamm MA, Nicholls RJ, and Phillips RKS. Topical glyceryl trinitrate in the treatment of chronic anal fissure. Br J Surg. 1996;83:771–5.
52. Loder PB, Kamm MA, Nicholls RJ, and Phillips RKS. Chemical sphincterotomy by local application of glyceryl trinitrate. Br J Surg. 1994;81:386–9.

53. Lund JN and Scholefield JH. Follow-up of patients with chronic anal fissure treated with topical glyceryl trinitrate. Lancet. 1998;352:1681.
54. Bacher H, Mischinger HJ, Werkgartner J, Cerwenka H, El-Shabrawi A, Pfeifer J, et al. Local nitroglycerin for treatment of anal fissures: an alternative to lateral sphincterotomy? Dis Colon Rectum. 1997;40:840–5.
55. Carapeti EA, Kamm MA, McDonald PJ, Chadwick SJD, Melville D, and Phillips RKS. Randomised controlled trial shows that glyceryl trinitrate heals anal fissures, higher doses are not more effective, and there is a high recurrence rate. Gut. 1999;44:727–30.
56. Kennedy ML, Sowter S, Nguyen H, and Lubowski DZ. Glyceryl trinitrate ointment for the treatment of chronic anal fissure. Dis Colon Rectum. 1999; 42:1000–6.
57. Beck D, Rafferty J, Yee L, Binderow S; Fissure Study Group. GTN paste as a treatment for anal fissure. Dis Colon Rectum. 2000;43:A35.
58. Altomare DF, Rinaldi M, Milito G, Arcana F, Spinelli F, Nardelli N, et al. Glyceryl trinitrate for chronic anal fissure-healing or headache? Results of a multicenter, randomised, placebo-controlled, double-blind trial. Dis Colon Rectum. 2000;43:174–9.
59. Richard CS, Gregoire R, Plewes EA, Silverman R, Burul C, Buie D, Reznick R, Ross T, Burnstein M, O'Connor BI, Mukraj D, and McLeod RS. Internal sphincterotomy is superior to topical nitroglycerine in the treatment of chronic anal fissure: results of a randomised, controlled trial by the Canadian Colorectal Surgical Trials Group. Dis Colon Rectum. 2000;43:1048–58.
60. Watson SJ, Kamm MA, Nicholls RJ, and Phillips RKS. Topical glyceryl trinitrate in the treatment of chronic anal fissure. Br J Surg. 1996;83:771–5.
61. Evans J, Luck A, and Hewett P. Glyceryl trinitrate vs lateral sphincterotomy for chronic anal fissure. Prospective randomized trial. Dis Colon Rectum. 2001;44:93–7.
62. Lysy J, Israelit-Yatzkan Y, Sestiere-Ittah M, Keret D, and Goldin E. Treatment of chronic anal fissure with isosorbide dinitrate: long term results and dose determination. Dis Colon Rectum. 1998;41:1406–10.
63. Schouten W, Zimmermann D, Briel J, and Hechtmann H. Effects of L-arginine on resting anal pressure. Dis Colon Rectum. 2000;43:A2.
64. Scott AB. Botulinum toxin injection into extraocular muscles as an alternative to strabismus surgery. Ophthalmology. 1980;87:1044–9.
65. Jost WH and Schimrigk K. Therapy of anal fissure using botulin toxin. Dis Colon Rectum. 1994;37:1321–4.
66. Jost WH. One hundred cases of anal fissure treated with botulin toxin: early and long term results. Dis Colon Rectum. 1997;40:1029–32.
67. Gui D, Cassetta F, Anastasio G, et al. Botulinum toxin for chronic anal fissure. Lancet. 1994;344:1127–78.
68. Jones OM, Moore JA, Brading AF, and Mortensen NJM. The site and mechanism of action of botulinum toxin in porcine anal sphincter. Colorect Dis. In press 2003.
69. Fernandez-Lopez F, Conde Freire R, Rios Rios A, Garcia Iglesias J, Cainzos Fernandez M, and Potel Lesquereux J. Botulinum toxin for the treatment of anal fissure. Dig Surg. 1999;16:515–8.
70. Madalinski M. Botox and dysport are distinct. Endoscopy. 2000;32:502–3.

71. Maria G, Brisinda G, Bentivoglio AR, Cassetta E, Gui D, and Albanese A. Botulinum toxin injections in the internal anal sphincter for the treatment of chronic anal fissure: long term results after two different treatment regimes. Ann Surg. 1998;228:664–9.
72. Minguez M, Melo M, Espi A, Garcia-Granero E, Mora F, Lledo S, et al. Therapeutic effects of different doses of botulinum toxin in chronic anal fissure. Dis Colon Rectum. 1999;42:1016–21.
73. Maria G, Brisinda G, Bentivoglio AR, Cassetta E, Gui D, and Albanese A. Influence of botulinum toxin site of injections on healing rate in patients with chronic anal fissure. Am J Surg. 2000;179:46–50.
74. Brisinda G, Maria G, Bentivoglio AR, Cassetta E, Gui D, and Albanese A. A comparison of injections of botulinum toxin and topical nitroglycerin ointment for the treatment of chronic anal fissure. N Engl J Med. 1999;341:65–9.
75. Keret D and Goldin E. Topical nitrates potentiates the effects of botulinum toxin in the treatment of patients with refractory anal fissure. Gut. 2001;48:221–4.
76. Chrysos E, Xynos E, Tzovaras G, Zoras OJ, Tsiaoussis J, and Vassilakis SJ. Effect of nifedipine on rectoanal motility. Dis Colon Rectum. 1996;39:212–6.
77. Antropoli C, Perrotti P, Rubino M, Martino A, De Stefano G, Migliore G, et al. Nifedipine for local use in conservative treatment of anal fissures: preliminary results of a multicenter study. Dis Colon Rectum. 1999;42:1011–5.
78. Knight JS, Birks M, and Farouk R. Topical diltiazem ointment in the treatment of chronic anal fissure. Br J Surg. 2001;88:553–6.
79. Monas M, Speake W, and Scholefield JH. Diltiazem heals glyceryl trinitrate resistant chronic anal fissures. Dis Colon Rectum. 2002;45:1091–5.
80. Carapeti EA, Kamm MA, and Phillips RKS. Topical diltiazem and bethanechol decrease anal sphincter pressure and heal anal fissures without side effects. Dis Colon Rectum. 2000;43:1359–62.
81. Pitt J, Craggs MM, Henry MH, and Boulos PB. Alpha-1 adrenoceptor blockade: potential new treatment for anal fissures. Dis Colon Rectum. 2000; 43:800–3.
82. Ojo-Aromokudo O, Pitt J, Boulos PB, Knight SL, and Craggs MD. A comparison of alpha and beta adrenoceptor function of the internal anal sphincter in people with and without chronic anal fissures. J Physiol (Lond). 1998;507:19P.
83. Pitt J, Dawson P, Hallan R, and Boulos P. Double-blind, randomised, placebo-controlled trial of oral indoramin to treat chronic anal fissure. Dis Colon Rectum. 2000;43:A32.
84. Eckhardt VF, Dodt O, Kanzler G, and Bernhard G. Treatment of proctalgia fugax with salbutamol inhalation. Am J Gastroenterol. 1996;91:686–9.
85. Jones OM, Brading AF, and Mortensen NJM. Phosphodiesterase inhibitors cause relaxation of the internal anal sphincter in vitro. A novel treatment for anal fissure? Dis Colon Rectum. 2002;45(4):530–6.
86. VanderWall KJ, Bealer JF, and Harrison MR. Cyclic GMP relaxes the internal anal sphincter in Hirschsprung's disease. J Pediatr Surg. 1995;30:1013–5.
87. Fawcett L, Baxendale R, Stacey P, McGrouther C, Harrow I, Soderling S, et al. Molecular cloning and characterization of a distinct human phosphodiesterase gene family: PDE11A. Proc Natl Acad Sci U S A. 2000;97:3702–7.

88. Ho YH, Seow-Chen F, Low JY, Tan M, and Leng AP. Randomised controlled trial of trimebutine (anal sphincter relaxant) for pain after haemorrhoidectomy. Br J Surg. 1997;84:377–9.
89. Gemsenjager E. Preserving Treitz's muscle in haemorrhoidectomy. Dis Colon Rectum. 1982;25:633–7.
90. Zbar AP, Kmiot WA, Aslam M, Williams A, Hider A, Audisio RA, Chiappa AC, and deSouza NM. Use of vector volume manometry and endoanal magnetic resonance imaging in the adult female for assessment of anal sphincter dysfunction. Dis Colon Rectum. 1999;42:1411–8.
91. Sangwan YP, Coller JA, Schoetz DJ, Roberts PL, and Murray JJ. Relationship between manometric anal waves and faecal incontinence. Dis Colon Rectum. 1995;38:370–4.
92. Leroi AM, Kamm MA, Weber J, Denis P, and Hawley PR. Internal anal sphincter repair. Int J Colorectal Dis. 1997;12:243–5.
93. Carapeti EA, Kamm MA, Evans BK, and Phillips RKS. Topical phenylephrine increases anal sphincter resting pressure. Br J Surg. 1999;86:267–70.
94. Carapeti EA, Kamm MA, Nicholls RJ, and Phillips RKS. Randomized, controlled trial of topical phenylephrine for faecal incontinence in patients after ileoanal pouch construction. Dis Colon Rectum. 2000;43:1059–63.
95. Cheetham MJ, Kamm MA, and Phillips RKS. Topical phenylephrine increases anal canal resting pressure in patients with faecal incontinence. Gut. 2001;48:356–9.
96. Jones OM, Mortensen NM, and Brading AF. L-erythro-methoxamine as a possible new means of treatment of faecal incontinence. Br J Surg. 2003;90(7):872–6.
97. Ooms LA, Degryse AD, and Janssen PA. Mechanisms of action of loperamide. Scand J Gastroenterol. 1984;96:145–55.
98. Read M, Read NW, Barber DC, and Duthie HL. Effects of loperamide on anal sphincter function in patients complaining of chronic diarrhea with faecal incontinence and urgency. Dig Dis Sci. 1982;27:807–14.
99. Musial F, Enck P, Kalveram KT, and Erckenbrecht JF. The effect of loperamide on anorectal function in normal healthy men. J Clin Gastroenterol. 1992;15:321–4.
100. Rattan S and Culver PJ. Influence of loperamide on the internal anal sphincter in the opossum. Gastroenterology. 1987;93:121–8.
101. Hallgren T, Fasth S, Delbro DS, Nordgren S, Oresland T, and Hulten L. Loperamide improves anal sphincter function and continence after restorative proctocolectomy. Dig Dis Sci. 1994;39:2612–8.
102. Sun WM, Read NW, and Verlinden M. Effects of loperamide oxide on gastrointestinal transit time and anorectal function in patients with chronic diarrhea and faecal incontinence. Scand J Gastroenterol. 1997;32:34–8.
103. Cheetham M, Brazzelli M, Norton C, and Glazener CM. Drug treatment for faecal incontinence in adults. Cochrane Database Syst Rev. 2003;CD002116.
104. Wasvary H, Hain J, Mosed-Vogel M, Bendick P, Barkel DC, and Klein SN. Randomized, prospective, double-blind, placebo-controlled trial of effect of nitroglycerin oinment on pain after hemorrhoidectomy. Dis Colon Rectum. 2001;44(8):1069–73.

Editorial Commentary

In vitro assessment of internal anal sphincter muscle strips has shown novel receptors which may result in relaxation including the central receptor status of nitric oxide as the putative non-adrenergic noncholinergic (NANC) neurotransmitter involved in rectoanal inhibition. This has led to an expanded primary use of topical therapies in the treatment of chronic anal fissure particularly when it has become evident that lateral internal anal sphincterotomy is associated in some patients with persistent fecal soiling which affects quality of life. The results of comparative studies of surgery versus topical therapy have shown a moderate recidivism in patients treated with local NO donors and more recently with calcium antagonists or diltiazem preparations. This approach has been transferred to the local treatment of fecal incontinence with agents such as phenylephrine, where further studies assessing chemical neurotransmitters in knockout mice have suggested a way forward for the development of novel treatments in patients with postoperative incontinence and intractable perianal pain.

AZ

Chapter 5
Anal and Perianal Pathology

Editorial Commentary

There has been an improved understanding of the development and structure of the anal transitional zone (ATZ) and its importance in anal intraepithelial neoplasia (AIN) as a precursor to invasive squamous cell carcinoma of the anus. Molecular biological techniques have shown a high prevalence of high-risk oncogenic human papillomavirus (HPV) subtypes and their persistence in immunocompromised patients who progress towards invasive cancer; an approach facilitated by specialized cytological assessment. The association between cervical intraepithelial neoplasia and invasive cervical cancer and AIN (and its invasive concomitant) is at present unclear as is the relationship between HPV persistence (or eradication) and the progression to invasive malignancy. At present the management of high-grade AIN field changes is uncertain with many adopting a "wait-and-see" policy given the morbidity of wide local excision and perineal resurfacing in these patients. The role of the immune response modifier Imiquimod is also not established and there is at present no evidence that there is resolution of high-grade AIN with the introduction of highly active antiretroviral therapy (HAART). Improved understanding of this problem will provide a better algorithm for management of extensive AIN (particularly in the HIV-positive patient) and the therapy and follow-up itself may secondarily impact on the natural history of the disease in high-prevalence AIN environments.

AZ

Chapter 5.1
Anal Histopathology

CLAUS FENGER

Introduction

Anorectal pathology comprises a number of common diseases such as hemorrhoids, anal polyps, and an occasional squamous carcinoma, and most diagnoses are relatively straightforward; therefore, this review will focus on pitfalls and differential diagnoses, with the main emphasis on more recent observations and controversial areas in anal pathology. As there has appeared through the ages a large number of definitions and eponyms for the different structures and their disorders, those terms as presently used will briefly be reviewed (1,2).

Definitions and Normal Histology

According to the World Health Organization (WHO), the anal canal is defined as the terminal part of the large intestine, beginning at the upper surface of the anorectal ring and passing through the pelvic floor to end at the anus, i.e., the junction with true skin at the anal margin. The latter—also called the perianal skin by some—is the region of puckered, pigmented skin surrounding the anus, and its lateral borders have not been strictly defined. The most important macroscopic landmark in the anal canal mucosa is the line composed of the anal valves and the bases of the anal columns called the dentate line (DL); however, in the past this has also been referred to as the pectenate line.

The epithelial ring of the anal canal can effectively be divided into three zones. The upper part is called the colorectal zone and is covered by colorectal-type mucosa identical with that of the rectum above. The middle part, which extends from the DL and about one centimeter upwards with a variation one to twenty millimeters, is called the anal transition(al) zone (ATZ) and shows a mixture of epithelial variants (3,4). The zone below the DL is called the squamous zone and is covered by non-keratinized squamous epithelium. At the anus, this is replaced by the perianal skin with keratinized squamous epithelium and skin appendages. These different zones are not always clearly distinguishable to the clinician and can show variations, particularly in cases with mucosal prolapse. It is therefore recommended that all biopsy material be forwarded to the pathologist with a description by the clinician of the location of the biopsy in relation to the DL.

Of these zones, the ATZ deserves particular comment. It is defined as the zone interposed between uninterrupted colorectal-type mucosa above and uninterrupted squamous epithelium below, irrespective of the type of epithelium found in the zone itself. Among the epithelial types found in the ATZ, the most prominent is usually the so-called ATZ-epithelium, which to some extent resembles the metaplastic epithelium found in the cervical transformation zone, consisting of four to nine cell layers. The basal cells are small, whereas the surface cells may be columnar, cuboidal, or flattened (Figure 5.1.1). The cytokeratin profile and the sparse mucin production of the ATZ epithelium is similar to that found in the anal glands, and their specialized epithelium also contains scattered endocrine- and melanin-producing cells (1). Knowledge by the histopathologist of this very varying picture is of importance when diagnosing precancerous changes.

Three special types of glands are found in this area. The anal (intramuscular) glands are mucin-producing and have their openings in the ATZ just above the DL from where they extend into the submucosa and sometimes even into the sphincter musculature. These structures traditionally have been implicated in the origin of perirectal abscess and fistula-in-ano, although the anatomy and histology in man is very variable (5). The perianal glands are apocrine and located in the anal margin. In addition to these, a third type of anogenital glands have been described—the so-called mammary-like glands—that are located around the anus, where the perianal skin begins (6).

Non-Neoplastic Pathology

Inflammation

Inflammatory bowel disease often involves the anal and perianal regions, and some pitfalls exist with regard to correct classification. The upper part of the anal mucosa is nearly constantly inflamed in ulcerative colitis, but normal mucosa does not exclude this diagnosis. Perianal complications are common in Crohn's colitis, but occasionally can be found in patients with ulcerative colitis. Tissue from fissures and fistulas, as well as from pouchitis, should therefore be examined histologically in search for granulomas and other features of Crohn's disease. However, granulomas also can be caused by foreign material, and rarely by tuberculosis, where, in the latter case, staining for acid-fast bacilli is not consistently positive (7). It also should be

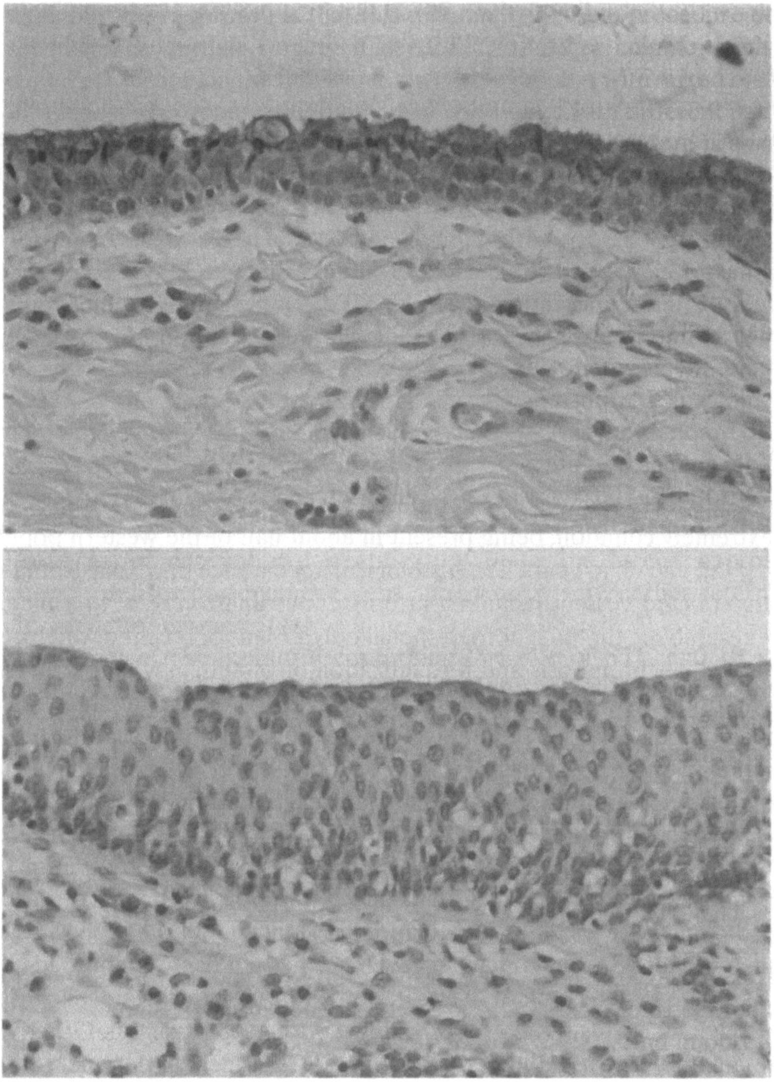

a

b

FIGURE 5.1.1. Normal variants of ATZ-epithelium. (a) Typical histology of the anal transition zone (ATZ). The basal cells are typically small with a progressive spread of columnar cells, which more superficially become flattened. Top layer consisting of mucus producing cells stained with Alcian Blue. (b) Top layer of polygonal cells, H&E.

remembered that inflammatory bowel disease might be found in children, but that this may be confused with eosinophilic inflammation secondary to allergic colitis (8).

Other inflammatory conditions encountered by the histopathologist include skin diseases such as lichen sclerosus et atrophicus and venereal diseases, such as syphilis, lymphogranuloma venereum, and granuloma inguinale, although these are uncommon in Western society. Anal ulcers may be due to infection with cytomegalovirus and herpesvirus, and the diagnosis may occasionally be missed by routine examination. In patients with increased risk for such infections (e.g., HIV/AIDS patients), clinical information is important because it can lead to the helpful use of specific immunohistochemistry (9).

Vascular Disorders

Hemorrhoids are excrescenses composed of vascular tissue and stroma. They are extremely common, being present in about half of the western population by the age of 50 years. The histological appearance may vary from that of large dilated vessels, including arteriovenous anastomoses, to a picture more resembling that of a fibroepithelial polyp. Signs of recent or old bleeding, as well as thrombosis and recanalization of vessels, may be prominent, and neuronal hyperplasia is not uncommon (10). The covering mucosa can be of colorectal, ATZ, or squamous type, depending on the location. Ulceration or squamous metaplasia is common and the mucosa may show all the signs typical for prolapse (11). Pathological examination of hemorrhoids is advisable as a few may show anal intraepithelial neoplasia (AIN) (12), rarely malignant tumors such as malignant melanoma (personal observation) or anal metastases (14). Hemorrhoids have traditionally been considered related to a low fiber diet, constipation, prolonged straining, obesity and portal hypertension, but convincing evidence has not been established (13). They seem to be the result of deterioration of the supporting and anchoring connective tissue, resulting in sliding down of the anal cushions. Other vascular changes occasionally seen by the pathologist include perianal thrombosis, rectal varices, and hemangiomas, each of which is rare.

Polyps

The fibroepithelial polyp—also called a fibrous anal polyp, hypertrophied anal papilla, or anal tag—is among the commonest anal lesions and may be found in up to half of all individuals. This lesion can be present as early as infancy, but it most often is found in the fourth decade (15,16), being located anywhere from the perianal skin up to the DL. Grossly, the polyp is spherical or elongated, the surface is white or grey, and the size can vary from a few millimeters to four centimeters in maximal diameter. Histologically, it consists of a fibrous stroma covered with squamous epithelium, which typically is slightly hyperplastic and may be keratinized or may show superficial ulceration. Anal intraepithelial neoplasia may be present in a few of these polyps (12). The stroma may contain atypical fibroblasts, mast cells, and proliferating peripheral nerves (10,17). The etiology is unknown, although some probably represent the end stage of hemorrhoids, whereas others are seen in Crohn's disease. Other polyps presenting in the anal canal include adenomas, hyperplastic polyps, juvenile polyps, and Peutz-Jegher polyps, all of which arise in colorectal-type mucosa. The "cloacogenic" polyp seen in prolapse and the inflammatory polyps found in long-standing inflammatory bowel disease are other lesions that occassionally may be submitted to the histopathologist.

Prolapse

Solitary rectal ulcer syndrome (SRUS) is the term commonly used for the mucosal changes in patients with rectal prolapse, but the term is largely a misnomer, for ulcers may be absent or multiple. Its clinical use by coloproctologists is different and is applied to a specific disorder of evacuation, which may or may not be associated with endoscopic evidence of frank ulceration, digitations, and response to rectopexy. The histological picture is quite characteristic with a mucosal thickening with edema of the lamina propria, a variable degree of fibrosis, hypertrophy of the muscularis mucosae, and vertically re-orientated extension of smooth muscle fibers upwards between the crypts with disturbance of the normal crypt architecture. Complications noted include crypt displacement under the muscularis mucosae (localized colitis cystica profunda), polypoid changes of the mucosa (inflammatory cloacogenic polyp), and ulceration or squamous metaplasia of the surface. Solitary rectal ulcer syndrome is probably underdiagnosed by some pathologists (18,19); it is most commonly a disease of the adult, but also may be found in children (20). The etiology of SRUS is unknown. Thickening of the muscularis propria is characteristic, and this is absent in complete rectal prolapse, where the mucosal changes are also less pronounced (21). The associated polypoid changes usually are found in the upper anal canal, but occasionally may be found in the sigmoid colon (22). Detailed histological examination of several biopsies is crucial because an identical picture can be seen in the vicinity of some malignant tumors and because some polyps may show AIN (23,24).

Neurological Disorders

The enteric nervous system is the largest and most complex division of the autonomic nervous system, and defects in its function are likely to occur in many, if not most, gastrointestinal diseases. Unfortunately, until now, pathological examination has only been useful in a few of these cases, most being examples of developmental disturbance. Comprehensive reviews of these disorders have recently been published (25,26). The introduction of laparoscopic biopsies opens up the possibility of investigating the musculature and the interstitial cells of Cajal, potentially providing new useful insight into their etiopathogenesis and diagnosis.

Hirschsprung's disease (HD) is a congenital abnormality characterized by the absence of ganglion cells in the myenteric as well as in the submucosal plexi, resulting in a sustained contraction of the aganglionic segment. The incidence is about one per 5 000 live births. A number of genes are involved and mutations are most commonly found in genes in the GDNF (Glial Cell Derived Neurotrophic Factor) or ET-3 (Endothelin–3) signaling systems. Mutations of these genes may result in dominant, recessive, or polygenic patterns of inheritance where HD is thought to be the result of failed migration of neuroblasts from the neural crest, although changes in the microenvironment may contribute to the pathogenesis (25,27).

Hirschsprung's disease generally is diagnosed shortly after birth, but occasionally not until adulthood in patients presenting with chronic obstipation. In classical HD, the aganglíosis starts at the DL and involves the rectum and varying lengths of colon. Short-segment HD is limited to a five to seven centimeter section above the DL, and ultra-short HD involves only a very short segment in the upper anal canal (29). Thus, a set of three large biopsies including submucosa taken at one to two, four, and nine centimeter levels above the dentate line should allow a correct diagnosis and classification. However, it must be remembered that there often is a transition zone of variable length with hypo- or hypergangliosis, and that cases of segmental aganglíosis above the rectum have been reported in children as well as in adults (28).

In these biopsies, the presence or absence of ganglion cells can be demonstrated by immunostaining for S-100 protein, which visualizes Schwann cells and hypertrophied nerves, leaving the ganglion cells unstained. Additional histochemical staining will show an increased number of acetylcholinesterase-positive nerve bundles and the absence of neuronal elements containing nitric oxide synthase, the latter being responsible for absent relaxation of the internal anal sphincter (29,30).

While the histological diagnosis of HD is usually straightforward, other disturbances in the enteric innervation can be impossible to diagnose on mucosal and submucosal biopsies. Isolated hypogangliosis is very rare and may be limited to the myenteric plexus, whereas intestinal neuronal dysplasia (IND) can be defined by the presence of giant ganglia in the submucosa showing many relatively hypogenetic (immature) nerve cells. Additional features include ectopic ganglion cells in the lamina propria and increased acetylcholinesterase activity in and around the submucosal plexus and vessels. However, there is a poor correlation between the histological and the clinical findings, presumably because some of the changes represent normal variations or stages in development or because the fundamental disorder is located in the myenteric plexus. This would explain why many of these patients do comparatively well on conservative treatment (31,32).

Neoplastic Pathology

Anal Intraepithelial Neoplasia and Bowen's Disease

A number of different terms have been used for the precursor for squamous carcinoma in this region, including anal dysplasia and carcinoma in situ (CIS), anal squamous intraepithelial lesion (ASIL), and, when located in the perianal skin, Bowen's disease. The term anal intraepithelial neoplasia (AIN) for anal canal lesions is now preferred by the WHO and will be used here (2).

Anal intraepithelial neoplasia may be an occasional finding in hemorrhoids, as outlined above, but otherwise can present as an eczematoid or papillomatous area or as papules or plaques. Induration or ulceration may indicate invasion. A more distinct picture can be obtained by high-resolution anoscopy with an operating microscope and topical application of 3% acetic acid. In cases of high-grade AIN, these will present as the corresponding cervical lesion with an aberrant vascular pattern, aceto-white changes, and the cells will not take up Lugol's iodine solution due to lack of glycogen (33,34). Histologically, AIN does not differ substantially from the corresponding cervical or vulvar lesion, and koilocytosis, as well as keratinization, may be present. In AIN, there appear to be different molecular mechanisms when compared with CIN or vulvar intraepithelial neoplasia (VIN), and the reader is referred to a recent review on the comparative molecular biological changes in these conditions where there are less chromosomal aberrations and genomic instability in AIN compared with CIN or VIN, and where there is less AIN-related reliance on changes in tumor suppression genes (such as p53) during the progression from AIN to invasive carcinoma (35). There also appears to be less reliance in AIN on oncogenic human papillomavirus (HPV) infection (and eradication) when compared with CIN and invasive cervical cancer, occasionally being associated with substantial spontaneous AIN regression (36). The entire clinical area of AIN surveillance, particularly in the HIV-positive patient, is extremely controversial, and is probably of value in patients with demonstrable AIN grade III, frankly exophytic or ulcerated areas with AIN changes, and in patients with CD4 T lymphocyte depletion or those on immunosuppressant therapy (e.g., post-transplant cases).

The appearance of the normal epithelial variants in the ATZ should, however, be kept in mind, so that not all cellular epithelia are classified as dysplastic. Anal intraepithelial neoplasia can be graded into grades I, II, and III, although the inter-observer variation of this grading is considerable and a two-grade system may be more appropriate (37). Histological examples of AIN (II and III) are shown in Figure 5.1.2. The finding of AIN should always be followed by an examination of the entire anogenital area, as AIN may be part of more widespread precancerous changes.

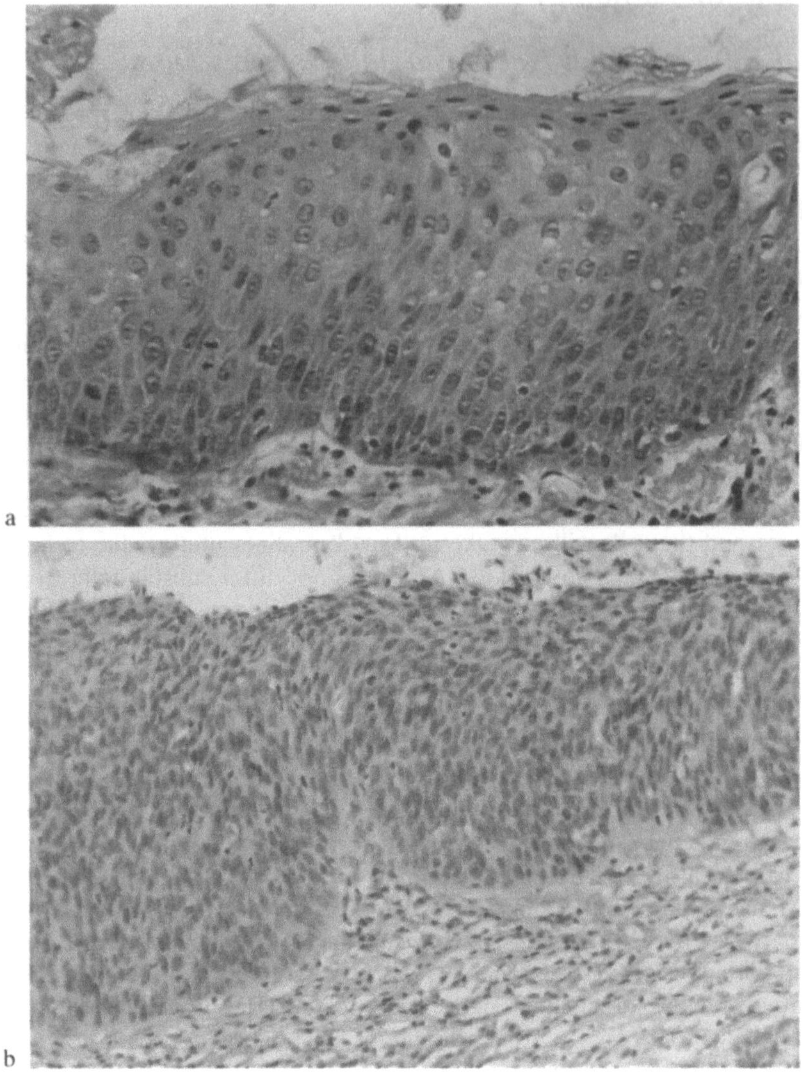

FIGURE 5.1.2. Variants of AIN. (a) AIN II with partly maturing top cells. (b) AIN III with no maturing cells at top.

In contrast, Bowen's disease tends to present as white or red areas and may rarely progress to squamous carcinoma (SCC). Bowenoid papulosis is histologically similar to Bowen's disease, but shows the clinical picture of multiple two to ten millimeter reddish-brown papules or plaques. It never progress to SCC, again underlining the importance of clinical information provided to the pathologist.

Condyloma Acuminatum

These not uncommon warty or papillary anal condylomata show the same histology as their genital counterparts, and flat lesions showing koilocytosis can also be found. Both types of lesions should be totally embedded and examined for the presence of HPV and for signs of AIN or SCC, which may occur, particularly in immunosuppressed patients (38). There appears to be progressive changes in the microvessel density between condylomata and preinvasive lesions progressing right through to frankly invasive carcinoma (39). Moreover, condylomata acuminata are associated with less oncogenic HPV subtypes than either AIN or SCC (40). When AIN is associated with anal condylomata in HIV-positive patients, there is an 80% incidence of AIN (mostly low-grade). High-grade lesions tend to recur more frequently than low-grade lesions, so although regression may be noted during follow-up, failure of topical therapies may indicate a later stage of the AIDS process (41).

Squamous Carcinoma

In the recently published WHO classification of anal tumors, it is recommended that the generic term "anal squamous cell carcinoma" (SCC) be used for all the previous subtypes of SCC; namely, basaloid (cloacogenic), large-cell keratinizing, and large-cell non-keratinizing carcinomas (2). There are four good reasons for this recommendation. Firstly, it has been shown that most anal SCCs show features of two or all of these histological patterns. Secondly, the reported proportion of basaloid carcinomas has varied from 10% to almost 70% in larger series, and there appears to be poor inter-observer and intra-observer agreement even amongst experienced pathologists with regard to histopathological subtyping (42). Thirdly, no significant correlation between subtypes and prognosis has been established (43), and finally, histological classification is nowadays nearly always performed on small biopsies with the subsequent risk of sampling error. This does not imply that different histological appearances are without any relation to the biology of the tumors, where it has been shown that poor keratinization, prominent basaloid features, and small tumor cell size are significantly related to infection with high-risk HPV (44).

The etiology of AIN and anal SCC has been extensively reviewed recently (35,45). High-risk human papillomavirus (hrHPV) has been demonstrated in 84% of anal SCC (45), and individuals seropositive for HPV 16 and 18 have an increased risk of developing anal and perianal SCC (46). In particular, men who have sex with men and individuals with HIV/AIDS, as well as immunosuppressed individuals, are at high risk. Patients who have had ileal pouch–anal anastomosis for inflammatory bowel disease may also rarely develop AIN in the spared ATZ, but this is usually self-limiting and may regress (47). No convincing relationship has been documented with regard to tobacco smoking or benign anal lesions such as hemorrhoids, fissures, fistulas, or Crohn's disease. In general, tumors located at the anal margin seem to have a slightly better prognosis, but this may be related to earlier diagnosis and tumor stage. Stage and nodal status are still the most important factors, and efforts to find useful molecular markers have failed (48). The role of a possible sentinel node biopsy technique is presently being investigated (49–51).

Variants of Tumors from Squamous Epithelium

A number of variants of tumors from squamous epithelium have been described, and pathologists still debate the relevance of these subgroups. As mentioned above, basaloid carcinoma is a variant of SCC and has a similar malignant behavior. In contrast, basal cell carcinoma is a skin tumor with a rather benign course, and the tumor is very rare in this location, but may histologically mimic SCC (2). Additionally, the benign keratoacanthoma—equally rare in this locale—can resemble SCC (52). Other rare tumors such as the mucoepidermoid carcinoma, SCC with mucinous microcysts, and small cell carcinoma (not to be confused with the neuroendocrine tumour bearing the same name!) all have a worse prognosis than ordinary SCC (43). The terms giant condyloma, verrucous carcinoma, and warty carcinoma all refer to variants of exophytic—often papillomatous—tumors of varying but low-grade malignancy. As the distinction between these subtypes may cause difficulties, and because these tumors occasionally contain components of standard SCC, a careful search by experienced pathologists for deep invasion and metastases is recommended in all cases (53).

Adenocarcinoma

Nearly all adenocarcinomas involving the anal canal have their origin in the colorectal zone and are identical with the common rectal adenocarcinomas. The very rare anal gland adenocarcinoma typically is located extramucosally, frequently leading to diagnostic delay. It is characterized by a different cytokeratin profile (54)—CK 20 negative/CK-7 positive (the reverse of colonic adenocarcinoma)—and typically has a poor prognosis (55). Malignant tumors from the perianal apocrine and mammary-like glands are extremely rare, but adenomas have been described (56).

Paget's Disease

Paget's disease can be found in the perianal region and up to the DL. It appears to represent at least two entities. Less than half are associated with a synchronous or metachronous malignancy, most often a colorectal adenocarcinoma, and the rest occur as isolated tumors. A distinction between the two types is therefore crucial. Immunohistochemical investigations have not given uniform results, but most cases with an underlying colorectal carcinoma show positive reactions for CK20 and gross cystic disease fluid protein-15 and negative reaction for CK7 (vide supra), while the others show the opposite pattern (57,58). Results from mucin investigations are conflicting. The histological diagnosis of Paget's disease is usually not difficult, but it must be kept in mind that pale intraepithelial cells may represent artifacts such as glycogen-rich cells, koilocytes, pagetoid dyskeratosis, pagetoid Bowen's disease, and pagetoid melanoma, in addition to spread of carcinoma cells (59). An example of the histological appearance of Paget's disease is shown with attendant cytokeratin immunohistochemistry in Figure 5.1.3.

Rare Tumors

One important reason for knowing about rare tumors is the fact that these can be mistaken for other conditions. Thus, malignant melanoma occasionally may look like a hemorrhoid and pigmented Bowen's disease may look similar to malignant melanoma (60). In anal melanoma, metastases are frequently present at the time of diagnosis and the five-year survival is less than 10% (61). Malignant lymphoma can present as a perianal abscess (62), and other typically extramucosal tumors, including gastrointestinal stromal tumor (GIST), neurofibroma, rhabdomyosarcoma, leiomyoma/sarcoma, granular cell tumor, and anorectal teratoma, may all present rarely in this region (63). This wide spectrum of mostly unsuspected neoplasms underlines the importance of histological examination of all anal lesions, no matter how benign their macroscopic appearance, along with the specialist requirement in these cases of a pathologist with particular experience and interest in the anorectal region.

Secondary Tumors

Metastases to the anal canal and perianal skin are extremely rare, but there are reports on tumors representing spread from carcinomas of the lung, breast, kidney, pancreas, and colon, as well as infiltrates in patients with malignant lymphoma, leukemia, and myeloma (2,62). Moreover, implantation metastases have been reported after endorectal stapling procedures (64) and rarely when there is a proximal carcinoma onto granulation tissue

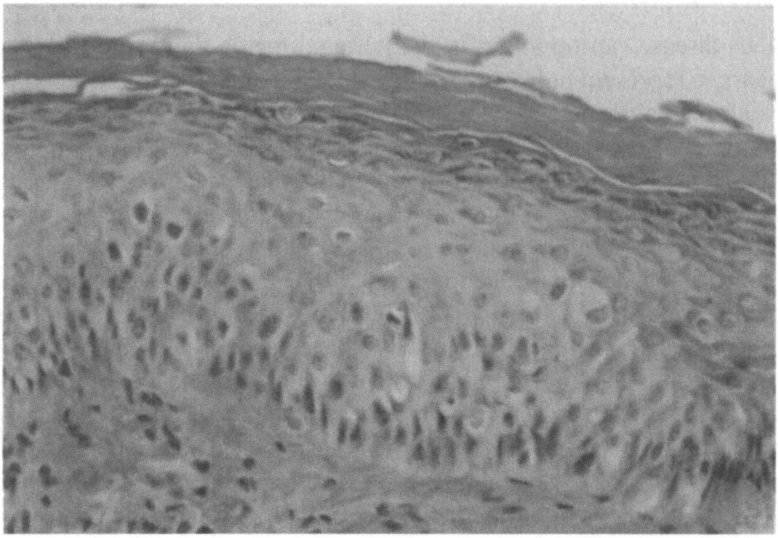
a

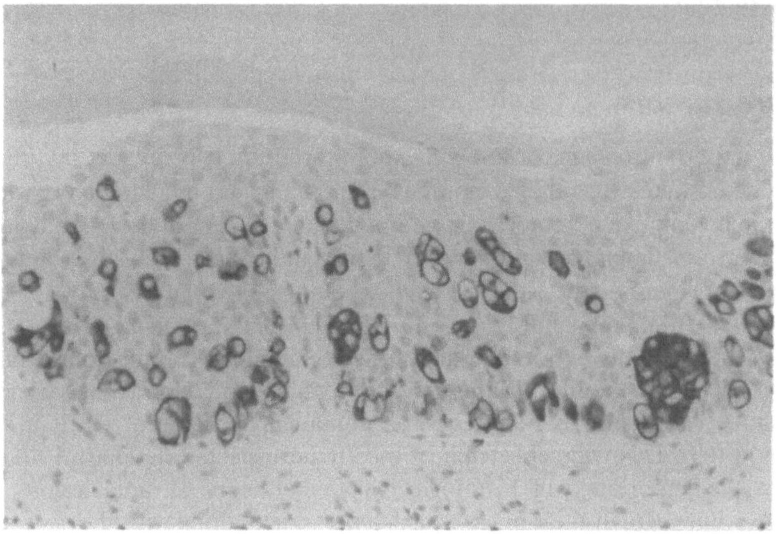
b

FIGURE 5.1.3. Paget's disease in perianal skin. (a) Clear cells scattered in keratinized squamous epithelium. H&E. (b) Paget cells stained with cytokeratin 7.

of preexisting long-standing fistulae-in-ano (65) (Figure 5.1.4). These tumors often are mucinous in type and may have a better overall prognosis that those developing as a malignant fistula transformation. The likelihood of this problem may be defined by the presence of detached carcinoma cells floating in mucinous lakes within fistula-in-ano biopsy material (66).

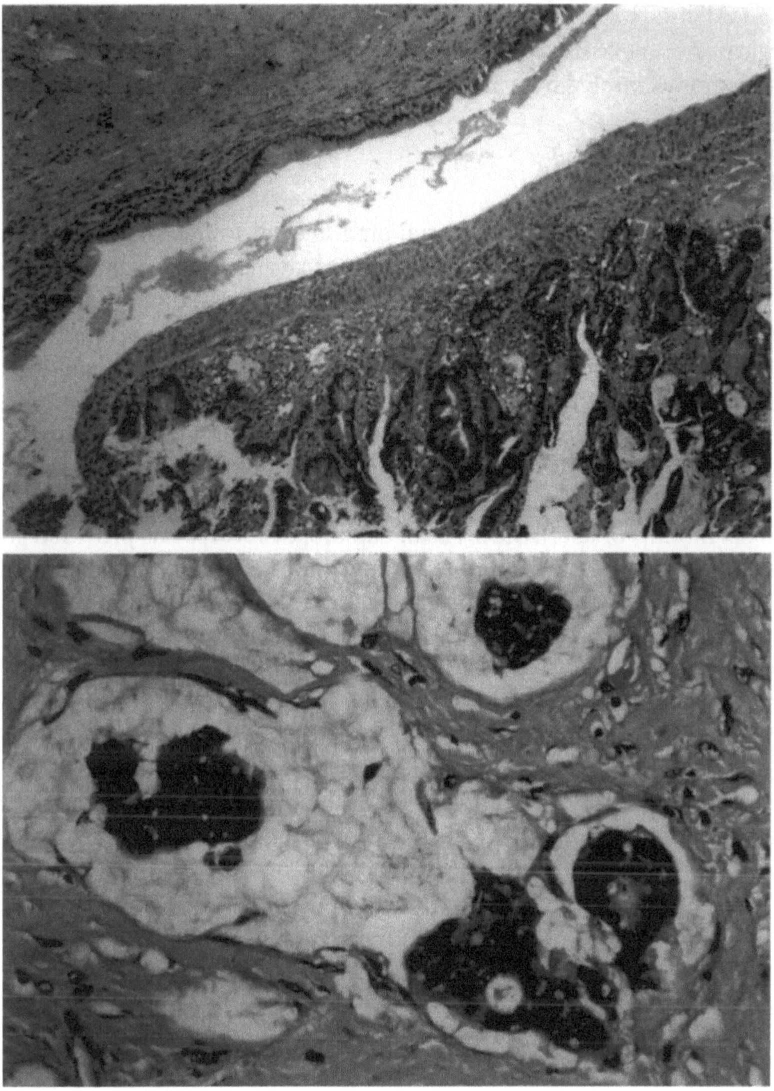

FIGURE 5.1.4. Section of an anal fistula track showing normal ductal epithelium (above) and infiltrating carinoma (below). The lower plate shows a high-power view of detached carcinoma cells floating within lakes of mucin. (Courtesy of Professor A.P. Zbar).

Handling the Surgical Specimen

Surgical specimens from the anal area include biopsies and local excisions, but nowadays rarely larger resections.

The Surgeon

Biopsies from the sensitive perianal area and up to the DL can be taken with a scalpel or scissors under local or general anesthesia. Mucosal lesions in the upper part of the anal canal can be biopsied with biopsy forceps, and it is often advisable to take several biopsies. Material from more deeply located processes can be obtained by needle biopsy or by ultrasound-guided fine needle aspiration.

In cases of suspected neurological disorders such as Hirschsprung's disease, it is necessary to investigate a larger part of the submucosa, and the use of large punch biopsies or suction biopsies is recommended. In children over six months of age, a Storz rectal cup biopsy forceps has provided good results (67). Irrespective of the technique, biopsies should be taken at several levels, as outlined above. In some children, an additional full-thickness rectal biopsy may be required for the correct diagnosis to be made.

Most material can be forwarded to the department of pathology fixed in neutral-buffered formalin, as this allows nearly all immunohistochemical and most of the more common molecular techniques to be performed accurately. Frozen sections for preoperative diagnosis are rarely necessary except for Hirschsprung's disease, but in the case of suspected lymphoma, biopsies should be forwarded fresh and by prompt transport. Any material should be followed by a request including a short history and clinical findings. In particular, a description of the exact location of the biopsy and the clinical macroscopic pathology is important. Small resections should be marked with a suture indicating the orientation of the specimen (e.g., at upper resection border) and should be pinned out on a small piece of cork or similar material in order to facilitate the judgment of resection lines.

The Pathologist

In the laboratory, it is most often possible to identify the smooth or wrinkled grayish squamous zone from the more glistening and slightly darker anal mucosa, even in small specimens. It is advisable to cut and embed the tissue along a longitudinal axis, as this allows a determination of the location and extent of the lesion with regard to the different mucosal zones of the anal canal. Small biopsies can be orientated with the use of a magnifying lamp. The pathologist's report should include a description of the location of the changes with regard to the different epithelial zones (as outlined), the histological character of the lesion, and, in cases of AIN, the lesional grade and possible signs of viral infection. Special attention should be paid to resection margins and signs of invasion.

It should be remembered that a correct diagnosis often rests on a combination of clinical and pathological observations, and that the therapeutic strategy therefore often is best determined by the surgeon and the pathologist in collaboration. Orientation and information by the surgeon for the histopathologist with specialist expertise in the anorectal area is necessary for the diagnosis and management of occasionally quite complex perirectal and perianal disorders.

References

1. Fenger C. Anal canal. In: Sternberg SS, editor. Histology for pathologists. 2nd ed. Philadelphia, PA: Lippincott-Raven; 1997. pp. 551–69.
2. Fenger C, Frisch M, Marti MC, and Parc R. Tumours of the anal canal. In: Hamilton SR and Aaltonen LA, editors. World Health Organization classification of tumours. Pathology and genetics of tumours of the digestive system. Lyon, France: IARC Press; 2000. pp. 146–55.
3. Fenger C. The anal transitional zone. Location and extent. Acta Pathol Microbiol Scand. 1979;87:379–386.
4. Thompson-Fawcett MW, Warren BF, and Mortensen NJ. A new look at the anal transitional zone with reference to restorative proctocolectomy and the columnar cuff. Br J Surg. 1998;85:1517–21.
5. McColl I. The comparative anatomy and pathology of anal glands. Ann R Coll Surg Engl. 1967;40:36–67.
6. van der Putte SCJ. Mammary-like glands of the vulva and their disorders. Int J Gynecol Pathol. 1994;13:150–60.
7. Sultan S, Azria F, Bauer P, Abdelnom M, and Atienza P. Anoperineal tuberculosis. Diagnostic and management considerations in seven cases. Dis Colon Rectum. 2002;45:405–10.
8. Chang J-W, Wu T-Z, Wang K-S, Huang I-F, Huang B, and Yu I-T. Colon mucosal pathology in infants under three months of age with diarrhea disorders. J Pediatr Gastroenterol Nutr. 2002;35:386–90.
9. Cohen SM, Schmitt SL, Lucas FY, and Wexner SD. The diagnosis of anal ulcers in AIDS patients. Int J Colorectal Dis. 1994;9:169–73.
10. Fenger C and Schrøder HD. Neuronal hyperplasia in the anal canal. Histopathology. 1990; 16:481–85.
11. Kaftan SM and Haboubi NY. Histopathological changes in haemorrhoid associated mucosa and submucosa. Int J Colorect Dis. 1995;10:15–18.
12. Fenger C and Nielsen VT. Dysplastic changes in the anal canal epithelium in minor surgical specimens. Acta Path Microbiol Scand Sect A. 1981;89:463–65.
13. Nelson RL, Abcarian H, Davis FG, Persky Y. Prevalence of benign anorectal disease in a randomly selected population. Dis Colon Rect. 1995;38:341–44.
14. Ravindranauth NS, Borkowski J, and Broaddus R. Metastatic renal cell carcinoma presenting as a hemorrhoid. Arch Pathol Lab Med. 2002;126:856–58.

15. Wienert Y, Albrecht O, and Gablen W. Haufigkeitsanalytische ergebnisse uber marisken [Results of incidence analyses in fibrous polyps]. Der Hautartz. 1978;29:536–40.
16. Gupta PJ and Kalaskar S. Removal of hypertrophied anal papillae and fibrous anal polyps increases patient satisfaction after anal fissure surgery. Tech Coloproctol. 2003;7:155–8.
17. Groisman GM and Polak-Charcon S. Fibroepithelial polyps of the anus. A histologic, immunohistochemical, and ultrastructural study, including comparison with the normal anal subepithelial layer. Am J Surg Pathol. 1998;22: 70–6.
18. Tsang P and Rotterdam H. Biopsy diagnosis of colitis: possibilities and pitfalls. Am J Surg Pathol. 1999;23:423–30.
19. Rex DK, Alikhan M, Cummings O, and Ulbright TM. Accuracy of pathological interpretation of colorectal polyps by general pathologists in community practice. Gastrointest Endosc. 1999;50:468–74.
20. Godbole P, Botterill I, Newell SJ, Sagar PM, and Stringer MD. Solitary rectal ulcer in children. J R Coll Surg Edinb. 2000;45:411–14.
21. Kang YS, Kamm MA, Engel AF, and Talbot IC. Pathology of the rectal wall in solitary rectal ulcer syndrome and complete rectal prolapse. Gut. 1996;38:587–90.
22. Tendler DA, Aboudola S, Zacks JF, O'Brien MJ, and Kelly CP. Prolapsing mucosal polyps: an under-recognized form of colonic polyp—a clinicopathological study of 15 cases. Am J Gastroenterol. 2002;97:370–6.
23. Li SC and Hamilton SR. Malignant tumors in the rectum simulating solitary rectal ulcer syndrome in endoscopic biopsy specimens. Am J Surg Pathol. 1998;22:106–12.
24. Jaworski RC, Biankin SA, and Baird PJ. Squamous cell carcinoma in situ arising in inflammatory cloacogenic polyps: report of two cases with PCR analysis for H PY DNA. Pathology. 2001;33:312–4.
25. Newgreen D and Young HM. Enteric nervous system: development and developmental disturbances—part 1. Pediatr Dev Pathol. 2002;5:224–47.
26. Newgreen D and Young HM. Enteric nervous system: development and developmental disturbances—part 2. Pediatr Dev Pathol. 2002;5:329–49.
27. Hofstra RMW, Osinga J, and Buys CHCM. Mutations in Hirschsprung disease: when does a mutation contribute to the phenotype. Eur J Hum Genet. 1997;5:180–5.
28. Fu CG, Muto T, Masaki T, and Nagawa H. Zonal adult Hirschsprung's disease. Gut. 1996;39:765–7.
29. Moore BG, Singiram C, Eckhoff DE, Gaumnitz EA, and Starling JR. Immunohistochemical evaluations of ultrashort-segment Hirschsprung disease. Dis Colon Rectum. 1996;39:817–22.
30. Qualman SJ, Jaffe R, Bove KE, and Monforte-Munoz H. Diagnosis of Hirschsprung disease using the rectal biopsy: multi-institutional survey. Pediatr Dev Pathol. 1999;2:588–96.
31. Koletzko S, Jesch I, Faus-Kessler T, et al. Rectal biopsy for diagnosis of intestinal neuronal dysplasia in children: a prospective multicentre study on interobserver variation and clinical outcome. Gut. 1999;44:853–61.
32. Gillick J, Tazawa H, and Puri P. Intestinal neuronal dysplasia: results of treatment in 33 patients. J Pediatr Surg. 2001;36:777–9.

33. Chang GJ, Berry MJ, Jay N, Palfsky JM, and Welton ML. Surgical treatment of high-grade anal squamous intraepithelial lesions. A prospective study. Dis Colon Rectum. 2002;45:453–8.
34. Jay N, Berry JM, Hogeboom CJ, Holly EA, Darragh TM, and Palefsky JM. Colposcopic appearance of anal squamous intraepithelial lesions. Relationship to histopathology. Dis Colon Rectum. 1997;40:919–28.
35. Zbar AP, Fenger C, Efron J, Wexner SD, and Beer-Gabel M. The pathology and molecular biology of anal intraepithelial neoplasia: comparisons with cervical and vulvar intraepithelial carcinoma. Int J Colorectal Dis. 2002;17:203–15.
36. Sobhani I, Vuagnat A, Walker F, Vissuzaine C, Mirin B, Hervatin F, Marmuse JP, Cremieux AC, Carbon C, Henin D, Lehy T, and Mignon M. Prevalence of high-grade dysplasia and cancer in the anal canal in human papilloma-virus infected individuals. Gastroenterology. 2001;120:857–66.
37. Carter PS, Sheffield JP, Shepherd N, et al. Interobserver variation in the reporting of the histopathological grading of anal intraepithelial neoplasia. J Clin Pathol. 1994;47:1032–4.
38. Byars RW, Poole GV, and Barber WH. Anal carcinoma arising from condyloma acuminata. Am Surg. 2001;67:469–72.
39. Mullerat J, Wong Te Fong LF, Davies SE, Winslet MC, Perrett CW. Angiogenesis in anal warts, anal intraepithelial neoplasia and anal squamous cell carcinoma. Colorectal Dis. 2003;5:353–7.
40. Sobhani I, Vuagnat A, Walker F, et al. Prevalence of high-grade dysplasia and cancer in the anal canal in Human Papillomavirus-Infected individuals. Gastroenterol. 2001;120:857–66.
41. Manzione CR, Nadal SR, and Calore EE. Postoperative follow-up of anal condylomata acuminata in HIV-positive patients. Dis Colon Rectum. 2003; 46:1358–65.
42. Fenger C, Frisch M, Jass JJ, Williams GT, and Hilden J. Anal cancer subtype reproducibility study. Virchows Arch. 2000;436:229–33.
43. Shepherd NA, Scholefield JH, Love SB, England J, and Northover JMA. Prognostic factors in anal squamous carcinoma: a multivariate analysis of clinical, pathological and flow cytometric parameters in 235 cases. Histopathology. 1990;16:545–55.
44. Frisch M, Fenger C, van den Brule AJC, et al. Variants of squamous cell carcinoma of the anal canal and perianal skin and their relation to human papillomaviruses. Cancer Res. 1999;59:753–7.
45. Frisch M. On the etiology of anal squamous carcinoma. Laegeforeningens Forlag. 2002;5–21.
46. Bjørge T, Engeland A, Luostarinen T, et al. Human papillomavirus infection as a risk factor for anal and perianal skin cancer in a prospective study. Br J Cancer. 2002;87:61–4.
47. Remzi FH, Fazio VW, Delaney CP, et al. Dysplasia of the anal transitional zone after ileal pouch-anal anastomosis. Results of prospective evaluation after a minimum of ten years. Dis Colon Rectum. 2003;46:6–13.
48. Fenger C. Prognostic factors in anal carcinoma. Pathology. 2002;34:573–8.
49. Keshtgar MRS, Amin A, Taylor I, and Ell PJ. The sentinel node in anal carcinoma. Euro J Surg Oncol. 2001;27:113–22.
50. Mistrangelo M, Mobiglia A, Mussa B, et al. The sentinel node in anal carcinoma. Tumori. 2002;88:S51–2.

51. Rabbitt P, Pathma-Nathan N, Collinson T, Hewett P, and Rieger N. Sentinel lymph node biopsy for squamous cell carcinoma of the anal canal. ANZ J Surg. 2002;72:651–4.
52. Kuppers F, Jongen J, Bock J-U, and Rabenhorst G. Keratoacanthoma in the differential diagnosis of anal carcinoma: difficult diagnosis, easy therapy. Report of three cases. Dis Colon Rectum. 2000;43:427–9.
53. Trombetta LJ and Place RJ. Giant condyloma acuminatum of the anorectum: trends in epidemiology and management. Report of a case and review of the literature. Dis Colon Rectum. 2001;44:1878–86.
54. Hobbs CM, Lowry MA, Owen D, and Sobin LH. Anal gland carcinoma. Cancer. 2001;92:2045–9.
55. Li SC, Waters BL, Simmonds-Arnold L, and Beatty BG. Cytokeratin 7 and 20 expressions in rectal adenomas, rectal adenocarcinomas, anal glands and functional rectal mucosa. Mod Pathol. 2001;14:90A.
56. Donati P and Amantea A. Adenoma of anogenital mammary-like glands. Am J Dermatopathol. 1996;18:73–6.
57. Nowak MA, Guierrere-Kovach P, Pathan A, Campbelle TE, and Deppisch LM. Perianal Paget's disease. Distinguishing primary and secondary lesions using immunohistochemical studies including gross cystic disease fluid protein-15 and cytokeratin 20 expression. Arch Pathol Lab Med. 1998;122:1077–81.
58. Ohnishi T and Watanabe S. The use of cytokeratins 7 and 20 in the diagnosis of primary and secondary extrammary Paget's disease. Br J Dermatol. 2000;142: 243–7.
59. Val-Bernal JF and Pinto J. Pagetoid dyskeratosis is a frequent finding in hemorrhoidal disease. Arch Pathol Lab Med. 2001:125:1058–62.
60. Krishnan R, Lewis A, Orengo IF, and Rosen T. Pigmented Bowen's disease (Squamous carcinoma in situ): a mimic of malignant melanoma. Dermatol Surg. 2001;27:673–4.
61. Cooper P, Mills SE, and Allen M. Malignant melanoma of the anus: report of 12 patients and analysis of 255 additional cases. Dis Colon Rectum. 1982;25: 693–703.
62. Bhama JK, Azad NS, and Fisher WE. Primary anorectal lymphoma presenting as a perianal abscess in an HIV-positive male. Eur J Surg Oncol. 2002;28:195–7.
63. Tan GY, Chong CK, Eu KW, and Tan PH. Gastrointestinal stromal tumor of the anus. Tech Coloproctol. 2003;7:169–72.
64. Norgren J and Svensson JO. Anal implantation metastasis from carcinoma of the sigmoid colon and rectum: a risk when performing anterior resection with the EEA stapler? Br J Surg. 1985;75:602.
65. Hyman N and Kida M. Adenocarcinoma of the sigmoid colon seeding a chronic anal fistula. Report of a case. Dis Colon Rectum. 2003;46:835–6.
66. Onerheim RM. A case of perianal mucinous adenocarcinoma arising in a fistula-in-ano. A clue to the early pathologic diagnosis. Am J Clin Pathol. 1988;89: 809–12.
67. Alizai NK, Batcup G, Dixon MF, Stringer MD. Rectal biopsy for Hirschprung's disease: what is the optimum method? Pediatr Surg Int. 1998;13:121–4.

Chapter 5.2
Anal Intraepithelial Neoplasia (AIN)

John H. Scholefield

Introduction

Squamous cell carcinoma (SCC) of the anus is the most common histological type of anal carcinoma, comprising over 80% of all anal cancers. They may arise from the perianal skin or from the anal canal itself, the other primary anal malignancies include anal gland adenocarcinoma, melanoma, and lymphoma (1). The variety of nomenclature used to describe histological subtypes of anal SCC reflects two facts: firstly, the changing epithelium of the anal region from the keratinized hair-bearing epithelium of the perianal skin through the modified squamous epithelium to the anal transition zone and rectal mucosa above, and secondly, the inconsistent use of a number of terms such as cloacogenic (2) and epidermoid (3) to refer to particular histological subtypes of anal SCC thought to arise from the transitional epithelium of the anal canal.

The term anal intraepithelial neoplasia (AIN) was first used by Fenger (1978) to describe the histological features of dysplasia in squamous epithelium (4). Some ten years later, when the etiology of anal squamous cancer was shown to be etiologically linked with human papillomavirus type 16 (HPV 16), the potential parallels between AIN, cervical intraepithelial neoplasia (CIN), and vulvar intraepithelial neoplasia (VIN) became apparent and colposcopic techniques were applied to the anal epithelium to determine whether gynecological diagnostic principles could be applied to the anus. The identification of dysplastic anal lesions colposcopically (5) led to the suspicion that there may be a number of "at-risk" groups for AIN. Further work identified women with previous genital intraepithelial and those individuals who were systemically immunosuppressed as being at increased risk for AIN (6). Despite the identification of "at-risk" groups, the natural history of the condition remains uncertain. The following account presents the development of our present state of knowledge about the etiology, pathogenesis and diagnosis of AIN, its relationship to CIN and VIN, the treatment options available, and some of the difficulties that arise in managing these patients. The role of cytology and "colposcopy" as it applies to advanced proctological practice is outlined.

Anatomy of the Anus

The anal canal is the most caudal part of the gastrointestinal tract; it is a short muscular tube about three centimeters in length situated between the rectum and perianal skin. Its boundaries are poorly defined; the upper border generally is quoted as the puborectalis sling, and the lower border is less well defined and merges with the perianal skin. The pectenate line lies between these areas and represents the fusion of the lower two-thirds of the anal canal (ectodermal in origin) and the upper one-third (endodermal in origin). The anal canal shares a common embryological origin with the endocervical canal from the proctodeum. The primary function of the anus is that of preserving continence, and to this end, the anal sphincter mechanisms are of great importance.

In the perianal skin, the epithelium is keratinized, hair-bearing squamous epithelium. In the lower anal canal, the keratinization is lost and the epithelium becomes thinner; further up the canal, at about the level of the pectenate line, the epithelium becomes transitional (cuboidal) and subsequently columnar (rectal epithelium).

The boundaries of the anal region are poorly defined, leading to confusion in the classification of anal tumors described by different authors. Despite discrepancies in definition, it is apparent that anal canal carcinoma is nearly three times more common than cancer of the anal margin in the population of England and Wales (7). The age distribution is the same for both canal and margin cancers (average 57 years), but anal canal cancers are said to be more common in women than in men (3:2), whereas anal margin cancers are more common in men (4:1) (1).

Pathological Features of AIN (See Chapter 5.1)

Histologically, AIN is characterized by a loss of epithelial cellular maturation with associated nuclear hyperchromasia, pleomorphism, cellular crowding, and abnormal mitoses within the anal epithelium. These features are identical to those of similar cervical and vulval lesions, and AIN lesions are classified according to the nomenclature used for genital intraepithelial neoplasia (8). Thus, in AIN I, cellular and nuclear abnormalities are restricted to the lower third of the epithelium; in AIN II and AIN III, the lower two-thirds and the full thickness of the epithelium, respectively, are affected. The histological features of AIN III are consistent with it being the precursor lesion of invasive squamous cancer, although this progression is not as certain as that evident with the cervix. Anal intraepithelial neoplasia III is synonymous with carcinoma in situ of the anus—sometimes termed Bowen's disease when applied to the perianal skin. Microinvasive carcinoma of the anus has been described and parallels similar lesions described on the cervix (i.e., a lesions in which the basement membrane has been breached by dysplastic epithelial cells). Careful orientation of the specimen in processing and examination must be enforced to avoid sections containing obliquely cut tissue, which can easily be misinterpreted as invasive. While the term AIN is used in most of the European literature on this subject, the terms used in the United States are slightly different. Thus, American authors describe HiSIL (or HSIL) and LoSil (or LSIL) (high-grade and low-grade squamous intraepithelial lesions). These are analogous to AIN III and AINI/II, respectively.

Natural History and Epidemiology of AIN

Anal intraepithelial neoplasia is a relatively recently described phenomenon, and at present, its natural history is unknown. In cervical cancer, rates of progression are well documented, but such data is lacking for anal dysplasia. Etiological parallels with CIN and the histological appearances of AIN III suggest that AIN III may have malignant potential (9–11). The molecular biological changes occurring with AIN and its comparison with CIN and VIN (vulvar intraepithelial neoplasia) are briefly outlined in Chapter 5.1 and covered in a recent review article by Zbar et al. (12) There also have been case reports of malignant change in anal condylomata (13–15). In the original report of Fenger and Nielsen (16), AIN was found incidentally in 19 patients undergoing minor anal surgery; 17 of these patients were alive five years after initial diagnosis, and none developed invasive disease. Nine of the lesions were graded as AIN III and were treated by local excision (4 lesions recurred). Foust et al. (17) reported 19 cases of AIN III in the anal canal mucosa of routinely excised hemorroidal tissue. In a mean follow-up period of 6 years, only one patient developed recurrent disease and none developed invasive disease. These reports suggest that incidentally discovered AIN III is a non-aggressive lesion. However, Fenger and Nielsen (18) also have reported the presence of AIN III in 81% (13 of 16) of cases of anal squamous carcinoma assessing abdominoperineal resection specimens. The lesions were found to be situated at the border of the invasive lesions, as well as in areas separated from the tumors by normal mucosa.

In the Sheffield series, 32 patients with AIN III, including nine anal cancers in a field change of AIN III, were identified (6,19,20). Of these, 5 (15.5%) developed invasive anal disease within a median follow-up period of 18 months (range 0.5 to 2 years). This strongly suggests that AIN, particularly AIN III, has malignant potential. This series of cases, however, was drawn from a unit with a reputation for its aggressive surgical approach to genital intraepithelial disease and may not represent the generality of AIN. The authors' subsequent experience in Nottingham is that only 2 of 26 patients with AIN III have progressed to invasive anal cancer over an 8-year period. It is the author's view that the latter series is more likely to represent the natural history of this condition. A figure of 10% progression for VIN III to invasive cancer is widely quoted, and it is the authors' impression that a similar progression rate for AIN III is likely. Nevertheless, more prospective cohort evidence is required to determine the proportion of AIN III lesions that progress to invasive disease or which indeed regress; the latter phenomenon having been quoted at about 5 percent (21).

Even less is known of the fate of low-grade AIN lesions (AIN I and II); however, Palefsky et al. (22) observed that progression of low-grade lesions to high-grade AIN lesions occurred in 6 out of 37 homosexual men with human immunodeficiency virus (HIV) disease over an average follow-up period to 17 months. However, these patients were immunosuppressed and the natural history of the condition may have been accelerated. In the same series, it was observed that 10.8% of low-grade lesions regressed, and in the Sheffield series, regression of low-grade lesions was observed in 13% (3 of 23) of cases over a median follow-up period of 7 months. There is an urgent need for longitudinal studies to determine the rates of progression to high-grade disease in the various risk groups. In this respect, it is unknown whether an "altered immunology" may be responsible either for progression (or regression) of AIN quite independently of HPV persistence or eradication. The immune responses in HIV-related AIN are complex and more studies are required to assess impaired lymphocytotoxic responsiveness in vitro to HPV-related transforming proteins such as E6 and E7 (23). The epidemiologic increase in anal cancer appears to predate the AIDS epidemic where immunosuppressed patients with AIN appear to have more progressive disease with higher chemotherapy-related morbidity and mortality. The impact of highly active antiretroviral therapy (HAART) on this immune effect is unclear, although there is evidence to suggest that high-grade lesions, once established, do not regress during treatment (24).

Invasive anal cancer is at present an uncommon malignancy in which only approximately 400 cases are registered in England and Wales each year, where it is five times less common than cervical cancer (7,25). This would suggest that the risk of progression from intraepithelial neoplasia to invasive cancer is lower for the anus than for the cervix. However, balanced against this, there is some evidence that the incidence of AIN is increasing. Wexner et al. (26) showed that the incidence of AIN and anal cancer, particularly in the anal canal, is rising, where, in this study, a three-fold increase in the incidence of anal cancers in both sexes between 1959 and 1986 was observed. This is supported by further data from the United States and Scandinavia, and this may be due in part to the increasing prevalence of anogenital HPV infections (27). If the natural history of AIN is similar to that of CIN (and there are clinical assumptions here that are yet unproven), then the development of anal cancer may occur several years after the diagnosis of AIN. This may account for the fact that although homosexual men with HIV are at increased risk of AIN, the incidence of anal cancer in this group, although increasing, is still relatively low. As stated above, the introduction of HAART will affect the overall prognosis, as well as the incidence, of recognizable invasive anal carcinoma and its complications.

Although there has been an increase in anogenital HPV infections in the UK, Office of Population Censuses and Surveys (OPCS) data do not show a similar increase in the incidence of anal cancer, as has been demonstrated in the United States and in Scandinavia (28–30). This is most likely due to under-registration resulting from difficulties in the classification of squamous anal canal cancers—where tumors have been variously classified as cloacogenic, basaloid, and epidermoid—and where anal cancers often are misclassified as rectal tumors, whereas anal margin and perianal tumors typically have been classified as skin tumors (18).

The Prevalence of AIN

The true prevalence of AIN is unknown. Although it initially was thought that AIN was a rare condition, the frequency of occurrence of unrecognized intraepithelial neoplasia encountered during minor surgery of the anal canal was reported as between 0.2% and 4.4% (16,31,32). However, in groups thought to be at risk—homosexual men who practice receptive anal intercourse, immunosuppressed HIV-positive individuals, renal allograft recipients, women with high-grade genital intraepithelial and invasive squamous neoplasia, and individuals of both sexes with anogenital condylomata—the prevalence of AIN is much higher. In these groups, the prevalence has been reported as between 15% to 53% in immunosuppressed HIV-positive individuals, 19% to 47% in women with high-grade genital intraepithelial or invasive neoplasia, and 24% in renal allograft recipients (22,33–38). In contrast, the prevalence of AIN in control populations is very low, being reported as less than 1%.

Etiology and Pathogenesis of AIN

Human papillomavirus 16 has been increasingly implicated as an etiological factor throughout the range of anogenital squamous cell carcinomas (SCCs). Human papillomavirus 16 is one of several sexually transmissible papillomavirus types (other common types are 6, 11, 18, and 31) associated with a spectrum of lesions from subclinical infection through condylomata to intraepithelial neoplasia and ultimately (and almost certainly involving co-carcinogens) to invasive SCC. Human papillomavirus 16 has been identified in 56% to 80% cases of SCC of the anus, and AIN lesions

(5,19,20,34,35,39,40). Anal intraepithelial neoplasia III lesions appear to contain HPV 16 more frequently than lower grades of AIN, with a similar relationship existing in cervical and vulval disease. A number of studies in gynecological and genitourinary medicine have shown that once one area of the anogenital epithelium becomes infected by human papillomaviruses, the adjacent areas become infected by direct spread of the papillomavirus, creating a large potential field of epithelium susceptible to neoplastic change (41). In many of these cases, however, the papillomavirus infection may be asymptomatic and only detectable by colposcopic examination or cytological sampling. Epidemiological studies of sexually transmissible papillomavirus infection in Scandinavia have suggested that up to 70% of the sexually active adult population have at some time encountered genital HPV infection, and that the vast majority of these infections are completely asymptomatic (42). Although it is cited frequently that anal intercourse is a prerequisite in the pathogenesis of anal condylomata or AIN or anal SCC, this concept is essentially unfounded in the heterosexual population.

Despite the strong causal relationship between HPV and anogenital neoplasia, it is unlikely that HPV on its own is sufficient for the production and maintenance of the neoplastic state. It is possible that HPV acts in a synergistic fashion with other factors, including viruses such as HIV, herpes simplex virus 2 (HSV-2), Epstein-Barr virus (EBV), and cytomegalovirus (CMV). Herpes simplex virus 2 has long been suggested as a co-factor in the etiology of cervical cancer (43), and among individuals without genital warts, a history of seropositivity for HSV-2 has been found to be associated with anal cancer. In the only such published study to date, Palefsky et al. (44), using the polymerase chain reaction, detected HSV-2 deoxyribonucleic acid (DNA) in anal cancer tissues of five of 13 patients and three of four patients with AIN III. This association between HSV-2 DNA detection and high-grade anal disease suggests that HSV-2 infection could play a role in the pathogenesis of AIN and anal cancer. Although EBV and CMV have been detected in cervical epithelium (normal and neoplastic), similar data on anal neoplasia have yet to be reported. With regard to the relationship between HIV and HPV, a number of reports suggest that HIV infection increases the risk of HPV infection and HPV related anogenital neoplasia (34,36,38). However, in a recent study, Surawicz et al. (45) observed no differences in the prevalence of anal HPV infection and AIN in immunosuppressed HIV-positive men compared with immunocompetent HIV-negative men.

Other factors that may be involved in the pathogenesis of anogenital neoplasia in general and anal neoplasia in particular include smoking and the interaction between HPV, oncogenes, and tumor-suppressor genes. As in the cervix, recent epidemiological studies have shown a significant increase in the risk of anal neoplasia related to heavy or prolonged smoking (34,46,47); however, the nature of this predisposition is unknown. Furthermore, there have been numerous reports on the possible interactions of HPV with the p53 tumor-suppressor gene, as well as the c-myc oncogene in the pathogenesis of anogenital neoplasia (48–51). Some of these reports suggest that the expression of the products of these genes may act as prognostic indicators of disease progression (52,53). This issue is complex, for example, in the relationship between the oncogene c-myc and AIN. It is expected that proto-oncogenic growth factors are required for the development of invasive anogenital malignancy, but the c-myc oncogene product, which is over expressed in CIN and which is partially integrated with HPV gene sequences close to its locus in some cervical cancer lines, does not appear to play a major role in AIN progression (54). This is despite in vitro studies showing higher c-myc expression in HPV 16-transformed cell lines and differentiation resistance in HPV-immortalized keratinocytes over-expressing c-myc protein and c-myc gene sequences (55).

The association between neoplasia and systemic immunosuppression is well established. Studies based primarily on organ-transplant recipients have demonstrated an overall 5% to 6% risk of developing a neoplasm after transplantation (56–58). These tumors—lymphoid system, skin, urogenital and anogenital tracts—are etiologically associated with oncogenic viruses, therefore non-Hodgkin's lymphoma with EBV, squamous tumors of the skin and anogenital tracts with HPV, and primary liver cancer with the Hepatitis B virus. Although the nature of this predisposition is unknown, immunosuppression in this group may reduce immunosurveillance by the lymphorcticular system (59). Reports from Cancer Registry data and controlled studies suggest that transplant patients show a four- to 14-fold increase in the incidence and prevalence of HPV-associated high-grade intraepithelial and invasive tumors of the cervix (57,58,60,61). Registry data also suggest a similar increase for the prevalence of invasive anal and vulval neoplasia. A prevalence rate of 24% (32 of 133) for anal HPV infection and associated AIN in renal transplant recipients has been reported (19,20). Of these, 18% (6 of 32) of patients had prior or synchronous high-grade intraepithelial or invasive genital lesions. Furthermore, a number of published reports on the prevalence of AIN in immunosuppressed HIV-positive patients also have demonstrated that a high prevalence of anal HPV infection and AIN is related to the degree of immunosuppression as determined by T-helper/T-suppressor cell ratios (34,35–38,62).

Systemic immunosuppression, however, does not appear to be a prerequisite for the development of multifocal HPV-associated neoplasia. In clinical studies on apparently immunocompetent women who had high-grade cervical or vulvar intraepithelial neoplasia or invasive vulval cancer, prevalence rates of 20%, 19%, and 47%, respectively, for AIN were reported (6,20). It is possible that HPV infection of the anogenital area causes changes in the local cellular immunity that facilitate progression to neoplastic change. Some evidence for this is available from a few studies on the cervix, which have shown a reduction in local T-lymphocyte subset numbers and activity in women with CIN (63,64). In immunocompetent homosexual men—in whom prevalence rates for AIN of up to 8% have been reported—it has been suggested that there may be subclinical immunosuppression, possibly due to the local immunosuppressive effects of seminal fluid, known to be rich in prostaglandins capabale of enhancing tumor promotion (34,65,66). Such immunosuppression might make homosexual men more susceptible to the development of anal HPV infection and neoplasia. Although this hypothesis may have some validity, it is equally possible that, since some homosexual men engage in large numbers of sexual encounters, they are at high risk of developing sexually transmitted diseases such as syphilis and HIV, which also may permit de novo infection or reactivation of dormant anal HPV infection. The epithelial abnormalities that subsequently occur may represent a consequence of actively replicating HPV with independent contributions from local or systemic immunosuppression, smoking, and other co-factors (67).

Diagnostic Techniques for AIN

The diagnostic techniques that may be used to identify AIN include histopathology, cytopathology, and "colposcopy."

Histopathology remains the "gold standard" of diagnosis, but obtaining material for histopathological examination is invasive and uncomfortable for the patient, as biopsy of the anal canal and perianal area can only be performed under anesthesia. The histopathological features of AIN have already been described above and are generally robust (68) (see Chapter 5.1).

Cytopathological examination is minimally invasive, requires no anesthesia, and is capable of repeatedly sampling a large area. Until recently, the application of this technique to the anus has yielded rather inconsistent results. Colposcopic examination of the anus is more invasive than cytopathology, although it does not require anesthesia and it can examine the entire anal canal. Anal colposcopy has a definite learning curve and requires considerable experience. Any abnormal areas must be biopsied for histopathological examination to confirm the diagnosis. Anal colposcopy has been used extensively in our practice to identify anal dysplastic lesions (69).

Cytology

The increasing clinical awareness of AIN and its association with genital intraepithelial neoplasia has provided an impetus for the development of a simple method of examining the malignant potential of the anal epithelium.

Anal cytology offers two main advantages over anal colposcopy—specimen collection is simple and sampling from a large area is possible. As such, a cytological test could play a major role in screening patients in high-risk groups for anal dysplasia.

Several studies have used anal cytology for the diagnosis of anal dysplasia. These studies reported a number of technical difficulties in obtaining adequate samples from the anus. Inadequate specimens were encountered in 15% to 30% of samples in published studies (70); however, there is a general trend in the manner of collection of anal cytological specimens that is producing results that are more consistent. Most early studies tried to sample the entire anal canal in every cytological preparation, and it was believed that, unless transitional type cells could be identified, the preparation should be labeled as inadequate. However, trying to sample the whole anal canal and anal transitional zone is uncomfortable for the patient, as no lubricant can be used on the collection device—as this reduces cell yield dramatically—and fecal contamination of the preparation is almost inevitable. Because the vast majority of anal intraepithelial lesions occur on or near the anal vergc—whcrc AIN rarely involves the anal transitional zone in the absence of perianal skin involvement—sampling the perianal area is appropriate in most cases (Figure 5.2.1). This area is also easily accessed, reduces fecal contamination, and cell collection does not cause discomfort to the patient. In the author's opinion, it is inappropriate to insist on sampling the anal transitional zone, particularly as attempting this greatly increases the likelihood of severe fecal contamination of the specimen, thus rendering adequate cytopathological examination impossible. The use of guidelines to provide a framework for the reporting of anal cytological has provided a sound basis for the interpretation of anal cytological

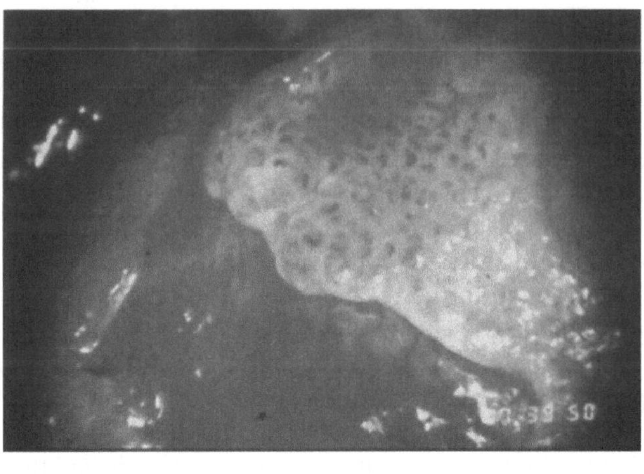

FIGURE 5.2.1. Cytological appearances of the normal anal canal.

preparations with consistent results among experienced cytopathologists (69). Further developments along these lines may make anal cytology a useful test in both the diagnosis and follow-up of patients "at risk" for anal dysplasia.

The technique of preparation of anal cytological smears is similar to that used for the cervix and vulva, and it is quick and easy to perform after initial instruction. The author's preferred technique is to use a small cotton swab moistened in 0.9% saline and then rubbed firmly against the perianal skin for 20 to 30 seconds, sampling a wide area of the perianal skin. The collected cells then are transferred to a labeled glass microscope slide and either air-dried of fixed according to the local cytopathologist's preference. If the cotton swab appears to be fecally contaminated, a second swab should be taken after wiping the perianal area to reduce the fecal load as much as possible.

It seems likely that the use of anal cytology probably will reduce the need for anal colposcopy, which has proved unpopular with both gynecologists and surgeons alike.

Anal Colposcopy Technique

In the author's practice, patients usually are examined in a modified lithotomy position, as this permits examination of the whole anogenital area without having to change the patient's position. Genital colposcopy usually is performed prior to anal colposcopy—genital colposcopy for female patients is an essential part of the assessment of these patients, but does not necessarily need to be a part of the anal colposcopy procedure. Colorectal surgeons using colposcopy should be familiar with genital colposcopy, and the classical saline and topical acetic acid techniques in anal colposcopy use essentially the same techniques. A combined clinic with a gynecological colposcopist is a good way of developing the necessary colposcopic skills.

Anal colposcopic examination as performed in the lithotomy position begins by parting the buttocks to examine the perianal skin. Firm traction on the perianal skin also permits examination of the lower anal canal. In general, relatively low magnification is required (6× is adequate). It is useful to begin anal colposcopy by examination of the perianal skin and lower anal canal before the application of 5% aqueous acetic acid. The perianal skin then is covered with swabs or cotton wool balls soaked in acetic acid for three minutes prior to further examination. Then the anal canal is examined using an oblique viewing Graham Anderson proctoscope, before and after application of aqueous acetic acid spray. Using this instrument, views of the upper anal canal, the transition zone, and the lower rectal mucosa are readily obtained. Spraying the anal canal with acetic acid is adequate, as the epithelium in the anal canal is less heavily keratinized than the perianal skin and therefore responds rapidly to the acetic acid spray.

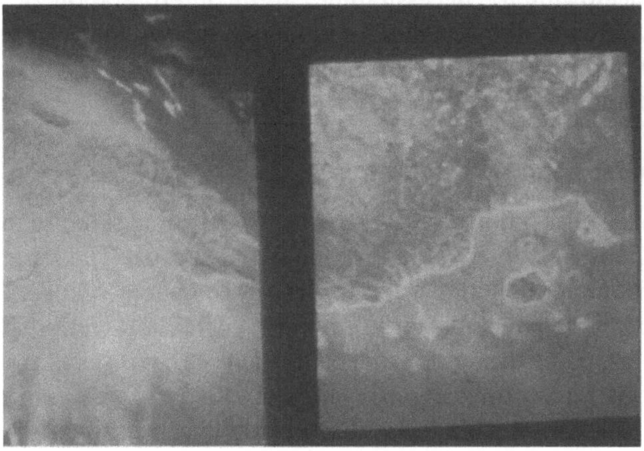

FIGURE 5.2.2. Colposcopic appearance of the normal cervical (left) and anal (right) transition zones after topical application of acetic acid.

The appearance of the anal transition zone is similar to that of the cervical transformation zone in its natural state and takes on a pearly appearance when sprayed with acetic acid. Gland openings in the anal transition zone are analogous to those seen in the cervix (Figure 5.2.2).

Colposcopic Identification of AIN

The clinical diagnosis of AIN using colposcopy is still evolving. The range of abnormalities that may occur includes papillomavirus-associated lesions occurring throughout the anal area, paralleling those seen in the cervix and vulva (5,6,69).

Normal Colposcopic Appearances of the Perianal Skin and Anal Canal

Since the boundaries of the anal canal and perianal epithelium are clinically and histologically poorly defined, these terms are used in their broadest sense, where the perianal skin is that which can readily be seen on parting the buttocks. The anal canal epithelium is that epithelium above this level and is limited above by the rectal epithelium, where this area is best examined using a proctoscope. As stated above, the author's preference is for the oblique-ended Graham Anderson pattern proctoscope for colposcopy.

Normal perianal skin is unremarkable on colposcopy, both before and after the application of acetic acid. Immature normal squamous epithelium tends to "acetowhiten," necessitating careful interpretation of anal colposcopy in patients who recently have undergone any anal surgery or who have anal symptoms such as pruritis ani.

The colposcopic features of AIN are described below.

Low Grade AIN and HPV Infection

The clinical features of low-grade AIN on the perianal skin are more difficult to diagnose accurately than those in the anal canal. The keratinization of the perianal epithelium results in dense acetowhite change, obscuring vessel patterns and making differentiation of HPV infection from low-grade dysplasia difficult. In the anal canal, however, the vessel patterns are more obvious; hence, the diagnosis of low-grade dysplasia is more reliable than on the perianal skin. In the author's experience, less than 10% patients with subclinical papillomaviral (SPI) or AIN I had anal canal disease in the absence of perianal SPI or AIN.

High Grade Anal Intraepithelial Neoplasia (AIN III)

High-grade perianal intraepithelial neoplasia (Figure 5.2.3) may be apparent on naked eye inspection as patchy, irregular pigmentation of the perianal skin. In the absence of pigmentation, a further clue to high-grade AIN may be thickening of the skin. Such areas may be single or multiple and may extend cephalad to the rectal mucosa or caudad onto the buttocks and thighs.

The normal perianal skin is heavily keratinized and responds slowly to acetic acid "soaks," where hyperkeratotic perianal epithelium becomes acetowhite very slowly. Capillary patterns are unusual on the perianal epithe-

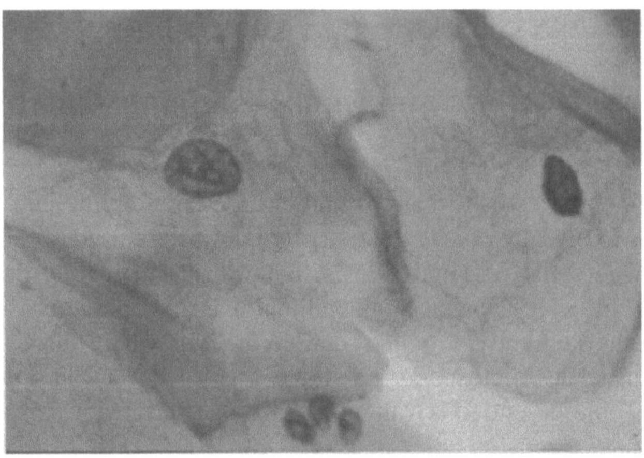

FIGURE 5.2.3. Characteristic colposcopic appearances of high-grade AIN (see text).

lium, even in high-grade disease, differentiating the technique from cervical colposcopy. In 3 of 6 cases in which perianal skin mosaicism was noted colposcopically (Figure 5.2.3), the histology was reported as early invasive squamous carcinoma in that area, suggesting that mosaicism in the perianal skin may be a marker of progression to invasive disease.

In the anal canal, dysplastic epithelium may appear hyperemic on examination prior to the application of acetic acid. However, such areas become more obvious after the application of acetic acid spray. The colposcopic appearances of anal canal intraepithelial neoplasia are similar to those seen on the cervix, namely acetowhite areas with punctation and mosaic vessel patterns. In keeping with the lack of a clear anatomical distinction between the anal canal and perianal skin, the colposcopic features of papillomavirus infection and dysplasia in the lower anal canal and perianal skin merge into each other.

In the author's experience, it is difficult to distinguish colposcopically invasive lesions from high-grade AIN.

Therapeutic Options

Possible treatment options for AIN III lesions include simple excision, excision with grafting, laser ablation, cryoablation, the application of cytotoxic creams (such as 5-fluorouracil), or the use of newer disease modifiers such as the retinoids and Imiquimod. Skinner et al. (71) reported the frequent occurrence of involvement of hair shafts and sweat glands in AIN III lesions and suggested that these may not be destroyed by ablative techniques. Surgical excision also has the great advantage of providing a specimen for complete histological assessment.

For large areas of AIN III involving more than 50% of the anal margin or anal canal, the risk of anal stenosis following excision is a major concern. Anal stenosis may be prevented by the application of split skin grafts to the anal canal and margin at the time of excision of the lesion. Scholefield et al. (72) reported their experience in local excision of AIN III lesions involving less than 50% of the anal circumference from 9 patients without any sequelae. An additional 5 patients with circumferential AIN III extending from the perianal skin to the dentate line underwent excision of the affected epithelium and split skin grafting. In these patients, a defunctioning sigmoid loop colostomy was performed some weeks prior to anal skin excision and was rewarded by improved survival of the skin grafts. Treatment of this type necessitates multiple surgical procedures with an inherent morbidity; such treatment can only be justifiable for a lesion with a high malignant potential.

Interestingly, treatment for invasive anal SCC is moving away from surgical intervention, sparing the patient a colostomy. This trend towards nonsurgical treatment for invasive disease adds to the difficulties in managing

AIN III, where an observational policy for AIN III has many attractions, particularly as the malignant potential of AIN III is uncertain and AIN lesions are often asymptomatic. A policy of observation requires repeated examination, and because patients find anal colposcopy unpleasant, compliance is a major problem in such a policy (twice yearly as a minimum seems reasonable). An observational policy of this type has become our practice in Nottingham over the last 8 years. While it is too early to determine whether this less aggressive approach will prove effective, our early results show only 2 invasive carcinomas developing in a group of 26 patients over eight years. One of the 2 patients whose AIN progressed to invasive disease was immunosuppressed for systemic lupus for over 5 years.

The retinoids and Imiquimod have been used to treat skin dysplasia and have been shown capable of impressive remission; however, once treatment ceases, there is a very high relapse rate. In addition, the retinoids have severe and unpleasant side effects, such as photosensitivity, liver dysfunction, and gastrointestinal disturbances. Their use needs to be supervised by a dermatologist experienced in their use. While they are interesting developments, treatments with these agents cannot be recommended for the treatment of AIN at present (73).

A Recommended Therapeutic Strategy

Low Grade AIN (AIN I and II)

In common with current gynecological practice, AIN I and II probably have minimal malignant potential, and therefore do not require definitive treatment. Biopsy of the visibly most abnormal area is essential for diagnosis with 6 monthly follow-ups for one year, with repeated colposcopic or cytological examination. After one year, if the worst affected area has not progressed, the patient is discharged from follow-up with a warning reminder to re-attend if the appearance of the lesions changes or if bleeding occurs.

Expectant treatment of low-grade AIN lesions seems appropriate for two reasons. Firstly, mild dysplasia is notoriously difficult to diagnose consistently and resolution of AIN I or II to subclinical papillomavirus infection may occur and therefore must be interpreted with some caution (72). Secondly, many AIN I and AIN II lesions are likely to be due to HPV types other than HPV 16, and therefore are much less likely to possess inherent malignant potential.

High Grade AIN (AIN III)

Excision of AIN III lesions parallels the policy adopted by many gynecologists for VIN III and CIN III along the lines of those described by Reynolds et al. (74), Kaplan et al. (75), and Schlaerth et al. (76). In the

Sheffield experience where the lesion occupied less than 50% of the area of the anal margin or canal, local excision with a margin of non-dysplastic tissue was performed. In those patients with extensive perianal and anal canal disease extending circumferentially and cephalad to the DL, complete excision of the affected epithelium with a margin required resurfacing of the anal canal and perianal area with split skin grafts taken from the medial aspect of the thigh. A sigmoid loop colostomy was performed several weeks before the skin grafting procedure. The loop colostomy was closed approximately two months after the grafting procedure.

The trend towards non-surgical treatment of invasive anal squamous cancer (77,78) and the lack of information concerning the rate of progression of AIN III to invasive cancer may lead to over treatment of AIN III; however, it may be difficult to exclude occult invasive disease in an area of AIN III, and histopathological assessment of the whole of such a high grade lesion is therefore desirable. Interestingly, by comparison, the incidence of occult invasion in extensive high-grade VIN treated by wide excision is only 7% to 10% (79).

Those who argue in favor of not treating AIN III do so on the basis that anal cancer is rare and that anal cancers may be treated non-surgically, avoiding the need for a stoma. Although OPCS figures do not show an increase in the incidence of anal cancer (7), the data may be incomplete due to the multitude of histological types reported and difficulties in defining the morphology of the anal canal. Recent epidemiological data show that there is an increasing incidence of anal cancer over the last ten years, particularly in women (29)—a factor that may affect this conservative view.

In order to answer these uncertainties, further longitudinal information is required. A multicenter study could randomize patients with AIN III lesions to treatment or observation only, and although such a study would be costly given the rarity of invasive anal cancer, such a trial seems unlikely to be conducted at the present time.

Therapeutic Dilemmas

The uncertainties surrounding the natural history of AIN III lead to difficult management decisions when faced with patients who have extensive areas of AIN III and appear to be at high risk of malignant progression.

Such patients are best managed by examination under anesthetic with multiple colposcopically guided punch biopsies, approximately 4 millimeters in diameter (a disposable corneal punch is ideal for this purpose), taken from each quadrant of the anal margin and the lower and upper anal canal, with the site of each biopsy carefully recorded. In so doing, the extent of the AIN can be mapped histologically. Where facilities for, or expertise in, anal colposcopy are lacking, it is even more important to take a large number of biopsies to thoroughly assess the extent of the disease. Localized segments of AIN III then can be excised, and where there are several adjacent lesions, several local excisional procedures with intraoperative mapping several months apart may allow healing of the previous sites of excision with healthy skin and thereby reduce the risk of anal stenosis. In patients with pan-anal disease, excisional treatment without grafting is likely to result in a severe anal stenosis, and thus is best managed by observation with a low threshold for biopsy of any lesion that appears to undergo change. Access to an experienced gynecological cytopathologist may reduce the need for repeated anal colposcopy, but a low threshold for biopsy is still recommended. Excision and split skin grafting with a defunctioning loop colostomy is probably best reserved for those with pan-anal disease with a micro-invasive or small invasive squamous carcinoma.

Conclusion

The natural history of AIN is at present unclear, although high-risk groups—with or without HIV-related disease and possibly with high-grade CIN who are oncogenic HPV-positive with high-risk HPV subtypes—should be regularly surveyed by "new" adapted cytologic and colposcopic techniques for the specific assessment of anal diseases using technology that has been translated from gynecologic practice. Such an approach requires the accrual of a multidisciplinary team experienced in anal "colposcopy" and anal cytopathological and histopathological assessment of this very specialized area.

References

1. Morson BC and Dawson IMP. In: Gastrointestinal pathology. Oxford: Blackwell Scientific; 1984.
2. Frost DB, Richards PC, Montague ED, et al. Epidermoid cancer of the anorectum. Cancer. 1984;53:1285–93.
3. Papillon J and Montbarbon JT. Epidermoid carcinoma of the anal canal: a series of 276 cases. Dis Colon Rectum. 1987;30:324–33.
4. Fenger C. The Anal Transitional Zone. A method for macroscopic demonstration. Acta Pathol Microbiol Scand [A]. 1978;86:225–30.
5. Scholefield JH, Sonnex C, Talbot IC, et al. Anal and cervical intraepithelial neoplasia: possible parallel. Lancet. 1989;ii:765–8.
6. Scholefield JH, Hickson WGE, Smith JHF, et al. Anal intraepithelial neoplasia: part of a multifocal disease process. Lancet. 1992;340:1271–3.
7. Office of Population Censuses and Surveys. Cancer statistics and registrations, 1986. Series MB1 no.8. London: Her Majesty's Stationary Office; 1991.
8. Richart R.M. Cervical intraepithelial neoplasia. In: Sommers ED, editor. Pathology annual. New York: Appleton-Century-Crofts; 1973. pp. 301–28.
9. Peters RK, Mack TM, and Bernstein L. Parallels in the epidemiology of selected anogenital carcinomas. J Natl Cancer Inst. 1984;72:609–15.

10. Sherman KJ, Daling JR, Chu J, et al. Multiple primary tumors in women with vulvar neoplasms: a case control study. Br J Cancer. 1988;57:423–7.
11. Melbye M and Sprogel P. Etiological parallel between anal cancer and cervical cancer. Lancet. 1991;338:657–9.
12. Zbar AP, Fenger C, Efron J, Beer-Gabel M, and Wexner SD. The pathology and molecular biology of anal intraepithelial neoplasia: comparisons with cervical and vulvar intraepithelial carcinoma. Int J Colorect Dis. 2002;17:203–15.
13. Siegal A. Malignant transformation of condyloma acuminatum: review of the literature and report of a case. Am J Surg. 1962;103:613–7.
14. Sturm JT, Christianson CE, Uecker JH, et al. Squamous cell carcinoma of the anus arising in a giant condyloma acuminatum: report of a case. Dis Colon Rectum. 1975;18:147–51.
15. Prassad ML and Abcarian H. Malignant potential of perianal condyloma acuminatum. Dis Colon Rectum. 1980;23:191–7.
16. Fenger C and Nielsen VT. Dysplastic change of the anal canal epithelium in minor surgical specimens. Acta Pathol Microbiol Scand. 1981;89:463–5.
17. Foust RL, Dean PJ, Stoler MH, et al. Intraepithelial neoplasia of the anal canal in hemorroidal tissue: a study of 19 cases. Hum Pathol. 1991;22:529–34.
18. Fenger C and Nielsen VT. Precancerous changes in the anal canal epithelium in resection specimens. Acta Pathol Microbiol Scand. 1986;94:63–9.
19. Ogunbiyi OA, Scholefield JH, Raftery AT, et al. Prevalence of anal human papillomavirus infection and intraepithelial neoplasia in renal allograft recipients. Br J Surg. 1994;8(1):365–7.
20. Ogunbiyi OA, Scholefield JH, Robertson G, et al. Anal human papillomavirus infection and squamous neoplasia in patients with invasive vulvar cancer. Obstet Gynaecol. 1994;82:212–6.
21. Cleary RK, Schaldebrand JD, Fowler JJ, Schuler JM, and Lampman RM. Perianal Bowen's disease and anal intraepithelial neoplasia. Dis Colon Rectum. 1999;42:945–51.
22. Palefsky JM, Holly EA, Gonzales J, et al. Natural history of, and aetiologic abnormalities and papillomavirus infection among homosexual men with Group IV H disease. J Acquir Immune Defic Syndr. 1992;5:1258–65.
23. Nakagawa M, Stites DP, Patel S, Farhat S, Scott M, Hills NK, Palefsky JM, and Moscicki AB. Persistence of human papillomavirus type 16 infection is associated with lack of cytotoxic T lymphocyte response to the E6 antigens. J Infect Dis. 2000;182:595–8.
24. Condra JH. Resisting resistance: maximizing the durability of antiretroviral therapy. Ann Intern Med. 1998;128:951–4.
25. Morson BC. The pathology and results of treatment of squamous cell carcinoma of the anal canal and anal margin. Proc R Soc Med. 1960;53:416–20.
26. Wexner SD, Milsom JW, and Dailey TH. Demographics of anal cancers are changing: identification of a high risk population. Dis ColonRectum. 1987; 30:942–6.
27. Department of Health and Social Security. Sexually transmitted diseases. In: On the state of public health: annual report of the Chief Medical Officer of the Department of Health and Social Security for the year 1978. London: HMSO; 1979. pp. 1–65.

28. Rabkin CS, Biggar PJ, Melbye M, et al. Second primary cancers following anal and cervical carcinoma: evidence of shared aetiologic factors. Am J Epidemiol. 1992;136:54–8.
29. Frisch M, Melbye M, and Moiler H. Trends in the incidence of anal cancer in Denmark. Br Med J. 1993;306:419–22.
30. Melbye M, Cote TR, Kessler L, et al. High incidence of anal cancer among AIDS patients. Lancet. 1994;343:636–9.
31. Grodsky L. Unsuspected anal cancer uncovered after minor anorectal surgery. Dis Colon Rectum. 1968;10:471–9.
32. Nash G, Allen W, and Nash S. Atypical lesions of the anal mucosa in homosexual men. JAMA. 1986;2:873–6.
33. Palefsky JM, Gonzales J, Greenblatt RM, et al. Anal intraepithelial neoplasia and anal papillomavirus infection in homosexual males with Group IV HIV disease. JAMA. 1990;263:2911–6.
34. Kiviat NB, Critchiow CW, Holmes KK, et al. Association of anal dysplasia and human papillomavirus with immunosuppression and HIV infection among homosexual men. AIDS. 1993;7:43–9.
35. Caussy D, Goedert JJ, Palefsky J, et al. Interaction of human immunodeficiency and papillomaviruses: association with anal epithelial abnormality in homosexual men. Int J Cancer. 1990;46:214–9.
36. Melbye M, Palefsky J, Gonzales J, et al. Immune status as a determinant of human papillomavirus detection and its association with anal epithelial abnormalities. Int J Cancer. 1990;46:203–6.
37. Williams AB, Darragh TM, Vranzian K, et al. Anal and cervical human papillomavirus infection and risk of anal and cervical epithelial abnormalities in human immunodeficiency virus-infected women. Obstet Gynecol. 1994;83: 205–11.
38. Frazer IH, Medley G, Crapper RM, et al. Association between anorectal dysplasia, human papillomavirus and human immunodeficiency virus infection in homosexual men. Lancet. 1986;ii:657–60.
39. Palmer JG, Scholefield JH, Coates PJ, et al. Anal cancer and human papillomaviruses. Dis Colon Rectum. 1989;32:1016–22.
40. zur Hausen H and Schneider A. The role of human papillomaviruses in human anogenital cancer. In: Howley PM and Salzman NP, editors. The papillomaviruses. New York: Plenum; 1987. pp. 245–63.
41. Goorney BP, Waugh MA, and Clarke J. Anal warts in homosexual men. Genitourin Med. 1987;63:216–8.
42. Syrjanen SM, von Krogh G, and Syrjanen K. Anal condylomas in men. Histopathological and virological assessment. Genitourin Med. 1989;65:216–24.
43. zur Hausen H. Herpes simplex virus in human genital cancer. Int Rev Exp Pathol. 1983;25:307–26.
44. Palefsky JM, Holly EA, Gonzales J, et al. Detection of human papillomavirus DNA in anal intraepithelial neoplasia and anal cancer. Cancer Res. 1991;51: 1014–9.
45. Surawicz CM, Kirby P, Critchlow C, et al. Anal dysplasia in homosexual men: role of anoscopy and biopsy. Gastroenterology 1993;105:658–66.
46. Holmes F, Borek D, Owen-Kummer M, et al. Anal cancer in women. Gastroenterology. 1988;95:107–11.

47. Daniell HW. Re: causes of anal carcinoma. JAMA. 1985;254:358.
48. Ocadiz R, Sauceda R, Cruz M, et al. High correlation between molecular alterations of the c-myc oncogene and carcinoma of the uterine cervix. Cancer Res. 1987;47:4173–7.
49. Dyson N, Howley PM, Munger K, et al. The human papillomavirus 16 E7 oncoprotein is able to bind to the retinoblastoma gene product. Science. 1989; 243:934–7.
50. Scheffner M, Wemess BA, Hulbregtse JM, et al. The E6 oncoprotein encoded by human papillomavirus types 16 and I8 promotes the degradation of p53. Cell. 1990;63:1129–36.
51. Werness BA, Levine AJ, and Howley PM. Association of human papillomavirus types 16 and I8 E proteins with p53. Science. 1990;248:76–9.
52. Riou G, Barrios M, Dutronquay V, et al. Presence of papillomavirus DNA sequences, amplification of c-myc and c-ras oncogenes and enhanced expression of c-myc in carcinomas of the uterine cervix. In: Hawley P and Brocke T, editors. Papillomaviruses: molecular and clinical aspects. New York: Alan R Liss; 1985. pp. 47–55.
53. Riou G, Barrios M, Le MG, et al. C-myc proto-oncogene expression and prognosis in early carcinoma of the cervix. Lancet. 1987;I:761–3.
54. Ogunbiyi OA, Scholefield JH, Rogers K, Sharp F, Smith JHF, and Polacarz SV. C-myc oncogene expression in anal squamous neoplasia. J Clin Pathol. 1993;46:23–7.
55. Crook T, Greenfield I, Howard J, and Stanley M. Alterations in growth properties of human papillomavirus type 16 immortalized human cervical keratinocyte cell line correlate with amplification and overexpression of c-myc oncogene. Oncogene. 1990;5:619 22.
56. Porreco R, Penn I, Droegemueller W, et al. Gynecologic malignancies in immunosuppressed organ homograft recipients. Obstet Gynecol. 1975;45:359–64.
57. Penn I. Cancers of the anogenital region in renal transplant recipients. Analysis of 65 cases. Cancer. 1986;58:611 6.
58. Penn I. Cancer is a complication of severe immunosuppression. Surg Gynecol Obstet. 1986;162:603–10.
59. Karpeh M and Portlock C. The immunology of lymphoproliferative disorders. In: Zbar AP, Guillou PJ, Bland KI, and Syrigos KN, editors. Immunology for surgeons. London: Springer Verlag; 2002.
60. Alloub MI, Barr BBB, McLaren KM, et al. Human papillomavirus infection and cervical intraepithelial neoplasia in women with renal allografts. Br Med J. 1989;298:153–6.
61. Halpert R, Butt KMH, Sedlis A, et al. Human papillomavirus infection and lower genital neoplasia in female renal allograft recipients. Transplant Proc. 1985;17:93–5.
62. Beckmann AM, Acker R, Christiansen AE, et al. Human papillomavirus infection in women with multicentric squamous cell neoplasia. Am J Obstet Gynecol. 1991;165:1431–7.
63. Tay SK, Jenkins D, Maddox M. et al. Subpopulation of Langerhans' cells in cervical neoplasia. Br J Obstet Gynaecol. 1987;94:10–5.
64. Tay SK, Jenkins D, Maddox M, et al. Tissue macrophage response in human papillomavirus infection and cervical intraepithelial neoplasia. Br J Obstet Gynaecol. 1987;94:1094–7.

65. Saxena S, Jha P, and Faroz A. Immunosuppression by human seminal plasma. Immunol Invest. 1985;14:255–69.
66. Fischer SM, Gleason GL, Bohrinan JS, et al. Prostaglandin enhancement of skin tumour irritation and promotion. Adv Prostagland Thromb Res. 1991;6:517–22.
67. Critchlow CW, Surawicz CM, Holmes KK, et al. Prospective study of high grade anal squamous intraepithelial neoplasia in a cohort of homosexual men: influence of HIV infection, immunosuppression and human papillomavirus infection. AIDS. 1995;9:1255–62.
68. Carter PS, Sheffield JP, Shepherd NA, et al. Interobserver variation in the reporting of the histopathological grading of anal intraepithelial neoplasia. J Clin Pathol. 1994;47:1032–4.
69. Scholefield JH, Ogunbiyi OA, Smith JHF, et al. Anal colposcopy and the diagnosis of anal intraepithelial neoplasia in high risk gynecological patients. Int J Gynecol Cancer. 1994;4:119–26.
70. de-Ruiter A, Carter PS, Katz DR, et al. A comparison between cytology and histology to detect anal intra-epithelial neoplasia. Genitourin Med. 1994;70: 20–1.
71. Skinner PP, Ogunbiyi OA, Scholefield JH, et al. Skin appendage involvement in anal intraepithelial neoplasia. Br J Surg. 1997;84:675–8.
72. Scholefield J, Ogunbiyi OA, Smith JHF, et al. Treatment of anal intra-epithelial neoplasia. Br J Surg. 1994;81:1238–40.
73. Stanley M. Genital human papillomavirus infections—current and prospective therapies. J Natl Cancer Inst Monogr. 2003;17(31):117–24.
74. Reynolds VH, Madden JJ, Franklin JD, et al. Preservation of anal function after total excision of the anal mucosa for Bowen's disease. Ann Surg. 1984;199:563–8.
75. Kaplan AL, Kaufman RH, Birken RA, et al. Intra-epithelial carcinoma of the vulva with extension to the anal canal. Obstet Gynecol. 1981;58:368–71.
76. Schlaerth JB, Morrow CP, Nalick RH, et al. Anal involvement with carcinoma in situ of the perineum in women. Obstet Gynecol. 1984;64:406–11.
77. UKCCCR Anal Cancer Trial Working Party. Epidermoid anal cancer: results from the UKCCCR randomised trial of radiotherapy alone versus radiotherapy, 5 fluouracil, and mitomycin. Lancet. 1996;348:1049–54.
78. Northover JMA. Epidermoid cancer of the anus—the surgeon retreats. J R Soc Med. 1991;84:389–90.
79. Rettenmaier MA, Berman ML, and Di Saia PJ. Skinning vulvectomy for the treatment of multifocal vulvar intraepithelial neoplasia. Obstet Gynecol. 1987;69:247–50.

Section 2
Clinical Anorectal Assessment

Chapter 6
Assessment of the Constipated Patient

Chapter 6.1
An Overview*

MICHELLE J. THORNTON and DAVID Z. LUBOWSKI

Clinical History

Definition of Constipation

Constipation comprises a number of diverse symptoms relating to frequency of bowel movement, consistency of stools, and the ease and completeness of defecation (1). The subjective complaint of constipation is influenced by social customs and expectations and has been shown to be neither sensitive nor specific compared with symptom-based criteria. Less than 50% of patients reporting constipation would be given the diagnosis of constipation when colonic transit studies and patient diaries are assessed (2). Symptoms of infrequent defecation—less than three stools per week—correlate better with gut dysfunction compared with symptoms of straining and incomplete evacuation (2).

The most common definition used in the literature is that of Drossman, described over twenty years ago whereby there are two or fewer stools per week and/or straining at stool more than 25% of the time (3). In 1992, this definition was expanded to include lumpy and /or hard stools more than 25% of the time and the sensation of incomplete evacuation more than 25% of the time. Patients are considered constipated if they have had two or more of these four symptoms in the preceding three months, while not using laxatives (4). More recently, most comparative studies have utilized the Rome II criteria (Table 6.1-1), although this scoring system has yet to be validated. Knowles et al. have validated an 11 point scoring system—KESS—that is able to demonstrate the discriminatory ability of multiple symptoms (5,6), but this has not been widely used.

*Editor's Note: This overview should be read in conjunction with other components of Chapter 6 as well as the chapters regarding ambulatory manometry, colonic transit and motility and biofeedback therapy.

Table 6.1-1. Rome criteria for functional constipation and irritable bowel syndrome.

Rome I Criteria
Constipation = Yes to 2 or more of answers 1,3,5,7
Excluding IBS (see below)
Rome II Criteria
Constipation = Yes to 2 or more of answers 1,3,5,7,10,11
No to answer 4
Excluding IBS
Question: Have you had any of the following symptoms at least one-fourth (1/4) of the time (occasions or days) in the last three months?

1. Fewer than three bowel movements in a week
2. More than three bowel movements a day
3. Hard or lumpy stools
4. Loose, mushy, or watery stools
5. Straining during a bowel movement
6. Having to rush to the toilet to have a bowel movement
7. Feeling of incomplete emptying after a bowel movement
8. Passing mucous (slime) during a bowel movement
9. Abdominal fullness, bloating, or swelling
10. A sensation that the stool cannot be passed (i.e., blocked) when having a bowel movement
11. A need to press on or around your bottom or vagina to try to remove stool to complete a bowel movement

Irritable bowel syndrome (IBS)
Abdominal pain at any site for at least three months in the prior year that was either relieved by defecation often (>25% of time) or was associated with looser or more frequent stool at its onset often; and three or more of:
a) altered stool frequency (<3 stools per week or >3 stools per day often)
b) altered stool form (hard or loose/watery stools often)
c) altered stool passage (straining or urgency or a feeling or incomplete evacuation often)
d) passage of mucous per rectum
e) visible abdominal distension

Quality of Life Assessment

The general well-being of patients with chronic constipation is lower than that of a comparable normal population, as assessed by quality of life scores. Constipation severity correlates inversely with the patient's perceived quality of life. Functional, constipation is associated with an increased reporting of frequent fatigue, severe headaches, and dizziness, which may account for work absenteeism in up to 75% of constipated patients (7). Interestingly, patients with normal transit constipation have lower quality of life scores than those with slow transit constipation (8), possibly reflecting the abdominal pain and bloating that occurs in the irritable bowel syndrome (IBS Rome II criteria—Table 6.1-1). Mason et al. have recently documented a correlation between pretreatment quality of life scores and a favorable response to biofeedback for constipation (9). Patients who did not experience lifestyle limitations due to emotional problems, pain, or lethargy had a statistically greater response to treatment.

Etiology of Chronic Constipation

The symptom of constipation has a broad range of causes (Table 6.1-2). The colon is subject to a number of intrinsic, as well as extrinsic, factors that may affect function.

Dietary fiber deficiency is the most common etiology of mild/moderate constipation. Social factors should always be considered carefully, particularly in the elderly. Endocrine causes, particularly hypothyroidism, should

TABLE 6.1-2. Etiology of constipation.

Dietary
Inadequate fiber
Social
Immobility
Environmental changes (hospitalization, vacation)
Ignoring call to stool
Elderly
Endocrine and Metabolic
Hypothyroidism, pregnancy, hypercalcemia, diabetes, hypokalemia, uremia, hypopituitarism, lead poisoning, porphyria
Central and Peripheral Nervous System Pathology
Autonomic neuropathy (diabetes), porphyria, Parkinson's disease
Drugs
Iron supplements, calcium channel blockers, anticholinergics, antidepressants, narcotic agents, non-steroidal anti-inflammatory drugs, laxative abuse
Psychiatric
Depression, psychoses, anorexia nervosa
Gastrointestinal
Structural
Colonic obstruction: neoplasm, diverticular disease, inflammatory bowel disease, volvulus, intussusception
Anal outlet obstruction: stenosis, fissure
Functional
Normal transit: constipation-predominant irritable bowel syndrome
Slow transit constipation
• Idiopathic
• Intestinal pseudo-obstruction
• Hirschsprung's disease
• Megacolon
Obstructed defecation
• Hypertonic internal sphincter
• Rectocele
• Pelvic floor weakness
• Anismus
• Idiopathic

not be overlooked. Slow transit constipation is a disorder of colonic motility characterized by a reduction in the frequency, amplitude, and duration of propulsive contractions in the colon. Several pathophysiological differences between normal transit and slow transit colonic function have been identified, which may account for the difference between these conditions. In slow transit, the colon is hypersensitive to cholinergic stimulation (10), more strongly innervated by non-cholinergic inhibitory nerves (11), and is associated post-prandially with an increased secretion of proximal gut hormones (12). The significance of these findings remains to be determined.

Obstructed defecation may be due to weakness or lack of coordination of the pelvic floor muscles involved in defecation. Paradoxical pelvic floor or sphincter contraction or inadequate relaxation during defecation may cause functional outlet obstruction (13), although the condition has been somewhat over-diagnosed (14,15). In many cases, the precise pathophysiology may not be clear, and importantly, in some patients, a more generalized colonic motility disorder is present (16).

Prevalence

The prevalence of constipation is dependent upon the definition used. Population-based studies are limited to subjective patient reporting, and therefore may over-estimate the true prevalence. Between 2% and 34% of Western populations report symptoms of constipation. Applying the Rome criteria, the prevalence of constipation is 4.6% for functional constipation and 4.5% for outlet obstruction (17). A gender association is debated where outlet delay (but not functional) constipation appears to be increased in women (7). Age often has been considered important, although in the age group over 65 years, functional constipation was found in 24.4% and outlet obstruction in 20.5%, which was not statistically increased compared with the general population (18).

Assessment of Constipation

Clinical Examination

A general physical examination is performed to search for evidence of systemic disease associated with constipation. Rectal examination should be performed to exclude the presence of an anal stricture, anal fissure, anorectal mass, or rectal blood. During rectal examination, perineal descent with straining can be estimated by palpating the ischial tuberosities. As the patient bears down, the examiner should perceive relaxation of the external anal sphincter (EAS) together with perineal descent. If this does not occur, obstructed defecation should be suspected.

Stool Diary

Self-reported constipation may be unreliable. When requested to record a stool diary, over 50% of patients who reported severe constipation did not meet the Drossman criteria (2). A stool diary is a simple and inexpensive means of assessing the patient's symptoms, and is particularly helpful when the symptoms do not match the clinical and radiological findings.

Biochemistry

Requests for laboratory investigations should be based on a clinical index of suspicion. They may include thyroid function tests, serum calcium and creatinine, full blood count, and glucose to help exclude systemic disease.

Psychological Assessment

Psychiatric illnesses such as depression, obsessive–compulsive disorder, and anorexia nervosa are independent risk factors for constipation (19). Several studies also have suggested that underlying emotional trauma may be associated with constipation and other pelvic floor disorders. A pretreatment psychological assessment may indicate those patients who are likely to benefit from behavioral intervention (20,21) and will assist in the referral of patients prior to surgery.

Flexible Sigmoidoscopy

Flexible sigmoidoscopy and biopsy, where appropriate, may aid in the diagnosis of the solitary rectal ulcer syndrome (SRUS), a colorectal mass lesion or intussusception. The presence of melanosis coli will help in diagnosing laxative abuse.

Imaging

Barium Enema

Barium enema examination is indicated in patients with longstanding constipation. The purpose is not to diagnose mucosal pathology, but to exclude megarectum or megacolon, and a single contrast study without bowel preparation should be performed because preparation of the colon or gas insufflation may respectively mask or artificially produce features of megacolon (Figure 6.1.1). In patients over 40 years of age with recent onset of constipation or iron deficiency, colonoscopy is the preferred investigation.

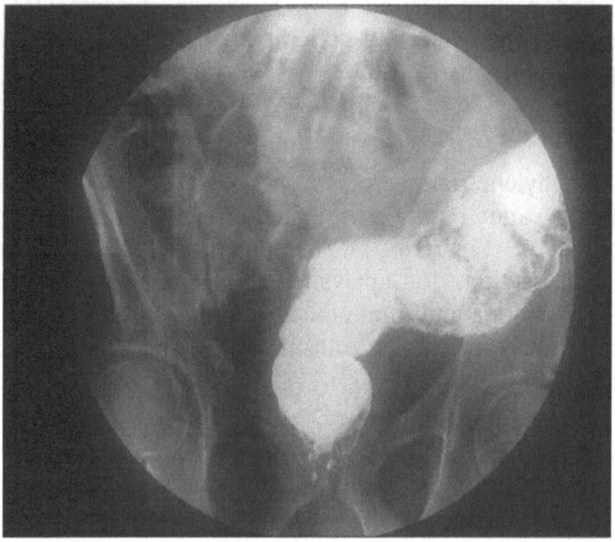

FIGURE 6.1.1. Single contrast unprepared barium study showing megacolon.

Defecating Proctography

A defecating proctogram provides information about anatomic pelvic floor changes and may be useful in the investigation of obstructed defecation (22). The test may demonstrate poor activation of the levator muscles, retention of barium, or a significant rectocele (significant implies failure to empty the rectocele despite otherwise emptying the rectum). It is important to recognize that some findings, such as internal intussusception, are secondary and not the cause of the obstructed defecation.

Colonic Transit Studies

Radiopaque Markers

This is a test of whole gut transit, which, when prolonged, usually reflects slow colonic transit because time through the colon forms a large component of whole gut transit time (23). Laxatives are ceased for 48 hours and 20 radiopaque markers are ingested. A single radiograph is taken on Day 5 where 14 markers (80%) will have been passed in normal subjects. Pelvic retention of the markers is consistent with pelvic outlet obstruction, whereas a diffuse scatter is more consistent with colonic inertia. Laxatives and enemas must be avoided for the duration of the study and patient compliance must be considered when interpreting the results.

Segmental transit can be calculated by taking daily X-rays for five days and dividing the abdomen into three segments reflecting the right colon, left colon, and rectum/sigmoid (24). However, if segmental transit is required, usually when selecting patients for colectomy, we prefer to use radioisotope scintigraphy.

Colonic Scintigraphy

Indium-111 diethylenetriamine pentaacetic acid (DTPA) is swallowed and the abdomen is scanned using a wide field-of-view gamma camera at 6, 24, 48, 72, and 96 hours (Figure 6.1.2). The colon is divided into right, left, and rectum/sigmoid sections for analysis. Segmental transport is measured by retention of isotope and total percent retention is calculated. This provides direct evidence of colonic transit, which is increased in slow transit constipation (25,26).

Physiological Studies

Anorectal Physiology

Anal manometry will diagnose a hypertonic internal anal sphincter (IAS). The presence of the rectoanal inhibitory reflex (RAIR) will exclude Hirschsprung's disease (HD). This is particularly useful with ultra short segment HD, where histology can be difficult to interpret. Manometry is also important to confirm normal sphincter tone when considering a patient for colectomy.

Rectal Balloon Distension Studies. Rectal sensation is impaired in two-thirds of patients with slow transit constipation (22). Loss of sensation may be a useful predictor of outcome of colectomy for constipation.

Pelvic Floor and Sphincter Electromyogram. The normal response to defecation straining is reduction of electrical activity in the EAS and puborectalis and increased activity in the pubococcygeus muscles, which contract and prevent excessive downward movement during defecation (27). In obstructed defecation, there is increased activity of the EAS and puborectalis during straining (28) due to anismus. These tests should be interpreted with caution because, in many cases, apparent anismus is due to a laboratory artifact, and testing under physiological conditions shows that anismus is not present in this setting (14,15).

Rectal balloon expulsion has been found to be impaired in patients with anismus (28) and was a popular, simple test of rectal evacuation. Recent careful studies have seriously challenged the validity of this test (29), and we no longer routinely use it.

Upper Gastrointestinal Motility Studies

It generally is accepted that patients with a generalized gastrointestinal disorder rather than an isolated disorder of colonic motility have poorer outcomes following surgery for slow transit constipation. Therefore, patients

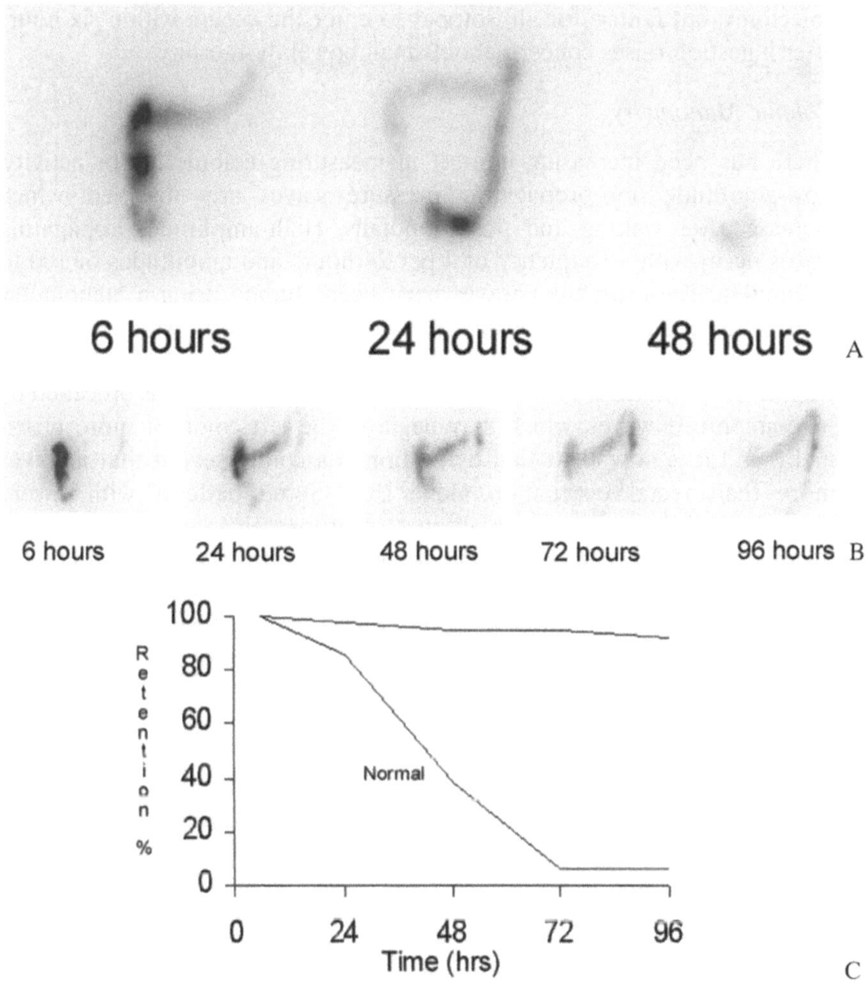

FIGURE 6.1.2. Radioisotope colon transit study. (A) Normal subject showing isotope in the right colon 6 hours after ingestion, and passage of isotope through the colon over 48 hours. (B) Patient with severe slow transit constipation showing prolonged retention of isotope. (C) Total percent retention of isotope in the patient with slow transit constipation (shown in the upper line). The upper range of normal values is represented by the lower line (McLean et al.) (26).

with slow transit constipation who have symptoms such as nausea, vomiting, and bloating within 30 minutes of eating, weight loss, and upper abdominal pain warrant further investigation prior to being considered for surgery (20). Esophageal manometry also may be indicated to exclude a global motility disorder. Gastric emptying studies may be helpful and a barium meal is the best means of excluding megaduodenum. Small bowel transit studies have not been proven to be a useful predictor of the outcome of colectomy, but failure for all isotopes to enter the cecum within six hours after ingestion raises concern about small bowel dysmotility.

Colonic Manometry

There has been increasing interest in measuring colonic motor activity. Low-amplitude non-propagating pressure waves are observed, which increase after waking and post-prandially. High-amplitude propagating waves occur with a frequency of 4 per 24 hours and amplitudes of 100 to 200 mmHg. These pressure waves have been studied using a manometry catheter placed colonoscopically (30), and more recently, we have studied the unprepared colon under physiological conditions using a soft 16-channel tube passed transnasally (31,32). Normal defecation is preceded by high-amplitude waves, which may begin in the left colon or more proximally, and it is now clear that defecation is a colonic event that involves more than rectal evacuation alone (33). Some patients with severe obstructed defecation have an absence of propagating colonic waves, and it would seem that rectal symptoms are due to a diffuse colonic motility disorder in these cases. These tests are evolving and will eventually find a place in the clinical investigation of patients with severe constipation. For further discussion, the reader is referred to Chapter 2.6 on ambulatory manometry and Chapter 2.7 on colonic motility and transit.

Approach to Management

Diet

An empirical trial of fiber supplementation (at least 25 grams of dietary fiber daily) in the form of unprocessed bran or psyllium should be considered at the initial presentation for all patients with functional constipation. A gradual increase in the dietary fiber content will reduce the side effects of bloating and flatulence. Many patients presenting to specialist Colorectal Units will already have been given additional dietary fiber and laxatives, and indeed may seem to have failed all forms of conservative therapy. However, it is important to be sure that compliance with diet and laxatives has been adequate. Failure to respond to fiber supplementation and initial simple laxative therapy should prompt investigation of pelvic floor function and colonic transit.

Lifestyle and Defecation

Although the place of exercise has not been proven, patients should be encouraged to take regular physical exercise. They should be asked to avoid suppressing the urge to defecate and to avoid spending excessive time on the toilet. Excessive straining may lead to pelvic nerve damage (34) and should be avoided.

Laxatives

A graduated progression from fiber supplements to laxatives should occur. Lubricants such as mineral oils (liquid paraffin) may be helpful, but may cause lipoid pneumonia and should be avoided in the elderly or patients with severe reflux. Osmotic laxatives are very effective, including Epsom salts (magnesium sulphate), sodium phosphate (Fleet™), or Lactulose, which may be used. Lactulose is a disaccharide that is metabolized in the colon to produce methane and hydrogen gas, and this may exacerbate bloating and flatulence. Stimulant laxatives include anthraquinones (senna, cascara segrada), castor oil, diphenylamines (bisacodyl, sodium picosulphate), and surface-active agents (docusate) may be considered for different specific uses and should be considered when other first-line laxatives have failed. There is experimental evidence to show that senna damages the colonic myenteric plexus and we do not use it except where all other combinations have failed, and generally only in cases where surgery may otherwise become indicated.

Biofeedback

There are no randomized trials confirming the efficacy of conditioning techniques for constipation. The mechanism of biofeedback is also poorly understood, and improvement may be due to the active behavioral intervention or a consequence of the attention to and better management of constipation (35). Outcome is also dependent on patient motivation (36). Nevertheless, there are a large number of nonrandomized trials that show that up to 80% of patients report symptom improvement with treatment (37,38). This symptom improvement correlates with decreased depression and anxiety scores and improved general health (9). The treatment is noninvasive, and we use it routinely in patients whose symptoms and physiological investigations suggest an abnormality of outlet obstruction. There is some evidence that biofeedback may improve colonic transit time (39), and some researchers also have advocated its use in patients with diffuse slow transit constipation, although this has not been our practice.

Botulinum Toxin

Botulinum toxin has been used selectively to weaken the EAS and puborectalis muscles in constipation. Initial results suggest that there may be some role for this treatment (40), but detailed prospective investigation of its efficacy and safety is required.

Sacral Nerve Stimulation

Although the study numbers are small and follow-up is currently short term, sacral nerve stimulation may prove to have a role in the treatment of intractable idiopathic constipation. The technique probably acts via parasympathetic nerve stimulation, but other factors, including modulation of rectal sensation, may be important. In one small study, stimulation produced an increased bowel frequency, improved ease of evacuation, and improved abdominal pain and bloating (41).

Surgery

Rectocele Repair

A rectocele is a defect in the rectovaginal fascia, formed as a condensation of the endopelvic fascia. Surgical intervention is recommended on the basis of rectocele size greater than three centimeters (although controversial), barium entrapment during the evacuation phase of defecating proctography (when the remainder of the rectal contents empties), and the need for manually assisted defecation. A rectocele may be repaired via a transanal, transvaginal, transperineal, or laparoscopic technique. There are numerous studies reporting results, particularly after transanal or transvaginal repair (42,43), but there are currently no published prospective comparative studies. The results of two randomized trials comparing transanal and transvaginal repair are awaited. Transanal repair appears to cause less pain than transvaginal repair, but interestingly, dyspareunia occurred with equal frequency in one study (44).

Incontinence associated with rectocele remains an area where more information is required. Recent magnetic resonance imaging (MRI) studies have suggested that although internal or external sphincter defects may contribute to incontinence in patients with a rectocele, there is also often global pelvic floor weakness involving ballooning of the puborectalis muscle and marked depression of the levator plate posteriorly and the levator muscles bilaterally (45).

Internal Sphincterotomy

Martelli et al. first reported strip myectomy for obstructed defecation in 1978 (46). More recent studies with longer-term follow-up have shown that the procedure has minimal efficacy except for short segment HD (47). Similarly, anal dilatation is not effective and is potentially dangerous. In rare cases, patients with a markedly hypertrophic or hypertonic IAS may require internal sphincterotomy (48), although recent developments in pharmacological relaxation of the sphincter with glyceryl trinitrate and botulinum toxin would obviate the need for surgery in some cases.

Surgery for Slow Transit Constipation

Antegrade Colonic Enema (ACE)

Antegrade irrigation of the colon may be used as an alternative to colectomy or a stoma in patients with severe laxative-resistant constipation. Malone modified the procedure described by Mitranoff for antegrade irrigation of the colon using the appendix in children (49,50), and several studies have shown good results (51). The ACE technique is particularly useful in patients with slow transit or severe obstructed defecation when sphincter weakness is also present, so that the use of laxatives is complicated by the resulting incontinence.

Colectomy (See Chapter 6.2)

Subtotal colectomy and ileorectal anastomosis will result in functional improvement in over 90% of patients in terms of frequency of defecation (52,53). Severe diarrhea will occur in up to 10% of cases, which may be associated with incontinence if the anal sphincter tone is reduced. Incomplete colectomy with ceco-rectal or ileo-sigmoid anastomosis is associated with recurrent constipation in up to 30% of cases. Exclusion of patients with proximal gut involvement is also critical in preventing failure due to recurrent constipation. Optimal functional outcome might be achieved by segmental colectomy after identifying the affected part of the colon, but current motility studies are not sufficiently sensitive to allow this distinction and segmental colectomy has a high rate of recurrent constipation (54). Although 50% of patients have persistent abdominal pain after colectomy and ileorectal anastomosis, the severity of the pain is usually significantly reduced (53). There are now a number of studies that report an overall patient satisfaction of 80% to 90%.

Conclusions

Functional constipation is a complex physiological interaction of the motor and sensory function of the colon, rectum, anus, pelvic floor, and higher centers. It is a symptom rather than a true diagnosis. This overview provides a broad outline of the assessment and management of patients presenting with intractable constipation not responsive to the usual remedies, where the patients' quality of life is affected and an overview of our unit's approach is presented, summarized in the algorithm at the end of this chapter (Figure 6.1.3). Several important aspects regarding the management of these complex patients are dealt with in detail in the chapters that follow in this section.

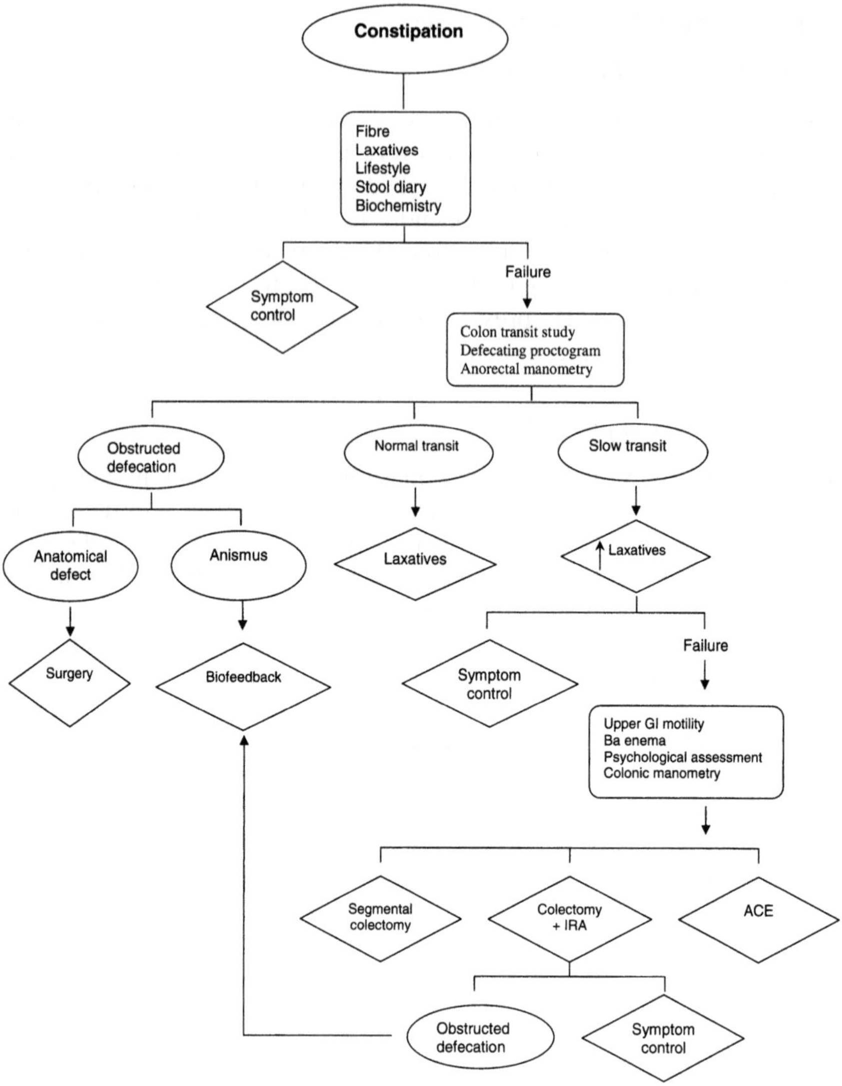

FIGURE 6.1.3. Management algorithm for the patient with constipation.

References

1. Thompson WG, Longsteth GF, Drossman DA, et al. Functional bowel disorders and functional abdominal pain. In: Drossman DA Corazziari E, and Talley NJ, editors. Functional gastrointestinal disorders. McLean, VA: Degnon; 2000. pp 351–432.
2. Ashraf W, Park F, Lof J, and Quigley EM. An examination of the reliability of reported stool frequency in the diagnosis of idiopathic constipation. Am J Gastroenterol. 1996; 91(1):26–32.

3. Drossman DA, Sandler RS, McKee DC, and Lovitz AJ. Bowel patterns among patients not seeking health care. Gastroenterology. 1982;83:529–34.
4. Thompson WG, Creed F, and Drossman DA. Functional bowel disorders and chronic functional abdominal pain. Gastroenterol Int. 1992;5:75–91.
5. Knowles CH, Eccersley AJ, Scott SM, Walker SM, Deeves B, and Lunnis PJ. Linear discriminant analysis of symptoms in patients with chronic constipation: validation of a new scoring system (KESS). Dis Colon Rectum. 2000;43(10): 419–26.
6. Knowles CH, Scott MS, Legg PE, Allison ME, and Lunniss PJ. Level of classification performance of KESS (symptom scoring system for constipation) validated in a prospective series of 105 patients. Dis Colon Rectum. 2002;45(6): 842–3.
7. Talley NJ, Weaver AL, Zinmeister AR, and Melton LJ. Functional constipation and outlet delay: A population-based study. Gastroenterology. 1993;105:781–90.
8. Glia A and Lindberg G. Quality of life in patients with different types of functional constipation. Scand J Gastroenterol. 1997;32:1083–9.
9. Mason HJ, Serrano-Ikkos E, and Kamm MA. Psychological state and quality of life in patients having behavioural treatment (biofeedback) for intractable constipation. Am J Gastroenterol. 2002;97(12):3154–9.
10. Slater BJ, Varma JS, and Gillespie JI. Abnormalities in the contractile properties of colonic smooth muscle in idiopathic slow transit constipation. Br J Surg. 1997;84:181–4.
11. Tomita R, Fujisaki S, Ikeda T, and Fukuzawa M. Role of nitric oxide in the colon of patients with slow transit constipation. Dis Colon Rectum. 2002;45(5):593–600.
12. Penning C, Delemarre JB, Bemelman WA, Biemond I, Lamers CB, and Masclee AA. Proximal and distal gut hormone secretion in slow transit constipation. Eur J Clin Invest. 2000;30(8):709–14.
13. Kuijpers HG and Bleijenberg G. The spastic pelvic floor syndrome. Dis Colon Rectum. 1985;28:669–72.
14. Duthie GS and Bartolo DCC. Anismus: the cause of constipation? Results of investigation and treatment. World J Surg. 1992;16:831–5.
15. Jones PN, Lubowski DZ, Swash M, and Henry MM. Is paradoxical contraction of puborectalis muscle of functional importance? Dis Colon Rectum. 1987;30:667–70.
16. Dinning PG, Bampton PA, Kennedy ML, et al. The manometric correlates of spontaneous defecation in patients with obstructed defecation. Gastroenterology. 1998;114(4):A716.
17. Pare P, Ferrazzi S, Thompson WG, Irvine EJ, and Rance L. An epidemiological survey of constipation in Canada: definitions, rates, demographics, and predictors of health care seeking. Am J Gastroenterol. 2001;96(11):3130–7.
18. Talley NJ, Fleming KC, Evans JM, et al. Constipation in an elderly community: A study of prevalence and potential risk factors. Am J Gastroenterol. 1996; 91(1):19–25.
19. Everhart JE, Go VLW, Johannes RS, Fitzsimmons SC, Roth HP, and White LR. A longitudinal study of self-reported bowel habits in the United States. Dig Dis Sci. 1989;34:1153–62.
20. Knowles CH, Scott M, and Lunniss PJ. Outcome of colectomy for slow transit constipation. Ann Surg. 1999;230(5):627–38.

21. Reiger NA, Wattchow DA, Sarre RG, et al. Prospective study of biofeedback for treatment of constipation. Dis Colon Rectum. 1997;40(10):1143–8.
22. Halverson AL and Orkin BA. Which physiological tests are useful in patients with constipation? Dis Colon Rectum. 1998;41(6):735–9.
23. Hinton JM, Lennard-Jones JE, and Young AC. A new method for studying gut transit times using radio-opaque markers. Gut. 1969;10:842–7.
24. Metcalf AM, Phillips SF, Zinsmeister AR, MacCarty RL, Beart RW, and Wolff BG. Simplified assessment of colonic transit. Gastroenterology. 1987;92:40–7.
25. Stivland T, Cammileri M, Vassalo M, et al. Scintigraphic measurement of regional gut transit in idiopathic constipation. Gastroenterology. 1991;101:107–15.
26. McLean RG, Smart RC, Lubowski DZ, King DW, Barbagallo S, and Talley NA. Oral colon transit scintigraphy using Indium-111 DTPA: variability in healthy subjects. Int J Colorectal Dis. 1992;7:173–6.
27. Lubowski DZ, King DW, and Finlay IG. Electromyography of the pubococcygeus muscles in patients with obstructed defaecation. Int J Colorectal Dis. 1992;7:184–7.
28. Preston DM, and Lennard-Jones JE. Anismus in chronic constipation. Dig Dis Sci. 1985;30:413–8.
29. Schouten WR, Briel JW, Auwerda JJ, et al. Anismus: fact or fiction? Dis Colon Rectum. 1997;40:1033–41.
30. Bassotti G, Gaburri M, Imbimbo BP, et al. Colonic mass movements in idiopathic constipation. Gut. 1988;29:1173–9.
31. Bampton PA, Dinning PG, Kennedy ML, Lubowski DZ, and Cook IJ. Prolonged multi-point recording of colonic manometry in the unprepared human colon: providing insight into the potentially relevant pressure wave parameters. Am J Gastroenterol. 2001;96(6):1838–48.
32. Lubowski DZ and Kennedy ML. Tests of anorectal physiology. In: Keighley MRB, and Williams NS, editors. Surgery of the anus, rectum and colon. 2nd ed. London: WB Saunders; 1999. pp. 33–6.
33. Lubowski DZ, Meagher AP, Smart RC, and Butler SP. Scintigraphic assessment of colonic function during defaecation. International J Colorectal Dis. 1995; 10:91–3.
34. Kiff ES, Barnes PRH, and Swash M. Evidence of pudendal neuropathy in patients with perineal descent and chronic straining at stool. Gut. 1984;25:1279–82.
35. Meagher AP, Sun WM, Kennedy ML, Smart RC, and Lubowski DZ. Biofeedback for anismus: has placebo effect been overlooked. Colorectal Dis. 1999; 1:80–7.
36. Gilliland R, Heymen S, Altomare DF, Park UC, Vickers D, Wexner SD. Outcome and predictors of success of biofeedback for constipation. Br J Surg. 1997;84: 1123–6.
37. Fleshman JW, Dreznik Z, Meyer K, Fry RD, Carney R, and Kodne IJ. Outpatient protocol for biofeed-back therapy of pelvic floor outlet obstruction. Dis Colon Rectum. 1992;35:1–7.
38. Wexner SD, Cheape JD, Jorge JMN, Heymen S, and Jagelman DG. Prospective assessment of biofeedback treatment of paradoxical puborectalis contraction. Dis Colon Rectum. 1992;35:145–50.

39. Emmanuel AV and Kamm MA. Response to a behavioural treatment, biofeedback, in constipated patients is associated with improved gut transit and autonomic innervation. Gut. 2001;49(2):214–9.
40. Maria G, Sganga G, Civello IM, and Brisinda G. Botulinum neurotoxin and other treatments for fissure in ano and pelvic floor disorders. Br J Surg. 2002;89(8):950–61.
41. Kenefick NJ, Nicholls RJ, Cohen RG, and Kamm MA. Permanent sacral nerve stimulation for treatment of idiopathic constipation. Br J Surg. 2002; 89(7):882–8.
42. van Dam JH, Ginai AZ, Gosselink MJ, et al. Role of defecography in predicting clinical outcome of rectocele repair. Dis Colon Rectum. 1997;40(2):201–7.
43. Ayabaca S, Zbar A, and Pescatori M. Anal continence after rectocele repair. Dis Colon Rectum. 2002;45(1):63–9.
44. Arnold MW, Stewart WRC, and Aguilar PS. Rectocele repair: four years experience. Dis Colon Rectum. 1990;33:684–7.
45. Steiner RA and Healy JC. Patterns of prolapse in women with symptoms of pelvic floor weakness: magnetic resonance imaging and laparoscopic treatment. Curr Opin Obstet Gynecol. 1998;10(4):295–301.
46. Martelli H, Devroede G, Arhan P, and Duguay C. Mechanisms of idiopathic constipation; outlet obstruction. Gastroenterology. 1978;75:623–31.
47. Pinho M, Yoshioka K, and Keighley MRB. Long-term results of anorectal myectomy for chronic constipation. Br J Surg. 1989;76:1163–4.
48. Kamm MA, Hoyle CVH, and Burleigh D. Hereditary internal anal sphincter myopathy causing proctalgia and constipation. Gastroenterology. 1991; 100:805–10.
49. Malone PS, Ransley PG, and Kiely EM. Preliminary report: the antegrade continence enema. Lancet. 1990;336:1217–8.
50. Malone PS, Curry JI, and Osborne A. The antegrade continence enema procedure, why, when and how? World J Urol. 1998;16:274–8.
51. Dick AC, McCallion WA, Brown S, and Boston VE. Antegrade colonic enemas. Br J Surg. 1996;83:642–3.
52. Nyam DCNK, Pemberton JH, Ilstrup DM, and Rath DM. Long-term results of surgery for chronic constipation. Dis Colon Rectum. 1997;40:273–9.
53. Lubowski DZ, Chen FC, Kennedy ML, and King DW. Results of colectomy for severe slow transit constipation. Dis Colon Rectum. 1996:39:525–9.
54. Lundin E, Karlbom U, Pahlman L, and Graf W. Outcome of segmental colonic resection for slow transit constipation. Br J Surg. 2002;89(10):1270–4.

Editorial Commentary

The assessment of patients with chronic severe constipation is highlighted throughout this book and the use of transit measurement broadly separates patients into potentially operable and conservative categories. Anal endosonography and its semiquantitative rôle in the dynamic contractile function of the puborectalis during straining (the puborectalis displacement and distance between its inner marking and the internal anal sphincter from rest to strain) may be a diagnostic aid in anismus. For those patients unresponsive to medical therapy, biofeedback, and toilet retraining, the surgical options revolve around subtotal colectomy and antegrade colonic enema lavage. For the latter procedure some selection of motivated patients is required. Recent data have shown a complex aetiology (and predictability) for postileorectal anastomosis diarrhoea where patients may benefit from preoperative small bowel transit assessment and a systemic assessment of serum PYY tyrosine peptide which can function as a circulating "ileal brake" on ileocaecal transport. Such an assessment may define the benefit in selected cases for the construction of an ileal reservoir and restorative proctectomy in complex cases presenting with combined megacolon and megarectum.

MP

Chapter 6.2
Managing Slow-Transit Constipation

JOHANN PFEIFER

History

In 1908, Sir Arbuthnot Lane published the first series of abdominal procedures for the treatment of chronic intractable constipation (1). He postulated that "autointoxication" (caused by chronic constipation) was responsible for a large number of diseases in the population of London, such as, "dilatation of the stomach, peptic ulceration, mobility of the kidney and degenerative changes of the breasts." His advocacy of colectomy for constipation is still a controversial issue among specialist surgeons dealing with this problem. Over recent decades, there have been a variety of physiological tests designed in part to improve our understanding of the pathophysiology of constipation, where it was realized that there is indeed a small group of patients with this chronic complaint who can benefit from surgery. The aim of this chapter is to summarize the indications for and results of surgery in adult patients presenting with severe and intractable slow-transit constipation.

Introduction

Constipation is one of the most frequent gastrointestinal symptoms and one of the most common reasons for medical consultation. Broadly, constipation can be related to intestinal motility disorders, pelvic floor disturbances, or a combination of both, although the exact origin of these disorders (and the interplay of factors responsible for their chronicity) is not yet fully understood.

The definition of constipation is sometimes difficult, as physicians and patients have different opinions about what constitutes constipation. Patients often include such subjective feelings as incomplete evacuation, abdominal or rectal pain, firm stool consistency, and the repeated need for straining. Probably the best definition for constipation was proposed by Whitehead and colleagues (2), where two or more of the following complaints must be present when the patient is not taking laxatives and where symptoms must have persisted for at least 12 months; namely:

1. Straining on ≥25% of bowel movements
2. Feeling of incomplete evacuation after ≥25% of bowel movements
3. Scyballous stools on ≥25% of bowel movements
4. Stools less frequent than two per week with or without other symptoms of constipation.

Objective scoring recently has been introduced to standardize the clinical presentation and severity of chronic constipation, and although these systems have been validated in specialized clinical practice, they have not yet been widely adopted or utilized as discriminants in the decision for surgery (3,4).

Initial Assessment

History

A detailed history addressing the specifics of bowel activities, as well as the medication profile, must be obtained from constipated patients. Extracolonic causes for constipation must be excluded systematically before applying terms such as "functional disorder" or "idiopathic constipation." Table 6.2-1 shows a veritable legion of extracolonic causes that may play a role in the patient's presentation with this symptom. The scoring systems (alluded to above) provide a much more detailed and objective assessment, as they include more variables than just stool frequency and stool consistency; however, it must be remembered that constipation is a symptom and not a disorder. Several authors report higher rates of constipation in patients after hysterectomy (5).

Physical Examination

The first step is inspection of the anus and the perianal area, as well as a digital examination. During rectal digitations, the patient should be asked to squeeze, push down, and to relax. With this simple test, it often is easy to diagnose pelvic outlet obstruction caused by non-relaxation of the pelvic floor muscles. The next step is a proctoscopy without any preliminary bowel preparation. As patients with slow-transit constipation typically complain of diffuse abdominal pain and bloating, the abdomen should be inspected and palpated. Examination also will reveal a rectocele by turning the examining digit through 180 degrees and inspecting the posterior vaginal wall (6), and bimanual examination in the standing position during a Valsalva maneuver will be suggestive of an attendant enterocele (7).

TABLE 6.2-1. Extracolonic causes for constipation.

Endocrine and metabolic:	Diabetes mellitus
	Glycagonoma
	Hypercalcemia
	Hyperparathyroidism
	Hypokalemia
	Hypopituitarism
	Hypothyroidism
	Milk—alkali—syndrome
	Pheochromocytoma
	Porphyria
	Pregnancy
	Uremia
Neurologic Cerebral	Parkinson's disease
	Stroke
	Tumors
Spinal	Cauda equina tumor
	Ischemia
	Iatrogenic
	Meningocele
	Multiple sclerosis
	Paraplegia
	Shy—Drager syndrome
	Tabes dorsalis
	Trauma
Peripheral	Autonomic neuropathy
	Chagas disease
	Multiple endocrine neoplasia, Type 2B
	Von Recklinghausen's disease
Drugs	Anesthetics
	Analgesic
	Antacids (calcium and aluminium compounds)
	Anticholinergics
	Anticonvulsants
	Antidepressants
	Anti-Parkinsonians
	Barium sulfate
	Calcium channel blockers
	Diuretics
	Ganglion blockers
	Hematinics (iron)
	Hypotensives
	Laxative abuse
	Monoamono oxidase (MAO) inhibitors
	Metals (arsenic, lead, mercury, phosphorus)
	Opiates
	Paralytic agents
	Psychotherapeutics
Myopathy	Amyloidosis
	Dermatomyositis
	Myotonic dystrophy
	Sclerodermia

Clinical Evaluation

A barium enema and/or a colonoscopy should be part of the general evaluation for constipated patients to rule out structural (mechanically obstructive) disorders such as strictures, polyps, or cancer. We also perform screening abdominal sonography to exclude other intra-abdominal diseases that might present clinically as constipation. Blood chemistry—especially serum calcium and potassium levels, as well as thyroxine levels—also should be performed. Defecography (see Chapter 3.1) has a specialized place in proctological practice to assess rectal evacuation for the specific diagnoses of rectocele, enterocele, rectoanal intussusception, and occult rectal prolapse.

Initial Therapy

Conservative Treatment

The initial treatment of chronic constipation is always conservative and involves three main elements: general health issues, high-fiber diet, and medications (laxatives and enemas). General health issues are physical training (e.g., jogging, hiking, and gymnastics) and enough fluid intake (at least 1.5 to 2 liters per day). Furthermore, patients should be informed that physiological bowel activity is high in the morning after getting up and they should be encouraged to invoke the "gastrocolic reflex" by providing enough time after breakfast for evacuation ("toilet training"). Sometimes suppositories that increase rectal contractility can augment this reflex.

One of the best therapy options for increasing colon transit time is a high-fiber diet, which, in some patients, may increase cramping and bloating. In patients with an irritable bowel syndrome, a low-fiber diet is preferred. Medication for constipation consists of laxatives and cathartics, stool softeners, and agents affecting neurotransmission. Long-term use of oral stimulant laxatives (bisacodyl, phenolphthalein, cascara, senna) is best avoided due to the risk of electrolyte disturbances and damage to the colon. Probably the best laxative for chronic constipation is Macrogol [polyethylene glycol (PEG) with a molecular mass exceeding 3000]. It is inert and practically nonabsorbable. Further advantages include its lack of intestinal enzymatic degradation or bacterial metabolism and its water-binding capacity, and even long-term therapy does not appear to result in any significant side effects—a feature that is especially advantageous in cardiac and renal patients (8).

Advanced Assessment

Only if all of these basic tests fail to reveal a specific diagnosis and if the above-mentioned conservative therapy fails to produce improvement is a more exact and time-consuming physiological work up required.

Colonic Motility Study (See Chapter 2.7)

A radiopaque marker study is the least expensive examination available and is the easiest to perform; it is also the most informative and most commonly used colonic motility test. The markers are ingested and the time to arrival in the rectum is evaluated by serial abdominal X-rays. In normal subjects, 80% of the markers are passed by the fifth post-ingestion day and all are expelled by Day 7. Intraluminal measurements of colonic myoelectrical and motor functions are still experimental.

Anorectal Manometry

With anorectal manometry, resting and squeeze pressures, as well as the length of the high-pressure zone (HPZ), and especially the rectoanal inhibitory reflex (RAIR), can be assessed. The absence of the latter is characteristic of some young adolescent patients presenting late with short-segment Hirschsprung's disease (HD) in the absence of previous rectal surgery. Furthermore, anal sensitivity, urge to evacuate, and rectal capacity can be estimated.

Defecography

Defecography, a dynamic study, is especially useful for diagnosing outlet obstructions; however, defecography reveals abnormalities in as many as 50% of asymptomatic individuals. Considering significant findings worthy of extensive conservative (biofeedback) or surgical treatment, defecographic findings are considered reliable and reproducible in 87.9% of patients (9).

Electromyography (EMG) and Pudendal Nerve Terminal Motor Latency (PNTML)

The most common technique comprises placement of fine wire electrodes into the external anal sphincter (EAS) and puborectalis muscle. In non-constipated individuals, decreased EMG activity is seen during straining and, conversely, increased firing of motor potentials is noted during squeezing. Paradoxical puborectalis contraction during straining can be seen in patients with functional pelvic outlet symptoms. A more elegant, less painful, and equally reliable method involving plug electrodes has recently been described (10). Complete sphincter studies also should include measurement of the PNTML as described by Swash and Henry (11); however, the interpretation of a prolonged PNTML as a prognostic marker in such patients still remains controversial (12).

Other Tests

For the evaluation of constipated patients, many other tests have been proposed, such as the balloon expulsion test (13,14), balloon proctography, ultrasonography, magnetic resonance imaging (MRI), perineometry, scintigraphic assessment of transit time and/or of rectal evacuation, mechanical and electrical stimulation of sensation, as well as evoked potentials by rectal or cerebral stimulation (15). It is worth mentioning that no single test alone is pathognomonic, and therefore the diagnosis of functional disorders must be based upon interpretation of several tests. Especially when surgery is considered, physiologic investigation is mandatory to achieve the desirable postoperative outcome (16).

Small bowel transit studies have recently demonstrated that there might be two different kinds of idiopathic slow-transit constipation (17). One involves just the colon and the other involves the entire gastrointestinal tract [gastrointestinal dysmotility (GID)]. Long-term surgical results after colectomy are much worse in patients with GID when compared with patients with solely colonic slow-transit constipation (17). Patients with a panenteric dysmotility may have either anatomical (morphological) (18,19) or functional disturbances. The latter include changes in gastric emptying and biliary function (20). Additional upper gastrointestinal (GI) evaluation should therefore be done when colon transit studies show colonic inertia to exclude this subgroup of patients with GID, as this may have a direct bearing on surgery. Figure 6.2.1 shows a recommended algorithm approach to this disorder.

Interpretation of Results

If no structural cause for constipation is identified, a transit study should be performed. If transit is normal, the pelvic floor should be evaluated. After diagnostic evaluation, constipation can be categorized for surgery as follows:

1. (a) Colonic inertia (CI) or slow-transit constipation with/without megabowel
   (b) Colonic inertia (CI) or slow-transit constipation as part of a comprehensive gut dysmotility syndrome (GID)

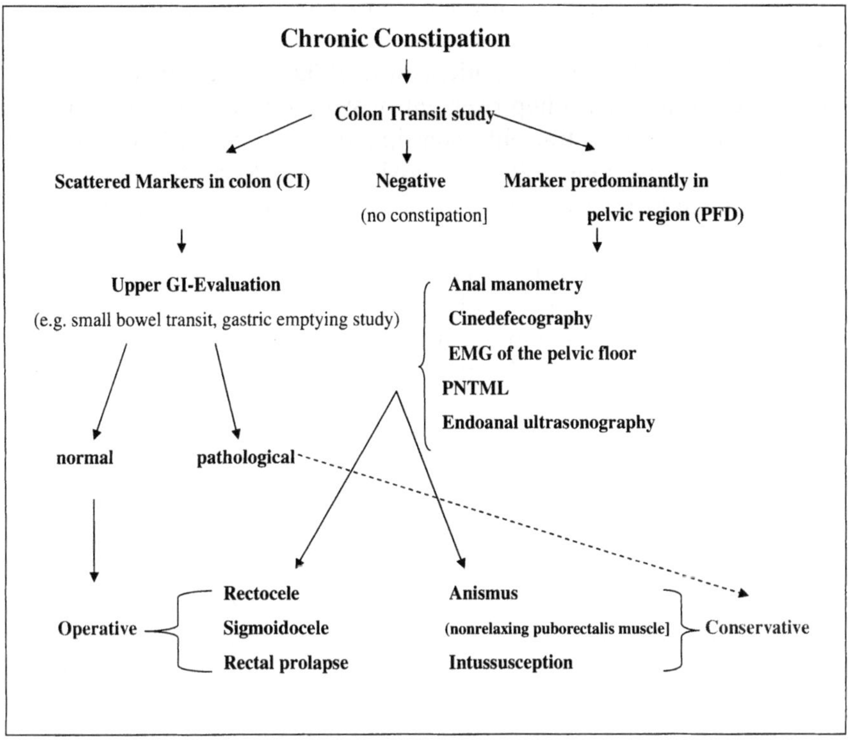

FIGURE 6.2.1. Algorithm for evaluation and treatment of chronic constipation. CI, colonic inertia; PFD, pelvic floor dysfunction; PNTML, pudendal nerve terminal motor latency.

2. (a) Pelvic floor dysfunction (PFD) with anatomical abnormalities (HD, perineal descent, rectocele, sigmoidocele, intussusception, rectal prolapse, etc.)
   (b) Pelvic floor dysfunction (PFD) without anatomical abnormalities (paradoxical puborectalis contraction, levator spasm, anismus, rectal pain)
3. Combined slow-transit constipation and PFD
4. Normal transit constipation [probably due to irritable bowel disease (IBS)]

Advanced Therapy

Conservative Treatment

If routine conservative therapy fails, a supervised diary of bowel habits during a regime including a high-fiber diet, fluid intake, and special medication can provide guidance for altering and adjusting the appropriate conservative treatment.

Biofeedback as therapy for patients with PFD is an accepted treatment tool. Recently, long-term improvement of symptoms also was reported in patients with severe intractable constipation. In a mixed group of 100 patients (65% slow transit; 59% paradoxical pelvic floor contraction), 55% felt that biofeedback had helped and 57% felt that their constipation was improved (21).

One cannot overlook the psychological component in many of these constipated patients. If an operation for a functional disorder is planned, there should be a preoperative psychiatric work up, including the Minnesota Multiphasic Personality Inventory (MMPI). Another interesting, semi-conservative approach recently published by the St. Mark's group is the use of sacral nerve stimulation. Eight women with proven slow-transit constipation were implanted with a temporary percutaneous stimulating S3 electrode for three weeks. Although colon transit time did not return to normal in any patient, two patients reported cessation or marked diminution of symptoms, including normalization of bowel frequency. In particular, rectal sensory threshold to distension was decreased (22).

Surgery should always be the last option in a highly selected group of patients suffering from pure CI. Surgery should never be performed on patients with GID. It must be stressed that the surgeon should not let him/herself be forced by the patient or relatives into performing an operation for pain and bloating, as surgery will not alleviate these disorders.

Recommendations and Indications

Surgical Treatment for Colonic Inertia with/without Megabowel

Antegrade Colonic Enema (ACE) (Malone Procedure)

In 1990, Malone described a washout technique for the colon in children using the appendix stump as a stoma sutured to the skin (23). There are only a few reports in the literature on the use of this technique in adult patients with intractable constipation. Hill reported 6 patients who received antegrade enemas with saline or phosphate enemas every 48 to 72 hours. The symptoms could be resolved in 4 patients and improved in 2 patients. The main problem was skin-level stenosis of the stoma in 50% requiring repeated dilatation. Hill concluded that this procedure might be especially suitable for patients with pelvic floor weakness who would be at risk of developing fecal incontinence if subtotal colectomy (STC) with ileorectal anastomosis (IRA) were performed (24).

Baeten and colleagues reported 12 patients (8 females) with intractable constipation in whom either the appendix or the distal ileum was used as the colon conduit. Although constipation scores could be markedly reduced (21.5 reduced to 5.5), 4 patients eventually required STC and IRA. The advantage of this approach is that this minimally invasive procedure does not compromise further surgery if needed (25). Other colonic conduits described are located in the transverse and sigmoid colon with mixed results (26). Gerharz, who applied this method to 16 patients with different pathologic conditions, concluded that, in adults, the Malone procedure is associated with a high failure rate due to stoma complications, wound infections, pain, and psychological problems (27).

Subtotal Colectomy

In megabowel, the dilated bowel caliber often precludes stapling of the distal rectal stump. Because of the size discrepancy between the dilated rectum and the small caliber small bowel, a hand-sutured anastomosis usually will be required. Subtotal colectomy with IRA is the standard operation for patients with colonic inertia with or without megabowel. The reported success rates are listed in Table 6.2-2 (17,28–45). In recent studies, an equivalent success rate was seen for a laparoscopic- (hand-) assisted approach as for conventional treatment, whereby the former approach resulted in shorter postoperative ileus and hospital stay, earlier return to work, and better cosmesis (41).

Assessment of the literature concerning the role of STC and IRA in chronic constipation reveals some salient points. A combination of functional colonic inertia and outlet obstruction seems to be associated with a poorer outcome in patients who have undergone surgery (46). Furthermore, a good postoperative outcome can be expected for patients with normal rectal sensation; however, Nyam et al., reporting the experience of the Mayo clinic, failed to identify any differences in the outcome in patients with (22 patients) or without (52 patients) concomitant PFD (40). In the study by Pluta and colleagues (36), 24 patients underwent STC and IRA for chronic constipation with an overall success rate of 71%, and all of the patients who complained of either pain or bloating before the operation noted continued postoperative persistence of these symptoms. Moreover, half of the patients had a documented psychiatric disorder and in only 2 of 12 patients in this subgroup were surgeries successful. Thus, the success rate was over 90% in patients without psychiatric disorders, but only 17% with such a history.

A recent report by FitzHarris addresses the problem of quality of life following STC for CI (45). Seventy-five patients out of 112 answered the quality of life questionnaire in this study. Even if the vast majority (93%) stated that they would undergo surgery again, 41% still complained of abdominal pain, 21% of incontinence, and 46% of occasional diarrhea after operation. A further interesting study by Redmond et al. (17) discussed 37 patients with CI. All patients underwent evaluation of the upper and lower GI tract. In this study, 21 patients (18 female, 3 male) were found to have abnormalities limited to the lower GI tract (CI). The 16 patients (all female)

TABLE 6.2-2. Subtotal colectomy (STC) with ileorectal anastomosis (IRA) with/without megacolon (MC).

Author	Year	*n*	Female %	Mean age	Follow up (years)	No megacolon	Success %	Megacolon	Success %
Preston (28)	1984	8	100	26	5.7	8	63	—	—
Barnes (29)	1986	6	43	38	5.0	—	—	6	67
Akervall (30)	1988	12	100	39	3.4	12	66	—	—
Kamm (31)	1988	33	100	34	2.0	33	50	—	—
Yoshioka (32)	1989	40*	98	35	3.0	32	58+	8	58+
Pena (33)	1992	105	91	43	8.0	78	89	—	—
Takahashi (34)	1994	38°	—	—	3.0	37	97	—	—
Redmond (17)	1995	34	92	43	7.5	34	90~,13#	—	—
Piccirillo (35)	1995	54	78	49	2.2	54	94	—	—
Pluta (36)	1996	24	—	—	—	—	71	—	—
Ghosh (37)	1996	21	90	46	8.0	—	29 &	—	—
Christiansen (38)	1996	12	—	—	—	—	83	—	—
De Graaf (39)	1996	24	83	47	—	—	33	—	—
Nyam (40)	1997	74	92	53	4.6	74	97	—	—
Schiedeck (41)	1999	3	100	60	2.0	3	66.6	—	—
Fan (42)	2000	24	79	37	1.9	24	87.5	—	—
Pikarsky (43)	2001	30	70	49	8.8	30	83	—	—
Athanasakis % (44)	2001	4	100	47	0.7	4	100	—	—
FitzHarris (45)	2003	112	97	n.a	n.a	112	93	—	—

* 34 IRA, 5 coecorectal, 1 ileosigmoidal anastomosis(ISA); + overall success; ° IRA or ISA; ~ for colonic inertia; # for gastrointestinal dysmotility; & not a single complication in the long run; % laparoscopic assisted colectomy.
n.a = not available.

with abnormalities in the lower and upper GI tract were thought to have gastrointestinal dysmotility with colonic predominance (GID).

Thirty-four patients underwent STC with IRA and three patients had a subtotal colectomy with an end ileostomy. At a mean follow-up of seven and a half years, there had been 3 deaths due to unrelated causes. Bowel frequency per week in the CI group increased from 1.7 per week preoperatively to 36 per week after 6 months. After one year, the frequency declined to 23 per week and remained constant for up to 10 years. Colonic inertia patients thus had a successful long-term outcome of 90%. In comparison, among patients with a mixed gastrointestinal dysmotility pattern, although after one year only 12% were constipated, within 5 years the prevalence had risen to 80%. Thus, the ultimate success in the GID group was only a rather unacceptable 13%.

Segmental Resections

Segmental resection of the colon has been associated with poor results. Partial resection of the colon usually is followed by recurrent constipation, which may in part be due to dilatation of the remaining colon. Idiopathic megasigmoid would seem to be the best indication for sigmoid resection (47,48). The procedure is especially promising when there is a long sigmoid colon with a likelihood of volvulus formation.

Isolated left-sided colectomy has usually produced poor results. However, DeGraaf et al. provided a recent update on segmental vs. subtotal colectomy (39). Based on segmental colon transit times, patients were foreseen either for segmental resection or STC. Twenty-four patients underwent STC and 18 underwent left-sided segmental resection. In this series, segmental resection was successful in 12 of 18 patients, but STC was only successful in 8 of 24. This report, however, fails to mention upper GI evaluation. Firstly, patients in the subtotal colectomy group may have had a comprehensive GID disorder rather than isolated CI. Moreover, both the 67% success rate after segmental resection and the 33% success rate after STC are far below expectations.

Lundin and Pahlman (49) presented another interesting work involving 28 patients. Their selection criteria for the type of surgery included a prolonged segmental transit time based on oral ^{111}In-labelled diethylenetriamine pentaacetic acid (DTPA) scintigraphic transit study. After a median of 50 months, 23 patients (81.1%) were pleased with the result. The conclusion of the authors was that impaired rectal sensation might predict poor outcome. Now, we find that segmental resection still has a limited role in the treatment of constipation and should not be offered to patients with inertia (Table 6.2-3).

In a limited number of patients, there has been a good success rate for proctocolectomy with formation of an ileoanal pouch (Table 6.2-4).

TABLE 6.2-3. Segmental colectomy with/without megacolon (MC).

Author	Year	n	Female %	Mean age	Follow up (years)	Success %
Jennings (50)	1967	8	—	—	—	13
Lane (51)	1977	2	—	—	8	50
		6*	—	—	—	16
Smith (52)	1977	1	0	16	2	100
McCready (47)	1979	13	—	—	—	85
		4*	—	—	9.2	75
Hughes (53)	1981	5	0	—	—	100
Belliveau (54)	1982	7	—	—	5.4	85
		1*	—	—	5.4	100
Preston (28)	1984	5	100	35	5	20
Jurvinen (55)	1985	1	0	36	—	100
Barnes (29)	1986	4	43	38	5	50
Gasslander (56)	1987	2	100	36	2	50
Coremans (48)	1990	2	100	34	3.2	100
Kamm (57)	1991	2	100	20	2.5	100
Keighley (58)	1992	2	—	—	—	50
Stabile (59)	1992	7	30	19	1	71
De Graaf (39)	1996	18	83	47		66
You (60)	1999	40	—	—	2	92
Lundin (49)	2002	28	93	52	4,2	82

* Megacolon.

Complications

While standard complications such as bleeding, wound infection, and anastomotic leakage may occur after any bowel operation, the most common complication in patients who have undergone bowel resection for constipation is small bowel obstruction. Pfeifer et al. reported in a summary of 25 publications an overall small bowel obstruction rate of 18%, 12% of whom required surgical therapy (46). Recent advances in adhesion prevention have included the development of Seprafilm® (Genzyme

TABLE 6.2-4. Ileoanal pouch operation for constipation.

Author	Year	*N*	Follow up (years)	Success (%)	Complications (%)
Nicholls (61)	1988	2	0.6	100	100
Yoshioka (32)	1989	6	—	70	50
Hosie (62)	1990	13	1.8	85	38
Keighley (63)	1993	6	—	83	17
		10	—	70	50
Stewart (64)	1994	18	6	78	17
		14	6	71	36
Brown (65)	1997	2	—	100	—
O'Suilleabhain (66)	2001	3	3.6	100	n.a.

n.a. = not available.

Corporation, Cambridge, MA), a composite bioresorbable membrane of sodiumhyalurinate and carboxymethylcellulose. In a prospective randomized surgeon-blinded series of 183 patients undergoing ileal pouch anal anastomosis, a 50% reduction in the incidence of adhesions was noted as compared to the control group (67). There was a similar significant decrease in the severity and extent of adhesions. Patients undergoing STL for constipation can receive Seprafilm at the time of fascial closure. In this way, complications due to adhesions could perhaps be diminished significantly in the future. The postoperative rate of recurrent constipation or fecal incontinence, as well as the use of laxatives or anti-diarrheal medication, is still unpredictable, but the complication rate after STC and IRA for various indications is generally acceptable (68).

Stoma

The potential result of surgery for constipation is the ultimate construction of a stoma. A stoma may be preferentially offered as an initial procedure to patients with psychiatric disorders, as well as to those with inertia combined with refractory pelvic outlet obstruction, or with significant pain and/or bloating. Patients who remain constipated after colectomy may well prefer a functioning stoma to a nonfunctioning anus.

Conclusion

Patients with intractable chronic constipation should be evaluated with physiological tests after structural disorders and extracolonic causes have been excluded. Conservative treatment options should be tried until they are exhausted. If surgery is indicated, STC with IRA is the treatment method of choice, although segmental resection may be a good option for isolated megasigmoid, sigmoidocele, or recurrent sigmoid volvulus. In general, patients with GID should not be offered any surgical options because of their anticipated poor results. Moreover, patients with psychiatric disorders should be actively discouraged from resection, as they tend to have a poorer prognosis. Patients must be counseled that preoperative pain and/or bloating will likely persist, even if surgery normalizes bowel frequency. Patients with associated problems may be served better by having a stoma without resection as both a therapeutic maneuver and a diagnostic trial. Colectomy is not a treatment option for pain and/or abdominal bloating.

References

1. Lane WA. Results of the operative treatment of chronic constipation. BMJ. 1908;1:1126–30.
2. Whitehead WE, Chaussade S, Corazziari E, and Kumar D. Report of an international workshop on management of constipation. Gastroenterol Int. 1991;4:99–113.

3. Agachan F, Chen T, Pfeifer J, Reissman P, and Wexner SD. A constipation scoring system to simplify evaluation and management of constipated patients. Dis Colon Rectum. 1996;39:681–5.
4. Knowles CH, Eccersley AJ, Scott SM, Walker S, Reeves B, and Lunniss PJ. Linear discriminant analysis of symptoms in patients with chronic constipation: validation of a new scoring system (KESS). Dis Colon Rectum. 2000;43:1419–26.
5. Martinelli E, Altomare DF, Rinaldi M, and Portincasa P. Constipation after hysterectomy: fact or fiction? Eur J Surg. 2000;166:356–68.
6. Heslop JH. Piles and rectoceles. Aust N Z J Surg. 1987;57:935–8.
7. Nichols DH and Randall CL. Enterocele. In: Nichols, DH, editor. Vaginal surgery. Baltimore: Williams & Wilkins; 1996. pp. 319–20.
8. Hammer H, Hammer J, and Gasche Ch. Polyäthylenglykol (Macrogol)—Übersicht über seine pharmakologischen Eigenschaften und seine Verwendung in der Diagnostik und Therapie gastroenterologischer Erkrankungen. Wien Klin Wochenschr. 2000;112:53–60.
9. Pfeifer J, Oliveira L, Park UC, Gonzales A, Agachan F, and Wexner SD. Are interpretation of video defecographies reliable and reproducible? Int J Colorectal Dis. 1997;12:67–72.
10. Pfeifer J, Teoh T-A, Salanga VD, Agachan F, and Wexner SD. Comparative study between intra-anal sponge and needle electrode for electromyographic evaluation of constipated patients. Dis Colon Rectum. 1998;41:1153–7.
11. Henry MM, Parks AG, and Swash M. The pelvic floor musculature in the descending perineum syndrome. Br J Surg. 1982;69:470–2.
12. Kiff ES, Barnes RPH, and Swash M. Evidence of pudendal nerve neuropathy in patients with perineal descent and chronic straining at stool. Gut. 1984; 25:1279–82.
13. Fleshman JW, Dreznik Z, Cohen E, Fry RD, and Kodner IJ. Balloon expulsion test facilitates diagnosis of pelvic floor outlet obstruction due to nonrelaxing puborectalis muscle. Dis Colon Rectum. 1992;35:1019–25.
14. Fleshman JW. Balloon expulsion. In: Smith LE, editor. Practical guide to anorectal testing. 2nd ed. New York: Igaku-Shoin; 1995. pp. 23–6.
15. Speakman CTM, Kamm MA, and Swash M. Cerebral evoked potentials—are they of value in anorectal disease? Gut. 1990;31:A1173.
16. Wexner SD, Daniel N, and Jagelman DG. Colectomy for constipation: physiologic investigation is the key to success. Dis Colon Rectum. 1991;34:851–6.
17. Redmond JM, Smith GW, Barofsky I, Ratych RE, Goldsborough DC, and Schuster M. Physiological tests to predict long term outcome of total abdominal colectomy for intractable constipation. Am J Gastroenterol. 1995;90:748–53.
18. Wedel T, Roblick UJ, Ott V, Eggers R, Schiedeck TH, Krammer HJ, and Bruch HP. Oligoneuronal hypoganglionosis in patients with idiopathic slow-transit constipation. Dis Colon Rectum. 2001;45:54–62.
19. Voderholzer WA, Wiebecke B, Gerum M, and Muller-Lissner SA. Dysplasia of the submucous nerve plexus in slow-transit constipation of adults. Eur J Gastroenterol Hepatol. 2000;12:755–9.
20. Altomare DF, Portincasa P, Rinaldi M, Di Ciaula A, Martinelli E, Amoroso A, Palasciano G, and Memeo V. Slow-transit constipation: solitary symptom of a systemic gastrointestinal disease. Dis Colon Rectum. 1999;42:231–40.

21. Chiotakakou-Faliakou E, Kamm MA, Roy AJ, Storrie JB, and Turner IC. Biofeedback provides long-term benefit for patients with intractable, slow, and normal transit constipation. Gut. 1998;42:517–21.
22. Malouf AJ, Wiesel PH, Nicholls T, Nicholls RJ, and Kamm MA. Short-term effects of sacral nerve stimulation for idiopathic slow transit constipation. World J Surg. 2002;26:166–70.
23. Malone PS, Ransley PG, and Kiely EM. Preliminary report: the antegrade continence enema. Lancet. 1990;336:1217–8.
24. Hill J, Stott S, and MacLennan I. Antegrade enemas for the treatment of severe idiopathic constipation. Br J Surg. 1994;81:1490–1.
25. Rongen MJ, van der Hoop AG, and Baeten CG. Cecal access for antegrade colon enemas in medically refractory slow-transit constipation: a prospective study. Dis Colon Rectum. 2001;44:1644–9.
26. Eccersley AJ, Maw A, and Williams NS. Comparative study of two sites of colonic conduit placement in the treatment of constipation due to rectal evacuatory disorders. Br J Surg. 1999;86:647–50.
27. Gerharz EW, Vik V, Webb G, Leaver R, Shah PJR, and Woodhouse RJ. The value of the MACE (malone antegrade colonic enema) Procedure in adult patients. J Am Coll Surg. 1997;185:544–7.
28. Preston DM, Hawley PR, Lennard-Jones JE, and Todd IP. Results of colectomy for severe idiopathic constipation in women (Arbuthnot Lane's disease). Br J Surg. 1984;71:547–52.
29. Barnes PR, Lennard-Jones JE, Hawley PR, and Todd IP. Hirschsprung's disease and idiopathic megacolon in adults and adolescents. Gut. 1986;27:534–41.
30. Akervall S, Fasth S, Nordgren S, Oreslund T, and Hulten L. The functional results after colectomy and ileorectal anastomosis for severe constipation (Arbuthnot Lane's disease) as related to rectal sensory function. Int J Colorectal Dis. 1988;3:96–101.
31. Kamm MA, Hawley PR, and Lennard-Jones JE. Outcome of colectomy for severe idiopathic constipation. Gut. 1988;29:969–73.
32. Yoshioka K and Keighley MR. Clinical results of colectomy for severe constipation. Br J Surg. 1989;76:600–4.
33. Pena JP, Heine JA, Wong WD, Christenson CE, and Balcos EG. Subtotal colectomy for constipation—a long term follow up study [abstr]. Dis Colon Rectum. 1992;35:P19.
34. Takahashi T, Fitzgerald SD, and Pemberton JH. Evaluation and treatment of constipation. Rev Gastroenterol Mex. 1994;59:133–8.
35. Piccirillo MF, Reissman P, and Wexner SD. Colectomy as treatment for constipation in selected patients. Br J Surg. 1995;82:898–901.
36. Pluta H, Bowes KL, and Jewell LD. Long-term results of total abdominal colectomy for chronic idiopathic constipation. Value of preoperative assessment. Dis Colon Rectum. 1996;39:160–6.
37. Ghosh S, Papachrysostomou M, Batool M, and Eastwood MA. Long-term results of subtotal colectomy and evidence of noncolonic involvement in patients with idiopathic slow-transit constipation. Scand J Gastroenterol. 1996;31:1083–91.
38. Christiansen J and Rasmussen OO. Colectomy for severe slow-transit constipation in strictly selected patients. Scand J Gastroenterol. 1996;31:770–3.

39. DeGraaf EJR, Gilberts LAM, and Schouten WR. Role of colonic transit time studies to select patients with slow transit constipation for partial left-sided or subtotal colectomy. Br J Surg. 1996;83:648–51.
40. Nyam DC, Pemberton JH, Ilstrup DM, and Rath DM. Long-term results of surgery for chronic constipation. Dis Colon Rectum. 1997;40:273–9.
41. Schiedeck TH, Schwandner O, and Bruch HP. Laparoscopic therapy of chronic constipation. Zentralbl Chir. 1999;124:818–24.
42. Fan CW and Wang JY. Subtotal colectomy for colonic inertia. Int Surg. 2000;85:309–12.
43. Pikarsky AJ, Singh JJ, Weiss EG, Nogueras JJ, and Wexner SD. Long-term follow-up in patients undergoing colectomy for colonic inertia. Dis Colon Rectum. 2001;44:179–83.
44. Athanasakis H, Tsiaoussis J, Vassilakis JS, and Xynos E. Laparoscopically assisted subtotal colectomy for slow-transit constipation. Surg Endosc. 2001; 15:1090–2.
45. FitzHarris GP, Garcia-Aguilar J, Parker SC, Bullard KM, Madoff RD, Goldberg SM, and Lowry A. Quality of life after subtotal colectomy for slow-transit constipation: the quality and quantity count. Dis Colon Rectum. 2003;46:433–40.
46. Pfeifer J, Agachan F, and Wexner SD. Surgery for constipation: a review. Dis Colon Rectum. 1996;39:444–60.
47. McCready RA, Grace RH, and Todd IP. Organic constipation in adults. Br J Surg. 1977;64:305–10.
48. Coremans GE. Surgical aspects of severe chronic non-Hirschsprung's constipation. Hepatogastroenterology. 1990;37:588–95.
49. Lundin E, Karlbom U, Pahlman L, and Graf W. Outcome of segmental colonic resection for slow-transit constipation. Br J Surg. 2002;89:1270–4.
50. Jennings PJ. Megarectum and megacolon in adolescents and young adults: results of treatment at St. Mark's hospital. J R Soc Med. 1967;60:805–6.
51. Lane RH and Todd IP. Idiopathic megacolon: a review of 42 cases. Br J Surg. 1977;64:305–10.
52. Smith B, Grace RH, and Todd IP. Organic constipation in adults. Br J Surg. 1977;64:313–4.
53. Hughes ES, McDermott FT, Johnson WR, and Polglase AL. Surgery for constipation. Aust N Z J Surg. 1981;51:144–8.
54. Belliveau P, Goldberg SM, Rothenberger DA, and Nivatvongs S. Idiopathic acquired megacolon: the value of subtotal colectomy. Dis Colon Rectum. 1982;25:118–21.
55. Järvinen HJ and Rintala R. Funnel anus and megacolon in adult. Dis Colon Rectum. 1985;28:957–9.
56. Gasslander T, Larsson J, and Wetterfors J. Experience of surgical treatment for chronic idiopathic constipation. Acta Chir Scand. 1987;153:553–5.
57. Kamm MA, van der Sijp JR, Hawley PR, Phillips RK, and Lennard-Jones JE. Left hemicolectomy with rectal excision for severe idiopathic constipation. Int J Colorectal Dis. 1991;6:49–51.
58. Keighley MR. Megacolon and megarectum. In: Keighley MR and Williams NS, editors. Surgery of the anus, rectum and colon. Vol 1. London: WB Saunders; 1993. pp. 658–73.
59. Stabile G, Kamm MA, Phillips RK, Hawley PR, and Lennard-Jones JE. Partial colectomy and coloanal anastomosis for idiopathic megarectum and megacolon. Dis Colon Rectum. 1992;35:158–62.

60. You YT, Wang JY, Changchien CR, Chen JS, Hsu KC, Tang R, Chiang JM, and Chen HH. Segmental colectomy in the management of colonic inertia. Am Surg. 1998;64:775–7.
61. Nicholls RJ and Kamm MA. Proctocolectomy with restorative ileoanal reservoir for severe idiopathic constipation. Report of two cases. Dis Colon Rectum. 1988;31:968–9.
62. Hosie KB, Kmiot WA, and Keighley MR. Constipation: another indication for restorative proctocolectomy. Br J Surg. 1990 Jul;77:801–2.
63. Keighley MR, Grobler S, and Bain I. An audit of restorative proctocolectomy.
64. Stewart J, Kumar D, and Keighley MR. Results of anal or low rectal anastomosis and pouch construction for megarectum and megacolon. Br J Surg. 1994;81:1051–3.
65. Brown SR and Shorthouse AJ. Restorative proctocolectomy for idiopathic megarectum: postoperative recovery of hypotonic anal sphincters. Report of two cases. Dis Colon Rectum. 1997;40:625–7.
66. O'Sulleabhain CB, Anderson JH, McKee RF, and Finlay IG. Strategy for the surgical management of patients with idiopathic megarectum and megacolon. Br J Surg. 2001;88:1392–6.
67. Becker JM, Dayton MT, Fazio VW, Beck DE, Stryker SJ, Wexner SD, Wolff BG, Roberts PL, Smith LE, Sweeney SA, and Moore M. Prevention of postoperative abdominal adhesions by a sodium hyaluronate-based bioresorbable membrane: a prospective, randomised, double-blind multicenter study. J Am Coll Surg. 1996;183:297–306.
68. Eu KW, Lim SL, Seow-Choen F, Leong AF, and Ho YH. Clinical outcome and bowel function following total abdominal colectomy and ileorectal anastomosis in the Oriental population. Dis Colon Rectum. 1998;41:215–8.

Editorial Commentary

The decision to commit a patient with constipation to surgery is not made lightly. Those with definitive rectal evacuatory dysfunction are probably best served by biofeedback therapy (or perhaps in selected cases neuromodulation protocols) and there should be a strong psychological input on these cases where failure is a particular feature of patients with preexisting psychiatric disorders. It should also be recognized that even when constipation is improved after surgery that many ancillary symptoms such as abdominal pain and distension are unaffected. The role of the ileal pouch-anal anastomosis (IPAA) in megarectum is currently unclear and little data exist to assess the emptying characteristics and the quality of life/functional analysis of reduction rectoplasty performed below an ileorectal anastomosis. Although these patients may have improvement in their physical (and social) functioning, pouch excision for intractable pain postoperatively has recently been reported.

MP

Chapter 6.3
Rectocele

Anders F. Mellgren, Jan Zetterström, and Annika López

A rectocele is an out pocketing of the anterior rectal and posterior vaginal wall into the lumen of the vagina. The vast majority of rectoceles are low, located just above the perineal body (1). The development of rectoceles is not completely understood, but it is assumed that factors associated with pelvic organ prolapse in general also are involved in the formation of rectoceles. Vaginal delivery with damage to the rectovaginal septum and obstructed defecation are probably the two most common underlying risk factors. The neuromuscular lesion is thought to induce muscle weakness and later pelvic floor incompetence with incontinence and prolapse. Mechanical risk factors are associated with vaginal delivery and soft-tissue damage, either as muscle tears or stretching of connective tissues (2). Other risk factors for development of rectoceles include age, pregnancy, estrogen deficiency, obesity, chronic constipation, chronic obstructive lung disease, or other conditions that increase intra-abdominal pressure.

The endopelvic fascia is important for supporting and suspending the pelvic organs, and an underlying abnormality of the connective tissue in this fascia may cause different types of pelvic organ prolapse. The relationship between the fibers and other matrix components is important, as the biomechanical properties are determined by structure and distribution of the various extracellular matrix components (3). Several factors, such as age, mechanical stress, hormones, enzymes and their inhibitors, growth factors, and cytokines, are involved in the regulation of connective tissue metabolism (4). Collagen turnover becomes slower with increasing age (5), but little is known about the impact of age on the endopelvic connective tissue fascia.

Defects within the integrity of the rectogenital (rectovaginal) septum—a homologue of the fascia of Denonvilliers—are postulated in the development of rectoceles, and it is suggested that specific defect repair (either endorectally or transvaginally) is required for correction (6–9). Although there is debate concerning the presence of the septum, recent examinations using histology and immunohistochemistry of plastinated adult and fetal specimens has confirmed its importance (9).

Patient Symptoms

Many rectoceles are asymptomatic; therefore, the prevalence of rectoceles is unknown. Rectoceles have been found in between 20% and 80% of women attending pelvic floor clinics, although these represent biased samples (10) with a high prevalence of a multiplicity of pelvic floor problems in rectocele patients including organ descensus and enterocele (11), particularly when these patients present post hysterectomy (12,13). The most common described symptom of a rectocele is evacuatory difficulty, often including the use of digital manipulation—transvaginally, transperineally, or transrectally—to correct the protruding rectocele to assist defecation during rectal evacuation. Other symptoms associated with rectocele are a feeling of a lump in the vagina, a sensation of rectal pressure or "something coming down," backache, and sexual dysfunction. Rectal pain, rectal bleeding, and anal incontinence also have been attributed to rectoceles (1), although it is recognized that there is a moderately high incidence of coincident anorectal pathology such as hemorrhoids and anterior mucosal rectal prolapse (14).

Emptying difficulties of the rectum and digitation are frequent symptoms in patients with rectoceles. Digital support of the perineum or the posterior wall of the vagina reduces the rectocele and facilitates emptying of stool.

Approximately 50% of women with prolapse seek medical attention with complaints of a sense that something is falling out or because of pelvic pressure (15). These symptoms frequently are reported to be accentuated during the day and relieved by bed rest.

Sexual dysfunction is common in women with pelvic organ prolapse, but the association is unclear, as sexual dysfunction increases with age (16). In a study by Weber et al. (17), the prevalence of sexual dysfunction was not different in a population with pelvic organ prolapse when compared with an age-matched population without prolapse. However, it is important to address this subject because elderly patients may feel embarrassed to bring up this subject with their physician.

Physical Examination

Patients with rectocele also may have other types of pelvic prolapse; therefore, it is important to include a physical examination of all vaginal compartments, as well as a digital rectal examination. It is important that all significant pelvic support defects be recognized and repaired at the same surgical event, even if the rectocele is considered the dominant pathology. It is important that the patient be examined not only in the supine position, but also in a more erect position or standing in order to examine the effect of gravity and pressure of intra-abdominal contents (18,19).

In 1996, the Pelvic Organ Prolapse Quantification (POP-Q) system was adopted for quantification of pelvic organ prolapse (20). Pelvic Organ Prolapse Quantification is easy to learn and it is reproducible (21,22). This system attempts to quantify the mean detectable prolapse score for the relative positions of the cervix and the posterior vaginal fornix, to assess the total vaginal length during provocative maneuvers, such as straining and squatting, and recently has been correlated with dynamic magnetic resonance imaging (MRI) (23).

Preoperative Evaluation

The preoperative evaluation of a woman with rectocele is based on history, physical examination, and defecography. A careful physical examination is important, but even an experienced clinician may have difficulties in making a correct diagnosis, especially if a coexisting enterocele is present (24).

Defecography may be an important help in making a correct diagnosis and may influence the surgical approach. Using contrast media in both the rectum and the vagina, this examination may provide dynamic information of the rectocele at defecation and about possible concomitant pathology such as enterocele (25–28). Defecography may provide information about rectocele size, the degree of emptying, and signs of obstructed defecation (13,24,29–31). The size of the rectocele is determined by measuring the maximum depth of the bulge beyond the projected line of the anterior rectal wall. Small rectoceles tend to be asymptomatic, but there are conflicting reports regarding the correlation between rectocele size or emptying and symptomatology (13,27,31,32). The value of defecography, dynamic MRI, and dynamic transperineal ultrasonography in the diagnosis and surgical decision-making of rectocele is discussed elsewhere in this book.

There is little evidence to suggest that preoperative physiological assessment can categorize adequately these rectoceles and predict where surgery is more likely to be successful (8). It had previously been suggested by Pucciani and colleagues that rectoceles could be divisible into Type I (distension rectoceles), where there was a normal position of the pelvic viscera, but where high resting anorectal pressures were recorded with associated pelvic floor dyssynergia, and Type II (displacement rectoceles) with coincident genital descensus, anal hypotonia, and fecal incontinence (33). Although it is very tempting to use physiology to stereotypically define rectocele patients and to correlate these with clinical rectocele types, there appears little available physiological evidence to support this view (34).

Treatment

Non-Surgical Treatment

Patients with constipation and rectal emptying difficulties may benefit from a high-fiber diet with intake of appropriate amounts of fluids. Paradoxical sphincter reaction (PSR), also called anismus or paradoxical puborectalis contraction, is a frequent finding in patients with rectocele (35). Patients with PSR have a lack of relaxation of the anal sphincters and the puborectalis muscle during straining and rectal evacuation, and this lack of relaxation may inhibit rectal emptying.

Several studies (36,37) have reported success using biofeedback in the treatment of patients with combined rectocele and PSR. Patients attend biofeedback sessions every one to two weeks for up to five sessions and they learn to evacuate the rectum with a normal physiologic response. The physiologic response frequently is measured with electromyography (EMG) or manometry. This subject is addressed in Chapter 6.4.

Paradoxical sphincter reaction also is found in non-constipated patients, and its significance in patients with rectocele is debated. According to some authors (38–40), a failure to recognize PSR might be a cause of poor functional result after rectocele repair. However, in a study by van Dam et al. (41), there was no difference found in symptomatic outcome after rectocele repair between patients with or without PSR. In our clinical practice, patients with a combination of rectocele and PSR usually are offered biofeedback therapy in the first instance before surgical intervention is proposed.

Injection of botulinum toxin also has been advocated for the non-surgical treatment of rectocele and difficult evacuation, but this requires further evaluation before a more consistent use in clinical practice can be advocated (42).

Surgical Treatment (See also Chapters 6.6 and 8)

There are several approaches described for the surgical treatment of rectocele (8). Traditionally, gynecologists have preferred the transvaginal approach, whereas colorectal surgeons have used a transanal or a transperineal approach.

Indications for surgical repair of rectocele vary between institutions, and there are several criteria suggested for selecting patients for surgical repair (38,43,44). Relief of symptoms with vaginal digitation has been suggested to predict a successful surgical outcome (38,44), and other criteria used include lack of emptying of rectocele at defecography and rectocele size larger than four centimeters at defecography (Table 6.3-1), although this latter sign is controversial (45,46).

TABLE 6.3-1. Criteria used for surgical treatment.

Need of rectal and/or vaginal digitation to facilitate rectal evacuation
Lack of emptying of rectocele at defecography.
Rectocele ≥4 cm in diameter at defecography.

Depending on the surgical approach and local traditions, different preoperative protocols for preoperative bowel preparation are used. Some advocate bowel cleansing with polyethylene glycol (PEG) solution or a sodium phosphate preparation, whereas others use a fleet enema or no bowel preparation at all. Preoperative antibiotic prophylaxis frequently is used, and postmenopausal patients may benefit from preoperative local estrogen treatment. Patients generally have a short hospital stay after rectocele repair; the vast majority of patients can be discharged within one to two days postoperatively. Rectocele repair also is performed in an ambulatory setting (47).

Transvaginal Repair

What is clear here is that a greater acceptance of the defect theory of the rectogenital septum in the development and pathogenesis of rectocele has prompted a defect-specific transvaginal repair approach akin to that used endorectally by coloproctologists (48). Traditional transvaginal repair—posterior colpoperineorrhaphy—includes plication of the levator muscles in the midline and redundant vaginal wall resection (14,43,49). A transverse or a rhomboid incision is made at the mucocutaneous border; thereafter, the posterior vaginal wall is incised in the midline to a point cranial to the rectocele and often to the apex of the vagina. The rectovaginal space is then identified and the rectal wall is then separated from the overlying connective tissue of the rectovaginal septum. The connective tissues and the levator muscles are identified, mobilized, and plicated in the midline. The redundant vaginal wall is excised, aiming at reconstructing a vaginal diameter of two to three fingers' width. It is important to avoid a too tight plication of the levator muscles and excessive excision of vaginal wall, as this may cause vaginal narrowing and dyspareunia. The exact role of levatorplasty here is somewhat unclear, where the gynecologic tradition is one of genital support with limited understanding of the effect levatorplasty/plication may have on anorectal function (50,51).

Recently, authors have advocated repair of discrete fascial defects in the rectovaginal septum instead of plicating the levator muscles in the midline (48,52,53). The vagina is separated from the underlying fascia, and the site of the defect in the rectovaginal fascia is defined by an anteriorly directed finger in the rectum. The fascial defect is repaired with plicating sutures and the vaginal epithelium is then re-approximated. However, discrete fascia repair may be associated with a higher recurrence rate and Cundiff et al. (48) reported an 18% anatomic recurrence rate at defecography.

A perineorrhaphy is frequently added to a transvaginal repair. Sutures are placed side-to-side in the lower portion of the reconstructed perineal body including the transverse perineal and the bulbocavernosus muscles. The aim of the perineorrhaphy is to restore an anatomically and physiologically adequate perineal body that in turn increases the distance between the vaginal introitus and the anus. Such an approach is essential when the perineal body is attenuated or if there is an associated anovaginal fistula.

Reported results of transvaginal repair of rectocele are quite good and improvement in defecation symptoms usually is achieved in 60% to 90% of patients (13,43,51,54). The durability of transvaginal rectocele repair is debated. In a study by Kahn and Stanton, 24% of women had recurrent rectoceles on clinical examination after a mean follow-up time of 42 months (51). In a prospective evaluation, our group found that 90% of the operated patients were symptomatically improved five years after the operation (29). Sexual dysfunction in particular frequently is improved after rectocele repair (13,48,51); however, dyspareunia has been identified as a postoperative complaint in 19% to 41% of patients following posterior colporrhaphy (29,43,51,55,56), and this may be attributed to the use of levator muscle plication as part of the procedure.

Rectocele repair is usually a limited procedure and the risk for complications is small. The most common complications are minor, such as hematoma formation, urinary tract infection, or superficial wound infection. Rectovaginal fistula is a serious complication, but it is rare and occurs in less than one percent of operated patients. We would recommend this transvaginal approach when a vaginal incision is being contemplated, such as when there is a concomitant cystocele or in association with a vaginal hysterectomy.

Transperineal Repair

Instead of incising the posterior vaginal wall, access to the rectovaginal septum also may be obtained with a transverse incision in the perineum and dissection in the plane between the external anal sphincter (EAS) and vaginal epithelium. The dissection can be carried out to the top of the rectocele, and then the rectovaginal septum can be strengthened with plication of the levators and/or use of mesh. This avoids the need for a second transperineal incision if an endorectal or transvaginal approach is used where a sphincteroplasty/levatorplasty is needed in the rectocele patient presenting with incontinence (57).

Rectocele Repair Using Artificial Mesh

Augmentation of rectocele repair with mesh or fascia has been used to reduce the risk of recurrence or postoperative dyspareunia. Both transvaginal (58) and transperineal techniques (59) have been used and both absorbable and nonabsorbable mesh have been recommended. A mesh is introduced through the incision used with transvaginal and transperineal repairs. The dissection is carried out in the plane between the EAS and the vaginal epithelium, and it is continued to the upper part of the vagina. The mesh is then placed over the rectovaginal septum and often sutured to fascial structures (sometimes to the levator muscles), and anchored to the perineal body. Some authors also have included approximation of the levator muscles, with dissection of the rectovaginal septum becoming progressively easier in the more rostral position (60).

Watson et al. (58) used Marlex mesh to strengthen the rectovaginal septum in nine women with obstructed defecation. They reported symptomatic improvement in eight of the nine women. Sand et al. (59) compared 73 patients operated with a polyglactin mesh and compared them with 70 patients operated without mesh. No differences in recurrence rates could be demonstrated. An anatomic cure rate of 93% was described recently by Kohli and Miklos (61); however, this study did not include any radiological or symptomatic evaluation.

Use of mesh carries a risk for mesh erosion, which is reported in up to 25% of the operated patients for cystocele (62,63). The use of mesh for rectocele repair still is limited, and further studies are needed to define the risk and the optimal mesh for this use.

Transanal Rectocele Repair

Transanal rectocele repair may be a procedure of lesser magnitude than the gynecologic approach, but the access of high rectoceles may be limited with this approach. The opportunity to address simultaneous vaginal pathology, such as a cystocele, also is limited. The transanal approach is preferred by many colorectal surgeons, as they are experienced operating in this area. Many of their patients also may have other anorectal pathology, such as hemorrhoids (38,64).

During transanal repair, the rectovaginal septum is plicated, while redundant rectal mucosa is resected (65–67). Patients usually are operated in the prone jackknife position with the buttocks taped apart. The rectum is cleaned and exposure achieved with a retractor. The size and location of the rectovaginal defect is confirmed by digital palpation. Frequently, the submucosal plane of the anterior wall is infiltrated with a solution containing epinephrine, and diathermy is used to improve hemostasis. Depending on the type of repair that is to be performed, the defect is plicated longitudinally or transversely with interrupted or continuous absorbable sutures (68–70).

Despite minor technical variations, reported results of this approach are similar and quite good (54,71). Improvement of anorectal symptoms ranges from 30% to 100% in reported series (64–71). There is a small risk of anal incontinence developing after surgery, probably because of distention of the anal canal with the anal retractors. Other complications include bleeding (9%), infection (6%), and rectovaginal fistula (1%–3%) (38,66).

Rectocele Repair Using Circular Stapler

Recently, Altomare et al. (72) described a new technique for rectocele repair using a circular stapler. The rectovaginal septum was opened with a transverse incision between the anus and vagina. The perineal wound and the anus were held open with retractors to control both sides of the rectocele. A transparent anoscope for stapled hemorrhoidectomy (Ethicon EndoSurgery, Cincinnati, OH) was introduced into the anus and two purse strings were prepared. The rectal wall was included anteriorly in the purse strings, whereas only the submucosa was included posteriorly. Then the stapler was fired, taking care to include the full rectal wall anteriorly. Before closing the perineal wound, a levatoroplasty was fashioned.

Eight female patients with symptoms of obstructed defecation and rectocele at defecography were treated. One minor complication was noted. Postoperative defecography showed correction of the rectocele, and all eight patients had significantly improved defecation after a median follow-up of one year.

Enterocele

An enterocele is defined as a peritoneum-lined sac herniating down between the vagina and rectum and filled with abdominal content, often small bowel (9). Enterocele frequently is associated with other anorectal and pelvic floor disorders, such as rectal intussusception, vaginal vault prolapse, cystocele, and rectocele (73).

Etiology

Nichols and Genadry (74) describe four etiologic types of enterocele that can be congenital or acquired. In the latter form, traction enterocele is associated with cystocele and rectocele; pulsion enterocele is associated with prolapse of the vaginal vault and results from increased intra-abdominal pressure. Iatrogenic enteroceles are common. Changes in pelvic anatomy after hysterectomy and changes of the vaginal axis after cystourethropexy may lead to enterocele formation.

It is well known that the peritoneum-lined cul-de-sac occasionally extends caudally between the posterior wall of the vagina and the rectum and sometimes may reach as deep as to the perineal body (9,75). It has been debated whether a deep cul-de-sac predisposes for development of enterocele. Kuhn and Hollyock (76) measured the depth of the cul-de sac in 44 women during laparoscopy. Five of the multiparous women had a clinically diagnosed enterocele. They found no direct relationship between enterocele formation and the depth of the cul-de sac.

However, the development and use of radiological examination techniques in the evaluation of anorectal and pelvic floor disorders have enabled visualization of the peritoneal outline and the alterations in the pelvic peritoneal cavity during defecation (77–79). During examination, the cul-de sac may sometimes be filled with abdominal content and sometimes not. With this knowledge, a common opinion is that a deep cul-de sac may predispose for enterocele formation.

Preoperative Assessment

Typical symptoms of enterocele include a bulge at the introitus, a feeling of pressure, a dragging sensation, or pelvic heaviness especially when standing, walking, or bearing down (80,81). The influence of enterocele on rectal emptying is debated (82), and recent studies have shown no direct relationship between enterocele and rectal emptying difficulties (83).

Enterocele can be diagnosed at gynecologic examination. With the patient in the supine position, a bulge emerging from the upper part of the posterior vaginal wall can be observed when asking the patient to bear down. To distinguish between a rectocele and an enterocele, a bimanual examination with the index finger in the rectum and the thumb in the vagina is performed. While asking the patient to bear down, the enterocele can be palpated, sliding down in between the vaginal and rectal wall. This also can be done with the patient in the standing position.

However, at clinical examination, there are often difficulties to detect an enterocele; therefore, radiological examination techniques are used. At defecography, contrast medium should be administered into the small bowel, vagina, and rectum. Small bowel filled with contrast can be seen between the vaginal and rectal contour. The technique has been developed further by adding contrast medium intraperitoneally, defeco-peritoneography. With this method, the peritoneal outline can be visualized and a deep cul-de-sac, a peritoneocele, with or without bowel can be diagnosed (25,77,84).

Treatment Options

When considering enterocele repair, it is important to evaluate the symptoms and to identify coexisting pelvic floor defects to be able to perform concomitant surgery. Enterocele repair is commonly performed abdominally or transvaginally. The peritoneum-lined sac (the peritoneocele) should be exposed, excised, or obliterated with high ligation (85).

One suture technique, described by Moschowitz (86), applies double purse string sutures placed circumferentially. There are, however, disadvantages with this technique. Suture slippage can leave a small hole centrally and herniation can occur. A risk for kinking the ureter also is described. An alternative method is vertical closure of the cul-de-sac using the technique described by Halban (87).

Enterocele combined with rectal intussusception or rectal prolapse can be corrected with Ripstein rectopexy (88). Recently, Gosselink et al. (85) have described treatment of enterocele by obliteration of the pelvic inlet using Mersilene mesh. Other modified techniques, including laparoscopic techniques, also have been described. Data on success rates are quite limited, and the investigation and treatment of enterocele continues to be a challenge for the physician.

References

1. Brubaker L. Rectocele. Curr Opin Obstet Gynecol. 1996;8:876–9.
2. Smith AR. Role of connective tissue and muscle in pelvic floor dysfunction. Curr Opin Obstet Gynecol. 1994;6:317–19.
3. Ruoslahti E. Proteoglycans in cell regulation. J Biol Chem. 1989;264:13369–72.
4. Kovacs EJ and DiPietro LA. Fibrogenic cytokines and connective tissue production. FASEB J. 1994;8:854–61.
5. Mays PK, McAnulty RJ, Campa JS, and Laurent GJ. Age-related changes in collagen synthesis and degradation in rat tissues. Importance of degradation of newly synthesized collagen in regulating collagen production. Biochem J. 1991;276:307–13.
6. Uhlenluth E, Wolfe WM, Smith EM, and Middleton EB. The rectovaginal septum. Surg Gynecol Obstet. 1948;86:148–63.
7. Ludwikowski B, Hayward IO, and Fritsch H. Rectovaginal fascia: an important structure in pelvic visceral surgery? About its development, structure and function. J Pediatr Surg. 2002;37:634–8.
8. Zbar AP, Lienemann A, Fritsch H, Berr-Gabel M, and Pescatori M. Rectocele: pathogenesis and surgical management. Int J Colorectal Dis. 2003;18:369–84.
9. Aigner F, Zbar AP, Ludwikowski B, Kreczy A, Kovacs P, and Fritsch H. The rectogenital septum: morphology, function and clinical relevance. Dis Colon Rectum. 2004;47:131–40.
10. Porter WE, Steele A, Walsh P, Kohli N, and Karram MM. The anatomic and functional outcomes of defect-specific rectocele repairs. Am J Obstet Gynecol. 1999;181:1353–9.
11. Olsen AL, Smith VJ, Bergstrom JO, Colling JC, and Clark AL. Epidemiology of surgically managed pelvic organ prolapse and urinary incontinence. Obstet Gynecol 1997;89:501–6.
12. DeLancey JO. Anatomic aspects of vaginal eversion after hysterectomy. Am J Obstet Gynecol. 1992;166:1717–24.
13. Kenton K, Shott S, and Brubaker L. The anatomic and functional variability of rectoceles in women. Int Urogynecol J Pelvic Floor Dysfunct. 1999;10:96–9.
14. Pitchford CA. Rectocele:a cause of anorectal pathological changes in women. Dis Colon Rectum. 1967;10:464–6.
15. Theofrastous JP and Swift SE. The clinical evaluation of pelvic floor dysfunction. Obstet Gynecol Clin North Am. 1998;25:783–804.

16. Diokno AC, Brown MB, and Herzog AR. Sexual function in the elderly. Arch Intern Med. 1990;150:197–200.
17. Weber AM, Walters MD, Schover LR, and Mitchinson A. Sexual function in women with uterovaginal prolapse and urinary incontinence. Obstet Gynecol. 1995;85:483–7.
18. Heslop JH. Piles and rectoceles. Aust N Z J Surg. 1987;57:935–8.
19. Nichols DH and Randall CL. Vaginal surgery. 4th ed. Baltimore: Williams & Wilkins; 1996.
20. Bump RC, Mattiasson A, Bo K, et al. The standardization of terminology of female pelvic organ prolapse and pelvic floor dysfunction. Am J Obstet Gynecol. 1996;175:10–17.
21. Hall AF, Theofrastous JP, Cundiff GW, et al. Interobserver and intraobserver reliability of the proposed International Continence Society, Society of Gynecologic Surgeons, and American Urogynecologic Society pelvic organ prolapse classification system [see comments]. Am J Obstet Gynecol. 1996;175:1467–70; discussion 1470–1.
22. Swift SE and Herring M. Comparison of pelvic organ prolapse in the dorsal lithotomy compared with the standing position. Obstet Gynecol. 1998;91:961–4.
23. Hodroff MA, Stolpen AH, Denson MA, Bolinger L, and Kreder KJ. Dynamic magnetic resonance imaging of the female pelvis: the relationship with the Pelvic Organ Prolapse quantification staging system. J Urol. 2002;167:1353–5.
24. Kelvin FM, Maglinte DDT, Hornback JA, and Benson JT. Pelvic prolapse: assessment with evacuation proctography (defecography). Radiology. 1992; 184:547–51.
25. Bremmer S, Mellgren A, Holmström B, Lopez A, and Udén R. Peritoneocele: Visualization with defecography and peritoneography performed simultaneously. Radiology. 1997;202:373–7.
26. Mellgren A, Bremmer S, Johansson C, et al. Defecography, results of investigations in 2816 patients. Dis Colon Rectum 1994;37:1133–41.
27. Kelvin FM, Maglinte DD, and Benson JT. Evacuation proctography (defecography): an aid to the investigation of pelvic floor disorders. Obstet Gynecol. 1994;83:307–14.
28. Kelvin FM, Maglinte DD, Hornback JA, and Benson JT. Pelvic prolapse: assessment with evacuation proctography (defecography). Radiology. 1992;184: 547–51.
29. Lopez A, Anzen B, Bremmer S, et al. Durability of success after rectocele repair. Int Urogynecol J Pelvic Floor Dysfunct. 2001;12:97–103.
30. Mimura T, Roy AJ, Storrie JB, and Kamm MA. Treatment of impaired defecation associated with rectocele by behavorial retraining (biofeedback). Dis Colon Rectum. 2000;43:1267–72.
31. van Dam JH, Ginai AZ, Gosselink MJ, et al. Role of defecography in predicting clinical outcome of rectocele repair. Dis Colon Rectum. 1997;40: 201–7.
32. Van Laarhoven CJHM, Kamm MA, Bartram CI, Halligan S, Hawley PR, and Phillips RKS. Relationship between anatomic and symptomatic long-term results after rectocele repair for impaired defecation. Dis Colon Rectum. 1999;42:204–11.
33. Pucciani F, Rottoli ML, Bologna A, Buri M, Cianchi F, Pagliai P, and Coretsini C. Anterior rectocele and anorectal dysfunction. Int J Colorect Dis. 1996; 11:1–19.

34. Zbar AP, Beer-Gabel M, and Aslam M. Rectoanal inhibition and rectocele: physiology vs. categorization. Int J Colorect Dis. 2001;16:307–12.
35. Mellgren A, Lopez A, Schultz I, and Anzen B. Rectocele is associated with paradoxical anal sphincter reaction. Int J Colorectal Dis. 1998;13:13–16.
36. Bleijenberg G and Kuijpers HC. Treatment of the spastic floor syndrome with biofeedback. Dis Colon Rectum. 1987;30:108–11.
37. Kuijpers JH and Bleijenberg G. Non-surgical treatment for constipation in adults: the place of biofeedback. Neth J Surg. 1991;43:218–21.
38. Sarles JC, Arnaud A, Selezneff I, and Olivier S. Endo-rectal repair of rectocele. Int J Colorectal Dis. 1989;4:167–71.
39. Johansson C, Nilsson BY, Holmström B, Dolk A, and Mellgren A. Association between rectocele and paradoxical sphincter response. Dis Colon Rectum. 1992;35:503–9.
40. Tjandra JJ, Ooi BS, Tang CL, Dwyer P, and Carey M. Transanal repair of rectocele corrects obstructed defecation if it is not associated with anismus. Dis Colon Rectum. 1999;42:1544–50.
41. van Dam JH, Schouten WR, Ginai AZ, Huisman WM, and Hop WC. The impact of anismus on the clinical outcome of rectocele repair. Int J Colorectal Dis. 1996;11:238–42.
42. Maria G, Sganga G, Civello IM, and Brisinda G. Botulinum neurotoxin and other treatments for fissure-in-ano and pelvic floor disorders. Br J Surg. 2002;89:950–61.
43. Mellgren A, Anzén B, Nilsson BY, et al. Results of rectocele repair, a prospective study. Dis Colon Rectum. 1995;38:7–13.
44. Karlbom U, Graf W, Nilsson S, and Pahlman L. Does surgical repair of a rectocele improve rectal emptying? Dis Colon Rectum. 1996;39:1296–302.
45. Ting KH, Mangel E, Eibl-Eibesfeldt B, and Muller-Lissner SA. Is the volume retained after defecation a valuable parameter at defecography? Dis Colon Rectum. 1992;35:762–8.
46. Halligan S and Bartram CI. Is barium trapping in rectoceles significant? Dis Colon Rectum. 1995;38:764–8.
47. Khubchandani IT, Clancy JP 3rd, Rosen L, Riether RD, and Stasik JJ Jr. Endorectal repair of rectocele revisited. Br J Surg. 1997;84:89–91.
48. Cundiff GW, Weidner AC, Visco AG, Addison WA, and Bump RC. An anatomic and functional assessment of the discrete defect rectocele repair. Am J Obstet Gynecol. 1998;179(6 Pt 1):1451–6.
49. Kahn MA and Stanton SL. Posterior colporrhaphy: its effect on bowel and sexual function. Br J Obstet Gynaecol. 1997;104:82–6.
50. Jeffcoate TN. Posterior colpoperineorrhaphy. Am J Obstet Gynecol. 1959;77: 490–502.
51. Kahn MA and Stanton SI. Posterior colporrhaphy: its effects on bowel and sexual function. Br J Obstet Gynaecol. 1997;104:882–6.
52. Glavind K and Madsen H. A prospective study of the discrete fascial defect rectocele repair. Acta Obstet Gynecol Scand. 2000;79:145–7.
53. Singh K, Cortes E, and Reid WM. Evaluation of the fascial technique for surgical repair of isolated posterior vaginal wall prolapse. Obstet Gynecol. 2003; 101:320–4.
54. Arnold MW, Stewart WR, and Aguilar PS. Rectocele repair. Four years' experience. Dis Colon Rectum. 1990;33:684–17.

55. Francis WJA. Dyspareunia following vaginal operations. J Obstet Gynaecol Br Comnwlth. 1961;68:1–10.
56. van Dam JH, Hop WC, and Schouten WR. Analysis of patients with poor outcome of rectocele repair. Dis Colon Rectum. 2000;43:1556–60.
57. Ayabaca SM, Zbar AP, and Pescatori M. Anal continence after rectocele repair. Dis Colon Rectum. 2002;45:63–9.
58. Watson SJ, Loder PB, Halligan S, Bartram CI, Kamm MA, and Phillips RK. Transperineal repair of symptomatic rectocele with Marlex mesh: a clinical, physiological and radiologic assessment of treatment. J Am Coll Surg. 1996; 183(3):257–61.
59. Sand PK, Koduri S, Lobel RW, et al. Prospective randomized trial of polyglactin 910 mesh to prevent recurrence of cystoceles and rectoceles.[comment]. Am J Obstet Gynecol. 2001;184:1357–62; discussion 1362–4.
60. Øster S and Astrup A. A new vaginal operation for recurrent and large rectocele using dermis transplant. Acta Obstet Gynecol Scand. 1981;60:493–5.
61. Kohli N and Miklos JR. Dermal graft-augmented rectocele repair. Int Urogynecol J Pelvic Floor Dysfunct. 2003 Jun:146–9.
62. Flood CG, Drutz HP, and Waja L. Anterior colporrhaphy reinforced with Marlex mesh for the treatment of cystoceles. Int Urogynecol J. 1998;9(4):200–4.
63. Migliari R and Usai E. Treatment results using a mixed fiber mesh in patients with grade IV cystocele.[comment]. J Urol. 1999;161(4):1255–8.
64. Murthy VK, Orkin BA, Smith LE, and Glassman LM. Excellent outcome using selective criteria for rectocele repair. Dis Colon Rectum. 1996;39(4):374–8.
65. Block IR. Transrectal repair of rectocele using obliterative suture. Dis Colon Rectum. 1986;29(11):707–11.
66. Khubchandani IT, Sheets JA, Stasik JJ, and Hakki AR. Endorectal repair of rectocele. Dis Colon Rectum. 1983;26(12):792–6.
67. Capps WF. Rectoplasty and perineoplasty for the symptomatic rectocele: a report of fifty cases. Dis Colon Rectum. 1975;18(3):237–44.
68. Sehapayak S. Transrectal repair of rectocele: an extended armamentarium of colorectal surgeons. A report of 355 cases. Dis Colon Rectum. 1985; 28(6):422–33.
69. Marks MM. The rectal side of the rectocele. Dis Colon Rectum. 1967; 10(5):387–8.
70. Sullivan ES, Leaverton GH, and Hardwick CE. Transrectal perineal repair: an adjunct to improved function after anorectal surgery. Dis Colon Rectum. 1968;11:106–14.
71. Janssen LW, van Dijke CF. Selection criteria for anterior rectal wall repair in symptomatic rectocele and anterior rectal wall prolapse. Dis Colon Rectum. 1994;37(11):1100–7.
72. Altomare DF, Rinaldi M, Veglia A, Petrolino M, De Fazio M, and Sallustio P. Combined perineal and endorectal repair of rectocele by circular stapler: a novel surgical technique. Dis Colon Rectum. 2002;45(11):1549–52.
73. Mellgren A, Johansson C, Dolk A, Anzén B, Bremmer S, Nilsson B-Y, et al. Enterocele demonstrated by defaecography is associated with other pelvic floor disorders. Int J Colorectal Dis. 1994;9:121–4.
74. Nichols DH and Genadry RR. Pelvic relaxation of the posterior compartment. Curr Opin Obstet Gynecol. 1993;5:458–64.

75. Zacharin RF. Chinese anatomy: The pelvic supporting tissues of the Chinese and Occidental female, compared and contrasted. Aust NZ J Obstet Gynaecol. 1977;17:1–11.
76. Kuhn RJ and Hollyock VE. Observations on the anatomy of the rectovaginal pouch and septum. Obstet Gynecol. 1982;59(4):445–7.
77. Bremmer S, Ahlbäck SO, Udén R, and Mellgren A. Simultaneous defecography and peritoneography in defecation disorders. Dis Colon Rectum. 1995;38: 969–73.
78. Halligan S, Nicholls RJ, and Bartram CI. Evacuation proctography in patients with solitary rectal ulcer syndrome: anatomic abnormalities and frequency of impaired emptying and prolapse. AJR Am J Roentgenol. 1995;164(1):91–5.
79. Sentovich SM, Rivela LJ, Thorson AG, Christensen MA, and Blatchford GJ. Simultaneous dynamic proctography and peritoneography for pelvic floor disorders. Dis Colon Rectum. 1995;38:912–15.
80. Kelvin FM, Maglinte DD, Hale DS, and Benson JT. Female pelvic organ prolapse: a comparison of triphasic dynamic MR imaging and triphasic fluoroscopic cystocolpoproctography. AJR Am J Roentgenol. 2000;174(1):81–8.
81. Brubaker LT and Saclarides TJ. The female pelvic floor, disorders of function and support. Philadelphia: F.A. Davis Company; 1996.
82. Chou Q, Weber AM, and Piedmonte MR. Clinical presentation of enterocele. Obstet Gynecol. 2000;96(4):599–603.
83. Walldén L. Defecation block in cases of deep rectogenital pouch. Acta Chir Scand. 1952;165:1–12.
84. Brodén B and Snellman B. Procidentia of the rectum studied with cineradiography: a contribution to the discussion of causative mechanism. Dis Colon Rectum. 1968;11:330–47.
85. Gosselink MJ, van Dam JH, Huisman WM, Ginai AZ, and Schouten WR. Treatment of enterocele by obliteration of the pelvic inlet.[comment]. Dis Colon Rectum. 1999;42(7):940–4.
86. Moschowitz AV. The pathogenesis, anatomy and cure of prolapse of the rectum. Surg Gynecol Obstet. 1912;15:7–21.
87. Halban J. Gynäkologische operationslehre. Berlin: Urban and Schwarzenberg; 1932.
88. Mellgren A, Dolk A, Johansson C, Bremmer S, Anzén B, and Holmström B. Enterocele is correctable using the Ripstein rectopexy. Dis Colon Rectum. 1994;37:800–4.

Editorial Commentary

The management of rectocele is controversial. Much of the literature has come from gynecological sources that traditionally have taken little account of the associated bowel dysfunction and which have incorporated such procedures as levatorplasty with colpoperineorrhaphy. Moreover, there are no available comprehensive prospective, randomized, controlled trials assessing the different approaches (transvaginal, transperineal, endorectal) for rectocele repair. The decision to perform rectocele repair is also hotly debated and surgical approaches are more a reflection of attendant pathology (cystocele, vaginal vault prolapse and haemorrhoids) than on objective evidence regarding predictability for successful outcomes. It would appear that improved understanding of the anatomy of the rectogenital septum (and its importance in the aetiopathogenesis of rectocele development) has confirmed the value of the septal defect repair whether performed via the vaginal or rectal route. It should always be remembered that the multiplicity of functional and organic occult lesions in these patients creates a set of "underwater rocks" for this "Iceberg syndrome." For this a crew of urogynecologists, coloproctologists and anorectal technicians may be required for the ship not to founder. The related condition of mucosal prolapsectomy (whether performed by hand or by stapler) is a particularly difficult problem where our group has noted considerable perioperative morbidity with a high requirement for postoperative laxative use particularly when surgery is utilized in patients with defineable preoperative anxiety and/or depression or if there is demonstrable non-relaxing puborectalis syndrome.

With regard to enterocele, failure to diagnose this condition when there is an associated rectocele will result in poor long-term results. Enteroceles are best diagnosed these days by dynamic magnetic resonance imaging or by the simpler technique of dynamic transperineal ultrasonography and they are potentially preventable following hysterectomy by attention to sacrocolpopexy.

MP

Chapter 6.4
Anismus

Kim F. Rhoads and Julio Garcia-Aguilar

Introduction

The term anismus was coined by Preston and Lennard-Jones in 1985 to describe the clinical conditions of 15 female patients with slow-transit constipation and a normal barium enema who were unable to expel a water-filled balloon, had markedly raised anal canal pressures during defecation, and an increase in the electrical activity of the external sphincter or puborectalis on straining effort (1). The authors concluded that the subjects had a disordered defecatory mechanism with failure of relaxation of the striated muscles of the pelvic floor during straining. They related the disorder to spasm of the pelvic floor muscles occurring in vaginismus; on this basis, they proposed the term anismus (1). Since then, the term anismus has been used to describe a syndrome characterized by obstructed defecation attributed to inappropriate contraction of the pelvic floor during attempted evacuation. Other terms for this condition include puborectalis syndrome (2), paradoxical puborectalis syndrome (3), spastic pelvic floor syndrome (4), and pelvic floor dyssynergia (5).

Anismus falls into the category of functional constipation and its symptoms include straining to pass fecal material, generally associated with lumpy or hard stool, the sensation of incomplete evacuation, a feeling of anorectal obstruction/blockage, and the use of manual maneuvers to facilitate defecation (6). Patients with anismus typically present with the symptom of incomplete rectal evacuation associated with the finding of lack of relaxation or paradoxical contraction of the pelvic floor musculature during defecation in the presence of adequate propulsive forces.

Encopresis is a well-known functional anorectal disorder among school-aged children in which fecal retention results in overflow incontinence. More than half of the children with encopresis share many of the symptoms of anismus and demonstrate paradoxical contraction of the external anal sphincter (EAS) and puborectalis muscle during defecation. Accordingly, in children, the term anismus often is associated with encopresis.

Constipation is a common complaint that affects between 2% and 28% of the adult population depending on the population sampled and the definition used (7–9). Constipation may be secondary to other colorectal or systemic conditions, but in most patients, no structural or biochemical cause can readily be identified. Functional constipation falls into one of two categories: colonic inertia and anismus. The prevalence of each one of these disorders has not been well documented because their diagnosis is often uncertain and because both conditions can coexist in the same individual; however, in some series, anismus accounts for between 36% and 52% of children with encopresis (10) and between 25% and 53% of constipated adults (11). Anismus—as with constipation in general—is more common in women than in men, and its prevalence increases with age (12).

Initially, it was felt that symptoms and physical examination were sufficient to make the diagnosis of anismus (2). A consensus panel has extended the diagnostic criteria by requiring manometric, electromyographic, or radiological evidence of failure of relaxation of the pelvic floor when attempting to defecate, along with evidence of incomplete evacuation despite adequate propulsive forces (6). The introduction of the diagnostic test to document the pathophysiologic changes associated with anismus has complicated the understanding of a relatively well-defined clinical entity. In recent years, not only has the diagnosis been questioned, but the clinical significance of anismus also has been questioned for a number of reasons. The symptoms are nonspecific and do not always correlate with the physiologic alterations detected (13,14), as the paradoxical sphincter contraction is a common finding in healthy controls and patients with other pelvic conditions (13,15). Here, the results of specialized diagnostic tests are nonspecific (13) and the response to treatment is variable (16,17). The uncertainty surrounding the diagnosis of this syndrome is caused by our imperfect understanding of the mechanisms of defecation, by the limitations of the methods currently available to reproduce the process of defecation, and by the divergent aspects of the defecatory process evaluated by each of the available diagnostic tests.

Etiology

The etiology of anismus is currently unknown. Anismus cannot be attributed to a neurological lesion because the symptoms and the pathophysiologic changes are often reversible with biofeedback.

Patients with symptoms of obstructive defecation and documented paradoxical contraction of the puborectalis during straining often have concomitant anatomical abnormalities of the rectoanal region. These include rectocele, rectal intussusception, enteroceles, excessive perineal descent, and solitary rectal ulcer syndrome (SRUS). Some of these specific disorders are discussed in other parts of this book. The role of excessive straining in the genesis of these anatomical abnormalities and their contribution of those anatomical abnormalities to the symptoms of obstructive defecation are not always obvious.

Patients with difficult evacuation have an increased prevalence of psychological traits such as hypochondriasis, hysteria, anxiety, depression, emotional conflict, social dysfunction, increased somatization, and less satisfaction in their sexual life when compared with healthy age-matched controls (18–23). In one series, patients with constipation and normal transit time had higher scores for psychological distress compared to patients with slow-transit constipation (18), suggesting that psychological distress may be particularly prevalent among patients with anismus. Whether psychological distress is the cause or a consequence of the gastrointestinal symptoms is unclear. Some authors have suggested that obstructed defecation represents somatization of a psychological conflict (19), and a history of physical and/or sexual abuse is common in patients with functional gastrointestinal illnesses (20). In one series, 40% of patients suffering from functional lower digestive disorders gave a history of having been victims of sexual abuse compared with 10% of patients with organic disease (21). The prevalence of sexual abuse was significantly higher among patients with constipation compared with patients presenting with upper gastrointestinal dysfunction (21). Leroi et al. found manometric findings consistent with anismus in 39 of 40 abused women compared with six of 20 healthy controls (21). These data suggest that a history of physical or sexual abuse may be an etiologic factor in some patients with chronic constipation and anismus. However, others consider that the psychological distress in constipated patients is determined, at least in part, by the underlying bowel condition (24). Whatever the etiological relationship, psychological distress is frequent in patients with anismus.

Clinical Evaluation

History

The overall assessment of the constipated patient is addressed by Michelle Thornton and David Z. Lubowski in Chapter 6.1. Patients with anismus are typically young or middle-aged females with classical symptoms of obstructed defecation. They describe an inability to defecate despite feeling the "call to stool," excessive and ineffective straining to empty the rectum, a sense of incomplete evacuation, and occasionally pelvic pain. Some patients digitally evacuate the rectum, whereas others apply pressure to the perineum or assume unusual postures to facilitate defecation. The frequency and duration of the symptoms is important in making the diagnosis (Table 6.4-1). Most of these patients have failed treatments with fiber supplements and/or a variety of laxatives.

TABLE 6.4-1. Diagnostic criteria for anismus [modified from Whitehead et al. (5)].

1. The patient must satisfy criteria for functional constipation consisting of at least 12 weeks—which need not be consecutive—in the preceding 12 months of two or more of:
   a. Straining in >1/4 defecations;
   b. Lumpy or hard stools in >1/4 defecations;
   c. Sensation of incomplete evacuation in >1/4 defecations;
   d. Sensation of anorectal obstruction/blockade in >1/4 defecations;
   e. Manual maneuvers to facilitate >1/4 defecations (e.g., digital evacuation, support of the pelvic floor); and/or
   f. <3 defecations/week
2. Loose stool are not present and there are insufficient criteria for irritable bowel syndrome (IBS).
3. There must be manometric, electromyographic, or radiologic evidence of inappropriate contraction or failure to relax the pelvic floor muscles during repeated attempts to defecate;
4. There must be evidence of adequate propulsive forces during attempts to defecate; and
5. There must be evidence of incomplete evacuation.

A complete physical examination is essential to identify anorectal pathology and structural abnormalities such as anal stricture, rectal prolapse, internal intussusception, rectocele, solitary rectal ulcer, excessive perineal descent, and pelvic or extrarectal tumors, which might impair defecation. Digital rectal examination can provide useful information about the resting tone and squeeze pressure of the EAS and the degree of relaxation of the sphincter during straining.

Patients describe constipation in a variety of ways, and the physician should clarify what the patient means by constipation. A detailed clinical history and physical examination may help ascribe patient complaints to specific pathophysiologic alterations (25). Others have questioned the value of clinical symptoms in the assessment of patients with chronic constipation (14). Glia et al. studied the prevalence of specific symptoms in four groups of constipated patients categorized by physiologic evaluation (14). They found that symptoms are good predictors of colonic inertia but poor predictors of pelvic floor dysfunction (14). This study suggests that history and physical examination alone cannot reliably make the diagnosis of anismus and underscores the importance of physiologic testing in the clinical assessment of patients with potential pelvic floor dysfunction.

Anorectal Testing Techniques

Several reviews on the evaluation of patients with constipation and the use of anorectal testing techniques have been published recently (25–27). The technical aspects of the anorectal testing techniques are covered in previous chapters of this book (Section 1). In this section, we will review the value of these techniques in the diagnosis of anismus.

Radiological Studies

A plain film of the abdomen can demonstrate the degree of fecal loading in the colon, providing a more objective idea of the severity of constipation. Barium enema helps exclude organic causes of constipation and provides information about the size and morphology of the colon and rectum.

Transit Studies

The diagnosis of anismus requires documentation of adequate propulsive forces; consequently, colonic transit studies should be part of the initial evaluation of every patient with severe idiopathic constipation. The most commonly used technique to measure colonic transit time involves having the patient swallow a capsule with a defined number of radiopaque markers with follow-up serial simple abdominal plates at established intervals (28,29). The colonic transit studies provide objective confirmation of the patient's subjective complaint of decreased bowel frequency and help determine whether the patient has generalized colonic inertia or a regional delay. Delayed transit through the rectosigmoid junction has been considered indicative of pelvic floor dysfunction, and segmental colonic transit time has been used to differentiate colonic inertia from hindgut dysfunction and pelvic outlet obstruction (28). However, whereas whole colonic transit studies are considered to be the gold standard in the diagnosis of colonic inertia, the value of segmental colonic transit time in the diagnosis of anismus has not been proven (30,31). Colonic transit studies are important in identifying patients with combination syndromes in which elements of colonic inertia and anismus coexist.

Manometry

Resting and squeeze anal pressures can be normal, elevated, or decreased in patients with anismus, and manometry does not always correlate with symptoms of chronic constipation (32,33). However, anal manometry provides useful information in the differential diagnosis of patients with obstructive defecation, particularly in children—where a normal rectoanal inhibitory reflex excludes the diagnosis of Hirschsprung's disease (HD) (34).

Anal manometry also can be used to document pelvic floor dyssynergia by simultaneously measuring the pressure in the intrarectal balloon—an indication of the intra-abdominal pressure generated during simulated defecation—and the pressure in the anal canal at rest, during squeezing, and straining effort (1). A non-relaxation or paradoxical increase of the anal canal pressure with a documented simultaneous increase in intrarectal pressure during simulated defecation is consistent with of the diagnosis of anismus (1,32). Borowitz et al. prospectively correlated the frequency and severity of symptoms with the manometric findings in children presenting with chronic constipation and encopresis. The degree of sphincter spasm during attempted defecation was the only manometric parameter that correlated with the frequency and duration of symptoms (35). Sutphen et al. used anal manometry to distinguish encopretic-constipated children from normal controls (36). They found no differences in resting and squeeze pressures in the anal canal or the rectum between patients and normal controls. The changes in sphincter pressure during simulated defecation and the pressure gradient between the rectum and the sphincters—both at rest and during straining—were the only two parameters that distinguished constipated patients from normal controls (36). However, despite these results, the value of these manometric findings in the diagnosis of anismus is limited because the correlation between anal manometry and other diagnostic tests is relatively low (37).

Electromyography

Electromyography (EMG) is considered the most informative test in the diagnosis of anismus. Electromyography provides an accurate assessment of the activity of the EAS and puborectalis by detecting the number of motor units firing at any given time. The EAS and the puborectalis maintain a tonic activity at rest that increases on demand by recruitment of additional motor units. The number of motor units recruited during external sphincter contraction correlates with anal canal squeeze pressures (38). The reflex relaxation of the EAS and the puborectalis muscle during defecation is registered as a decreased recruitment of motor units, where patients with anismus typically have a stable or a paradoxical increase in motor potentials during defecation.

Electromyography of the EAS and puborectalis can be performed with concentric needle, fine needle, or anal sponge electrodes (39–41). A comparative study has demonstrated that in constipated patients surface EMG recorded within the intra-anal sponge electrode is as accurate, but less painful, than concentric needle electromyography (CNEMG).[41] Consequently, surface EMG by intra-anal sponge electrodes is now the method of choice for the electromyographic evaluation of the EAS and puborectalis in patients with anismus.

The significance of anal EMG in the diagnosis of anismus has been questioned because its results are influenced by the environment in which the test is conducted, by patient position, and by the degree of distension of the rectum during the test. Duthie and Bartolo recorded anal and rectal pressures and sphincter electrical activity using an ambulatory system in a group of 11 patients diagnosed with anismus based on defecography and EMG recordings obtained in the anorectal physiology laboratory (15). All but three of the 11 patients investigated had appropriate relaxation of the puborectalis during the home recordings (15). Mayo et al. studied recruitment of the anal sphincter in the sitting and the supine position in a group of 61 patients diagnosed with anismus. They found substantial differences in anal recruitment in those two positions. Neither measurement correlated with the results of the balloon expulsion test, the defecographic findings, or with a favorable clinical outcome after biofeedback treatment (42). Lopez et al. performed needle EMG in 14 constipated patients during attempted defecation of a rectal balloon filled with different volumes; 13 patients had paradoxical sphincter contraction with an empty balloon as compared with eight patients with a 150-milliliter balloon (43). In addition, the electromyographic findings are not specific for anismus, with paradoxical recruitment frequently being found in normal individuals and non-constipated patients (3,13). Finally, paradoxical EMG recruitment does not always correlate with the results of others tests frequently used for the diagnosis of anismus. Whereas some authors have found a correlation between paradoxical recruitment of the puborectalis during EMG and impaired rectal evacuation on defecography (44–46), others have found a poor correlation between both tests (39,40,47). Consequently, although EMG recruitment provides useful information about the activity of the puborectalis and EAS during simulated defecation, the diagnosis of anismus cannot be based solely on electromyographic data.

Defecography

Imaging of the rectum with viscous contrast material to observe the process, rate, and completeness of evacuation during simulated defecation is one of the tests most commonly used in the diagnosis of anismus (48). Common findings described in patients with anismus include a marked impression of the puborectalis muscle, persistent or accentuated puborectalis impression during evacuation, failure to increase the anorectal angle during straining, accentuated perineal descent, reduced anal canal width, prolonged initiation and evacuation time, and incomplete evacuation (44,49–56). Halligan et al. have recently reviewed the proctographic findings in a group of patients diagnosed with anismus based on a long history of difficult rectal evacuation, excessive straining, paradoxical recruitment of the puborectalis on EMG, and an inability to expel a 50-milliliter water-filled balloon. The subjects were compared with a control group of asymptomatic patients. They found no differences in structural measurements such as the anorectal angle, anal canal width, or the presence of rectocele between patients with anismus and control subjects. However, patients with anismus had a delayed initiation of evacuation, prolonged evacuation time, and a lower percentage of contrast material evacuated compared with normal controls (56). The authors concluded that measurement of the anorectal angle in the diagnosis of anismus should be abandoned, but that impaired evacuation during defecography is highly predictive of the diagnosis of anismus (56).

The value of defecography in the diagnosis of anismus has been criticized on several grounds. The methodology used to conduct the test, such as the volume and composition of the contrast material, varies significantly between institutions (56–58). Moreover, some of the parameters assessed during defecography are rather subjective and therefore susceptible to interpretation bias (58). The forceful evacuation of contrast material instilled into the rectum with a syringe does not recapitulate the process of natural defecation, where response to a physiological reflex is integrated with the electromuscular events of the entire gastrointestinal tract. Defecography typically is conducted in an unnatural environment that can cause embarrassment to the patient and falsely influence the results (59). Some of the abnormalities described in patients with anismus also have been described in patients with other anorectal conditions, and even in asymptomatic patients (60). Finally, as is the case with EMG and manometry, the proctographic findings of anismus do not always correlate with the patient's symptoms and the findings of other diagnostic tests (11,45,61). Consequently, some authors have questioned the value of defecography in the clinical diagnosis or the selection of therapy in patients with anismus (61,62).

Defecography is useful to diagnose anorectal structural causes of obstructed defecation such as rectocele, internal intussusception, and enterocele often present in patients with anismus (54,58,63). Defecography also has been conducted using scintigraphic techniques by labeling the stool-like paste with technetium-99m (^{99m}Tc) and using a gamma camera to register the images (64–67). Scintigraphic defecography provides accurate images of anatomical abnormalities of the pelvic floor and allows quantitative assessment of rectal evacuation (65). Rectal emptying of the isotope-labeled artificial stool tends to be slower in constipated patients than in normal controls, but there is a wide overlap between both groups (65,67). The main advantage over conventional defecography is in radiation safety because radiation exposure is reduced compared with conventional defecography (67); however, prolonged retention of radionuclide in severely constipated patients presents a theoretical health hazard. In addition, scintigraphic methods provide less-detailed rectoanal anatomy compared with conventional defecography. Thus, scintigraphic protography provides no overall advantage over conventional defecography and is currently not widely used or available.

Magnetic Resonance Imaging

Magnetic resonance imaging (MRI) is used in the evaluation of patients with pelvic floor pathology because of its high soft tissue resolution, multiplanar capabilities, and simultaneous visualization of all pelvic anatomical structures surrounding the rectum and the anal canal (68). Dynamic fast sequence MRI has been used to directly visualize structures comprising the functional pelvic floor during straining and defecation (69). The sagittal views of the pelvis provide similar information to conventional defecography; however, dynamic MRI in closed configuration scanners is considered non-physiologic because the defecatory efforts are made while the patient is lying in the supine position. Closed-scanner dynamic MRI has been compared with conventional defecography in patients with chronic constipation. Healy et al. found good correlation between the two techniques for the change in anorectal angle, anorectal junction descent, rectocele depth, and the position of the rectal angle on maximal straining (70), although others have reported a significant discrepancy in those same measurements (71). In addition, Matsuoka et al. found that closed MRI only detected one of 12 anterior rectoceles, none of 4 rectoanal intussusceptions, and 9 of 12 sigmoidocoeles (71). Therefore, some authors consider that closed-configuration dynamic MRI does not provide enough additional information in the evaluation of the constipated patient as compared with defecography to justify the higher cost (71).

Dynamic MRI using open-design systems allows imaging in the sitting position with rapid scans in real-time, thus allowing for analysis of the anorectal angle, anal canal length, puborectalis muscle, and perineal floor descent in a fashion similar to the more physiologic proctographic testing (72–75). However, open-configuration MRI is only available in a few institutions, and its impact on the management of anismus has not been assessed fully.

Balloon Expulsion Testing

The inability to expel a balloon filled with a variable volume of water from the rectum is considered an indication of paradoxical puborectalis contraction (76,77). However, the specificity of this test is low because normal controls and patients with pelvic conditions other than anismus frequently are unable to expel the water balloon. Furthermore, the ability to expel the balloon depends on the position of the patient during the test, where patients unable to expel the water balloon in the left lateral position often are able to do so in the sitting position. The results of the test also depend on the volume of water within the balloon. In the study by Lopez et al. (43), six of 18 patients with chronic constipation and electromyographic evidence of anismus were able to expel a 50-milliliter water-filled balloon, but only one of them was unable to expel a 150-milliliter balloon. This discrepancy has been attributed to a decrease in the activity of EAS with progressive rectal distension.

The results of balloon-expulsion testing, however, have been found to predict the response to biofeedback in patients with anismus. In the series by Fleshman et al. (37), patients with anismus who were able to expel the balloon were more likely to benefit from biofeedback training when compared with patients unable to expel the balloon. Despite these results, the balloon-expulsion test is not routinely used for diagnostic evaluation or in the selection of therapy in patients with anismus.

Diagnosis

The diagnostic criteria for anismus have bee established by a consensus panel in gastrointestinal functional disorders and are summarized in Table 6.4-1 (5,78). Anismus is a functional disorder defined primarily based on symptoms of functional constipation (6). As clinical symptoms cannot reliably distinguish colonic inertia from anismus, anorectal physiology testing is recommended to confirm the diagnosis of the different pathophysiological types of functional constipation. The diagnosis of anismus requires evidence of incomplete evacuation in the presence of normal propulsive forces and manometric, electromyographic, or proctographic documentation of failure to relax the pelvic floor when attempting defecation (6). The accuracy of the different diagnostic tests required for the diagnosis of anismus varies significantly between series (Table 6.4-2), and no single test has demonstrated 100% sensitivity or specificity for diagnosis. Furthermore, the concordance between different tests is relatively low. These discrepancies reflect the lack of a gold standard to document paradoxical puborectalis contraction. Therefore, the diagnosis of anismus cannot be based on the results of a single diagnostic test.

Treatment

Medical Therapy

By the time patients undergo physiologic evaluation, most patients with anismus have been treated empirically with a variety of laxatives. Still, it is important that patients with anismus follow the standard recommendations for all constipated patients; namely, fiber supplementation, bulking agents, sufficient fluid intake, and regular exercise. Surface-active stool softeners may be necessary in patients with hard stools despite ample fiber and water intake. Stimulant laxatives may be necessary in some patients. Behavior modification—avoidance of prolonged sitting on the toilet and excessive straining—based on the investigation of the defecatory habits also should be recommended.

Most therapeutic approaches specific to patients with anismus have been based on the premise that the condition is the result of a paradoxical contraction of an otherwise normal puborectalis muscle. The initial approach to this condition was to surgically weaken the muscle. Subsequently, biofeedback therapy gained widespread acceptance because of its superior safety and efficacy compared with surgery. Botulinum toxin injection and

TABLE 6.4-2. Accuracy of different tests in the diagnosis of anismus.

Author	Year	#	Mean age	Diagnosis[1]	Manometry[2]	Defecography[3]	EMG[4]	Colonic transit[5]	Balloon expulsion[6]
Womack (44)	1985	16	41	Symptoms Manometry		56%			
Turnbull (77)	1986	13	28.4	Symptoms transit time		54%, 100%	85%		77%
Jones (3)	1987	50	46	EMG			44%		81%
Pemberton (6)	1991	37	36	Various tests			56%		81%
Fink (40)	1991	96	41.3	Symptoms			20%		
Fleshman (37)	1992	21	53	Defecography				38%	57%
Ger (32)	1993	116	60	Symptoms	63%	36%	38%		
Jorge (47)	1993	112	59	Symptoms CD, EMG		37%			
Schouten (13)	1995	121	51	EMG, BET			60%		66%
Halligan (55)	1995	24	37	Symptoms EMG, BET		67%, 71%			
Halligan (55)	1995	74	NS	Proctography					53%
Rao (97)	1997	69	NS	Various tests		48%			
Sutphen (36)	1997	88	8.7	Symptoms					15%
Halverson (138)	1998	98	48	Symptoms	12.5%			20%	
Karlbom (45)	1998	136	51	Manometry, transit time EMG		29%	83%		
Rao (139)	1998	35	44	Symptoms	51%				88%
Glia (14)	1999	134	52	Symptoms		41%, 59%	44%	9%	
Prokesch (31)	1999	30	44	Defecography					
Gosselink (140)	2001	100	50	Symptoms		44%	31%	4%	
Halligan (56)	2001	31	48	Symptoms EMG, BET		90%			

[1] Test used to confirm the diagnosis (EMG, electromyography; BET, balloon expulsion test.
[2] Percentage of patients with failed relaxation of the EAS and puborectalis.
[3] Percentage of patients with prolonged initiation and incomplete evacuation during defecation.
[4] Percentage of patients with paradoxical puborectalis contraction.
[5] Percentage of patients with distal marker retention.
[6] Percentage of patients unable to expel a water-filled balloon.

sacral nerve stimulation are new and promising alternatives that are currently under investigation for the treatment of patients with symptoms refractory to biofeedback.

Surgery

In 1964, Wasserman described a syndrome characterized by progressive constipation, pelvic pain, difficult defecation, and incomplete evacuation. He attributed these symptoms to hypertrophy of the puborectalis with constriction of the rectal lumen and elongation of the anal canal. He and his colleagues reported on three patients treated by excision of a posterior segment of the puborectalis muscle using a postanal perineal approach. The patients were all immediately relieved of their symptoms and none developed incontinence (2). Based on this encouraging experience, Wallace and Madden treated 33 adults and 13 children with posterior resection of the puborectalis muscle. They reported excellent emptying and fecal continence in all but one of their patients. Complications were few and the procedure was subsequently recommended (79); however, it was only adopted at few specialized institutions.

Barnes et al. reported the St. Mark's experience with the surgical treatment of 9 women with intractable constipation, electromyographic evidence of paradoxical contraction of the puborectalis, and an inability to expel a water-filled rectal balloon. The operation was performed through a curved incision posterior to the anus, close to the anal verge. The intersphincteric plane was dissected and the internal sphincter was retracted anteriorly. The puborectalis and upper one centimeter of the external sphincter were divided under direct vision from above downwards. Two of 9 patients benefited from the operation and were able to expel a water-filled balloon, although 7 patients reported no symptomatic improvement. None of their patients developed fecal incontinence for solid stools, but 4 patients developed incontinence for liquid and five patients complained of soiling. They attributed these disappointing results to persistence of the external sphincter activity or to extensive lateral attachments of the puborectalis to the rectal wall (80). Consequently, they modified the surgical technique to perform a unilateral or bilateral division of the puborectalis and the upper half of the external sphincter. The modified operation was performed through an intersphincteric approach using the same technique described for the posterior operation. They reported on 12 patients with unilateral and 6 with bilateral division of the puborectalis. Of the 18 patients, 4 (3 with bilateral division) experienced symptomatic improvement. Symptomatic improvement did not correlate with change in the puborectalis EMG or the ability to expel the balloon. Four patients developed mucous soiling or urgency, but no patient developed incontinence to solid stool (81). These disappointing results, combined with the higher success rates and safety of biofeedback, discouraged further use of puborectalis division in the surgical treatment of anismus.

Martelli et al. proposed a different approach to the surgical treatment of patients with chronic constipation. In 1978, the authors reported their experience with the use of anorectal myectomy in 62 patients with symptoms attributed to ineffective colonic motility. All except 2 of their patients had abnormal transit studies and the rectoanal inhibitory reflex was abnormal in 12 of the 13 patients. None of their patients underwent EMG, defecography, or balloon-expulsion testing. Surgery consisted of submucosal resection in the posterior midline of a strip of internal anal sphincter (IAS) and the rectal wall musculature up to six centimeters above the dentate line (DL). Four patients developed complications and 16% of patients became incontinent following surgery. One year later, 62% of patients considered themselves cured of their constipation (28).

Despite the remarkable results reported by Martelli et al., anorectal myectomy never gained widespread acceptance. In the mid 1980s, Yoshioka and Keighley used anorectal myectomy for the treatment of patients with outlet obstruction documented by an inability to expel a water-filled balloon, increased electrical activity of the puborectalis, or inability to open the anorectal angle and evacuate contrast during videoproctography. Their initial results were encouraging, with 18 of 29 (62%) of the patients able to adequately defecate after surgery. Eight patients were found to have HD, and all improved with the procedure (82). The same authors conducted a controlled randomized trial comparing anorectal myectomy with anal dilatation in patients with outlet obstruction. Seven of 13 patients were able to defecate spontaneously more than three times a week in the surgical arm compared with zero of the 10 patients in the anal dilatation group. They reported no postoperative incontinence. Anorectal myectomy resulted in a significant fall in anal canal pressure and improvement of rectal emptying. Patients with a favorable outcome had a significantly shorter history of constipation and normal colonic transit compared with patients who saw no benefit from the operation (83); however, the improvement with anorectal myectomy was transient, where 50% of patients reported normal evacuation at 8 to 12 weeks compared with 17% at 30 months (84). Based on these disappointing results, anorectal myectomy was abandoned for the treatment of obstructed defecation. Consequently, neither anorectal myectomy nor the division of the puborectalis and external sphincter has any role today in the treatment of anismus.

Biofeedback

The use of operant conditioning of rectosphincteric responses originally was introduced by Engel for the treatment of fecal incontinence (85). The demonstration that constipation could be caused by functional outlet obstruction led to the speculation of using biofeedback in patients with anismus (86). Olness et al. were the first to report their experience with the use of biofeedback for the purpose of achieving anal sphincter control in children and adolescents with encopresis secondary to functional constipation (87). They used manometric tracings to teach pelvic muscle relaxation to 40 patients with functional constipation and soiling. After 2 to 5 sessions, 24 patients developed normal bowel habits and stopped soiling, whereas 14 had persistent minor soiling but overcame the requirement for enemas to induce bowel movements. These promising results sparked interest in the use of biofeedback for the treatment of patients with constipation due to functional outlet obstruction (87). Since then, multiple authors have reported on the use of biofeedback in the treatment of anismus in children and adults (88). A detailed description of biofeedback techniques is provided in Chapter 6.5 of this book.

The results of some of the case series on the use of biofeedback in patients with anismus are presented in Table 6.4-3 with a reported rate of success varying from 18% to 100%. The variability in the success rate may be explained by differences in patient selection, small sample size, the method of biofeedback used, the number of sessions employed, the definition of success, and the length of follow-up.

Patient Selection

Some of the differences in patient selection between series are due in part to the lack of uniformity in the diagnostic criteria for anismus. The original report from Olness et al. included children with encopresis and constipation. Their initial physiologic assessment was limited to the evaluation of the rectoanal inhibitory reflex (RAIR), but paradoxical puborectalis contraction was not documented fully in this series (87). Recent series have restricted the use of biofeedback to patients with normal colonic transit and paradoxical contraction of the puborectalis documented by manometry, the balloon-expulsion test, EMG, and defecography (89–91). Others have included patients who also have prolonged colonic transit time (92,93) and structural causes of obstructed defecation such as rectoceles, abnormal perineal descent, rectoanal intussusception, and even pelvic pain (94).

Children with encopresis share some of the same pathophysiologic alterations of anismus as in the adult population, but the clinical characteristics and the goals of the treatment in both age groups are different. Despite these differences, many series reporting the results of biofeedback in the treatment of anismus include both children and adults (89,95).

Biofeedback Methods

Two main types of biofeedback training have been used for the treatment of anismus. The most widely used method operates by providing the patient with feedback about the activity of the pelvic floor muscles during simulated defecation. Different monitoring instruments can be used to provide feedback to the patient about the activity of the pelvic floor muscles. Olness et al. used a manometric system with two small balloons placed at the level of the internal and external anal sphincters (87), whereas others have used manometric systems with water-filled balloons (96), strain-gauge transducers (97), or water-perfused capillaries (17). As the isometric muscular tension of striated muscle correlates with its electrical activity, many biofeedback protocols have used EMG to register the activity of the striated muscle of the pelvic floor (98,99). Some series have used rectal balloon training in addition to EMG or manometry in order to improve sensory awareness of rectal distension during training of the external sphincter (16,17,59,89,90,96,100–102). However, the additional value of using a rectal balloon during biofeedback training has not been proved. For example, Heymen et al. compared EMG biofeedback training with or without intrarectal balloon use in patients with anismus and found that the addition of a rectal balloon does not improve outcomes when compared with EMG biofeedback alone (103).

The second type of biofeedback operates by practicing the process of defecation with a water-filled balloon. Bleijenberg and Kuijpers prospectively compared both methods of biofeedback—electromyography and balloon expulsion—in the treatment of patients with anismus (104). Twenty-one patients diagnosed with spastic pelvic floor syndrome on the basis of clinical and electromyographic findings were allocated randomly to either EMG-based biofeedback using an anal plug electrode ($n = 11$) or balloon biofeedback ($n = 10$). With the balloon biofeedback treatment, the patients place a balloon in the rectum and inflate it with 20 milliliters of air. First, they learn to pull the balloon without straining. Successful pulling of the balloon requires relaxation of the puborectalis. Later, the patients help pulling the balloon by straining while maintaining the relaxation of the pelvic floor muscles (104). Patients were assessed by standard EMG, a self-observation diary, constipation score, a visual analog scale of complaints, and a psychopathology symptoms checklist before, during, and after treatment (104). To compare overall success rates between the two forms of biofeedback, improvement scores for each parameter were calculated. There were no differences between the two groups in the pretreatment assessment. The number of patients improved with the EMG-based biofeedback (8 out of 11) compared with patients treated with balloon biofeedback (2 of 9). Furthermore, 5 of the 7 patients in the balloon biofeedback group who failed to improve were later treated with EMG biofeedback and four of them had a good result (104). Glia et al. also compared the efficacy of EMG and manometry biofeedback in 26 consecutive patients with anismus. Six patients were unable to complete the treatment, 10 were retrained using manometry and 10 using EMG. Six patients in the manometry group and 9 in the EMG group experienced an overall improvement of symptoms (105). Based on these studies, EMG has become the biofeedback method of choice in patients with anismus.

Koutsomanis et al. investigated whether the visual feedback signal during muscle training is necessary to help the patient to learn pelvic floor muscular relaxation (106). They randomized 60 consecutive patients with obstructive defecation to muscular coordination training with or without visual display. The authors found that training of the abdominal muscle contraction with pelvic floor relaxation was equally effective when performed with or without visual feedback to the patient about the state of muscle contraction or relaxation (106). Despite this provocative result, pelvic floor muscle relaxation exercises usually are performed with some audio or visual feedback.

Although at one time it was performed in the in-patient setting requiring lengthy hospital admission, professional expertise, and extensive psychotherapy (107), biofeedback is now a relatively simple office procedure in which the patient has a very active role. Some series also included additional home training to practice the learned exercises during daily situations in a familial environment (59,90,101,108).

Combination with Psychotherapy

A number of patients with anismus have increased psychological morbidity, and in some centers, biofeedback is associated with a variety of psychological interventions. Turnbull et al. combined anal biofeedback with instructions in general relaxation based on meditation techniques in 7 women with intractable constipation. The treatment was successful in improving bowel function and abdominal symptoms with results maintained at 2 to 4 years of follow-up (16). Leroi et al. found that, in women with anismus and a history of physical or sexual abuse, biofeedback combined with psychotherapy is more effective than biofeedback alone (109). In other series, psychometrically defined psychological distress-anxiety, somatic symptoms, and social dysfunction level did not predict response to biofeedback. However, patients with pain, emotional problems, or low vitality interfering with daily living were less likely to respond to therapy (24). These data suggests that some of the differences in the results of biofeedback can be attributed to the biopsychosocial profile of the patient population and to the addition of specific psychological interventions to the standard biofeedback therapy.

Number of Sessions

Gilliland et al. have reported a strong correlation between clinical improvement and the number of sessions attended (110). In their series, 18% of patients attending between 2 and 4 sessions versus 44% of those attending more than 4 sessions had complete success (110). The number of sessions attended was a better predictor of success than patient age, gender, or duration of symptoms (110). Despite these compelling data, the number of biofeedback sessions varies significantly between series, and even between patients in the same series (Table 6.4-3).

Definition of Success

In some series, success with biofeedback therapy is defined based on patient perception of subjective improvement (93,93,111,112), whereas in others, success was based on objective improvement of specific symptoms (97,99,102) or normalization of specific tests such as EMG recruitment or the balloon-expulsion test (90,113).

Length of Follow Up

Most series reporting the results of biofeedback on the treatment of anismus had a short follow-up, rarely extending beyond 6 months. Information regarding the long-term benefits is limited. Karlbom et al. reported a 43% success rate in a group of 28 constipated patients with any evidence of paradoxical activity of the puborectalis measured on needle EMG (93). In their series, the treatment effect lasted at least one year (93). Chiotakakou-Faliakou et al. reported 55% symptomatic improvement at a median follow-up of 23 months in a group of 100 consecutive patients with idiopathic constipation (92). Patients with anismus were as likely to be improved as patients with colonic inertia (92). Wiessel et al. reported symptomatic improvement and patient satisfaction after biofeedback in 85% with anismus, where satisfaction was maintained after a mean follow-up of 2 years in 79% of the patients (112). In contrast to these series, Ferrara et al. have reported a time-related decay of the benefits of biofeedback in adults (114). All 9 patients with anismus in this study had good or excellent initial responses to biofeedback, but the benefit decayed in all cases after a mean follow-up of 35 months (114). The same controversy about the long-term effect of biofeedback exists for patients treated for fecal incontinence (115,116).

Loening-Baucke compared the long-term outcome in children with anismus and encopresis treated by conventional therapy versus children treated with conventional treatment plus biofeedback. They found that at one year of follow-up more patients treated with biofeedback improved (50%) compared with conventionally treated patients (16%). However, after 5 years of follow-up there was no difference in the proportion of patients improved between biofeedback (50%) and conventionally treated (62%) groups. These data suggested that in children with anismus and encopresis the symptomatic improvement obtained with biofeedback persists over time. More importantly, at least in the pediatric population, most patients improved long-term independent of the basic type of treatment (117).

TABLE 6.4-3. Biofeedback in the treatment of anismus.

Author	Year	Patient number	Mean age	Type of Biofeedback	Setting[2]	# Sessions	Outcome[3]	F/U[4]	Improved[5]	Cured[5]
Olness (87)	1980	40	4–18	Manometry	outpatient	ns	ns	ns	95	ns
Weber (95)	1987	42	20:5[1]	Manometry	outpatient	4	ns	6	64	ns
Bleijenberg (107)	1987	10	32	EMG	inpatient	10	Stool frequency	14	70	ns
Dahl (89)	1991	14	9:5[1]	EMG	inpatient	5	Laxative use	6	93	ns
Lestar (90)	1991	16	42	Manometry	ambulatory	1	Successful BET	12	69	56
Kawimbe (59)	1991	15	45	EMG	ambulatory	2/day	Stool frequency	3–6	87	ns
Fleshman (113)	1992	9	49	EMG	outpatient	4–8	Successful BET	6	100	89
Wexner (91)	1992	18	68	EMG	outpatient	9	Laxative use	9	89	72
Turnbull (16)	1992	6	37	Manometry	outpatient	9	Stool frequency	24–54	100	83
Papachysostomou (101)	1994	22	42	EMG	outpatient ambulatory	2–5	Anismus index	12	86	27
Keck (17)	1994	12	62	Manometry	outpatient	3	Laxative use	8	30	9
Ho (96)	1996	62	48	Manometry	outpatient	4	Stool frequency Laxative use	15	90	90
Rao (97)	1997	25	50	Manometry	outpatient	6	Anorectal function Successful BET	6	76	76
Patankar (108)	1997	86	73	EMG	ambulatory	8	Unassisted BM	ns	84	ns
Gilliland (110)	1997	178	69	EMG	outpatient	2–10	Unassisted BM	ns	48	35
Ko (99)	1997	15	50	EMG	outpatient	4	Normal EMG Unassisted BM	ns	80	ns
Rieger (94)	1997	19	63	EMG	outpatient	6	Symptoms index	6–12	32	11
Karlbom (93)	1997	28	46	EMG	outpatient	8	Stool frequency Symptom index	14	43	63
McKee (102)	1999	28	35	Manometry	outpatient	3–4	Relaxation of EAS Successful BET	12	32	ns
Dailianas (111)	2000	11	43	Manometry	outpatient	2	Symptoms index Improved PPC	6	63	45
Wiesel (112)	2001	41	41	Manometry	outpatient	5	Symptoms index Laxative use	24	63	51

[1] Children to adult ratio.
[2] Setting in which the biofeedback was conducted.
[3] Criteria used to define outcome (BET, balloon expulsion test; BM, bowel movement; EAS, external anal sphincter; PCP, paradoxical puborectalis contraction).
[4] Length of follow-up in months.
[5] Percentage of patients with partial improvement.
[6] Percentage of patients considered "cured" of their main symptoms.

Physiological Changes After Biofeedback

An approach frequently used to demonstrate the efficacy of biofeedback in the treatment of anismus has been to establish a correlation between clinical improvement and a reversal of the physiological alterations detected in the pretreatment evaluation. Some authors have reported a correlation between clinical improvement and the normalization of the paradoxical contraction of the puborectalis assessed by manometry (89,90) or EMG (89,100,101,113), the ability to expel a rectal balloon (90,97,100), the normalization of the defecographic findings (59,90), and improvement in rectal sensation (16,97,101,118). However, other series have found a dissociation between the clinical improvement and the change in physiological parameters (17,59,96,99). Kawimbe et al. found a strong correlation between clinical improvement and normalization of balloon-expulsion tests, but poor correlation with the patient ability to expel a barium potato mixture (59). In the series of Keck et al., all 12 patients with anismus learned to reduce anal canal pressure and "silence" the electromyographic tracing with biofeedback, but only 4 patients reported a clinical improvement (17). Ho et al. reported a clinical improvement in defecation habits after 4 sessions of biofeedback in 56 of 62 (90%) consecutive patients with anismus (96); however, the number of patients with paradoxical puborectalis contraction defined by anal manometry and fine needle EMG was only reduced from 41 to 31. In their series, the presence of inappropriate puborectalis contraction did not affect response to biofeedback (96). Ko et al. also reported an 80% clinical improvement with biofeedback therapy without significant change in electromyographic values in a series of 17 patients with constipation and pelvic floor dysfunction (99).

Although the correlation between clinical improvement and the reversal of the physiological alterations is not perfect, the experience accumulated over the years demonstrates that relaxation of the puborectalis can be taught, and that learning to relax the pelvic floor during straining is correlated with symptomatic improvement. The lack of perfect correlation reported in some series may be the result of differences in patient selection and the limitations of the studies in reproducing the process of defecation rather than a specific lack of effect of biofeedback.

Prospective Randomized Trials

Biofeedback therapy entails a close relationship between the patient and therapist, and such interaction could lend itself to a placebo effect. Consequently, the symptomatic improvement may be the result of the care received rather than a true change in the underlying paradoxical contraction of the puborectalis. The most direct way to address this concern has been through prospective randomized trials comparing patients treated with biofeedback with patients receiving sham biofeedback. To date, no placebo-controlled studies have been conducted in the adult patient population. However, several prospective randomized studies have investigated the efficacy of biofeedback therapy in children with encopresis.

Wald et al. randomized 18 patients with encopresis and abnormal defecation patterns to conventional or biofeedback therapy. Patients were evaluated at 3-, 6-, and 9-month intervals for frequency of defecation, gross fecal incontinence, soiling, and parental perception of clinical status. They found no difference between the two groups at 3, 6, or 12 months. Children with an abnormal defecation pattern responded better to biofeedback treatment than to conventional treatment; however, the number of patients with an abnormal defecation pattern in both groups was too small to assess adequately and the differences did not reach statistical significance (119). Loening-Baucke studied the effect of biofeedback in a group of children with chronic constipation, encopresis, and abnormal defecation dynamics. Patients were randomized to conventional therapy alone or conventional therapy plus biofeedback. At 7 months, 55% of biofeedback-treated patients had improved clinically compared with only 5% of those in the conventional arm. In addition, 77% of patients treated with biofeedback had normalized their defecation dynamics compared with 13% of patients who received conventional treatment alone. In this study, the learning of normal defecation was correlated with clinical recovery (120).

Van der Plas et al. randomized 192 patients with encopresis to conventional treatment with or without biofeedback. The proportion of patients with abnormal defecation dynamics before treatment was similar in both treatment groups. At one year, the treatment was successful in 50% of patients who received biofeedback compared with 59% of patients who received conservative treatment alone. More patients treated with biofeedback improved defecation dynamics compared with patients who received conventional treatment alone, but the authors found no correlation between normalization of defecation dynamics and clinical success—defined as improvement of soiling and incontinence (121). The authors also investigated the behavioral problems in this patient population using a validated checklist (122). They observed abnormal behavioral scores in 35% of children. Total behavioral scores, internalizing problems, withdrawal and thought, and attention problem scores were observed between children treated successfully and those who failed therapy; however, no differences were found between children treated with biofeedback and those treated with conservative treatment alone (122). The authors concluded that biofeedback had no additional effect on clinical improvement, defecation dynamics, or behavioral scores over conventional treatment alone in children with encopresis (122).

Nolan et al. randomized 29 children with encopresis and anismus to conventional medical therapy with or without biofeedback (123). All but one of the 14 biofeedback-treated patients demonstrated relaxation of the EAS and were able to expel a rectal balloon by the time of their final biofeedback session (123). They found a transient clinical improvement, but no lasting clinical benefit for patients who received biofeedback compared with patients who received conventional treatment alone (123). Similar results have been reported by Borowitz et al., who found no benefit with biofeedback over maximal medical therapy and intensive toilet training in children with encopresis (124).

The combined experience of these trials indicated that biofeedback improves defecation dynamics in children with encopresis, but this functional improvement is not always paralleled with a similar improvement in continence, the main criterion used to assess clinical success in this patient population. These results have been interpreted as an argument against the effectiveness of biofeedback in children with encopresis (121–124). It is possible that while anismus may be a frequent finding in children with encopresis, it may not be the principal or basic underlying etiological mechanism of incontinence in this patient population (123). Consequently, the results of biofeedback therapy in children with encopresis and fecal incontinence may not be applicable to the adult population in whom constipation is the clinical manifestation of anismus.

Predicting Response to Biofeedback

Many studies have tried to identify patient characteristics associated with improved response to biofeedback therapy. Gilliland et al. looked retrospectively at 178 patients undergoing biofeedback with a successful clinical outcome after biofeedback treatment. They also looked at electrical activity of the puborectalis as a measure of success. In their series, 70% of the patients quit therapy before the therapist thought they were ready. Although they did not clearly define how the therapist made this determination, the authors used the high attrition rate to make a prediction about successful retraining. They found no correlation between age, gender, or duration of symptoms and successful outcome. What strongly correlated with successful biofeedback was the number of sessions the patient attended; 44% of patients attending five or more sessions had successful outcome compared with 18% of patients attending between two and four sessions. In total, 63% of patients completing the training protocol had complete success compared with 25% of those patients who self-discharged (110). However, in other series, the duration of symptoms was a predictor of outcome (93,125), whereas the number of session attended was not (125). Therefore, whereas completion of the treatment and practice of the techniques learned are associated with prognosis, the number of biofeedback sessions necessary for a successful outcome may vary from one individual to another.

Park et al. identified two patterns of anismus in a cohort of 68 patients with anismus defined by manometric, electromyographic, and colonic transit studies. The first type, called type A, had a wide anorectal angle and appropriate puborectalis activity during defecation, but failed to relax the anal canal. The second type, called type B, was characterized by paradoxical puborectalis activity and a narrow anorectal angle. Patients with type B anismus had an 86% response to biofeedback compared with 25% of patients with type A anismus (98). The association between results of anorectal testing and biofeedback outcomes has been reported in some series (95,102,126), but not in others (92,93,96). Consequently, the results of the physiologic testing cannot currently be used to select patients to biofeedback therapy.

Many patients with anismus also have structural causes of obstructed defecation that may affect the results of biofeedback. Lau et al. have investigated the prognostic significance of rectocele, intussusception, and abdominoperineal descent in a group of 108 patients with anismus who completed a course of biofeedback. None of the structural causes of anismus, alone or in combination, adversely affected the outcome of biofeedback treatment (127). In the series of Karlbom et al., patients who improved with biofeedback had less perineal descent compared with the unimproved group, but intussusception did not influence outcome (93). Therefore, biofeedback therapy also can be recommended to patients with anismus and structural causes of obstructed defecation.

Some authors also have investigated whether the psychological distress frequently associated with functional constipation is predictive of response to biofeedback. Nehra et al. found psychological disorder in 39 of the 60 patients with constipation related to rectal evacuation (22). Psychological impairment had a negative impact on the outcome of biofeedback treatment (22). Mason et al. investigated the psychological state and quality of life before and after biofeedback for intractable constipation (24). Twenty-two of their 31 patients felt subjectively improved. The symptomatic improvement produced by biofeedback is associated with an improvement in the psychological state and quality of life (24). Pretreatment physiologic measures did not predict who would benefit from treatment, but patients with pain, emotional problems, or low vitality were less likely to respond to therapy (24). Similar results have been reported by Loening-Baucke in children with encopresis in whom psychological factors such as social competence and behavior problems were not predictors of clinical outcomes (100). Given the conflicting results, biofeedback also should be recommended to constipated patients with psychological distress.

In spite of the lack of uniformity in almost all aspects of biofeedback treatment in patients with anismus, biofeedback is the initial treatment of choice for patients with this principal disorder. More than half of patients who complete the treatment experience a significant symptomatic improvement that is associated with improved quality of life (24). An even larger proportion of patients experience satisfaction with the procedure (108,112,128).

Botulinum Toxin

Intramuscular injection of Botulinum toxin—which inhibits release of acetylcholine—produces localized paralysis at the injection site. Complete recovery of muscle function occurs over 6 to 12 weeks in a dose-related manner. It has been used successfully in the treatment of a variety of spastic conditions. Hallan et al. were the first to investigate the use of Botulinum toxin A in the treatment of 6 patients diagnosed with anismus based on EMG and dynamic proctography. They injected the toxin into the puborectalis muscle bilaterally, initially under monopolar EMG guidance and later by anatomic guidance. The first patient was injected with five nanograms (100 units) of Botulinum toxin A into each side of the puborectalis muscle and became temporarily incontinent to formed stool. Subsequent clinical results improved, with 4 out of 5 patients successfully treated. The symptomatic improvement was attributed to a reduction in maximum voluntary squeeze pressure and widening of the anorectal angle on maximal straining (129).

Joo et al. (130) used Botulinum toxin in the treatment of 4 patients with anismus who had failed a minimum of three sessions of biofeedback therapy. Between 6 and 15 units (0.3–0.75 ng) of Botulinum toxin A were injected bilaterally under EMG guidance. All patients improved between one and three months after injection, but only two patients had a sustained improvement lasting up to a year. Similar results were reported by Maria et al. using a dose of 30 units (1.2 ng) of Botulinum toxin A injected under endoanal ultrasound guidance (131).

In a more recent and larger cohort of patients, Ron et al. showed manometric relaxation after one injection of the puborectalis muscle in 75% of patients (132). The effects persisted during 24 weeks of follow-up. None of the patients in either cohort suffered significant side effects. Pain at the injection site occurred in the latter study; however, there were no reported cases of fecal incontinence. Although preliminary studies appear to be promising, more studies are required to determine standard and safe dosages to obtain therapeutic effect while avoiding adverse side effects.

Sacral Nerve Stimulation

Tanagho et al. were the first to describe the use of low-amplitude chronic stimulation to the sacral nerve in order to modify the electrical activity of the pelvic floor (133). It originally was used in the treatment of detrusor irritability and urinary retention. The observation that some patients with stimulators implanted for bladder dysfunction experience improvement of concurrent constipation suggested a possible use of the technique for modulation of bowel function. Further evidence for modulation or anorectal function comes from successful treatment of fecal incontinence using permanent sacral nerve stimulation (134).

Temporary electrodes are initially placed under local anesthesia as an out-patient procedure. A 20-gauge spinal needle is inserted bilaterally into the S2, S3, and S4 foramina. A portable stimulator is used to find the best physical response of the pelvic floor and great toe to the lowest stimulus and is used to position electrodes in the optimal neural foramina. The percutaneous electrode is connected to a portable stimulator and screening is performed for a period of three weeks. The permanent electrodes are then placed surgically in the optimal foramina with the patient under general anesthesia. The stimulator is placed subcutaneously on the ipsilateral buttock (135).

Kenefick et al. (136) reported their experience with the use of permanent sacral nerve stimulation in 4 patients with severe idiopathic constipation who failed conservative medical treatment, including biofeedback. Eligible patients had two or fewer bowel movements per week and strained more than 25% of the time for a minimum of one year. At a median follow-up of 8 months, 3 out of 4 patients had improved bowel frequency, greater ease of evacuation, less time with abdominal pain and bloating, a lower constipation score, and an improved quality of life. Permanent sacral stimulation resulted in an improvement in the maximum anal resting and squeeze pressure and increased rectal sensitivity to distension and electrical stimulation (136).

To rule out a placebo effect, the same authors conducted a double-blind placebo-controlled crossover study of sacral nerve stimulation in two patients with severe idiopathic constipation. The study consisted of two two-week intervals with stimulation either "on" or "off." There was a marked improvement in the symptoms and quality of life when the stimulators were "on" compared with the time when stimulators were "off." This data suggests that sacral nerve stimulation may be a therapeutic option for patients with anismus who have failed conventional therapy and biofeedback; however, the long-term effects of sacral nerve stimulation remain to be established (137).

Conclusions

Anismus is a relatively common syndrome characterized by symptoms of obstructed defecation including excessive straining, a sensation of incomplete evacuation, and manual facilitation of defecation. Patients with anismus commonly demonstrate lack of relaxation or paradoxical contraction of the pelvic floor muscles during defecation. The diagnosis is confirmed by manometric, electromyographic, and defecographic demonstration of lack of relaxation of the pelvic floor muscles and delayed rectal emptying during simulated defecation in the presence of normal propulsive forces. However, the results of these tests are often inconsistent and add confusion to the diagnosis of an otherwise well-defined clinical entity. Some of these tests—particularly defecography—are useful to exclude structural causes of obstructed defecation such as internal rectal intussusception, rectocele, solitary rectal ulcer, anterior rectal prolapse, and descending perineum syndrome, each of which often is associated with anismus. The condition is more common in females and the prevalence increases with age. A history of psychosocial morbidity is common among patients with anismus.

Patients with anismus should aim to pass soft stools by drinking enough fluid and taking fiber supplements and surface-active stool softeners. Biofeedback should the first-line therapeutic approach. Compliance with the treatment is important for a successful outcome that can be achieved in more than half of the patients. Patients with psychological morbidity may benefit from psychological treatment. For patients failing biofeedback, Botulinum toxin injection of the puborectalis or sacral nerve stimulation should be given consideration. Surgery does not appear to have any substantial role in the treatment of anismus.

References

1. Preston DM and Lennard-Jones JE. Anismus in chronic constipation. Dig Dis Sci. 1985;30:413–18.
2. Wasserman IF. Puborectalis syndrome (rectal stenosis due to anorectal spasm). Dis Colon Rectum. 1964;7:87–98.
3. Jones PN, Lubowski DZ, Swash M, and Henry MM. Is paradoxical contraction of puborectalis muscle of functional importance? Dis Colon Rectum. 1987; 30:667–70.
4. Kuijpers HC and Bleijenberg G. The spastic pelvic floor syndrome. A cause of constipation. Dis Colon Rectum. 1985;28:669–72.
5. Drossman DA RJ, Talley NJ, Thompson WG, Corazziari, and Whitehead WE, editors. The functional gastrointestinal disorders: diagnosis, pathophysiology, and treatment: a multinational consensus. Boston: Little, Brown and Co.; 1994.
6. Whitehead WE, Wald A, Diamant NE, Enck P, Pemberton JH, and Rao SS. Functional disorders of the anus and rectum. Gut. 1999;45 Suppl 2:II55–9.
7. Sonnenberg A and Koch TR. Epidemiology of constipation in the United States. Dis Colon Rectum. 1989;32:1–8.
8. Drossman DA, Li Z, Andruzzi E, et al. U.S. householder survey of functional gastrointestinal disorders. Prevalence, sociodemography, and health impact. Dig Dis Sci. 1993;38:1569–80.
9. Stewart WF, Liberman JN, Sandler RS, et al. Epidemiology of constipation (EPOC) study in the United States: relation of clinical subtypes to sociodemographic features. Am J Gastroenterol. 1999;94:3530–40.
10. Wald A, Chandra R, Chiponis D, and Gabel S. Anorectal function and continence mechanisms in childhood encopresis. J Pediatr Gastroenterol Nutr. 1986;5:346–51.

11. Wald A, Caruana BJ, Freimanis MG, Bauman DH, and Hinds JP. Contributions of evacuation proctography and anorectal manometry to evaluation of adults with constipation and defecatory difficulty. Dig Dis Sci. 1990;35:481–7.
12. Stewart RB, Moore MT, Marks RG, and Hale WE. Correlates of constipation in an ambulatory elderly population. Am J Gastroenterol. 1992;87:859–64.
13. Schouten WR, Briel JW, Auwerda JJ, et al. Anismus: fact or fiction? Dis Colon Rectum. 1997;40:1033–41.
14. Glia A, Lindberg G, Nilsson LH, Mihocsa L, and Akerlund JE. Clinical value of symptom assessment in patients with constipation. Dis Colon Rectum. 1999;42:1401–8; discussion 1408–10.
15. Duthie GS and Bartolo DC. Anismus: the cause of constipation? Results of investigation and treatment. World J Surg. 1992;16:831–5.
16. Turnbull GK and Ritvo PG. Anal sphincter biofeedback relaxation treatment for women with intractable constipation symptoms. Dis Colon Rectum. 1992; 35:530–6.
17. Keck JO, Staniunas RJ, Coller JA, et al. Biofeedback training is useful in fecal incontinence but disappointing in constipation. Dis Colon Rectum. 1994;37: 1271–6.
18. Wald A, Hinds JP, and Caruana BJ. Psychological and physiological characteristics of patients with severe idiopathic constipation. Gastroenterology. 1989;97:932–7.
19. Devroede G, Girard G, Bouchoucha M, et al. Idiopathic constipation by colonic dysfunction. Relationship with personality and anxiety. Dig Dis Sci. 1989;34: 1428–33.
20. Drossman DA, Talley NJ, Leserman J, Olden KW, and Barreiro MA. Sexual and physical abuse and gastrointestinal illness. Review and recommendations. Ann Intern Med. 1995;123:782–94.
21. Leroi AM, Bernier C, Watier A, et al. Prevalence of sexual abuse among patients with functional disorders of the lower gastrointestinal tract. Int J Colorectal Dis. 1995;10:200–6.
22. Nehra V, Bruce BK, Rath-Harvey DM, Pemberton JH, and Camilleri M. Psychological disorders in patients with evacuation disorders and constipation in a tertiary practice. Am J Gastroenterol. 2000;95:1755–8.
23. Mason HJ, Serrano-Ikkos E, and Kamm MA. Psychological morbidity in women with idiopathic constipation. Am J Gastroenterol. 2000;95:2852–7.
24. Mason HJ, Serrano-Ikkos E, and Kamm MA. Psychological state and quality of life in patients having behavioral treatment (biofeedback) for intractable constipation. Am J Gastroenterol. 2002;97:3154–9.
25. Locke GR 3rd, Pemberton JH, and Phillips SF. AGA technical review on constipation. American Gastroenterological Association. Gastroenterology. 2000;119:1766–78.
26. Diamant NE, Kamm MA, Wald A, and Whitehead WE. AGA technical review on anorectal testing techniques. Gastroenterology. 1999;116:735–60.
27. Locke GR 3rd, Pemberton JH, and Phillips SF. American Gastroenterological Association medical position statement: guidelines on constipation. Gastroenterology. 2000;119:1761–6.
28. Martelli H, Devroede G, Arhan P, and Duguay C. Mechanisms of idiopathic constipation: outlet obstruction. Gastroenterology. 1978;75:623–31.

29. Metcalf AM, Phillips SF, Zinsmeister AR, MacCarty RL, Beart RW, and Wolff BG. Simplified assessment of segmental colonic transit. Gastroenterology. 1987;92:40–7.
30. Klauser AG, Voderholzer WA, Heinrich CA, Schindlbeck NE, and Muller-Lissner SA. Behavioral modification of colonic function. Can constipation be learned? Dig Dis Sci. 1990;35:1271–5.
31. Prokesch RW, Breitenseher MJ, Kettenbach J, et al. Assessment of chronic constipation: colon transit time versus defecography. Eur J Radiol. 1999;32:197–203.
32. Ger GC, Wexner SD, Jorge JM, and Salanga VD. Anorectal manometry in the diagnosis of paradoxical puborectalis syndrome. Dis Colon Rectum. 1993;36:816–25.
33. Rasmussen OO, Sorensen M, Tetzschner T, and Christiansen J. Dynamic anal manometry in the assessment of patients with obstructed defecation. Dis Colon Rectum. 1993;36:901–7.
34. Tobon F, Reid NC, Talbert JL, and Schuster MM. Nonsurgical test for the diagnosis of Hirschsprung's disease. N Engl J Med. 1968;278:188–93.
35. Borowitz SM, Sutphen J, Ling W, and Cox DJ. Lack of correlation of anorectal manometry with symptoms of chronic childhood constipation and encopresis. Dis Colon Rectum. 1996;39:400–5.
36. Sutphen J, Borowitz S, Ling W, Cox DJ, and Kovatchev B. Anorectal manometric examination in encopretic-constipated children. Dis Colon Rectum. 1997;40:1051–5.
37. Fleshman JW, Dreznik Z, Cohen E, Fry RD, and Kodner IJ. Balloon expulsion test facilitates diagnosis of pelvic floor outlet obstruction due to nonrelaxing puborectalis muscle. Dis Colon Rectum. 1992;35:1019–25.
38. Sorensen M, Tetzschner T, Rasmussen OO, and Christiansen J. Relation between electromyography and anal manometry of the external anal sphincter. Gut. 1991;32:1031–4.
39. Wexner SD, Marchetti F, Salanga VD, Corredor C, and Jagelman DG. Neurophysiologic assessment of the anal sphincters. Dis Colon Rectum. 1991;34:606–12.
40. Fink RL, Roberts LJ, and Scott M. The role of manometry, electromyography and radiology in the assessment of intractable constipation. Aust N Z J Surg. 1992;62:959–64.
41. Pfeifer J, Teoh TA, Salanga VD, Agachan F, and Wexner SD. Comparative study between intra-anal sponge and needle electrode for electromyographic evaluation of constipated patients. Dis Colon Rectum. 1998;41:1153–7.
42. Mayo SW, Jensen L, Park DK, and Congilosi S. Is any puborectalis evaluation technique predictive of success with biofeedback? Proceedings of the American Society of Colon and Rectal Surgeons Annual Meeting; 2001 Jun 2–7; San Diego, CA.
43. Lopez A, Holmstrom B, Nilsson BY, Dolk A, Johannson C, Schultz I, Zetterstrom J, and Mellgren A. Paradoxical sphincter reaction is influenced by rectal filling volume. Dis Colon Rectum. 1998;41:1017–22.
44. Womack NR, Williams NS, Holmfield JH, Morrison JF, and Simpkins KC. New method for the dynamic assessment of anorectal function in constipation. Br J Surg. 1985;72:994–8.

45. Karlbom U, Edebol Eeg-Olofsson K, Graf W, Nilsson S, and Pahlman L. Paradoxical puborectalis contraction is associated with impaired rectal evacuation. Int J Colorectal Dis. 1998;13:141–7.
46. Roberts JP, Womack NR, Hallan RI, Thorpe AC, and Williams NS. Evidence from dynamic integrated proctography to redefine anismus. Br J Surg. 1992; 79:1213–15.
47. Jorge JM, Wexner SD, Ger GC, Salanga VD, Nogueras JJ, and Jagelman DG. Cinedefecography and electromyography in the diagnosis of nonrelaxing puborectalis syndrome. Dis Colon Rectum. 1993;36:668–76.
48. Mahieu P, Pringot J, and Bodart P. Defecography: I. Description of a new procedure and results in normal patients. Gastrointest Radiol. 1984;9:247–51.
49. Mahieu P, Pringot J, and Bodart P. Defecography: II. Contribution to the diagnosis of defecation disorders. Gastrointest Radiol. 1984;9:253–61.
50. Kuijpers HC and Strijk SP. Diagnosis of disturbances of continence and defecation. Dis Colon Rectum. 1984;27:658–62.
51. Turnbull GK, Bartram CI, and Lennard-Jones JE. Radiologic studies of rectal evacuation in adults with idiopathic constipation. Dis Colon Rectum. 1988; 31:190–7.
52. Bartolo DC, Roe AM, Virjee J, Mortensen NJ, and Locke-Edmunds JC. An analysis of rectal morphology in obstructed defaecation. Int J Colorectal Dis. 1988;3:17–22.
53. Kelvin FM, Maglinte DD, and Benson JT. Evacuation proctography (defecography): an aid to the investigation of pelvic floor disorders. Obstet Gynecol. 1994;83:307–14.
54. Agachan F, Pfeifer J, and Wexner SD. Defecography and proctography. Results of 744 patients. Dis Colon Rectum. 1996;39:899–905.
55. Halligan S, Bartram CI, Park HJ, and Kamm MA. Proctographic features of anismus. Radiology. 1995;197:679–82.
56. Halligan S, Malouf A, Bartram CI, Marshall M, Hollings N, and Kamm MA. Predictive value of impaired evacuation at proctography in diagnosing anismus. AJR Am J Roentgenol. 2001;177:633–6.
57. Karlbom U, Nilsson S, Pahlman L, and Graf W. Defecographic study of rectal evacuation in constipated patients and control subjects. Radiology. 1999; 210:103–8.
58. Wiersma TG, Mulder CJ, Reeders JW, Tytgat GN, and Van Waes PF. Dynamic rectal examination (defecography). Baillieres Clin Gastroenterol. 1994; 8:729–41.
59. Kawimbe BM, Papachrysostomou M, Binnie NR, Clare N, and Smith AN. Outlet obstruction constipation (anismus) managed by biofeedback. Gut. 1991;32:1175–9.
60. Goei R. Anorectal function in patients with defecation disorders and asymptomatic subjects: evaluation with defecography. Radiology. 1990;174:121–3.
61. Hiltunen KM, Kolehmainen H, and Matikainen M. Does defecography help in diagnosis and clinical decision-making in defecation disorders? Abdom Imaging. 1994;19:355–8.
62. Ott DJ, Donati DL, Kerr RM, and Chen MY. Defecography: results in 55 patients and impact on clinical management. Abdom Imaging. 1994;19:349–54.
63. Jones HJ, Swift RI, and Blake H. A prospective audit of the usefulness of evacuating proctography. Ann R Coll Surg Engl. 1998;80:40–5.

64. O'Connell PR, Kelly KA, and Brown ML. Scintigraphic assessment of neorectal motor function. J Nucl Med. 1986;27:460–4.
65. Wald A, Jafri F, Rehder J, and Holeva K. Scintigraphic studies of rectal emptying in patients with constipation and defecatory difficulty. Dig Dis Sci. 1993;38:353–8.
66. Papachrysostomou M, Stevenson AJ, Ferrington C, Merrick MV, and Smith AN. Evaluation of isotope proctography in constipated subjects. Int J Colorectal Dis. 1993;8:18–22.
67. Hutchinson R, Mostafa AB, Grant EA, et al. Scintigraphic defecography: quantitative and dynamic assessment of anorectal function. Dis Colon Rectum. 1993;36:1132–8.
68. Kruyt RH, Delemarre JB, Doornbos J, and Vogel HJ. Normal anorectum: dynamic MR imaging anatomy. Radiology. 1991;179:159–63.
69. Healy JC, Halligan S, Reznek RH, et al. Magnetic resonance imaging of the pelvic floor in patients with obstructed defaecation. Br J Surg. 1997;84:1555–8.
70. Healy JC, Halligan S, Reznek RH, et al. Dynamic MR imaging compared with evacuation proctography when evaluating anorectal configuration and pelvic floor movement. Am J Roentgenol. 1997;169:775–9.
71. Matsuoka H, Wexner SD, Desai MB, et al. A comparison between dynamic pelvic magnetic resonance imaging and videoproctography in patients with constipation. Dis Colon Rectum. 2001;44:571–6.
72. Schoenenberger AW, Debatin JF, Guldenschuh I, Hany TF, Steiner P, and Krestin GP. Dynamic MR defecography with a superconducting, open-configuration MR system. Radiology. 1998;206:641–6.
73. Lamb GM, de Jode MG, Gould SW, et al. Upright dynamic MR defaecating proctography in an open configuration MR system. Br J Radiol. 2000;73:152–5.
74. Law PA, Danin JC, Lamb GM, Regan L, Darzi A, and Gedroyc WM. Dynamic imaging of the pelvic floor using an open-configuration magnetic resonance scanner. J Magn Reson Imaging. 2001;13:923–9.
75. Bertschinger KM, Hetzer FH, Roos JE, Treiber K, Marincek B, and Hilfiker PR. Dynamic MR imaging of the pelvic floor performed with patient sitting in an open-magnet unit versus with patient supine in a closed-magnet unit. Radiology. 2002;223:501–8.
76. Barnes PR and Lennard-Jones JE. Balloon expulsion from the rectum in constipation of different types. Gut. 1985;26:1049–52.
77. Turnbull GK, Lennard-Jones JE, and Bartram CI. Failure of rectal expulsion as a cause of constipation: why fibre and laxatives sometimes fail. Lancet. 1986;1:767–9.
78. Drossman DA. The functional gastrointestinal disorders and the Rome II process. Gut. 1999;45 Suppl 2:II1–5.
79. Wallace WC and Madden WM. Experience with partial resection of the puborectalis muscle. Dis Colon Rectum. 1969;12:196–200.
80. Barnes PR, Hawley PR, Preston DM, and Lennard-Jones JE. Experience of posterior division of the puborectalis muscle in the management of chronic constipation. Br J Surg. 1985;72:475–7.
81. Kamm MA, Hawley PR, and Lennard-Jones JE. Lateral division of the puborectalis muscle in the management of severe constipation. Br J Surg. 1988; 75:661–3.

82. Yoshioka K and Keighley MR. Anorectal myectomy for outlet obstruction. Br J Surg. 1987;74:373–6.
83. Yoshioka K and Keighley MR. Randomized trial comparing anorectal myectomy and controlled anal dilatation for outlet obstruction. Br J Surg. 1987; 74:1125–9.
84. Pinho M, Yoshioka K, and Keighley MR. Long term results of anorectal myectomy for chronic constipation. Br J Surg. 1989;76:1163–4.
85. Engel BT, Nikoomanesh P, and Schuster MM. Operant conditioning of rectosphincteric responses in the treatment of fecal incontinence. N Engl J Med. 1974;290:646–9.
86. Almy TP and Corson JA. Biofeedback—the light at the end of the tunnel? Gastroenterology. 1979;76:874–6.
87. Olness K, McParland FA, and Piper J. Biofeedback: a new modality in the management of children with fecal soiling. J Pediatr. 1980;96:505–9.
88. Enck P. Biofeedback training in disordered defecation. A critical review. Dig Dis Sci. 1993;38:1953–60.
89. Dahl J, Lindquist BL, Tysk C, Leissner P, Philipson L, and Jarnerot G. Behavioral medicine treatment in chronic constipation with paradoxical anal sphincter contraction. Dis Colon Rectum. 1991;34:769–76.
90. Lestar B, Penninckx F, and Kerremans R. Biofeedback defaecation training for anismus. Int J Colorectal Dis. 1991;6:202–7.
91. Wexner SD, Cheape JD, Jorge JM, Heymen S, and Jagelman DG. Prospective assessment of biofeedback for the treatment of paradoxical puborectalis contraction. Dis Colon Rectum. 1992;35:145–50.
92. Chiotakakou-Faliakou E, Kamm MA, Roy AJ, Storrie JB, and Turner IC. Biofeedback provides long-term benefit for patients with intractable, slow and normal transit constipation. Gut. 1998;42:517–21.
93. Karlbom U, Hallden M, Eeg-Olofsson KE, Pahlman L, and Graf W. Results of biofeedback in constipated patients: a prospective study. Dis Colon Rectum. 1997;40:1149–55.
94. Rieger NA, Wattchow DA, Sarre RG, Saccone GT, Rich CA, Cooper SJ, Marshall VR, and McCall JL. Prospective study of biofeedback for treatment of constipation. Dis Colon Rectum. 1997;40:1143–8.
95. Weber J, Ducrotte P, Touchais JY, Roussignol C, and Denis P. Biofeedback training for constipation in adults and children. Dis Colon Rectum. 1987; 30:844–6.
96. Ho YH, Tan M, and Goh HS. Clinical and physiologic effects of biofeedback in outlet obstruction constipation. Dis Colon Rectum. 1996;39:520–4.
97. Rao SS, Welcher KD, and Pelsang RE. Effects of biofeedback therapy on anorectal function in obstructive defecation. Dig Dis Sci. 1997;42:2197–205.
98. Park UC, Choi SK, Piccirillo MF, Verzaro R, and Wexner SD. Patterns of anismus and the relation to biofeedback therapy. Dis Colon Rectum. 1996;39:768–73.
99. Ko CY, Tong J, Lehman RE, Shelton AA, Schrock TR, and Welton ML. Biofeedback is effective therapy for fecal incontinence and constipation. Arch Surg. 1997;132:829–33; discussion 833–4.
100. Loening-Baucke V. Persistence of chronic constipation in children after biofeedback treatment. Dig Dis Sci. 1991;36:153–60.

101. Papachrysostomou M and Smith AN. Effects of biofeedback on obstructive defecation—reconditioning of the defecation reflex? Gut. 1994;35:252–6.
102. McKee RF, McEnroe L, Anderson JH, and Finlay IG. Identification of patients likely to benefit from biofeedback for outlet obstruction constipation. Br J Surg. 1999;86:355–9.
103. Heymen S, Wexner SD, Vickers D, Nogueras JJ, Weiss EG, and Pikarsky AJ. Prospective, randomized trial comparing four biofeedback techniques for patients with constipation. Dis Colon Rectum. 1999;42:1388–93.
104. Bleijenberg G and Kuijpers HC. Biofeedback treatment of constipation: a comparison of two methods. Am J Gastroenterol. 1994;89:1021–6.
105. Glia A, Gylin M, Gullberg K, and Lindberg G. Biofeedback retraining in patients with functional constipation and paradoxical puborectalis contraction: comparison of anal manometry and sphincter electromyography for feedback. Dis Colon Rectum 1997;40:889–95.
106. Koutsomanis D, Lennard-Jones JE, Roy AJ, and Kamm MA. Controlled randomised trial of visual biofeedback versus muscle training without a visual display for intractable constipation. Gut. 1995;37:95–9.
107. Bleijenberg G and Kuijpers HC. Treatment of the spastic pelvic floor syndrome with biofeedback. Dis Colon Rectum. 1987;30:108–11.
108. Patankar SK, Ferrara A, Larach SW, et al. Electromyographic assessment of biofeedback training for fecal incontinence and chronic constipation. Dis Colon Rectum. 1997;40:907–11.
109. Leroi AM, Duval V, Roussignol C, Berkelmans I, Peninque P, and Denis P. Biofeedback for anismus in 15 sexually abused women. Int J Colorectal Dis. 1996;11:187–90.
110. Gilliland R, Heymen S, Altomare DF, Park UC, Vickers D, and Wexner SD. Outcome and predictors of success of biofeedback for constipation. Br J Surg. 1997;84:1123–6.
111. Dailianas A, Skandalis N, Rimikis MN, Koutsomanis D, Kardasi M, and Archimandritis A. Pelvic floor study in patients with obstructive defecation: influence of biofeedback. J Clin Gastroenterol. 2000;30:176–80.
112. Wiesel PH, Dorta G, Cuypers P, et al. Patient satisfaction after biofeedback for constipation and pelvic floor dyssynergia. Swiss Med Wkly. 2001;131:152–6.
113. Fleshman JW, Dreznik Z, Meyer K, Fry RD, Carney R, and Kodner IJ. Outpatient protocol for biofeedback therapy of pelvic floor outlet obstruction. Dis Colon Rectum. 1992;35:1–7.
114. Ferrara A, De Jesus S, Gallagher JT, et al. Time-related decay of the benefits of biofeedback therapy. Tech Coloproctol. 2001;5:131–5.
115. Enck P, Daublin G, Lubke HJ, and Strohmeyer G. Long-term efficacy of biofeedback training for fecal incontinence. Dis Colon Rectum. 1994;37:997–1001.
116. Guillemot F, Bouche B, Gower-Rousseau C, et al. Biofeedback for the treatment of fecal incontinence. Long-term clinical results. Dis Colon Rectum. 1995;38:393–7.
117. Loening-Baucke V. Biofeedback treatment for chronic constipation and encopresis in childhood: long-term outcome. Pediatrics. 1995;96:105–10.
118. Benninga MA, Buller HA, and Taminiau JA. Biofeedback training in chronic constipation. Arch Dis Child. 1993;68:126–9.

119. Wald A, Chandra R, Gabel S, and Chiponis D. Evaluation of biofeedback in childhood encopresis. J Pediatr Gastroenterol Nutr. 1987;6:554–8.
120. Loening-Baucke V. Modulation of abnormal defecation dynamics by biofeedback treatment in chronically constipated children with encopresis. J Pediatr. 1990;116:214–22.
121. van der Plas RN, Benninga MA, Buller HA, et al. Biofeedback training in treatment of childhood constipation: a randomised controlled study. Lancet. 1996; 348:776–80.
122. van der Plas RN, Benninga MA, Redekop WK, Taminiau JA, and Buller HA. Randomised trial of biofeedback training for encopresis. Arch Dis Child. 1996;75:367–74.
123. Nolan T, Catto-Smith T, Coffey C, and Wells J. Randomised controlled trial of biofeedback training in persistent encopresis with anismus. Arch Dis Child. 1998;79:131–5.
124. Borowitz SM, Cox DJ, Sutphen JL, and Kovatchev B. Treatment of childhood encopresis: a randomized trial comparing three treatment protocols. J Pediatr Gastroenterol Nutr. 2002;34:378–84.
125. Siproudhis L, Dautreme S, Ropert A, et al. Anismus and biofeedback: who benefits? Eur J Gastroenterol Hepatol. 1995;7:547–52.
126. Rhee PL, Choi MS, Kim YH, et al. An increased rectal maximum tolerable volume and long anal canal are associated with poor short-term response to biofeedback therapy for patients with anismus with decreased bowel frequency and normal colonic transit time. Dis Colon Rectum. 2000;43:1405–11.
127. Lau CW, Heymen S, Alabaz O, Iroatulam AJ, and Wexner SD. Prognostic significance of rectocele, intussusception, and abnormal perineal descent in biofeedback treatment for constipated patients with paradoxical puborectalis contraction. Dis Colon Rectum. 2000;43:478–82.
128. Patankar SK, Ferrara A, Levy JR, Larach SW, Williamson PR, and Perozo SE. Biofeedback in colorectal practice: a multicenter, statewide, three- year experience. Dis Colon Rectum. 1997;40:827–31.
129. Hallan RI, Williams NS, Melling J, Waldron DJ, Womack NR, and Morrison JF. Treatment of anismus in intractable constipation with botulinum A toxin. Lancet. 1988;2:714–17.
130. Joo JS, Agachan F, Wolff B, Nogueras JJ, and Wexner SD. Initial North American experience with botulinum toxin type A for treatment of anismus. Dis Colon Rectum. 1996;39:1107–11.
131. Maria G, Brisinda G, Bentivoglio AR, Cassetta E, and Albanese A. Botulinum toxin in the treatment of outlet obstruction constipation caused by puborectalis syndrome. Dis Colon Rectum. 2000;43:376–80.
132. Ron Y, Avni Y, Lukovetski A, et al. Botulinum toxin type-A in therapy of patients with anismus. Dis Colon Rectum. 2001;44:1821–6.
133. Tanagho EA and Schmidt RA. Bladder pacemaker: scientific basis and clinical future. Urology. 1982;20:614–19.
134. Matzel KE, Bittorf B, Stadelmaier U, and Hohenberger W. Sacral nerve stimulation in the treatment of fecal incontinence. Chirurg. 2003;74:26–32.
135. Malouf AJ, Wiesel PH, Nicholls T, Nicholls RJ, and Kamm MA. Short-term effects of sacral nerve stimulation for idiopathic slow transit constipation. World J Surg. 2002;26:166–70.

136. Kenefick NJ, Nicholls RJ, Cohen RG, and Kamm MA. Permanent sacral nerve stimulation for treatment of idiopathic constipation. Br J Surg. 2002;89:882–8.
137. Kenefick NJ, Vaizey CJ, Cohen CR, Nicholls RJ, and Kamm MA. Double-blind placebo-controlled crossover study of sacral nerve stimulation for idiopathic constipation. Br J Surg. 2002;89:1570–1.
138. Halverson AL, and Orkin BA. Which psychological tests are useful in patients with constipation? Dis Colon Rectum. 1998;41:735–9.
139. Rao SSC, Welcher KD, Leistikow JS. Obstruction defecation: a failure of rectoanal coordination. Am J Gastroenterol. 1998;93:1042–50.
140. Gosselink MJ and Schouten WR. Rectal sensory perception in females with obstructed defecation. Dis Colon Rectum. 2001;44:1337–44.

Editorial Commentary

One of the most difficult and vexing conditions encountered on a daily basis by the colorectal surgeon is anismus. The mere existence of the myriad of terms such as "paradoxical puborectalis contraction," "incomplete puborectalis relaxation," "spastic pelvic floor," "pelvic dyssynergia," and other such appellations attest to our failure to comprehend the ideology and appropriate therapy for these conditions. In this chapter, Drs. Rhodes and Garcia-Aguilar expertly outline the evaluation and the possible therapeutic alternatives for this challenging condition. Much of the debate centers on whether the condition represents a pathologic aberration or a normal variant. Regardless of which view is accepted, biofeedback is an innocuous enough technique that it can be safely offered to patients with findings of failure of the puborectalis muscle to relax during attempted evacuation. Numerous series have shown varying success rates contingent upon the methodology of biofeedback employed as well as the length of follow-up. Other factors that may help determine success include coexistent conditions such as rectoanal intussusception, rectocele, solitary rectal ulcer, rectal prolapse, and descending perineal syndrome. When biofeedback fails, other therapies such as botulinum toxin injection and possibly sacral nerve stimulation may be indicated. Despite the lack of uniformity regarding definitions, the challenge of appropriate diagnostic methodologies and the lack of any universally successful treatment, Drs. Rhodes and Garcia Aguilar have expertly dealt with a very challenging subject in a comprehensive and comprehensible manner.

SW

Chapter 6.5
Biofeedback for Constipation and Fecal Incontinence

DAWN E. VICKERS

Introduction

Biofeedback for Constipation

Constipation and associated symptoms are the most common chronic gastrointestinal complaints, accounting for 2.5 million physician visits per year with a prevalence of 2% in the United States population (1,2). The Rome II Diagnostic Criteria for the Definition of Constipation as a Symptom Complex is specified in Table 6.5-1 (3). After identification and exclusion of extracolonic or anatomic causes, many patients respond favorably to medical and dietary management. However, patients unresponsive to simple treatment may require further physiologic investigation to evaluate the pathophysiologic process underlying these symptoms. Physiologic investigation generally includes a colonic transit time study, cinedefecography, anorectal manometry, and electromyography (EMG) (4), which allows for definitive diagnosis of treatable conditions including anismus, colonic inertia, rectocele, and sigmoidocele (5).

Anismus—also termed pelvic floor dyssynergia, spastic pelvic floor syndrome, paradoxical puborectalis contraction, and nonrelaxing puborectalis syndrome—accounts for an estimated 50% of patients with symptoms of chronic constipation (6). The Rome II Diagnostic Criteria for a Diagnosis of Pelvic Floor Dyssynergia are specified in Table 6.5-2 (3). This disorder of unknown etiology is characterized by a failure of the puborectalis muscle to relax during defecation. Invasive surgical therapies or injection of botulinum neurotoxin (7) may be associated with an unacceptable incidence of incontinence in this disorder, and in 1993, Enck's critical review summarized the role for biofeedback, which has become widely accepted as the treatment of choice for anismus (8) (see Chapter 6.4).

Biofeedback for Fecal Incontinence

Fecal incontinence—the involuntary passage of stool through the anus—can have a devastating psychologic and social impact on otherwise

Table 6.5-1. Rome 2 Criteria for Diagnosis of Constipation.*

- Straining >25% of defecations;
- Lumpy or hard stools >25% of defecations;
- Sensation of incomplete evacuation >25% of defecations;
- Sensation of anorectal obstruction/blockage >25% of defecations.
- Manual maneuvers to facilitate >25% of defecations (e.g., digital evacuation, support of the pelvic floor): and/or
- <3 defecations per week.
- Loose stools are not present, and there are insufficient criteria for irritable bowel syndrome

* Based on 12 weeks, which need not be consecutive, in the preceding 12 months of two or more of.

functional persons, causing fear, anxiety, and perceived shame, often leading to progressive isolation and depression. It is estimated that 7.15% of the general population experiences fecal soiling and 0.7% experienced gross incontinence (9). Because of the perceived shame, incontinence is not often spontaneously reported by patients.

Fecal incontinence is a complex and challenging dilemma of multifactorial etiology. A careful history, physical examination, and selected objective test of the continence mechanisms are recommended so that appropriate therapy can be instituted. Continence depends on the presence of a series of anatomic barriers to the movement of feces through the anus. These barriers include the puborectalis muscle of the pelvic floor and the internal and external anal sphincters. Continence requires normal sensation of rectal distension, intact innervation of the muscles, and adequate reservoir capacity of the rectum. Although the pelvic floor muscles and external anal sphincter (EAS) are tonically active, entry of stool into the rectum or upper anal canal calls for heightened contraction of these muscles to preserve continence (9). Anal sphincter weakness has long been associated with fecal incontinence. Although attention usually is focused on EAS weakness, dysfunction of the internal anal sphincter (IAS) also contributes to incontinence (9). Enck's critical review concluded that rehabilitation of the pelvic floor muscles utilizing biofeedback applications for the treatment of fecal incontinence has shown to improve anorectal function in the majority of patients (8).

Table 6.5-2. Rome 2 Criteria for Pelvic Floor Dyssynergia.

- The patient must satisfy diagnostic criteria for functional constipation in Diagnostic Criteria listed in Table 6.5–1.
- There must be manometric, EMG, or radiological evidence for inappropriate contraction or failure to relax the pelvic floor muscles during repeated attempts to defecate;
- There must be evidence of adequate propulsive forces during attempts to defecate, and
- There must be evidence of incomplete evacuation.

Biofeedback Defined

Schwartz defined the biofeedback process as "a group of therapeutic procedures that utilizes electronic instruments to accurately measure, process and feed back to persons and their therapists, meaningful physiological information with educational and reinforcing properties about their neuromuscular and autonomic activity, (both normal and abnormal), in the form of analog, binary, auditory and/or visual feedback signals" (10). This process helps patients develop a greater awareness of, confidence in, and an increase in voluntary control over physiological processes. This is achieved best with a competent biofeedback professional. Employing biofeedback instruments without proper cognitive preparation, instruction, and guidance is not appropriate biofeedback therapy. As with all forms of therapy, the therapist's skill, personality, and attention to the patient all affect the outcome (10).

It has been suggested that when researchers understand the essential components of biofeedback training, research studies are often successful. These components include (1) the fact that the biofeedback instrument is no more and no less than a mirror. Like a mirror, it feeds back information, but has no inherent power to create change in the user. (2) To maximize results, biofeedback training, like any type of complex skill training, involves clear goals, rewards for approximating the goals, ample time and practice for achieving mastery, proper instruction, a variety of systematic training techniques, and feedback of information. (3) The person using the feedback must have a cognitive understanding of the process and goals, positive expectations, positive interaction with the trainer, and must be motivated to learn (11).

Practical Aspects of Biofeedback Therapy for Fecal Incontinence and Constipation

Practical aspects of biofeedback therapy for pelvic floor muscle (PFM) dysfunction to treat symptoms of constipation and fecal incontinence include the technical, therapeutic, behavioral, and the pelvic muscle rehabilitation (PMR) components. The technical component involves the instrumentation used to provide meaningful information or feedback to the user. There are several technical systems available and the advantages of any one device have not been tested scientifically. Devices include surface electromyography (sEMG), water-perfused manometry systems, and the solid-state manometry systems with a latex balloon. Although each system has inherent advantages and disadvantages, most systems provide reproducible and useful measurements. The choice of any one system depends on many factors, including cost and the goals of training. A solid-state system is preferable to a water-perfused system because there is no distraction or embarrassment from leakage of fluid and the patient can be moved to a sitting position without adversely affecting calibration. Although this instrumentation is of proven effectiveness, this method is relatively cumbersome, complicated, and expensive (12). Surface EMG instrumentation is widely used and has proven effective for biofeedback training. Although not suitable for coordination training or sensory conditioning for fecal incontinence (13), sEMG is more cost-effective and suitable for office use (12). Patients are able to remain fully clothed during the session and position changes are accomplished easily to assist with functional maneuvers. The therapeutic component involves the clinician taking an active role by establishing a rapport with the patient; listening to concerns; reviewing the patient's medical history, including current medications, as well as over-the-counter and herbal preparations; reviewing bowel and bladder habits; educating the patient; and interpreting data. Clinicians must have a complete understanding of bowel and bladder functioning considering the coexistence of multifactorial concomitant PFM dysfunction in a patient with symptoms of urinary stress incontinence, nocturia, and difficulty voiding. Figure 6.5.1 shows the dysfunctional voiding pattern on the cystometrogram (CMG). The increase in sEMG activity is indicative of outlet obstruction inhibiting the detrusor contraction, thus requiring excessive straining by increasing intra-abdominal pressure to empty the bladder. This consequently produces a dysfunctional defecation pattern and contributes to

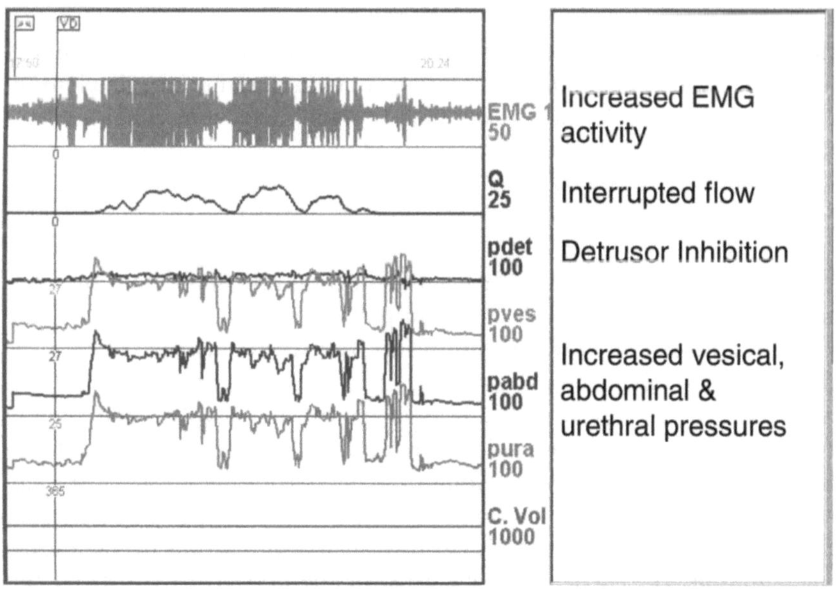

FIGURE 6.5.1. Voiding phase cystometrogram (CMG) recording.

symptoms of constipation. Chronic straining with stool is another source of PFM denervation that contributes to PFM weakness and incontinence (14). Patients with fecal incontinence may complain of multiple daily bowel movements and a feeling of incomplete evacuation resulting in post-defecation seepage (10). Many patients who present with fecal incontinence frequently have concomitant symptoms of urinary incontinence (see Chapter 7.3). For these reasons, it is difficult to offer a specific standard biofeedback therapy protocol that is beneficial for all patients. Therefore, the clinician must address all bowel and bladder symptoms and develop an individualized program for each patient with progressive realistic goals. The behavioral component is aimed towards systematic changes in the patient's behavior to influence bowel and bladder function. Operant conditioning utilizing trial and error as an essential part of learning is merely one aspect of the learning process. Treatment is aimed at shaping the patient's responses towards a normal model by gradually modifying the patient's responses through positive reinforcement of successive approximations to the ideal response (10). As a behavioral program, the patient's active participation is paramount in achieving subjective treatment goals, which include symptom improvement, quality of life improvement, and patient satisfaction. The PMR component involves designing an exercise program suitable for each patient to achieve the ultimate goal of efficient PFM function (Table 6.5-3).

sEMG Instrumentation

There is no standardization for sEMG recordings among manufacturers of biofeedback instrumentation; therefore, it is important for clinicians to understand basic technical aspects such as signal detection, signal processing, data acquisition, and display.

Signal Detection

Surface electrodes summate the electrical action potentials from the contracting muscle and establish electrical pathways from skin contact of the monitored muscle site (10) (Figure 6.5.2). The sEMG instrument receives and processes this electrical correlate of a muscle activity measured in microvolts (μV) (Figure 6.5.3). Muscle contraction involves the pulling together of the two anchor points; therefore, active electrodes should be placed between anchor points along the long axis of the muscle (10). The inter-electrode distance determines the volume of muscle monitored. Various types of electrodes are used with sEMG devices for pelvic muscle rehabilitation. The most direct measure of the sEMG activity from the pelvic musculature occurs when using internal sensors. Binnie et al. compared fine-wire electrodes to sensors with longitudinal electrodes and

TABLE 6.5-3. Components of PMR utilizing sEMG instrumentation.

- **sEMG Instrumentation**
  - Signal detection
  - Signal processing
  - Data acquisition and display
- **sEMG Evaluation**
  - Abdominal muscles
  - Pelvic Floor muscles
- **Pelvic muscle exercise principals**
  - Overload principal
  - Specificity principal
  - Maintenance principal
  - Reversibility principal
- **Biofeedback treatment goals**
  - Short-term goals
  - Long-term goals
- **Behavioral strategies**
  - Patient education
  - Dietary modification
  - Habit training for difficult, infrequent, or incomplete evacuation
  - Urge suppression for urinary and fecal incontinence
- **Biofeedback-assisted pelvic muscle exercises**
  - Kegel exercises—Isolated pelvic muscle contractions
  - Beyond Kegel exercises—Obturator and adductor assist
  - Quick contractions
- **Valsalva or push maneuver**
- **Physiological quieting techniques**
  - Diaphragmatic breathing
  - Progressive relaxation techniques—Hand warming

circumferential electrodes during rest, squeeze, and push. Internal sensors with longitudinal electrodes correlated better with fine-wire electrodes in all three categories (Figure 6.5.4) (15). Current internal sensors may detect one or two channels of sEMG activity. The two-channel multiple electrode probe(MEP) anal EMG sensor (Figure 6.5.5) allows discrimination between proximal and distal EAS activity, thereby allowing the clinician to target specific areas of EAS inactivity in the rehabilitation process.

Signal Processing

The majority of the sEMG signal from the pelvic floor musculature is less than 100 Hertz (Hz). The instrumentation should have the ability to filter noise interference, allowing a clear signal to be displayed. In order to detect the majority of the pelvic musculature signal, the instrumentation should have a wide bandwidth filter of 30 to 500 Hz. As muscle encounters fatigue, a shift to the lower frequencies (Hz) occurs; therefore, a wide bandwidth allows signal detection of low amplitude contractions (10). A 60 Hz "notch"

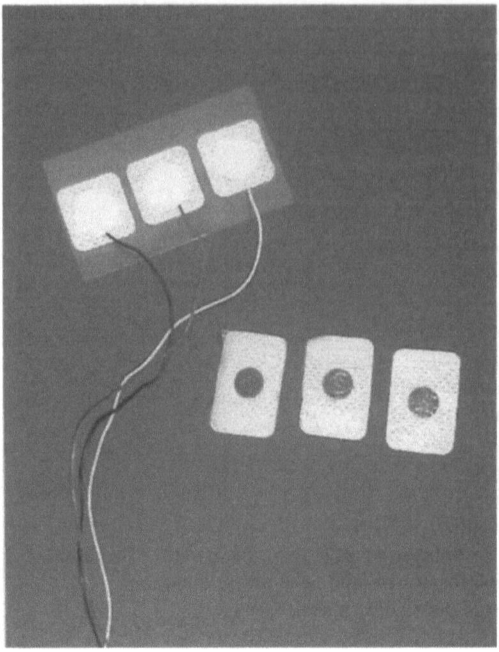

FIGURE 6.5.2. Disposable surface EMG electrodes.

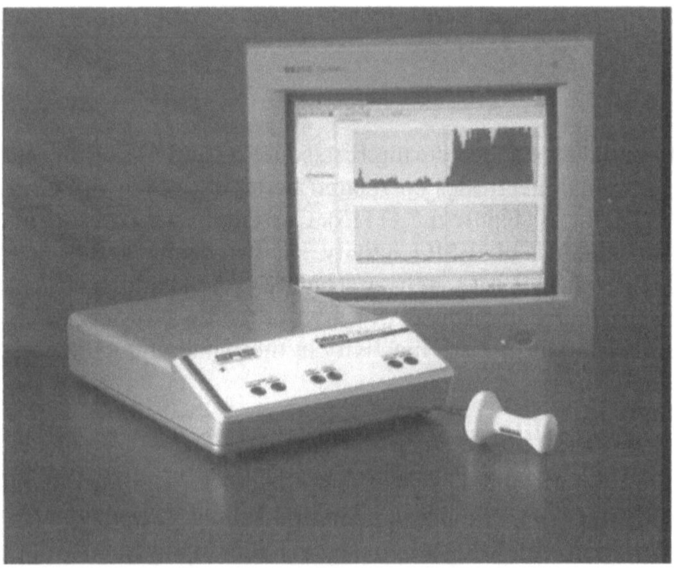

FIGURE 6.5.3. The Orion Platinum multimodality biofeedback system showing a typical display during a PFM contraction. (Photo courtesy of SRS Medical, Redmond, WA, USA.)

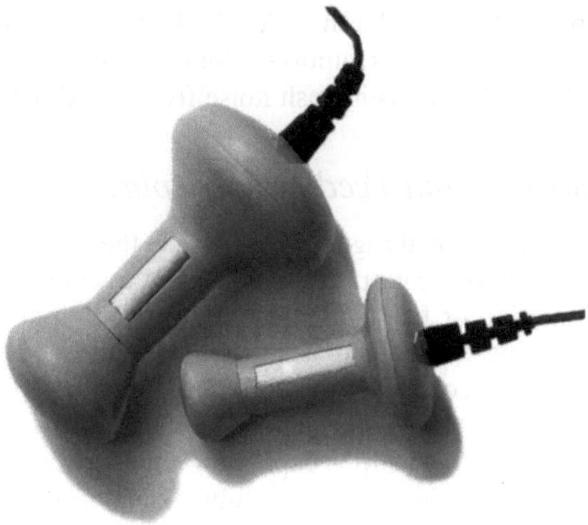

FIGURE 6.5.4. The SenseRx internal vaginal and anal sensors with longitudinal electrodes that maintain proper orientation to muscle fiber for accurate EMG monitoring. (Photo courtesy of SRS Medical, Redmond, WA, USA.)

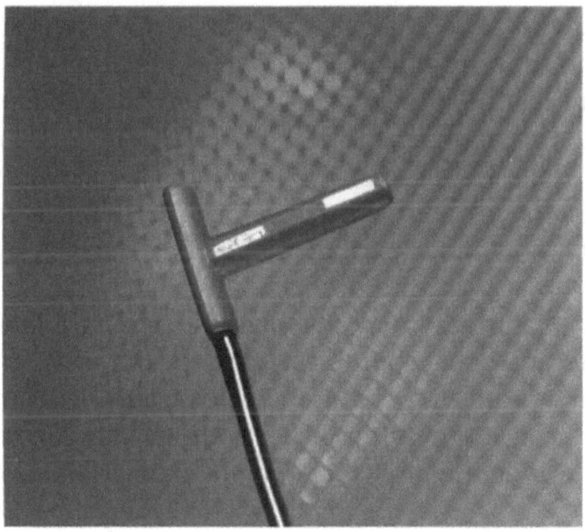

FIGURE 6.5.5. The multiple electrode probe (MEP) internal sensor. (Photo courtesy of SRS Medical, Redmond, WA, USA.)

filter rejects power-line interference. As all electronic instrumentation has internally generated noise, it is important for the clinician to know the internal noise level in order to distinguish noise from the sEMG signal.

Data Acquisition and Feedback Display

The sEMG instrument is designed to separate the electrical correlate of muscle activity from other extraneous noise and to convert this signal into forms of information or feedback meaningful to the user (10). Adjusting the sensitivity settings of the feedback display permits the clinician to tailor the shaping process according to the patient's ability to perform an isolated pelvic muscle contraction. For example, if the sensitivity setting of the feedback display is zero to 20 μV, expanding the display to a scale of zero to 10 μV provides reinforcement for submaximal contractions of weak muscles to help differentiate between these and abdominal contractions.

sEMG Evaluation

Abdominal and pelvic floor musculature—the two channels of sEMG muscle activity—should be monitored simultaneously during the sEMG evaluation and the sEMG biofeedback-assisted pelvic muscle exercise training. Interpretative problems arise when monitoring only pelvic floor muscles without controlling for changes in the intra-abdominal pressure. The transmission of abdominal artifact to perineal measurements invalidates changes in the PFM measurements and can inadvertently reinforce maladaptive abdominal contractions (10). The recommended surface electrode placement for monitoring abdominal muscle activity is along the long axis on the lower right quadrant of the abdominal oblique muscles. Perianal placement of surface electrodes may be used to monitor the PFMs when internal sensors are inappropriate, as in pediatric patients. Placing the active electrodes in the ten and four o'clock positions around the anal opening and placing the reference electrode on the gluteus maximus or coccyx reduces artifact (Figure 6.5.6). To obtain an evaluation, patients are

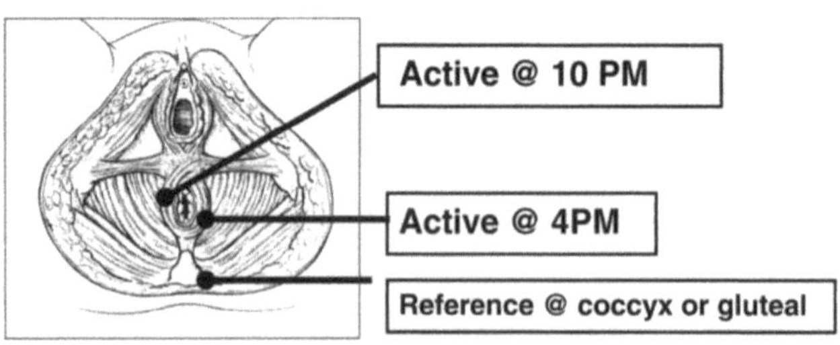

FIGURE 6.5.6. Surface perianal placement.

TABLE 6.5-4. Abdominal and pelvic floor muscle sEMG evaluation.

- sEMG resting baseline
- sEMG peak amplitude the contraction
- sEMG mean amplitude of the contraction during a 10-second period
- Duration of the contraction—0 if <5 s, 1 if 5 s, 2 if >5 s, 3 if >10 s.
- sEMG muscle recruitment scale: 0 = slow, 10 = fast
- Plevic muscle isolation during contraction: 0 = none, 10 = good
- Valsalva maneuver
- Progress this week: 0 = worse to 10 = excellent.

instructed to simply relax, then to perform an isolated pelvic muscle contraction over a ten-second period, followed by performing a Valsalva maneuver; this sequence is repeated two to four times for accuracy (Table 6.5-4). During contraction, the abdominal muscle activity should remain relatively low and stable, indicating the patient's ability to isolate PFM contraction from abdominal contraction (Figure 6.5.7). During the Valsalva maneuver, PFM activity should drop below the resting baseline to less than two microvolts, whereas the abdominal sEMG activity increases with elevated intra-abdominal pressure (Figure 6.5.8). These objective measurements are documented and reviewed with the patient. This also provides

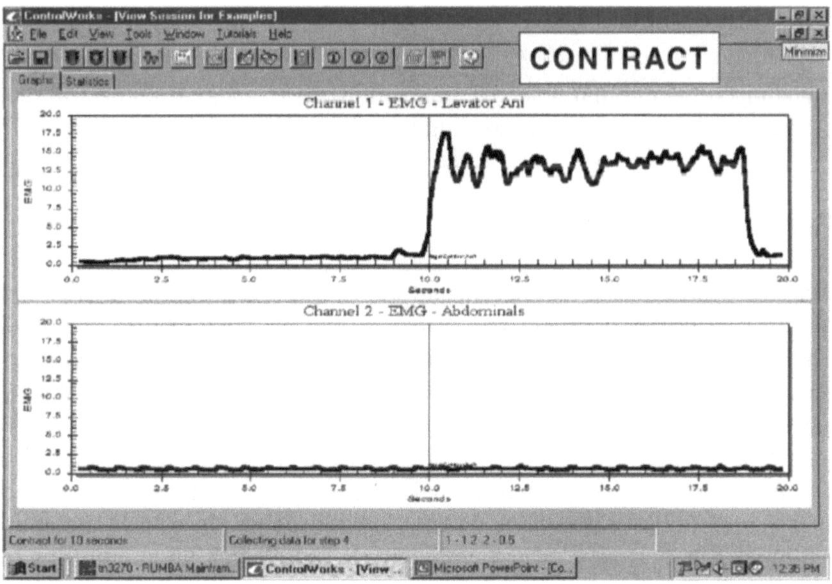

FIGURE 6.5.7. Channel 1: sEMG tracing of the PFM during contraction. Note the quick recruitment of appropriate PFM, ability to maintain the contraction, and ability to return to a normal resting tone. Channel 2: Abdominal sEMG tracing. Note the stability of the abdominal muscle acitivity.

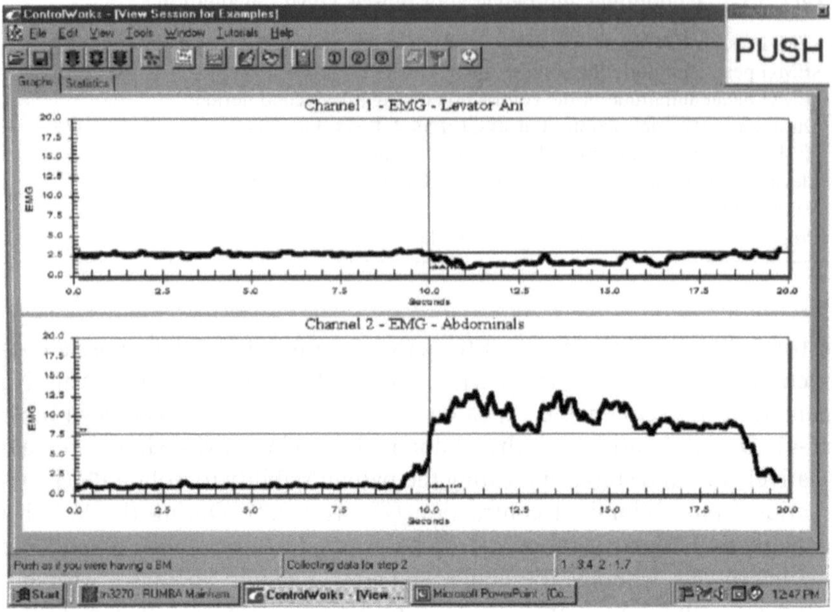

FIGURE 6.5.8. Channel 1: sEMG tracing of the PFM during a Valsalva maneuver. Note the decreased muscle activity. Channel 2: Abdominal sEMG tracing.

the clinician with initial objective measurements to gauge training and recommended home practice according to individual capabilities.

Pelvic Muscle Exercise Training Principals

Training principles that are important in any exercise program include the overload principle, the specificity principle, and the maintenance principal. The overload principle states that for pelvic muscles to strengthen, they must be pushed to the limit and just a little beyond. If muscles are underexercised, they are not challenged enough to increase in strength, endurance, or speed; therefore, length and resting tone remain constant. The specificity principle states that the pelvic muscles are composed of fast and slow twitch fibers in roughly a 35%:65% ratio; some fibers have a combination of fast and slow twitch components. Fast twitch fibers improve in speed and strength with quick contractions, whereas slow twitch fibers strengthen and gain optimal resting length and tone with longer "hold" contractions. Fast twitch fibers fatigue quickly, whereas slow twitch fibers are designed for endurance and postural tone; therefore, repetitions are low for fast twitch fibers and higher for slow twitch fibers. The maintenance principal describes exercising for continence as a lifelong endeavor. The pelvic muscle strength is maintained by one daily seven- to ten-minute session. The reversibility principle states that if after exercising and symptomatic improvement, discontinuing exercises will result in symptom reoccurrence over time (16).

Biofeedback Treatment Goals

After identifying functional problems and sEMG abnormalities, the clinician should prepare a treatment plan with specific short-term and long-term goals. Short-term goals describe the training components by which the patient may achieve the functional changes, whereas long-term goals refer to the expected functional outcomes (Table 6.5-5) (10).

Behavioral Strategies

Patient Education and Behavior Modification

Many misconceptions can be dispelled as patients gain a better understanding of their disorder. This begins with reviewing the anatomy of the pelvic floor musculature along with a review of normal bowel and bladder function with the use of visual aids. This is followed by reassurance that irregular bowel habits and other defecatory symptoms are common in the

Table 6.5-5. sEMG PRM treatment goals.

Short-term goals
- Reinforce pelvic floor muscle contractions isolated from abdominal and gluteal contraction.
- Reinforce pelvic floor muscle contractions toward greater amplitude and duration to improve strength and tone.
- Improve the coordination of pelvic floor muscle by shaping pelvic floor muscle contractions with short repose latency and immediate recovery to baseline after voluntary contraction ceases.
- Reduce chronically elevated PFM activity if implicated in perineal muscle pain, voiding dysfunction, or associated bowel disorders.
- Reduce straining pattern by reinforcing pelvic floor relaxation during defecation or micturation.
- To generalize skills learned in the office to the home situation.

Long-term goals
- Decrease laxative, enema, or suppository use
- Increase number of spontaneous bowel movements
- Decrease frequency of incontinent episodes
- Improved symptoms of incomplete evacuation
- Decreased straining

healthy general population. Patients may exhibit a variety of behavioral patterns, thus requiring tailored education specific to the underlying functional disorder. Some patients feel they need to have daily bowel movements and resort to laxative and enema misuse. Some patients may make several daily attempts, straining to evacuate, whereas others may postpone the urge or make hurried attempts for convenience. Another frequently observed behavioral pattern common among elderly women with symptoms of urinary incontinence is the restriction of fluid intake to avoid leakage; in fact, this may worsen symptoms of constipation, as well as symptoms of urinary incontinence.

Habit Training

Habit training is recommended for patients with symptoms of incomplete, difficult, or infrequent evacuation. Patients are encouraged to set aside 10 to 15 minutes at approximately the same time each day for unhurried attempts to evacuate. The patient should not be overly concerned with any failure, as another attempt later in the day is acceptable. This is best initiated after a meal, which stimulates the gastrocolic reflex (17).

Most commodes are approximately 35 to 40 centimeters in height; if a patient's feet or legs hang free or dangle above the floor while sitting, simulation of the squatting position will not be accomplished. Flexion of the hips and pelvis provides the optimal body posture. Full flexion of the hips stretches the anal canal in an anteroposterior direction and tends to open the anorectal angle, which facilitates rectal emptying. This may be achieved by the use of a footstool to elevate the legs and flex the hips (17).

Patients who have difficulty evacuating do not tolerate the symptoms of gas and bloating associated with fiber intake. Once emptying improves, these patients are encouraged to slowly begin weaning their laxative use and slowly add fiber.

Dietary Modification

Dietary information is reviewed with all patients to assist in improving bowel function. Patients are provided with written informational handouts regarding foods that are high in fiber or foods that stimulate or slow transit. Offering creative fiber alternatives that may be more appealing for the individual to incorporate easily into their daily diet regime assists with compliance. Such alternatives include unrefined wheat bran that can be mixed easily with a variety of foods, cereals, and muffins, as well as over-the-counter bulking agents. Adequate fluid intake and limiting caffeine intake is essential for normal bowel and bladder function; therefore, patients are encouraged to increase their fluid intake to 64 ounces per day unless otherwise prescribed by their physician. Patients who are incontinent of liquid stools may benefit from an anti-diarrheal medication. However, these medications typically slow colonic transit time. Therefore, this is contraindicated in patients with overflow incontinence from impaction or post-defecation seepage due to incomplete evacuation (10).

Urge Suppression Strategies for Incontinence

Burgio and colleagues (18) noted that suppression strategies assist with maintaining bowel and bladder control by educating patients to respond adaptively to the sensation of urgency. Rather than rushing to the toilet, which increases intra-abdominal pressure and exposes patients to visual cues that can trigger incontinence, patients were encouraged to pause, sit down if possible, relax the entire body, and contract their PFMs repeatedly to diminish urgency, inhibit detrusor contraction, and prevent urine loss. When urgency subsides, patients are instructed to proceed to the toilet at a normal pace. Patients with mixed urinary incontinence also are taught stress strategies, which consist of contracting the PFMs just prior to and during any physical activities, such as coughing or sneezing, that may trigger stress incontinence (18). These strategies—although intended for urinary incontinence—are quite helpful in maintaining control for patients with fecal incontinence. Norton reported that enhanced ability to contract the anal sphincter is likely to diminish large bowel peristalsis and may even induce retrograde peristalsis, or may simply allow continence to be preserved until the urge (bowl contractions) ceases. This appears to relate to the ability of biofeedback treatment to modify urgency (19).

Pelvic Muscle Exercise—Kegel Exercises

In the late 1940s, Arnold Kegel developed a vaginal balloon perineometer to teach pelvic muscle exercises for poor tone and function of the genital muscles. He was instrumental in developing a standardized program for treating urinary stress incontinence. Kegel's program included evaluation and training utilizing visual feedback for patients to receive positive reinforcement as they monitored improvements in the pressure readings. Kegel also recommended structured home practice with the perineometer along with symptom diaries. His clinical use of these techniques showed muscle re-education and resistive exercises guided by sight sense to be a simple and practical means of restoring tone and function of the pelvic musculature. This perineometer was developed before the word biofeedback was coined in the late 1960s (20).

Unfortunately, clinicians taught Kegel exercises without the use of instrumentation. Bump et al. showed that verbal or written instructions alone are not adequate, concluding that 50% of patients performed Kegel exercises incorrectly (21). Here, there are disadvantages to teaching Kegel exercises without specific feedback from muscle contractions. There is a strong tendency to substitute abdominal and gluteal contractions for weak PFMs. This incorrect manner of performing Kegel exercises is reinforced by sensory proprioceptive sensations, giving faulty feedback for the desired contraction and, in effect, rendering the Kegel exercise useless (10). For patients with fecal or urinary incontinence, abdominal contractions raise intra-abdominal pressure, thus increasing the probability of an accident. For patients to begin performing isolated pelvic muscle contractions, patients are instructed to contract their PFMs without contracting abdominal, gluteal, or leg muscles, and to hold this contraction to the best of their ability. This is done while using the instrumentation display of the simultaneous sEMG activity of the abdominal and pelvic floor muscles for feedback. The patient must tighten the pelvic diaphragm (levator ani) in a manner similar to stopping the passage of gas or to stopping the flow of urine. Patients should be advised that the initial aim of treatment is not to produce a contraction of maximum amplitude, but to contract the PFM in isolation from other muscles without undue effort. In order to build muscle endurance, training proceeds with gradual increases in the duration of each contraction, along with gradual increases in the number of repetitions. Rhythmic breathing patterns during contractions should be encouraged.

Recommended home practice is tailored according to the patient's ability and the degree of muscle fatigue observed during the session. At each stage of treatment, patients are encouraged to practice these exercises daily without instrumentation feedback. While Kegel asked patients to perform approximately 300 contractions daily during treatment and 100 during maintenance, there is no known optimal specific number of exercise sets. The goal of Kegel exercises is to facilitate rehabilitation of the PFMs to achieve efficient muscle function. This includes normal resting tone, quick recruitment of the PFMs, sustained isolated pelvic muscle contraction, quick release to a normalized resting tone, and appropriate relaxation during defecation or micturition.

Pelvic Muscle Exercise—Beyond Kegels

The Beyond Kegels—a complete rehabilitation program for pelvic muscle dysfunction developed by Hulme—is based on the principle that the support system for the pelvic organs includes more than just the PFMs. This support system, called the pelvic muscle force field (PMFF), includes the obturator internus, the pelvic diaphragm (levator ani), the urogenital diaphragm, and the adductor muscles. In summary, these muscles function as an interdigitated and interrelated synergistic unit rather than as separated entities to support abdominal organs, stabilize the lumbopelvic and sacroiliac region, and reflexively act for continence. Thus, as the obturator internus muscle contracts, it acts as a pulley, lifting the pelvic diaphragm and facilitating closure of the urogenital diaphragm. As the adductor contracts, it lifts the pelvic diaphragm through overflow (proprioceptive neuromuscular facilitation) principles via the close approximation of their attachments on the symphysis pubis. The balance and work–rest cycle of the obturator and adductor muscles function as an integral part of the urogenital continence system to maintain bladder and bowel continence and to facilitate effective and efficient elimination.

One portion of the Beyond Kegel protocol includes resistive exercises namely:

(1) The obturator assist—Roll knees out against an elastic band and hold for a count of ten seconds. Release for a count of ten seconds. Practice ten repetitions three times daily (Figure 6.5.9)
(2) Adductor assist—Roll knees inward on a soft ball and hold for a count of ten seconds. Release for a count of ten seconds. Practice ten repetitions three times daily (Figure 6.5.10).

This is a simple and effective beginning exercise for patients who are unable to perform isolated pelvic muscle contractions. As the pelvic muscles become more efficient, patients can progress to performing pelvic muscle contractions during the obturator assist and adductor assist ten-second hold. The Beyond Kegels protocols provide a detailed progressive pelvic

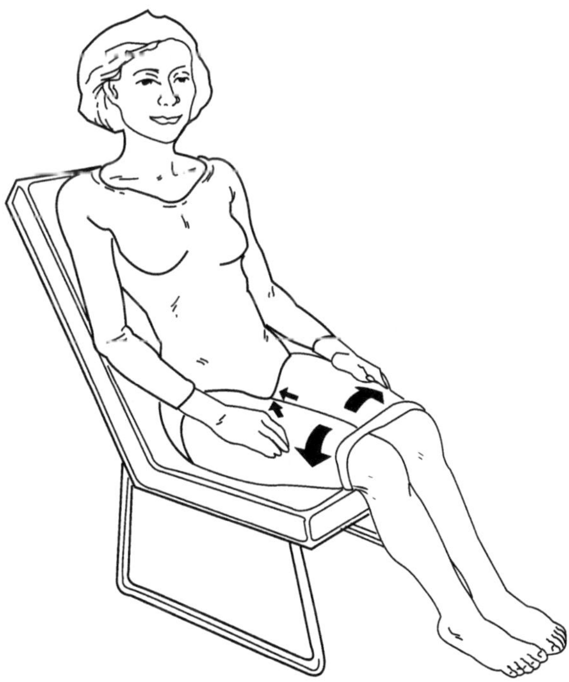

FIGURE 6.5.9. Beyond Kegels obturator assisted resistive exercise.

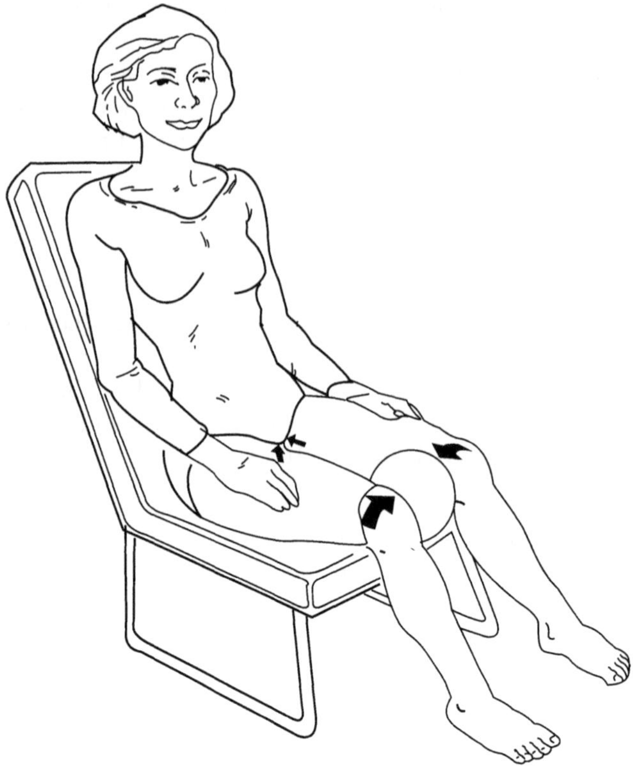

FIGURE 6.5.10. Beyond Kegels adductor assisted resistive exercise.

muscle rehabilitative exercise program that has shown to significantly improve and expedite the pelvic muscle rehabilitation process to achieve efficient muscle function (16).

Quick Contract and Relax Exercises

This exercise improves the strength and function of the fast twitch muscle fibers, primarily of the urogenital diaphragm and the EAS muscles. These fast twitch muscle fibers are important for the prevention of accidents caused by increased intra-abdominal pressure exerted during lifting, pulling, coughing, or sneezing. Once the patient has learned to perform isolated pelvic muscle exercises, they are instructed to perform quick contract and release repetitions five to ten times at the beginning and end of each exercise session they practice at home (16).

Physiological Quieting

Diaphragmatic Breathing

The breathing cycle is connected intimately to both sympathetic and parasympathetic action of the autonomic nervous system (ANS) (22). Bowel and bladder function is also mediated by the ANS (10). Conscious deep diaphragmatic breathing is one of the best ways to "quieten" the ANS. This effectively initiates a cascade of visceral relaxation responses. The aim of this exercise is to make the shift from thoracic breathing to abdominal breathing (22), Patients are instructed to inhale slowly through the nose while protruding the abdomen outward, as if the abdomen is a balloon being inflated, or allowing the abdomen to rise. This is followed by slow exhalation through the mouth as the abdominal balloon deflates or as the abdomen falls. Patients are encouraged to practice this in a slow, rhythmical fashion.

Hand Warming

The basic strategy for stress management is to be able to achieve and eventually maintain warm hands. This is accomplished by lowering sympathetic nervous system tone, promoting quiet emotions and relaxed muscles, and ultimately promoting a "quiet body" (22). Visualization and progressive relaxation techniques in conjunction with diaphragmatic breathing may be used to achieve hand warming.

Anorectal Coordination Maneuver

Patients with symptoms of difficult, infrequent, or incomplete evacuation or those with increased muscle activity while performing the Valsalva maneuver during the initial evaluation are taught the anorectal coordination maneuver.

The goal is to produce a coordinated movement that consists of increasing intra-abdominal (intrarectal) pressure while simultaneously relaxing the pelvic muscles. During the initial sEMG evaluation of the Valsalva maneuver, patients are asked to bear down or strain as if attempting to evacuate, which may elicite an immediate pelvic muscle contraction and closure of the anorectal outlet (Figure 6.5.11). This correlates with symptoms of constipation, including excessive straining and incomplete evacuation. The results of the sEMG activity observed on the screen display must first be explained and understood by the patient before awareness and change can occur. Change begins with educating the patient on diaphragmatic breathing, proper positioning, and habit training. Relaxation and quieting the muscle activity while observing the screen is reviewed. Initially,

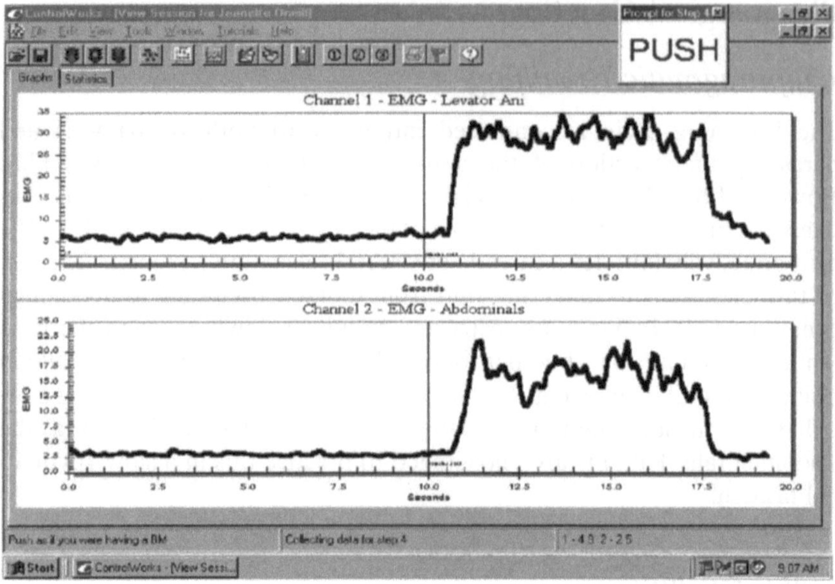

FIGURE 6.5.11. Channel 1: sEMG tracing of the PFM during a valsalva maneuver. Note the increase muscle activity indicative of a paradoxical contraction. Channel 2: Abdominal sEMG tracing.

patients are instructed to practice these behavioral strategies; however, some patients may continue to feel the need to "push" or strain to assist with expulsion. While observing the sEMG muscle activity on the screen, they are instructed to inhale slowly and deeply while protruding the abdominal muscles to increase the intra-abdominal pressure. They then are asked to exhale slowly through pursed lips. The degree of the abdominal and anal effort is titrated to achieve a coordinated relaxation of the PFMs. Patients are encouraged to reproduce this maneuver during defecation attempts.

Biofeedback Sessions

The initial session at the Cleveland Clinic Florida begins with a history intake. The learning process begins with a description of the anatomy and physiology of the bowel and pelvic muscle function using anatomical diagrams and visual aids. Verbal and written instructions are simplified for easy comprehension using layman's terminology. This is followed by a description of the biofeedback process, instrumentation, and PMR exercises. Patients should be aware that physicians cannot make muscles stronger, nor can they change muscle behavior. However, patients can learn to improve symptoms and quality of life by active participation and commitment to making changes. Results are not immediate; as with any exercise program, muscle improvement requires time and effort. Beginning goals of isolated pelvic muscle contractions are established and an example of a sEMG tracing showing efficient muscle function is reviewed. Patients are given instructions on proper insertion of the internal sensor and remain fully clothed during the session. They are placed in a comfortable semi-recumbent position for training; however, internal sensors work in a variety of positions for functional maneuvers, such as standing while reviewing urge suppression or sitting while performing the Valsalva maneuver. Then surface electrodes are placed on the right abdominal quadrant along the long axis of the oblique muscles and below the umbilicus (used to monitor abdominal accessory muscle use). The cables are attached to the SRS Orion PC/12 (SRS Medical Systems, Inc.; Redmond, Washington) multimodality instrumentation that provides the ability to monitor up to four muscle sites simultaneously (Figure 6.5.3). Electromyography specifications include a bandwith of 20 to 500 Hz and 50/60 Hz notch filter.

Training for dyssynergia, incontinence, or pain begins with the systematic shaping of isolated pelvic muscle contractions. Observation of other accessory muscle use such as the gluteals or thighs during the session is discussed with the patient. Excessive pelvic muscle activity with an elevated resting tone greater than two volts may be associated with dyssynergia, voiding dysfunction, and pelvic pain. Jacobson's progressive muscle relaxation strategy implied that after a muscle tenses, it automatically relaxes more deeply when released (23). This strategy is used to assist with hypertonia, placing emphasis on awareness of decreased muscle activity viewed on the screen as the PFM becomes more relaxed. This repetitive contract–relax sequence of isolated pelvic muscle contractions also facilitates discrimination between muscle tension and muscle relaxation. Some patients—usually women—have a greater PFM descent with straining during defecation associated with difficulty in rectal expulsion. Pelvic floor weakness may result in intrarectal mucosal intussusception or rectal prolapse, which contribute to symptoms of constipation. Furthermore, the PFM may not have the ability to provide the resistance necessary for extrusion of solid stool through the anal canal (17). Multifactorial concomitant PFM dysfunction accounts for the rationale to initiate all patients with isolated pelvic muscle rehabilitative exercises. Home practice recommendations depend on the observed decay in the duration of the contraction accompanied by the abdominal muscle recruitment (Figure 6.5.12). The number of contractions the patient is able to perform before notable muscle fatigue occurs gauges the number of repetitions recommended at one time. Fatigue can be observed in as few as three to four contractions seen in patients with weak PFMs. An example of home practice might be the patient performing an isolated pelvic floor muscle contraction, holding for a five-second duration, relaxing for ten seconds and repeating three to ten times (one set). One set is performed three to five times daily at designated intervals, allowing for

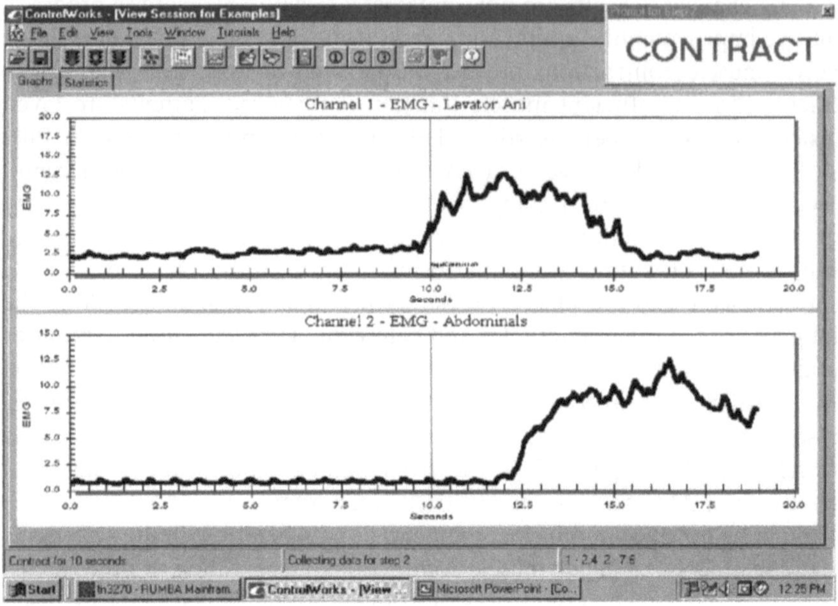

FIGURE 6.5.12. Channel 1: sEMG tracing of the PFM. Note slow recruitment and fatigue. Channel 2: Abdominal sEMG tracing. Note increased muscle activity.

extended rest periods between sets. The lower the number of repetitions, the more frequent interval sets should be performed daily. Excessive repetitions may overly fatigue the muscle and exacerbate symptoms. If patients are unable to perform an isolated contraction on the initial evaluation, they are given instructions for the Beyond Kegel exercises. The goal for patients is to be able to perform isolated pelvic muscle contractions alternating with the Beyond Kegel exercises to ultimately achieve efficient PFM function. All patients are requested to keep a daily diary of bowel habits, laxative, enema or suppository use, fluid intake, number of home exercises completed, fiber intake, and any associated symptoms of constipation or incontinence.

Subsequent sessions begin with a diary review and establishing further goals aimed towards individualized symptom improvement. This is followed by a sEMG evaluation that may include the addition of quick contract and release repetitions, the Valsalva maneuver, or Beyond Kegel exercises depending on the patient's progress. These objective measurements gauge improvements in muscle activity that should be seen with each visit and occur prior to symptomatic improvement; this provides positive reinforcement for the patient to continue treatment. To assist with compliance, additional tasks should be limited to no more than three at any given time. These tasks, tailored to the individual needs, may include increasing the duration and number of PFM exercises; alternating Beyond Kegel exercises, habit training, physiological quieting, and anorectal coordination maneuvers; increasing fiber and fluid intake; increasing activity and/or modifying laxative use or other methods of evacuatory assistance. Although the ideal goal may be to abolish all symptoms, this may not always be accomplished due to underlying conditions; however, patients' individual goals are significantly important, where some patients may be satisfied simply with the ability to leave home without fear of a significant relative fecal accident. Improved quality of life and patient satisfaction should be considered a treatment success.

Session Duration and Frequency

At the onset of biofeedback therapy, it may be difficult to ascertain how many sessions are required for successful training. The number of biofeedback training sessions should be customized for each patient depending on the complexity of their functional disorder, as well as the patient's ability to learn and master a new skill. They are commonly scheduled from 60 to 90 minute visits once or twice weekly. Additionally, periodic reinforcement is recommended to improve long-term outcome (24).

Adjunctive Treatment Methods

Various adjunctive biofeedback treatment methods have been employed throughout the years. Balloon expulsion has been used as an objective diagnostic tool and reportedly enhances sensory awareness in patients with outlet obstruction. It remains unclear which of the three components—sphincter training, sensory conditioning, or rectoanal coordination—is most useful in the treatment for fecal incontinence (6). However, most practitioners agree that additional treatment methods may be helpful with symptomatic improvement depending on the underlying condition.

Balloon Expulsion for Constipation

This training technique involves inserting a balloon into the rectum and inflating it with 50 milliliters of air so that the patient has the sensation of the need to defecate. Adherent perianal placement of surface electrodes allows the patient to see the resultant sEMG pattern made by voluntary sphincter contraction. The patient then is asked to expel the balloon, and if there is an increased, rather than decreased, sphincter activity, the patient is instructed on straining without increasing sphincter activity (25).

Sensory Discrimination Training for Fecal Incontinence

The sensory discrimination training technique involves a series of brief balloon inflations, noting the volume that induces a sensation of the urge to defecate, thereby establishing a current sensory threshold. The volume is subsequently reduced by 25% and a series of insufflations are repeated until the patient is able to promptly recognize the new stimuli (26). Once patients learn to associate the rise in intrarectal pressure with balloon inflation, the patient is encouraged to recognize sequentially smaller volumes of distention. Thus, after each session, new sensory thresholds are established (24). The mechanisms by which biofeedback training improves rectal perception are unclear. It is suggested that biofeedback training may recruit sensory neurons adjacent to damaged afferent pathways. However, the speed with which sensory thresholds improve during biofeedback suggests that patients use existing afferent pathways, but learn to pay more attention to weak sensations and to recognize their significance (discrimination training) (27).

Coordination Training for Fecal Incontinence

The aim of coordination training is to achieve a maximum voluntary squeeze in less than one to two seconds after inflation of the rectal balloon and to control the reflex anal relaxation by consciously contracting the sphincter muscles. This maneuver mimics the arrival of stool in the rectum and prepares the patient to react appropriately by using the relevant muscle group. With each balloon insufflation, the patient is asked to signal when they have perceived rectal distension and react to this distension by promptly contracting the PFM and maintaining this contraction without increasing intra-abdominal pressure. This maneuver is performed while the patient observes changes on the visual display, and the key element is to condition the EAS responses to improve the squeeze profile and the ability to respond to progressively smaller degrees of rectal distension (6).

Efficacy of Biofeedback—Literature Review

When interpreting the clinical outcome of the studies listed (Tables 6.5-6 and 6.5-7), one should keep in mind that there are no established guidelines regarding the number of sessions, teaching methods, clinician qualifications, type of equipment used, patient inclusion criteria, nor subjective or objective data used to establish success, all of which vary considerably. Hyman's critical review reports that, perhaps most importantly, there is no identified standard for training biofeedback clinicians to treat pelvic floor disorders. As with any therapy, the competence of the clinician is likely to have a significant impact on the outcome of treatment (28). Norton and

TABLE 6.5-6. Biofeedback studies in constipation.

First author	N	Pre-evaluation	DX	Mean age	Feedback method	Sessions	Follow-up	Evaluation assessment	Percent improved	Defined Success	Reference #
Emmanuel 2001	49	BE, EMG, CTT, CRAFT, Rectal Laser Doppler Flowmetry	IC	39	EMG + BD	4–7	28 months	Diary, Rectal Laser Doppler, BE, CTT Cardio respiratory autonomic function testing	59%	Pre- vs post-biofeedback: <3 BM/week (27 sv 9) Need to stain (26 vs 9) Laxative or suppository (34 vs 9) Slow transit (22 vs 9) Rectal mucosal blood flow: Improved vs not improved) (29% vs 7%)	25
Dailianas 2000	11	CTT, MN, DF, EMG	PPC	43	MN	2	6 months	Diary	54.5%	Symptom improvement	41
Lau 2000	173	DF	PPC	67	EMG	4–7	4–7	Diary	55%	Improved bowel function	42
Mollen 1999	7	CTT, DF, BE, MN	PPC	30	NR	10	NR	MN	NR	Effects rectocolonic inhibitory reflex	43
McKee 1999	30	DF, CTT, BEN, Colo, EMG, MN	PPC	35	MN	3–4	12 months	Diary, BE	30%	Symptom improvement	33
Chiotakakou 1998	100	CTT, MN, EMG	PPC + IC	40	EMG	4–5	23 months	Phone Interview	57%	Symptom improvement	34
Rieger 1997	19	MN, DF, CTT, EMG, BE	IC	63	EMG + BD	6	6 months	Interview	12.5%	>50% Symptom reduction at 6 months.	35
Glia 1997	26	MN, DF, CTT, EMG, BE	PPC	55	EMG, MN	1–2/week <10 weeks	6 months	Diary	58% 75% patients completed therapy	Symptom improvement	44

TABLE 6.5-6. *Continued*

First author	N	Pre-evaluation	DX	Mean age	Feedback method	Sessions	Follow-up	Evaluation assessment	Percent improved	Defined Success	Reference #
Ko 1997	32	EMG, DF, CTT, BE	PPC	50	EMG	4 (2–9)	7 months	Diary	80%	Symptom improvement	45
Patankar 1997	116	EMG, DF, MN, CTT, DF, AUS,	IC	73	EMG	8 (2–14)		Diary	73%	Satisfaction rate	46
Gilliland 1997	194	EMG, DF, MN	PPC	71	EMG	11 (5–30)	72 months	Return to normal (>3 unassisted BM/week)	35% overall (63% patients completed therapy	Normal bowel habits	29
Karlbom 1997	17	EMG, DF, MN, CTT	PPC	46	EMG, BE	8	14 months	Questionnaire	43%	Improved rectal emptying	47
Rao 1997	25	MN, DF, CTT, BE		50	MN, BE	2–10	<2 months	Diary MN, BE	92%	>% Anal relaxation >Intra rectal pressure >Defecation index <BE time <Laxative use <Straining	38
Patankar 1997	30			65.3	EMG	5–11	No	Diary EMG	84%	>Frequency of spontaneous BM >2/wk >EMG endurance and Net strength of external anal sphincter.	48
Park 1996	68	MN, DF, CTT, EMG	PPC	65.9	EMG	11	No	Diary and Questionnaire	25/85%	Improve or Unimproved	32

Ho 1996	62	MN, DF, CTT, EMG	PPC	48	MN, BE	4	14.9	Diary	90.3%	>Frequency of Spontaneous BM <Laxative and enema use >Symptom improvement	49
Leroi 1996	15	MN, EMG,	PPC	41.2	Psychotherapy, MN, EMG	16	6–10 months	Not reported (NR)	66.7%	Complete recovery of symptoms	50
Siproudhis 1995	27	MN, DF, BE	PPC	46	MN, BE	1–10	1–36 months	NR	51.8%	Complete disappearance of symptoms	51
Koutsomanis 1995	60	CTT, EMG, BE	PPC	40.5		1–7	2–3 months	Diary	50%	<EMG activity with Valsalva >Anismus index	52
Koutsomanis 1994	20	MN, DF, CTT, BE,	IC	34		2–6	6–12 months	Diary	50%	>BM Frequency <Staining >Symptom Improvement	53
Bleijenberg 1994	21	MN, EMG, DF, BE	PPC	37	EMG vs Balloon	8–11	No	Diary Constipation score	EMG—73% BE—22%	Symptom improvement	54
Papachrysostmou 1994	22	MN, DF, CTT, EMG, BE	PPC	42	EMG	>3	No	MN, DF, EMG Clinical Improvement	89% vs 86%	<EMG activity >Improved DF >Rectal Sensation	55
Keck 1994	12	MN, DF, CTT, EMG, BE	IC	62	EMG	3	1–8 months	Tel interview	58%	Symptom improvement	56
Trunbull 1992	7	MN, DF, CTT, EMG	PPC	35.7	MN, Relax	4–5	2–4 years	Diary	85.7%	Stool Frequency <Symptoms bloating and pain	57

TABLE 6.5-6. *Continued*

First author	N	Pre-evaluation	DX	Mean age	Feedback method	Sessions	Follow-up	Evaluation assessment	Percent improved	Defined Success	Reference #
Fleshman 1992	9	MN, DF, CTT, ENG, BE	PPC	49.4	EMG, BE, Relax	2 × 6	>6 months	BE, EMG	100%	<EMG activity during strain BE 60CC Eliminate psyllium slurry.	58
Wexner 1992	18	MN, DF, CTT, EMG	PPC	67.7	EMG	9	1–17	Diary	88.9%	Spontaneous BM Frequency <Laxative use	59
Dahl 1991	9	MN, DF, CTT, EMG, BE	IC	41	EMG	5	6	Diary	77.8%	BM frequency <Laxative use	60
Kawimbe 1991	15	MN, BE	PPC	45	EMG	2 per day	6.2	DF, Diary	86.7%	<Anismus index >anorectal angel straining BM frequency	
Lestar 1991	16	MN, DF, BE, CTT, EMG	PPC	42.5	Defecometer	1	0	Defecometer	68.7%	Ability to expel balloon	61
Webber 1987	22	MN	IC		MN	2–4	0	NR	18.2%	Daily spontaneous BM	62
Bleijenberg 1987	10	DF, CTT, EMG	PPC	32	EMG, BE	Daily	7	NR	70%	Spontaneous BM'S	63

MN, Manometry; CTT, Colon transit time; Colo, Colonoscopy; IC, Idopathic constipation; BE, Balloon expulsion; DF, Cinidefocography; BEN, Barium enema; PPC, Paradoxical puborectalis contraction.

TABLE 6.5-7. Biofeedback studies in fecal incontinence.

First author/Year	N	Age	Pre-evaluation	Post-evaluation	Feedback method	Treatment method	Sessions	Defined success	Percent improved	Reference
Engel 1974	7	40.7 (6–54)	MN	MN	MN	Coordination	1–4	Subjective	57%	64
Cerulli 1979	50	46 (5–97)	No	MN	MN	Coordination Sensitivity	1	>90%	72%	65
Goldenberg 1980	12	12	MN	No	MN	Sensitivity	>1	Subjective	83%	66
Wald 1981	17	47 (10–79)	MN	No	MN	Coordination Sensitivity PME	1–2	>75%	71%	67
Whitehead 1985	18	73 (65–92)	MN	MN	MN	PME	8	>75%	77%	68
Buser 1986	13	53.6	MN	MN	MN	Sensitivity PME	1–3	Subjective	92%	69
McLeod 1987	113	56 (25–88)	No	EMG	EMG	PME	3.3	>90%	63%	12
Enck 1988	19	47 (10–80)	MN	MN	MN	Coordination	5–10	Subjective	63%	70
Berti Riboli 1988	21	61 (14–84)	MN	MN	MN	Coordination Sensitivity PME	12	>90%	86%	71
Miner 1990	25	54 (17–76)	MN	MN	MN	Coordination Sensitivity PME	3	Subjective	76%	26
Loeing-Baucke 1990	8	63 (35–78)	MN	MN	MN	Coordination Sensitivity PME	3	>75%	50%	72
Keck 1994	15	39 (29–65)	MN	MN	EMG	Sensitivity PME	1–7	Subjective	53%	56
Guillemot 1995	24	(39–78)	MN	MN	MN	PME	4	Incontinence Score (IS)	Improved IS 19%	73

Table 6.5-7. *Continued*

First author/Year	N	Age	Pre-evaluation	Post-evaluation	Feedback method	Treatment method	Sessions	Defined success	Percent improved	Reference
Sangwan 1995	28	52 (30–74)	MN	MN	MN	Sensitivity PME	1–7	Complete Continence to solid stool	46% Excellent 29% Good 25% Bad	74
Ho 1996	13	62.1	MN	MN	MN	PME	11	>90%*	76.9%	75
Rao 1996	19	50 (17–78)	MN EMG	MN EMG	MN	Coordination Sensitivity PME	4–13	>67%	53%	76
Jensen 1997	28	34 (23–57)	MN		EMG	PME	3–4	>80% + Incontinence score	89%	77
Reiger 1997	30	68 (29–85)	MN	MN	EMG	PME	6	Incontinence score	67% Incontinence score	78
Ko 1997	25	63 (31–82)	MN EMG	EMG	EMG	PME	2–13	Subjective	92%	79
Pantankar 1997	25	34 (23–57)	EMG	EMG	EMG	PME	5–11	>75%	83%	46
Gila 1998	26	61 (32–82)	MN	MN	MN	Sensitivity PME	4–10	>50% Decrease in soiling episodes	23% Excellent 41% Good 36% No improvement	80
Leroi 1998	27	53 (29–74)	MN, PNTML USG	MN	MN	Coordination Sensitivity PME	4–14	Subjective	29.6%	81

MN, manometry; EMG, electromyography; PNTML, pudendal nerve terminal motor latency; PME, Pelvic muscle exercises.
* Decrease in frequency of incontinent episodes.

colleagues also reported that many patients lack the motivation or are unconvinced about the possible value of what they perceive to be simple exercises; therefore, the results of treatment are largely patient dependent, unlike drug or surgical therapy (19). Gilliland et al. from our group reported that patient motivation and willingness to comply with treatment protocols was the most important predictor of success (29).

Although feedback of information is essential for learning, the information itself—and the instrument providing the information—has no inherent power to create psychophysiological changes in humans. Therefore, to establish a double-blind placebo-controlled research protocol for biofeedback therapy based on the principle used for medication trials is inherently difficult. In 1991, Dahl defined his teaching methods of sensory awareness, shaping by teaching patients the correct sphincter responses, home practice, physiological quieting methods, generalization, and weaning from equipment. There was a reported symptom-improvement success rate of 78% for patients with anismus (30). Rao and colleagues' study is another example of defined teaching methods employing the essentials of biofeedback training and reporting 100% success, their defined success being greater than 50% symptomatic improvement whereby they concluded that biofeedback therapy effectively improves objective and subjective parameters of anorectal function in patients with fecal incontinence. They noted that customizing the number of sessions and providing periodic reinforcement might improve success (24).

Constipation

The many variants in these clinical trials may account for the wide range of success rates for biofeedback therapy ranging from 30% to 100% (Table 6.5-6). The number of treatment sessions varies significantly from one session of out-patient training to two weeks of daily in-patient training, followed by additional subsequent home training. Rao and colleagues' review noted that the end-point for successful treatment has not been clearly defined and the duration of follow-up has been quite variable (6). Enck pointed out that comparing clinical symptoms prior to and after treatment usually assesses treatment efficacy; however, other studies have reported formal evaluation of sphincter performance during physiological testing. Outcome sometimes was assessed by diary cards; however, reviews, telephone interviews, and questionnaires were used more often. These evaluation techniques are unreliable when the recorded event, such as defecation, is infrequent in nature (31). Furthermore, diagnostic data from physiologic testing beyond confirmation of spastic pelvic floor syndrome is often not reported. Patients' concomitant conditions disclose a significant variance in inclusion criteria (e.g., presence of rectoceles, rectal sensory thresholds, previous surgery), which presumably also contributes to the success of treatment (31). Park described two varieties of anismus—anal canal hypertonia and nonrelaxation of the puborectalis muscle—that appear, at least superficially, to correlate with the success of biofeedback, where anal canal hypertonia may be responsible for some cases of failure of biofeedback therapy (32).

McKee concluded that biofeedback for outlet obstruction constipation is more likely to be successful in patients without evidence of severe pelvic floor damage (33). Biofeedback is a conservative treatment option for patients with idiopathic constipation, although some studies have been shown to have less favorable results. The most recent study by Emmanuel and Kamm (25) in 2001 reported on 49 patients with idiopathic constipation pre- and post-biofeedback using objective measurements, as well as patient symptom diaries; symptomatic improvement occurred in 59% of patients. Twenty-two patients had slow transit before treatment, of which 14 reported symptomatic improvement and 13 developed normal colonic transit. There was a significant increase in rectal mucosal blood flow in patients who subjectively improved. These authors concluded that successful response to biofeedback for constipation is associated with specifically improved autonomic innervation to the large bowel and improved transit time. In 1998, Chiotakakou's study of 100 patients treated with biofeedback reported that 65% had slow transit and 59% had paradoxical puborectalis contraction on straining. Long-term follow-up at 23 months revealed that 57% of patients had felt their constipation improved (34). Reiger and colleagues evaluated the results of biofeedback to treat 19 patients with intractable constipation of nonspecific etiology and concluded that biofeedback had little therapeutic effect (35). In these cases, Wexner reported that patients remained symptomatic, requiring the inconvenience and expense of the use of cathartics (36). Engel and Kamm have also shown that excessive straining has both acute and chronic effects on pudendal nerve latencies, where long symptom duration with intense straining would result in significant nerve damage (14). It also has been reported that the chronic use of laxatives induces changes in the myenteric nerve plexi (37). In this respect, Wexner has suggested an alternate course of action, which would be to explain to patients that, although a success rate of only 40% to 60% with biofeedback can be anticipated, the success rate is determined by their willingness to complete the course of therapy. Patients should be counseled that biofeedback therapy is effectively the only recourse other than the continued use of laxatives and cathartics (36).

Fecal Incontinence

Enck's critical review summarized 13 clinical studies published between 1974 and 1990 using biofeedback therapy for the treatment of fecal incontinence (Table 6.5-6). He reported that weighting the number of patients included in each study yielded an overall success rate for this treatment of 79.8%. Despite the variety in almost all criteria used to compare these studies, the therapeutic outcome appears relatively consistent, ranging between 50% and 90% (8). In a review of 14 biofeedback studies performed between 1988 and 1997, Rao et al. reported that 40% to 100% of patients overall were improved (38). The mechanism by which training effects are achieved, however, is somewhat controversial (27). Some have argued that the most important ingredient is sensory discrimination training in which patients are taught to recognize and respond to increased intrarectal pressure (39) or to squeeze more quickly in response to rectal distension (26). Others believe that biofeedback works primarily by strengthening the EAS muscles (in conjunction with Kegel exercises) (40). In this regard, on one hand, sensation consistently improves with biofeedback. As this improvement occurs rapidly, it is likely to be associated with relearning of neurophysiologic patterns that are essentially intact but not in use because of "faulty" sensation. On the other hand, it is unlikely that short-term sensory discrimination training and coordination training will alter muscle tone or strength them sufficiently to modify a condition where muscle weakness is the primary contributor to the incontinence. Thus, when the muscles are weak but sensation is intact, symptom reduction would depend on changing muscle strength through an extended and well-designed exercise protocol (10). This approach has been shown clearly by Chiarioni (27) and Rao (24), who outlined specific goals to improve the strength of the anal sphincter, improve rectoanal coordination, and improve rectal sensory thresholds. Visual and verbal feedback techniques were used to reinforce their appropriate responses as they were being performed (24). In general, most experts believe that all components are useful and that the treatment program should be customized for a given patient depending on the underlying dysfunction (24).

Summary

Despite the many variables involved in the clinical trials reported for biofeedback, most experts agree that biofeedback is an attractive outpatient conservative treatment option that is cost-effective, relatively noninvasive, easy to tolerate, and morbidity free and that does not interfere with any future treatment options that may be recommended by the physician. It is gratifying to note that this simple technique can ameliorate symptoms and improve the quality of life in many patients with functional bowel and bladder symptoms attributed to pelvic muscle dysfunction. Its exact position in the treatment algorithm for subgroups with severe constipation and anismus or who present with fecal incontinence where there is not a demonstrable EAS defect is still being defined, as are the statistically significant prognostic factors predictive of success.

With the profusion of "newer" hemorrhoidectomy techniques (e.g., Ligasure hemorrhoidectomy, stapled hemorrhoidectomy) and procedures that are more minimalist for hemorrhoids (Doppler-guided hemorrhoid artery ligation), there appears to be a greater propensity for IAS damage because no operative attempt is made to separate the hemorroidal complex from the IAS muscle (82). In this context, there is little evidence that biofeedback therapy is effective once patients experience such isolated IAS damage with attendant passive fecal incontinence (19). This kind of troublesome soiling is also unresponsive to IAS muscle plication (83,84), silicone implantation (85), or autologous fat interposition (86). It has also been suggested by Kamm and colleagues (87) that biofeedback may be used with some success as a first-line therapy in the treatment algorithm when fecal incontinence is associated with a primary defect in the EAS muscle.

References

1. Sonnenberg A and Koch TR. Physician visits in the United States for constipation: 1958–1986. Dig Dis Sci. 1989;34:606–11.
2. Sonnenberg A and Koch TR. Epidemiology of constipation in the United States. Dis Colon Rectum. 1989;32:1–8.
3. Thompson WG, Longstreth GF, Drossman DA, Heaton KW, Irvien EJ, and Muller-lissner SA. Functional bowel disorders and functional abdominal pain. Gut. 1999;45:1143–54.
4. Jorge JMN and Wexner SD. Physiologic evaluation. In: Wexner SD and Vernava AM, editors. Clinical decision making in colorectal surgery. New York: IGAKU-Shoin: 1995. p. 11–22.
5. Wexner SD and Jorge JMN. Colorectal physiological tests: Use or abuse of technology? Eur J Surg. 1994;160:167–74.
6. Rao SSC, Welcher KDP, and Leistikow JS. Obstructive defecation: a failure of rectoanal coordination. Am J Gastroenterol. 1998:93:1042–50.
7. Hallan RI, Williams NS, Melling J, Walron DJ, Womack NR, and Morrison J. Treatment of anismus in intractable constipation with botulinum toxin. Lancet. 1988;2:714–7.
8. Enck P. Biofeedback training in disordered defecation: a critical review. Dig Dis Sci. 1993;38:1953–9.
9. Schiller LR. Fecal incontinence. In: Feldman M, Friedman L, and Sleisenger MH, editors. Slesinger and Fordtan's gastrointestinal and liver disease: pathophysiology/diagnosis/management. 7th ed. Philadelphia: Saunders; 2002. p.164–80.
10. Schwartz MS, and Associates. Biofeedback: a practitioner's guide. 2nd ed. New York: Guilford; 1995.
11. Shellenberger R and Green JA. From the ghost in the box to successful biofeedback training. Greeley, CO: Health Psychology Publication; 1986.
12. MacLeod JH. Management of anal incontinence by biofeedback. Gastroenterology. 1987;93:291–4.
13. Rao SSC. The technical aspects of biofeedback therapy for defecation disorders. The Gastroenterologist. 1998;6:96–103.
14. Engel AF amd Kamm MA. The acute effect of straining on pelvic floor neurological function. Int J Colorectal Dis. 1994;9:8–12.

15. Binnie NR, Kawimbe BM, Papachrysotomou M, Clare N, and Smith AN. The importance of the orientation of the electrode plates in recording the external anal sphincter EMG by non-invasive anal plug electrodes. Int J Colorectal Dis. 1991;6(5):8–11.
16. Hulme JA. Beyond kegels. Phoenix: Phoenix Publishing Co.; 1997.
17. Lennard-Jones JE. Constipation. In: Feldman M, Friedman L, and Sleisenger MH, editors. Slesinger and Fordtan's gastrointestinal and liver disease: pathophysiology / diagnosis / management. 7th ed. Philadelphia: Saunders; 2002. p. 181–209.
18. Burgio KL, Goode PS, Locher JL, Umlauf MG, Roth DL, Richter HE, Varner RE, and Lloyd LK. Behavioral training with and without biofeedback in the treatment of urge incontinence in older women. JAMA. 2002;288:2293–9.
19. Norton C and Kamm MA, Outcome of biofeedback for faecal incontinence. Br J Surg. 1999;86:1159–63.
20. Kegel A. The physiologic treatment of poor tone and function of the genital muscles and of urinary stress incontinence. West J Surg Obstet Gynecol. 1949;57:527–35.
21. Bump RC, Hurt WG, Fantl JA, and Wyman JF. Assessment of kegel pelvic muscle exercise performance after brief verbal instruction. Am J Obstet Gynecol. 1991;165:322–9.
22. Basmajian JV. Biofeedback: principles and practice for clinicians. Baltimore: Williams & Wilkins; 1989.
23. Charlesworth EA and Nathan RG. Stress management: A comprehensive guide to wellness. New York: Ballantine; 1985.
24. Rao SSC, Welcher KD, and Happel J. Can biofeedback therapy improve anorectal function in fecal incontinence? Am J Gastroenterol. 1996;91:2360–5.
25. Emmanuel AV and Kamm MA. Response to a behavioral treatment, biofeedback in constipated patients is associated with improved gut transit and autonomic innervation. Gut. 2001;49:214–9.
26. Miner PB, Donnelly TC, and Read NW. Investigation of mode of action of biofeedback in treatment of fecal incontinence. Dig Dis Sci. 1990;35:1291–8.
27. Chiarioni G, Bassotti G, Stegagnini S, Vantini I, and Whitehead WE. Sensory retraining is key to biofeedback therapy for formed stool fecal incontinence. Am J Gastroenterol. 2002;97:109–17.
28. Hyman S, Jones KR, Ringel Y, Scarlett Y, and Whitehead WE. Biofeedback treatment of fecal incontinence. Dis Colon Rectum. 2001;44:728–36.
29. Gilliland R, Heymen S, Altomare DF, Park UC, Vickers D, and Wexner SD. Outcome and predictors of success of biofeedback for constipation. Br J Surg. 1997;84:1123–6.
30. Dahl J, Lindquist BL, Leissner P, Philipson L, and Jarnerot G. Behavioral medicine treatment in chronic constipation with paradoxical anal sphincter contraction. Dis Colon Rectum. 1991;34:769–76.
31. Enck P and Musial F. Biofeedback in pelvic floor disorders. In: Pemberton JH, Swasch M and Henry MM, editors. The pelvic floor: its function and disorders. London: W.B. Saunders; 2002. p. 393–404.
32. Park UC, Choi SK, Piccirillo MF, Brezaro R, and Wexner SD. Patterns of anismus and the relation to biofeedback therapy. Dis Colon Rectum. 1996; 39:768–73.

33. McKee RF, McEnroe L, Anderson JH, and Finaly IG. Identification of patients likely to benefit from biofeedback for outlet obstruction constipation. Br J Surg. 1999;86:355–9.
34. Chiotakakou-Faliakou E, Kamm MA, Roy AJ, Storrie JB, and Turner IC. Biofeedback provides long term benefit for patients with intractable slow and normal transit constipation. Gut. 1998;6:517–21.
35. Rieger NA, Wattchow DA, Sarre RG, et al. Prospective study of biofeedback for treatment of constipation. Dis Colon Rectum. 1997;40:1143–8.
36. Wexner SD. Biofeeback for constipation. Dis Colon Rectum. 1998;41:670–1.
37. Smith B. Effect of irritant purgatives on the myenteric plexus in man and the mouse. Gut. 1968;9:139–43.
38. Rao SSC, Welcher KD, and Pelsan RE. Effects of biofeedback therapy on anorectal function in obstructive defecation. Dig Dis Sci. 1997;42:2197–205.
39. Latimer PR, Campbell D, and Dasperski J. A component analysis of biofeedback in the treatment of fecal incontinence. Biofeedback Self Regul. 1984;9:311–24.
40. Whitehead WE, Burgio KL, and Engel BT. Biofeedback treatment of fecal incontinence in geriatric patients. J Am Geriatr Soc. 1985;33:320–4.
41. Dailianas A, Skandalis N, Rimikis MN, Koutsomanis D, Kardasi M, and Archimandritis A. Pelvic floor study in patients with obstructive defecation. J Clin Gastroenterol. 2000;30(2):176–80.
42. Lau C, Heymen S, Albaz O, Iroatulam AJN, and Wexner SD. Prognostic significance of rectocele, intussusception, and abnormal perineal descent in biofeedback treatment for constipated patients with paradoxical puborectalis contraction. Dis Colon Rectum. 2000;43:478–82.
43. Mollen RMHG, Salvioli B, Camilleri M, Burton D, Kost L, Phillips SF, and Pemberton JH. The effects of biofeedback on rectal sensation and distal colonic motility in patients with disorders of rectal evacuation: Evidence of an inhibitory rectocolonic reflex in humans. Am J Gastroenterol. 1999;94:751–6.
44. Gila A, Gylin M, Gullberg K, and Lindberg G. Biofeedback retraining in patients with functional constipation and paradoxical puborectalis contraction. Dis Colon Rectum. 1997;40:889–95.
45. Ko CY, Tong J, Lehman RE, Shelton AA, Schrock TR, and Welton ML. Biofeedback is effective therapy for fecal incontinence and constipation. Arch Surg. 1997;132:829–34.
46. Patankar SK, Ferrara A, Larach SW, et al. Electromyographic assessment of biofeedback training for fecal incontinence and chronic constipation. Dis Colon Rectum. 1997;40:907–11.
47. Karlbohm U, Hallden M, Eeg-Olofssson, Pahlman L, and Graf W. Result of biofeedback in constipated patients. A prospective study. Dis Colon Rectum. 1997;40:1149–55.
48. Patankar SK, Ferrara A, Levy JR, Larach SW, Williamson PR, and Perozo SE. Biofeedback in colorectal practice. A multi center, statewide, three-year experience. Dis Colon Rectum. 1997;40:827–31.
49. Ho YH, Tan M, and Goh HS. Clinical and physiologic effects of biofeedback in outlet obstruction defecation. Dis Colon Rectum. 1996;39:520–4.
50. Leroi AM, Duval V, Roussignol C, Berkelmans I, Reninque P, and Denis P. Biofeedback for anismus in 15 sexually abused women. Int J Colorectal Dis. 1996;11:187–90.

51. Siproudhis L, Dautreme S, Ropert A, et al. Anismus and biofeedback: who benefits? Eur J Gastroenterol Hepatol. 1995;7:547–52.
52. Koutsomanis D, Lennard-Jones JE, Roy AJ, and Kamm MA. Controlled randomized trial of visual biofeedback versus muscle training without a visual display for intractable constipation. Gut. 1995;37:95–9.
53. Koutsomanis D, Lennard-Jones JE, and Kamm MA. Prospective study of biofeedback treatment for patients with slow and normal transit constipation. Eur J Gastroenterol Hepatol. 1994;6:131–7.
54. Bleijenberg G and Kuijpers HC. Biofeedback treatment of constipation: Comparison of two methods. Am J Gastroenterol. 1995;89:1021–6.
55. Papachrysostomou M and Smith AN. Effects of biofeedback on obstructed defecation—reconditioning of the defecation reflex. Gut. 1994;35:252–6.
56. Keck JO, Staniunas RJ, Coller JA, et al. Biofeedback training is useful in fecal incontinence but disappointing in constipation. Dis Colon Rectum. 1995; 37:1271–6.
57. Turnbull GK and Ritivo PG. Anal sphincter biofeedback relaxation treatment for women with intractable constipation symptoms. Dis Colon Rectum. 1992; 35:530–6.
58. Fleshman JW, Dreznik Z, Meyer K, Fry RD, Carney R, and Kodner IJ. Outpatient protocol for biofeedback therapy of pelvic floor outlet obstruction. Dis Colon Rectum. 1992;35:1–7.
59. Wexner SD, Cheape JD, Jorge JMN, Heyman SR, and Jagelman DG. Prospective assessment of biofeedback for the treatment of paradoxical puborectalis contraction. Dis Colon Rectum. 1992;35:145–50.
60. Kawimbe BM, Papachrysostomou M, Clare N, and Smith AN. Outlet obstruction constipation (anismus) managed by biofeedback. Gut. 1991;32:1175–9.
61. Lestar B, Penninckx F, and Kerremans R. Biofeedback defecation training for anismus. Int J Colorectal Dis. 1991;6:202–7.
62. Weber J, Ducrotte P, Touchais JY, Roussignol C, and Denis P. biofeedback training for constipation in adults and children. Dis Colon Rectum. 1987;30:844–6.
63. Bleijenberg G and Kuijpers HC. Treatment of the spastic pelvic floor syndrome with biofeedback. Dis Colon Rectum. 1987;30;108–11.
64. Engel BT, Nikoomanesh P, and Shcuster MM. Operant conditioning of rectosphincteric responses in the treatment of fecal incontinence. N Engl J Med. 1974;290:646–9.
65. Cerullli M, Nikoomanesh P, and Schuster MM. Progress in biofeedback conditioning for fecal incontinence. Gastroenterology. 1979;76:742–6.
66. Goldenberg DA, Hodges K, Hersh T, and Jinich H. Biofeedback therapy for fecal incontinence. Am J Gastroenterol. 1980;74:342–5.
67. Wald A. Biofeedback therapy for fecal incontinence. Ann Intern Med. 1981; 95:146–9.
68. Whitehead WE, Burgio KL, and Engel BT. Biofeedback treatment of fecal incontinence in geriatric patients. J Am Geriatr Soc. 1985;33:320–4.
69. Buser WE and Miner PB. Delayed rectal sensation with fecal incontinence. Gastroenterology. 1986;91:1186–91.
70. Enck P, Kranzle U, Schwiese J, et al. Biofeedback training in fecal incontinence. Dtsch Med Wochenschr. 1988;113:1789–94.
71. Riboli EB, Frascio MD, Pitto G, Reboa G, and Zanola R. Biofeedback conditioning for fecal incontinence. Arch Phys Med Rehabil. 1988;69:29–31.

72. Loening-Baucke V, Desch L, and Wolraich M. Biofeedback training for patients with myelomeningocele and fecal incontinence. Dev Med Child Neurol. 1988; 30:781–90.
73. Guillemot F, Bouche B, Gower-Rousseau C, et al. Biofeedback for the treatment of fecal incontinence: long-term clinical results. Dis Colon Rectum. 1995; 38:393–7.
74. Sangwan YP, Coller JA, Barrett RC, Roberts PL, Murray JJ, and Schoetz DJ Jr. Can manometric parameters predict response to biofeedback therapy in fecal incontinence? Dis Colon Rectum. 1995;38:1021–5.
75. Ho YH and Tan M. Biofeedback therapy for bowel dysfunction following low anterior resection. Ann Acad Med Singapore. 1997;26:299–302.
76. Rao SS, Welcher KD, and Happel J. Can biofeedback therapy improve anorectal function in fecal incontinence? Am J Gastroenterol. 1996;91:2360–6.
77. Jensen LL and Lowry AC. Biofeedback improves functional outcome after sphincteroplasty. Dis Colon Rectum. 1997;40:197–200.
78. Rieger NA, Wattchow DA, Sarre RG, et al. Prospective trial of pelvic floor retraining in patients with fecal incontinence. Dis Colon Rectum. 1997;40:821–6.
79. Ko CY, Tong J, Lehman RE, Shelton AA, Schrock TR, and Welton ML. Biofeedback is effective therapy for fecal incontinence and constipation. Arch Surg. 1997;132:829–34.
80. Glia A, Gylin M, Akerlund JE, Lindfors U, and Lindberg G. Biofeedback training in patients with fecal incontinence. Dis Colon Rectum. 1998;41:359–64.
81. Leroi AM, Dorival MP, Lecouturier MF, et al. Pudendal neuropathy and severity of incontinence but not presence of anal sphincter defect may determine the response to biofeedback therapy in fecal incontinence. Dis Colon Rectum. 1999;42:762–9.
82. Zbar AP, Beer-Gabel M, Chiappa A, and Aslam M. Fecal incontinence after minor anorectal surgery. Dis Colon Rectum. 2001;44:1610–23.
83. Deen KI, Kumar D, Williams JG, Grant EA, and Keighley MR. Randomized trial of internal anal sphincter plication with pelvic floor repair for neuropathic faecal incontinence. Dis Colon Rectum. 1995;38:14–8.
84. Leroi AM, Kamm MA, Weber J, Denis P, and Hawley PR. Internal anal sphincter repair. Int J Colorectal Dis. 1997;12:243–5.
85. Kenefick NJ, Vaizey CJ, Malouf AJ, Norton CS, Marshall M, and Kamm MA. Injectable silicone biomaterial for faecal incontinence due to internal anal sphincter dysfunction. Gut. 2002;51:225–8.
86. Cervigni M, Tomiselli G, Perricone C, and Panei M. Endoscopic treatment of sphincter insufficiency with autologous fat injection. Arch Ital Urol Androl. 1994;66(4 Suppl):219–24.
87. Kamm MA Personal communication (1997).

Editorial Commentary

Dawn Vickers has very simply described the methods of biofeedback employed for constipation and fecal incontinence. What is not stated in exact terms within this comprehensively referenced and authoritatively written yet user-friendly chapter is that the person who performs the therapy is as important, (if not more important), than the therapy itself. Specifically, the ability of the therapist to effectively communicate with the patient frequently and for prolonged periods of time is probably the most important factor for success. Although difficult to quantify, the therapist probably has as important a role, if not a more important role that the type of equipment and/or the setting where biofeedback therapy is undertaken. Ms. Vickers has presented a very easy to follow descriptive methodology for the application of biofeedback training for both constipation and fecal incontinence.

SW

Chapter 6.6
Evacuatory Dysfunction Following Gynecologic Surgery

THEODORE J. SACLARIDES and LINDA BRUBAKER

Introduction

The care of women with pelvic floor disorders is multidisciplinary and involves specialists who are skilled and knowledgeable in all anatomical and functional disorders. It is rare for a single specialist to have the necessary knowledge and skill to treat all of these problems. A multidisciplinary group of interested clinicians working together in a pelvic floor center may improve patient care. These centers typically include urologists, gynecologists, urogynecologists, and general or colorectal surgeons, as well as allied specialists including radiologists, pain specialists, neurologists, physical therapists, mental health specialists, and gastroenterologists.

This interrelationship between different entities is reflected in the very conditions being treated. For example, women who present for the evaluation of either fecal or urinary incontinence frequently will report flatus incontinence as well. Vaginal support problems are almost always combined disorders, and failure to recognize and treat all of the defects virtually ensures that the patient will be dissatisfied with the result. In short, one cannot treat women with pelvic floor problems without adopting a "whole pelvis" viewpoint.

This chapter will focus on anorectal abnormalities following gynecologic surgery. These abnormalities may be secondary to physiologic changes alone, anatomic changes, or a combination of the two. For example, while alterations in urinary function after radical hysterectomy have been widely documented, anorectal function may be changed as well after this operation, yet this has not received quite the same attention nor is it as well understood. These changes may represent a neurophysiologic alteration with preservation of the anatomy of the affected organ. Anatomic changes affecting the anus and rectum may occur following correction of vaginal prolapse or rectoceles. Combined anatomic and physiologic changes can affect the anus and rectum following obstetrical injuries.

Nervous System of the Pelvic Viscera

A review of the autonomic nervous system anatomy is essential in understanding the physiologic changes that may accompany surgical procedures in the pelvis. The sympathetic nervous system originates from preaortic nerve fibers that coalesce in the vicinity of the sacral promontory to form the superior hypogastric plexus. This plexus is a fenestrated group of nerve fibers anterior to the lower abdominal aorta; it divides into easily recognizable right and left hypogastric nerve trunks that traverse the lateral pelvic side wall to the deeper regions of the pelvis. Therefore, the hypogastric nerves carry sympathetic nerve fibers to the pelvic plexus, which is found in the vicinity of the lateral rectal stalks and which contain the middle rectal arteries. In some reports, the pelvic plexus has been called the inferior hypogastric plexus. The parasympathetic nervous system originates from the second, third, and fourth sacral nerve roots; thus, the nerves formed are called the nervi erigentes, which travel to the pelvic plexus. Fibers leaving the pelvic plexi contain both sympathetic and parasympathetic fibers, which then are distributed to the various pelvic viscera such as the bladder, prostate, seminal vesicles, urethra, rectum, and anal canal.

Mundy performed an elegant study involving 12 cadaveric dissections in order to understand why bladder dysfunction follows rectal and uterine surgery. His work confirmed that the pelvic parasympathetics come primarily from the S3 and S4 nerve roots, which lie deep to the parietal fascia covering the piriformis muscle. At the ischial spine, the nerves pierce this fascia and enter the visceral pelvic fascia, which encircles the rectum, ultimately joining the hypogastric nerves to form the pelvic plexus. In women, the pelvic plexus is very close to the anterolateral aspect of the lower rectum and some of the plexus is situated on the lateral wall of the upper one-third of the vagina. The bulk of the plexus is below the broad ligament, although some of its fibers extend into the cardinal ligament, hence its propensity for injury during radical hysterectomy. In men, the medial aspect of the pelvic plexus is situated more closely to the rectum than in women. The posterior one-half of the plexus lies close to the anterolateral wall of the lower rectum. The anterior half of the plexus is found on the posterolateral aspect of the prostate (1).

Regarding the bladder, parasympathetic nerves innervate the detrusor, which receives relatively few sympathetic fibers. The parasympathetic fibers also innervate the bladder neck and the urethral sphincter muscle. Sympathetic fibers provide a rich nerve network to the smooth muscle of the bladder neck. The rectal vault is composed of an inner circular and an outer longitudinal muscle layer. As the rectum descends through the levator hiatus, the circular muscle continues into the anal canal as the internal anal sphincter (IAS), a tight and uniform circle of smooth muscle. The longitudinal muscle continues caudally as the conjoined muscle layer. The levator ani consist of the pubococcygeus and iliococcygeus. The puborectalis muscle is an important determinant of fecal continence and, in some literature, is included in the levator ani complex; however, it functions more closely with the external anal sphincter (EAS) despite being separable from the deep component of the EAS (2). The IAS provides 50% to 85% of the resting tone of the anal canal and is in a state of constant tonic contraction. The IAS relaxes only when induced to do so by the presence of a bolus of air or solid material within the rectal lumen. This effect is called the rectoanal inhibitory reflex (RAIR) and can be demonstrated and measured manometrically with either a closed balloon or water-perfused anal manometry catheter. Resting tone within the anal canal—a reflection of the IAS—is measured when a balloon is inflated within the rectal vault. Relaxation of the IAS allows the bolus of material to descend into the anal canal and reach the sensory rich area of the anus, where anorectal sampling and sensory discrimination may occur. The IAS is stimulated by the sympathetic nervous system through the hypogastric nerves, and parasympathetic activity inhibits the IAS, inducing relaxation.

The EAS is an oval-shaped bundle of striated muscle fibers. It differs from other striated muscles in that, like the IAS, it is in a state of continuous tonic activity at rest and during sleep. By its bulk, it partially contributes to the resting tone of the anal canal and impedes the passage of air, liquid, and solid material. In fact, changes in the basal tone of the EAS pressure can be detected with postural changes, as well as increases in intra-abdominal pressure and during straining. The EAS is innervated by the inferior rectal branch of the pudendal nerve (S2, S3) and by its perineal branch (S4). When the RAIR is elicited with small volumes, there is some reflex contraction of the EAS when the IAS relaxes. With increasing volumes, the EAS ultimately relaxes as well.

The subject of the RAIR is discussed in Chapter 2.3. The neural pathways of the RAIR are not completely understood. The EAS response is mediated through the spinal cord, where both the afferent and efferent pathways are located in the pudendal nerve. The EAS response is abolished in the presence of cauda equina lesions and rarely by tabes dorsalis. The RAIR response of the IAS is separate and distinct and may be maintained through an intramural process whereby receptors within the wall of the rectum detect the presence of a bolus and then transmit this information to the IAS, resulting in relaxation. The IAS component of the RAIR is not present in cases of Hirschsprung's disease (HD) and may be abolished following proctectomy for cancer or inflammatory bowel disease, return of which after anterior resection appears to correlate with improvement in reported function and a reduction in nocturnal fecal urgency. Here, Lubowski et al. have shown that the RAIR is maintained after bilateral hypogastric nerve blockade and following complete isolation of the rectum from its extrinsic nerve supply. The reflex is absent when the rectum is distended above a circumferential myotomy and the response of the IAS is assessed within the anal canal. This report has demonstrated conclusively that the pathways for the RAIR are entirely within the wall of the rectum and the anal canal (3).

The pudendal nerve is a mixed motor and sensory nerve and is variably derived from the somatic components of the second, third, and fourth sacral nerves. The fibers typically coalesce to form nerve trunks superior to the sacrospinous ligaments and lateral to the coccyx. The pudendal nerves enter the ischiorectal space by passing through Alcock's canal close to the obturator internus. Their function is independent of the nervi erigentes, and the nerve usually is spared from injury during pelvic surgery because it is covered by dense pelvic fascia (4). The significance of pudendal nerve latency in clinical coloproctology is discussed in Chapter 2.9.

Changes Accompanying Pelvic Surgery

Damage to the superior hypogastric plexus, hypogastric nerves, and pelvic plexus may occur during abdominoperineal resection (APR) for rectal cancer. These alterations are less likely to occur during proctectomy for inflammatory bowel disease because the dissection in these cases is carried out in close proximity to the bowel wall, where injury to the laterally located nerves is less frequent. During APR, damage to the pelvic nerves can occur at several points, and caution should be exercised during the dissection when these critical areas are reached. These areas include the preaortic region (sympathetic fibers), the sacral promontory in delineation of the mesorectal plane (superior hypogastric plexus, hypogastric nerves), the lateral rectal stalks in dissection of the lateral ligaments of the rectum (pelvic plexus, parasympathetic, and sympathetic), and around each viscus (mixed nerve injury). In males, injury to the superior hypogastric plexus or hypogastric nerves causes retrograde ejaculation (30%–40%), whereas injury to the pelvic plexus is manifested primarily by impotence (up to 100%). If nerve-sparing surgery is performed, normal sexual function can be preserved in the vast majority of men who had normal function prior to surgery (5). Frequently, urinary retention is initially encountered after surgery, although the need for long-term bladder catheterization after abdominoperineal resection varies widely in the literature. There has equally been greater emphasis recently on the incidence and treatment of sexual dysfunction after rectal resection (6), with a high rate of success using Sildanefil for erectile difficulty after this procedure (7).

The technique of hysterectomy has evolved substantially and is tailored to the pathology being addressed and the local conditions within the pelvis. Simple hysterectomy is associated with a low incidence of nerve-related complications; however, the progressively more radical hysterectomy techniques require extensive lateral dissection with resulting nerve damage. A Wertheim (or modified radical) hysterectomy involves removal of the central portion of the parametrial tissue while minimizing disruption to ureteral and vesical vasculature. The cardinal ligaments are removed and the uterine artery is ligated medial to the point where it crosses the ureter. Radical hysterectomy removes as much parametrial tissue as possible and the cardinal ligaments are excised widely. Pelvic and para-aortic node dissections are frequently added to the procedure. Injury to the pelvic nerves during radical hysterectomy has been well described and probably occurs during division of the cardinal ligaments where the pelvic plexus can be found. The addition of pelvic radiotherapy produces an additive effect that results in deterioration in function or may cause overt nerve injury (8–10). Bladder catheter drainage initially after surgery is common, although normal function is seen in the majority of patients by two to three weeks, as evidenced by normal post-voiding urinary residual volumes without strain voiding (typically less than $100 cm^3$). However, long-term bladder problems are observed in approximately 5% of patients, although new techniques, including neuromodulation, may be an effective treatment for such refractory patients. The constellation of bladder-related problems stems from abnormal parasympathetic, sympathetic, and somatic nerve function and includes reduced bladder compliance, abnormal bladder sensation (usually decreased), detrusor hypo- or "acontractility," and urinary stress incontinence (11).

Anorectal dysfunction following hysterectomy has not been studied as extensively as bladder problems. The few reports that exist are limited in sample size, with reporting of inexact and nonspecific symptoms such as bloating and colic. Indeed, a lack of "state-of-the-art" means for assessing anorectal physiology is a hallmark of most of these small series. Small sample size is particularly a problem in trying to determine whether bowel symptoms are secondary to the surgery itself or result from the effects of pre- or postoperative irradiation (12). There is no question that bowel dysfunction follows radical hysterectomy in many patients, but the reported symptoms seem to be all-inclusive and vary from constipation to incontinence depending on the particular study. Whereas the disturbances in bladder function are understandable based on our knowledge of the pelvic nervous anatomy, such is not the case with anorectal dysfunction. Division of the cardinal ligaments and injury to the pelvic plexus should not affect IAS relaxation during the RAIR because this is an intramural reflex. Similarly, injury to the pelvic plexus should not affect the pudendal nerve because this nerve functions independently of the nervi erigentes and is protected from injury by its thick overlying fascia. (vide supra) Nevertheless, as the following reports show, anorectal dysfunction affects many women following radical hysterectomy.

Here, Barnes et al. studied anorectal function in 15 women with stage 1 cervical cancer treated with radical hysterectomy. Anal manometry was performed before surgery and again one week after. Various parameters were studied and bowel function surveys were conducted. Resting (IAS function) and squeeze (EAS function) pressures did not change significantly;

however, 9 patients had diminished relaxation of the IAS when the RAIR was elicited. Twelve patients needed increased volumes of air insufflated into the rectum in order to feel a sense of fullness. Clinically, 12 patients had worsening bowel function following surgery, where symptoms included a loss of the urge to defecate and excessive straining. These symptoms usually subsided within a period of 12 weeks. None of the patients experienced incontinence (13). These findings are somewhat hard to explain in light of our current knowledge of the pelvic nervous system. If the pelvic plexus was injured, one might expect lower anal resting pressures. Normal squeeze pressures are to be expected because these are a reflection of intact pudendal nerves. As expected, the RAIR was present, although the volumes of rectal air needed to elicit it were higher after surgery.

In a study by Sood et al. (14), 11 women with early stage cervical cancer undergoing radical hysterectomy were studied with anal manometry and a bowel symptom survey. The assessment was performed before surgery and again 6 months postoperatively. The findings were somewhat different from those of Barnes and colleagues in that diminished resting and squeeze pressures were detected. The authors noted that the rectum became more compliant following surgery, but that smaller volumes of intrarectally administered saline were needed to cause leakage (14). Furthermore, the maximum tolerated volume of saline was reduced, which seems at odds with the observation that the rectum became more compliant. Another confusing finding in this study was that pudendal nerve conduction times were bilaterally prolonged. Clinically, 6 patients experienced incontinence for flatus, with 2 women reporting incontinence for stool.

Regarding colonic motility, Vierhout et al. (15) have reported profound constipation in 2 patients following radical hysterectomy. One patient felt the first urge to defecate only after 180 milliliters of air had been instilled into the rectum, although she had completely normal manometry. In the second patient, colonic transit studies noted delayed transit in the sigmoid colon, where symptoms improved following segmental left hemicolectomy. During manometry, in this case, reduced squeeze pressures were noted.

In summary, radical hysterectomy is associated with potential complications as a consequence of injury to each pelvic plexus when the cardinal ligaments are resected widely. Bladder dysfunction has been well described and is understandable based on our knowledge of the pelvic autonomic nervous system. Anorectal dysfunction has been noted as well, but the conflicting manometric findings and clinical symptoms are neither consistently reported nor completely explainable. Perhaps the findings are due to factors not limited to autonomic nerve injury, as evidenced by the fact that EAS function and the RAIR should not be affected by an injury to the pelvic plexus, yet such observations have frequently been made. Rectal compliance, emptying, and the overall mechanics of defecation may be affected by a loss of anterior support following hysterectomy, where patients undergoing simple or subtotal hysterectomy rarely have bowel-related symptoms after surgery. In fact, the effect on bowel function and anorectal manometry following hysterectomy has been poorly studied, although there is a consensus that preexisting constipation in such patients is often considerably worsened (16). The reasons for this finding are complex and multifactorial, with little correlation between symptoms and anorectal manometry, although it is likely that pelvic autonomic and pudendal nerve injury play a part along with alteration of paravaginal support mechanisms, which may precipitate vaginal vault descensus and rectocele/perienocele development (17).

Dysfunction Following Repair of Vaginal Support Defects

A variety of surgical procedures has been developed to correct vaginal support defects. Symptoms stemming from rectoceles and enteroceles include evacuatory difficulty, vaginal pressure, and bulging and coital problems secondary to discomfort or fear of losing stool during intimacy. For the most part, selected surgical repair of these defects is successful; however, many women remain symptomatic and present to either their initial surgeon or another specialist for correction of persistent—or even new—symptoms.

Constipation is a frequently reported complaint; however, the treating physician must determine the exact type of problem the patient is experiencing. This subject is discussed extensively in other parts of this book. Constipation generally falls into two categories, each having a different physiologic basis, constellation of symptoms, and treatment. The first pattern is one of colonic inertia, whereby the patient does not feel the urge to defecate despite the passage of several days or even weeks. Progressive abdominal distension and bloating are noted, which frequently force the patient to possess two sets of clothing—one set for wear on the days immediately following defecation, the other set as constipation worsens. Diagnosis of this pattern of altered colonic motility rests upon measurement of colonic transit time. Radiopaque markers placed within gelatin capsules are ingested; their progress is followed with serial plain abdominal radiographs and transit time is calculated.

The second type of constipation is characterized by the sensation that stool has reached a certain point within the rectum beyond which it will not pass. Evaluation and treatment of stool consistency is the primary intervention; however, when symptoms persist despite normal stool consistency, further evaluation may be necessary. Typically, defecatory urges are present, but manual or digital assistance or positional gyrations on the toilet are required to evacuate. Conditions that may cause obstructed defecation include rectoceles, rectal intussusception, enteroceles, and sigmoidoceles. To evaluate fully the pelvic floor and the extent to which these entities are present and interfere with defecation, one must obtain a defecating proctogram, also known as defecography (see Chapter 3.1).

Defecography is a fluoroscopic evaluation of the pelvic floor and relies on opacification of the viscera with barium sulfate or a water-soluble contrast agent for the bladder. Oral contrast is ingested to facilitate identification of enteroceles; bladder contrast is given if there are coexisting bladder complaints or abnormal physical findings, and vaginal and rectal contrast are given as well. A dedicated radiologist is mandatory for successful completion and interpretation of the test. Once the contrast has reached its desired location, the patient sits on an upright commode specifically designed for this procedure, which is secured to a fluoroscopic table. Views of the pelvis are obtained at rest, and then the patient is instructed to squeeze her pelvic floor muscles and to expel the rectal contrast as though defecating. Rapid film sequences are obtained at two frames per second. The relationships of the pelvic viscera to each other can then be determined. This procedure is especially useful in the workup of patients with obstructed defecation, where the contours of rectoceles, enteroceles, and sigmoidoceles can be seen.

Defined as any outpouching beyond the normal confines of the rectum, rectoceles vary widely in their appearance and the degree to which they are responsible for symptoms. Many vaginally parous women have anatomic findings of distal vaginal support defects and even defecographic findings consistent with rectocele. It has been a research challenge to link the anatomical findings to the symptoms experienced by these patients. Most rectoceles are found low in the rectovaginal septum; however, if prior repairs were not extended sufficiently cephalad, then defects will persist higher in the septum. In addition to a feeling of obstructed defecation, rectoceles can cause a sudden and unanticipated loss of stool in up to one-third of cases (18). This occurs as a result of rapid delivery of previously sequestered stool to the anus, and there may be insufficient time for recognition, sampling of contents, and deferment of defecation until a socially acceptable time and place. Rectoceles can be found in asymptomatic patients; therefore, caution must be exercised before one attributes constipation to their presence. Certainly, the need for assisted defecation, a sense of incomplete evacuation, and the presence of a posterior vaginal bulge all point to the rectocele as the potential culprit. This is supported further by the finding during defecography of retention of contrast and an inability to completely expel the contrast despite maximum straining, although these matters are very controversial (19,20).

Enteroceles are defined as a herniation or abnormally low descent of the pelvic peritoneum below the normal confines of the cul-de-sac. Enteroceles normally are found posterior to the vagina. Here, the small bowel descends into this space and may cause outward bulging of the vagina, pelvic pressure, compression of the anterior wall of the rectum, and impaired evacuation of stool. In his landmark article, Burch noted that following cystourethropexy, that 7.5% of patients developed enteroceles (21). Enteroceles also may appear after hysterectomy as a component of vaginal vault prolapse where there is an inadequate culdosuspension (22). The principles of enterocele repair involve identification of coexisting defects, excision (or obliteration) of the hernia sac, high ligation of the sac, and support along the levator plate (levatorplasty). The axis of the upper vagina must be restored by pulling the apex posteriorly and superiorly—a procedure that may be performed at open surgery or laparoscopically (23,24).

Sigmoidoceles are defined as prolapse of redundant portions of the sigmoid colon into an abnormally deep cul-de-sac. The physical findings and symptoms are essentially the same as for enteroceles; however, the distinction between these two entities may not be possible unless defecography is performed (25). Rectoanal intussusception is considered a precursor of full-thickness rectal prolapse. During defecography, the rectum assumes a funnel-shaped configuration during straining. The intussusceptum may remain in the rectal vault, descend to the anal opening, or descend externally, as one would see with overt rectal prolapse. The significance of finding intussusception during defecography is controversial because it can be demonstrated in asymptomatic individuals, and the degree to which symptoms can be attributed reliably to its presence is debatable. Moreover, when surgical procedures originally designed to treat overt rectal prolapse have been applied to intussusception, the results have been less than satisfactory. This may stem from the fact that evacuatory problems may in fact have been principally due to other causes.

Dynamic magnetic resonance imaging (MRI) may be an alternative to defecography in the investigation of certain patients. In the only study directly comparing these two techniques, Kelvin et al. found that defecography was superior for the demonstration of rectoceles (26). It is likely that this represents an effect of position on principal diagnosis and categorization during simulated evacuation (27). Rentsch et al. confirmed that MRI is capable of detecting combined defects so commonly found in patients with pelvic floor dysfunction (28).

Symptoms of altered defecation and pelvic pressure may persist following seemingly successful repairs of vaginal support defects, although this has received comparatively little attention in the literature. In order to avoid this pitfall, preoperative recognition and identification of all defects is essential. Isolated defects are uncommon, and surgery should not be undertaken until one makes a concerted effort to fully study all of the pelvic viscera. Physical examination alone may not be accurate and the preoperative assessment must at least include defecography. Here, in a study by the authors, defecography changed the physical examination diagnosis in 75% of women studied by opacification of the pelvic viscera. Interestingly, 26% of clinically presumed cystoceles, 36% of enteroceles, and 25% of rectoceles were not present on defecography. In contrast, when physical examination was negative for these defects, 63% of patients were found to have cystoceles, 46% enteroceles, and 73% rectoceles. One could argue that many of these radiographic abnormalities are not clinically significant; however, only 61% of women with posterior vaginal eversions that either reached or went beyond the introitus were diagnosed correctly by physical examination. In the remainder, either the diagnosis was changed completely or additional unsuspected abnormalities were found. The larger the posterior vaginal support defect, the more likely physical examination was incorrect (29). This would certainly help explain why bowel evacuatory symptoms might persist following initial attempts at repair, although it is somewhat unclear why they become symptomatically more relevant when they presumably have predated surgery.

Bowel Dysfunction Following Repair of Obstetrical Injuries

Fortunately, most third- and fourth-degree obstetrical lacerations heal satisfactorily following prompt repair at the time of delivery, with only a small portion failing to heal adequately. However, symptoms of fecal and flatus incontinence occur frequently, even with prompt recognition and repair of anal sphincter injuries. These disorders can occur even without vaginal delivery, as demonstrated by Lal et al. (30) and by the group headed by O'Connell (31).

Two complications of non-healing include rectovaginal fistula formation and incontinence secondary to disruption of the anal sphincter muscle. Symptoms referable to the former include the passage of vaginal gas or stool, fecal soilage, chronic vaginitis, and social and sexual embarrassment. Incontinence may be for gas, liquid stool, or solid matter. When questioning a patient with incontinence, it is important to determine the extent to which she is symptomatic and what measures are used to control the symptoms. In other words, the physician should ascertain whether the patient is incontinent of solid stool, the frequency with which the episodes occur, whether pads are frequently needed, and whether the problem leads to social and sexual limitations.

If a rectovaginal fistula is suspected, the diagnosis can be confirmed by bi-digital examination or by a vaginal speculum examination. If the diagnosis is still in doubt, an examination under anesthesia is indicated. Once a fistula is found, surgery should be delayed for two reasons. Firstly, the strength and integrity of the local tissues may not be immediately suitable for reconstruction, and secondly, many fistulas may heal spontaneously. If a fistula has not healed within three months, it is not likely to do so and surgical repair may be undertaken if local inflammation and infection have subsided. If one considers the mechanism of injury—namely tearing or cutting of the rectovaginal septum, including the sphincter muscle—an assessment of clinical symptoms and the health of the sphincter muscle must be obtained preoperatively. In this regard, the authors feel that anal ultrasound imaging of the sphincter must be performed prior to repair of obstetrically induced rectovaginal fistulas. Failure to recognize a sphincter injury may lead to persistent symptoms of fecal soilage, or even gross incontinence if only the fistula is repaired. It is also not infrequent that a secondary perineoplasty is required in many cases to bolster an attenuated perineal body (32).

Anal ultrasound has had a tremendous impact in the diagnosis and management of patients complaining of incontinence. Routine postpartum ultrasound in asymptomatic primiparous women may reveal evidence of sphincter injuries in as many as 30% of patients. Later studies have cast some doubt on this high rate and suggested that there may be a normal "gap" in the anterior portion of the anal sphincter complex (33,34). Although initially asymptomatic, these women may develop problems later in life. A second vaginal delivery in a woman with an asymptomatic anal sphincter defect significantly increases her risk of symptoms. Ultrasound is capable of demonstrating injuries of either the internal sphincter, external sphincter, or both. If the ultrasound is normal, incontinence may be due to a stretch injury of the pudendal nerve or alterations in rectal sensory thresholds. It also is clear that there is a time-related deterioration in clinical and functional outcome after initially successful EAS repair (35). This may be due in part to an inadequacy in the rostral extent of repair a suggested by recent three-dimensional endoanal reconstructed ultrasonography (36) or, conversely, overzealous repairs that partially denervate and/or devascularize the sphincter ends.

Summary

Rather than considering it a loose association of independently functioning organs, the pelvis should be looked upon as an organ system unto itself, composed of subdivisions that rely on each other for normal function. The anterior and posterior compartments share a common nervous system and provide structural support for each other. Therefore, it is easy to see that surgical treatment of one subdivision may have functional impact on the others. In this chapter, we have discussed how radical hysterectomy has been associated with alterations in anorectal function, although an adequate and comprehensive explanation for these findings is currently lacking. Persistent evacuation symptoms may follow surgery for vaginal support defects if there was an incomplete assessment of the pelvic floor before surgery. Similarly, fecal incontinence may persist following repair of a rectovaginal fistula if one did not assess the anal sphincter preoperatively. A multidisciplinary approach to pelvic floor problems is truly required in order to optimize patient care.

References

1. Mundy AR. An anatomical explanation for bladder dysfunction following rectal and uterine surgery. Br J Urol. 1982;54:501–4.
2. Fucini C, Elbetti C, and Messerini L. Anatomic plane of separation between external sphincter and puborectalis muscle: clinical implications Dis Colon Rectum. 1999;42:374–9.
3. Lubowski DZ, Nicholls RJ, Swash M, and Jordan MJ. Neural control of internal anal sphincter function. Br J Surg. 1987;74:668–70.
4. Barber MD, Bremer RE, Thor KB, Dolber PC, Kuehl TJ, and Coates KW. Innervation of the female levator ani muscles. Am J Obstet Gynecol. 2002;187:64–71.
5. Havenga K, Enker WE, McDermott K, Cohen AM, Minsky BD, and Guillem J. Male and female sexual and urinary function after total mesorectal excision with autonomic nerve preservation for carcinoma of the rectum. J Am Coll Surg. 1996;182:495–502.
6. Kim NK, Aahn TW, Park JK, Lee KY, Lee WH, Sohn SK, and Min JS. Assessment of sexual and voiding function after total mesorectal excision with pelvic autonomic nerve preservation in males with rectal cancer. Dis Colon Rectum. 2002;45:1178–85.
7. Lindsey I, George B, Kettlewell M, and Mortensen N. Randomized, double-blind, placebo-controlled trial of Sildanefil (Viagra) for erectile dysfunction after rectal excision for cancer and inflammatory bowel disease. Dis Colon Rectum. 2002;45:727–32.
8. Kottmeier HL. Complications following radiation therapy in carcinoma of the cervix and their treatment. Am J Obstet Gynecol. 1964;88:854–66.
9. Farquharson DI, Shingleton HM, Sanford SP, Soong SJ, Varner RE Jr, and Hester S. The short-term effect of pelvic irradiation for gynecologic malignancies on bladder function. Obstet Gynecol. 1987;70(1):81–4.
10. Ferrigno R, dos Santos Novaes PE, Pellizzon AC, Maia MA, Fogorelli RC, Gentil AC, and Salvajoli JV. High-dose-rate brachytherapy in the treatment of uterine cervix cancer: Analysis of dose effectiveness and late complications. Int J Radiat Oncol Biol Phys. 2001;50(5):1123–35.
11. Lin HH, Sheu BC, Lo MC, and Huang SC. Abnormal urodynamic findings after radical hysterectomy or pelvic irradiation for cervical cancer. Int J Gynaecol Obstet. 1998;63:169–74.
12. Iwamoto T, Nakahara S, Mibu R, Hotokezaka M, Nakano H, and Tanaka M. Effect of radiotherapy on anorectal function in patients with cervical cancer. Dis Colon Rectum. 1997;40:693–7.
13. Barnes W, Waggoner S, Delgado G, Maher K, Potkul R, Barter J, and Benjamin S. Manometric characterization of rectal dysfunction following radical hysterectomy. Gynecol Oncol. 1991;42:116–19.
14. Sood AK, Nygaard I, Shahin MS, Sorosky JI, Lutgendorf SK, and Rao SS. Anorectal dysfunction after surgical treatment for cervical cancer. J Am Coll Surg. 2002;195:513–19.
15. Vierhout ME, Schreuder HW, and Veen HF. Severe slow transit constipation following radical hysterectomy. Gynecol Oncol. 1993;51:401–3.
16. Kell JL, O'Riordain DS, Jones E, Alawi E, O'Riordain MG, and Kirwan WO. The effect of hysterectomy on ano-rectal physiology. Int J Colorect Dis. 1998;13:116–18.

17. Thakar R, Ayers S, Clarkson P, Stanton S, and Manyonda I. Outcome after subtotal versus total hysterectomy. N Engl J Med. 2002;347:1318–25.
18. Marti M-C, Roche B, and Déléval J. Rectoceles: value of video-defaecography in selection of treatment policy. Colorectal Dis. 1999;1:324–9.
19. Ting KH, Mangel E, Eibl-Eibesfeldt B, and Muller-Lissner SA. Is the volume retained after defecation a valuable parameter at defecography. Dis Colon Rectum. 1992;35:762–8.
20. Halligan S and Bartram CI. Is barium trapping in rectoceles significant? Dis Colon Rectum. 1995;38:764–8.
21. Burch JC. Cooper's ligament urethrovesical suspension for stress incontinence. Nine years' experience—results, complications, technique. Am J Obstet Gynecol. 1968;100:764–74.
22. Cruickshank SH. Sacrospinous fixation—should this be performed at the time of vaginal hysterectomy? Am J Obstet Gynecol. 1991;164:1072–6.
23. Backer MH. Success with sacrospinous suspension of the prolapsed vaginal vault. Surg Gynecol Obstet. 1992;175:419–20.
24. Nezhat CH, Nezhat F, and Nezhat C. Laparoscopic sacral colpopexy for vaginal vault prolapse. Obstet Gynecol. 1994;84:885–8.
25. Fenner DE. Diagnosis and assessment of sigmoidoceles. Am J Obstet Gynecol. 1996;175:1438–42.
26. Kelvin FM, Maglinte D, Hale DS, and Benson JT. Female pelvic organ prolapse: A comparison of triphasic dynamic MR imaging and triphasic fluoroscopic cystocolpoproctography. AJR Am J Roentgenol. 2000;174:81–8.
27. Schoenberger AW, Debatin JF, Guldenschuh I, Hany TF, Steiner P, and Krestin GP. Dynamic MR defecography with a superconducting open-configuration MR system. Radiology. 1998;206:641–6.
28. Rentsch M, Paetzel C, Lenhart M, Feuerbach S, Jauch KW, and Furst A. Dynamic magnetic resonance imaging defecography: A diagnostic alternative in the assessment of pelvic floor disorders in proctology. Dis Colon Rectum. 2001;44:999–1007.
29. Smith C, Brubaker L, and Saclarides T. Fluoroscopic evaluation of the pelvic floor. In: Brubaker L and Saclarides T, editors. The female pelvic floor: disorders of function and support. Philadelphia: F.A. Davis; 1996. p. 88.
30. Lal M, Mann C, Callender R, and Radley S. Does Cesarean delivery prevent anal incontinence? Obstet Gynecol. 2003;101:305–12.
31. Fynes M, Donnelly VS, O'Connell PR, and O'Herlihy C. Caesarean delivery and anal sphincter injury. Obstet Gynecol. 1998;92(4 Pt1):496–500.
32. Draganic B, Eyers AA, and Solomon MJ. Island flap perienoplasty decreases the incidence of wound breakdown following overlapping anterior sphincter repair. Colorectal Dis. 2001;3:387–91.
33. Fritsch H, Brenner E, Lienemann A, and Ludwikowski B. Anal sphincter complex: reinterpreted morphology and its clinical relevance. Dis Colon Rectum. 2002;45:188–94.
34. Bollard RC, Gardiner A, Lindow S, Phillips K, and Duthie GS. Normal female anal sphincter: Difficulties in interpretation explained. Dis Colon Rectum. 2002;45:171–5.
35. Karoui S, Leroi AM, Koning E, Menard JF, Michot F, and Denis P. Results of sphincteroplasty in 86 patients with anal incontinence. Dis Colon Rectum. 2000;43:813–20.

36. Gold DM, Bartram CI, Halligan S, Humphries KN, Kamm MA, and Kmiot WA. Three-dimensional endoanal sonography in assessing anal canal injury. Br J Surg. 1999;86:365–70.

Editorial Commentary

Dynamic magnetic resonance imaging and transperineal sonography have both shown that the vast majority of female patients with evacuatory dysfunction have multicompartment disease needing a multidisciplinary approach to surgical and/or rehabilitative therapy. Moreover, preexisting evacuatory difficulty may be exacerbated by gynecological surgeries including hysterectomy and colpoperinneorhaphy. The etiology of this problem at the present time is somewhat unclear but it is likely to be secondary to an autonomic neuropathy consequent on cardinal ligament disruption as well as distortion of the posterior vaginal supporting mechanisms. Enterocele is a particular consequence of a failure of vaginal vault suspension after hysterectomy which may frequently be associated with vault prolapse itself, necessitating secondary sacrospinous fixation. Recently, more minimalist operative support techniques for patients with concomitant urinary incontinence have been employed and these appear to be associated with less postoperative anorectal dysfunction, given that about one-quarter of patients with faecal incontinence and one-third with full-thickness rectal prolapse will have associated genital prolapse.

AZ

Chapter 7
Assessing the Patient with Fecal Incontinence

Chapter 7.1
An Overview

Marc A. Gladman, S. Mark Scott, and Norman S. Williams

Definition and Epidemiology of Fecal Incontinence

Fecal incontinence may be defined as the "involuntary loss of stool or soiling at a socially inappropriate time or place" (1), or more formally by the Rome II criteria as the "recurrent uncontrolled passage of fecal material for at least one month, in an individual with a developmental age of at least 4 years" (2). It is common, affecting all ages and both sexes, and is estimated to affect approximately 2% of the adult population with an equal prevalence in males and females (3–6), increasing to up to 15% in the elderly (7,8). However, the prevalence is much higher in specific groups, in that 50% of nursing home residents (9) and patients with multiple sclerosis (10) and 20% of patients with diabetes mellitus (11) and irritable bowel syndrome (IBS) (12) suffer with fecal incontinence.

Fecal incontinence is a devastating condition and has a major impact on quality of life (13). Not only does it constitute a physical and psychological disability, but it also may lead to social isolation and loss of independence (14). In addition to individual suffering, it constitutes a substantial economic burden to individual patients and health care resources (15). The social embarrassment experienced by sufferers means that patients often are unwilling to admit to symptoms, and doctors are reluctant to embarrass patients by asking about it (14,16). Consequently, this means that we are likely to grossly underestimate the true prevalence of this condition.

Etiology of Fecal Incontinence

Fecal incontinence may occur as a consequence of congenital or acquired disorders (see Table 7.1-1). Acquired fecal incontinence may occur secondary to local organic pathology of the hindgut, and it is essential for such pathology to be excluded when patients are assessed. However, in the majority of cases, fecal incontinence occurs secondary to disordered function of the anorectum.

TABLE 7.1-1. Etiology of fecal incontinence.

Congenital		
Congenital anorectal anomalies		
Spina bifida		
Hirschsprung's disease		
Acquired		
Local organic pathology of the anorectum	Proctitis	
	Neoplasm	
		Carcinoma
		Adenoma
	Stricture	Radiation
		Inflammatory
		Iatrogenic
	Fistulae	
Functional disorders of the anorectum	Anatomical	Prolapse
		Rectocoele
	Physiological (see below)	Abnormal stool consistency
		Sphincter dysfunction
		Neuropathy (pudendal)
		Reservoir dysfunction
		Sensory dysfunction
		CNS/cognitive disorders

Pathophysiology of Fecal Incontinence

The normal continence mechanism is dependent on, amongst other factors, a complex physiological interaction between motor and sensory components of the anorectum. Thus, abnormalities of one or more of the components that maintain continence may result in fecal incontinence. It is far more useful in clinical practice to classify incontinence according to underlying pathophysiology, as this dictates appropriate management (see below). However, it is accepted that pathophysiology is often multifactorial.

Abnormal Stool Consistency

Fecal incontinence most commonly occurs as overflow secondary to fecal impaction, particularly in institutionalized older patients (17). Incomplete rectal emptying can result from disorders of rectal evacuation, which must be excluded, and if present, adequately addressed. Conversely, the arrival of copious quantities of liquid stool may overwhelm an otherwise normally functioning continence mechanism in patients with diarrhea (18). Rapid hindgut transit, as present in certain patients with the IBS, together with abnormalities of gastrointestinal secretion and/or absorption will affect stool consistency and volume.

Sphincter Dysfunction

In our practice, sphincter dysfunction accounts for the majority of cases of fecal incontinence. As in other tertiary referral centers (19), trauma to the anal sphincter during childbirth, followed by iatrogenic injury after anal surgery are the most common identifiable causes of sphincter injury.

Internal anal sphincter dysfunction may arise as a consequence of structural damage, usually during childbirth or anal surgery (19) or in the absence of structural damage either due to primary idiopathic degeneration (20) or secondary to tissue disorders such as scleroderma (21).

The contribution of other pelvic floor muscles to the continence mechanism may be underappreciated; it has recently been shown that levator ani weakness is strongly associated with severity of incontinence (22).

Pelvic Floor Denervation

The branches of the pudendal nerve, which provide efferent and afferent pathways to the external anal sphincter (EAS) and perineum, are vulnerable to stretch injury, which may result in muscle weakness and consequently incontinence. Such injury may occur during childbirth (23–26), with chronic straining at stool (27–29), or secondary to rectal prolapse (30). Prior to the advent of endoanal ultrasound, the majority of cases of idiopathic or "neurogenic" fecal incontinence were believed to be as a result of pudendal nerve injury (31). However, it is now recognized that structural damage to the anal sphincters rather than pudendal neuropathy is the underlying pathogenic mechanism in most patients (19,32–35), and true isolated neuropathy may be rare (36). Nevertheless, there is an association between pudendal neuropathy and EAS weakness in patients with fecal incontinence, which supports the theory that a pathological process affecting pudendal nerve conduction impairs anal sphincter function (37).

Rectal "Reservoir" Dysfunction

The mechanism of rectal compliance—the ability of the rectum to adapt to an imposed stretch—enables rectal contents to be accommodated, which allows defecation to be delayed. Under normal conditions, the viscoelastic properties of the rectal wall allow it to maintain a low intraluminal pressure during filling so that continence is not threatened. Alterations in rectal compliance, however, may result in decreased rectal capacity and heightened sensory perception (hypocompliance; i.e., a "stiffer" rectal wall) or increased rectal capacity and blunted sensory perception (hypercompliance; i.e., more "elastic" rectal wall). In patients with incontinence, the rectum is often poorly compliant (38,39), leading to reduced reservoir function/capacity and symptoms of urgency/frequency of defecation (40). Reduced compliance may be associated with inflammation, fibrosis, surgery, or reinnervation following anorectal injury (41–45), although the true cause–effect relationship is, as yet, unclear.

Anorectal Sensory Dysfunction

Anorectal sensation is conveyed via the pelvic nerves, although the location of the receptors mediating rectal sensory function is still unknown. Although mechanoreceptors are present in the rectal wall, the rectum itself is not essential for certain sensations, as patients with a coloanal anastomosis or ileal pouch can appreciate the desire to defecate (46). Therefore, it is likely that stretch receptors located in the puborectalis, levator ani, and sphincteric musculature contribute to sensory discrimination (47). Injury to the afferent nerve pathways will disturb sensory perception; this may be associated with fecal incontinence, as intact sensory function is an integral part of the continence mechanism. Both impaired (blunted) and heightened rectal sensation have been reported in patients with incontinence (14,40,48–51).

Neurological/Cognitive Dysfunction

Common neurological diseases (e.g., multiple sclerosis, dementia, stroke, diabetes mellitus) or traumatic CNS injury, which may affect function (efferent and afferent neural pathways) at any level of the nervous system, are likely to disturb continence. Both upper and lower motor neuron lesions have been shown to be associated with fecal incontinence. In addition, psychobehavioral factors will have an impact upon function of the anorectum. Patients often have a mixed clinical presentation (i.e., frequency and urgency of defecation/urge incontinence, or infrequency of defecation with blunted call to stool/overflow incontinence).

Risk Factors for the Development of Fecal Incontinence

Most individuals acquire fecal incontinence as a result of some form of insult, with obstetric trauma, anal surgery, neurological disease, and pelvic surgery being reported as risk factors (5,19,52–56). In some cases, the cause–effect relationship is clear in that a temporal relationship is evident; the sufferer ascribes the event to onset of symptoms (e.g., 5%–13% incidence of new onset fecal incontinence post-vaginal delivery in primiparous females) (57,58), and the pathophysiology is demonstrable on anorectal function testing (57). Symptoms, however, may not develop until many years after the event (59), and thus the clarity of association may be lost to both sufferer and practitioner. It is known that the incidence of occult anal sphincter damage following vaginal delivery (even those deemed "uneventful") is much higher than the incidence of immediate post-partum incontinence (60), and that unsuspected anal sphincter defects occur following various "minor" anal surgical procedures (53). Such pathophysiology provides the potential for subsequent development of incontinence in combination with other factors—namely, ageing (61).

Clinical Approach to Fecal Incontinence

Comprehensive clinical evaluation of patients, with integration of the findings from clinical history, physical examination, and investigations, allows the etiology of the incontinence to be deduced, coexisting pathology to be excluded, and a decision regarding choice of suitable, rather than empirical therapy to be made on an individual basis.

A detailed and careful clinical history will reveal important information relating to three key areas: (a) severity of the incontinence, (b) likely etiology, and (c) impact of symptoms on quality of life. An assessment of the severity of symptoms may be made by recording details relating to the frequency and amount of leakage of solid and liquid stool and to flatus. Indeed, several incontinence severity scales that take account of such features, together with the use of pads, anal plugs, and/or the use of constipating medications, have been devised in an attempt to objectively quantify the severity of the incontinence (52,62–64). However, such scales assign arbitrary weights to individual events and make no formal assessment of impact of symptoms on quality of life (14). Furthermore, no one system has been universally adopted.

The impact of symptoms on quality of life, along with the severity of the incontinence, is a major consideration when planning patient management, particularly when contemplating surgery. Consequently, present physical, social, and psychological function and the restriction imposed by symptoms must be assessed in detail. Details relating to lower gastrointestinal symptoms, and in particular anorectal function, may provide important clues regarding the underlying etiology and pathophysiology, and on the basis of associated presenting symptoms, it is frequently possible to make a differentiation between incontinence related to local organic pathology of the anorectum and that related to disordered function (Table 7.1-1).

In the absence of associated symptoms suggestive of organic bowel disease (e.g., inflammatory bowel disease, neoplasia, etc.), clues relating to potential pathophysiological abnormalities should be sought. For example, the nature of the incontinence may reveal clues as to the underlying pathophysiology in that passive and urge fecal incontinence tend to be related to internal and external anal sphincter dysfunction, respectively (65). Information relating to the consistency of the stools and the presence and degree of urgency or reduced sensory loss may be helpful. Similarly, a history of constipation or rectal evacuatory difficulties may indicate that the incontinence is secondary to overflow. The presence of neurological disorders, lumbosacral trauma, and features suggestive of rectal or hemorroidal prolapse should be noted.

A comprehensive history of past medical events should be taken, specifically searching for evidence of diabetes mellitus, alcohol abuse, and other conditions that may result in neuropathy. Particular attention should be paid to a history of past surgical procedures of the pelvis and anorectum, and in women, events relating to previous childbirth (parity, length of second stage, birth weights, instrumental delivery, perineal trauma) should be noted.

A thorough general and abdominal examination should be performed. Of particular relevance to the assessment of fecal incontinence is the examination of the neurological system and the anorectum. With respect to neurological evaluation, attention should be focused on somatic lumbosacral spinal cord function; an assessment of gait and neurological function of the lower limbs should be performed in all cases. If neurological disease is likely, clearly, more detailed examination is warranted.

When examining the anorectum, the patient usually is positioned in the left lateral position with the hips flexed, although the "jack-knife" position also is used. The examination begins with inspection of the anus and perineum. Evidence of congenital anomalies should be noted. The normal perianal skin has a corrugated appearance and, together with the surrounding area, should be checked for the presence of fecal soiling, mucus or purulent discharge, and excoriation. Any skin tags, external hemorrhoids, fistulae, etc. should be noted and clearly documented. The anal canal usually is closed at rest; a patulous anus may suggest underlying sphincter dysfunction. The "anocutaneous reflex" is a reflex retraction of the anus, secondary to contraction of the EAS, in response to stimulus of the perianal skin. Loss of the reflex is suggestive of a neuropathic process and requires more formal evaluation. Next, the patient is asked to bear down and the degree of perineal descent is noted, together with any hemorroidal, rectal, or utero-vaginal prolapse. Finally, the patient is asked to cough and any leakage of feces or urine is noted.

The examination proceeds with digital examination of the anorectum. A basic idea of resting tone and strength of voluntary contraction of the EAS and puborectalis can be gained, although this is not necessarily accurate (66). The sphincter complex is palpated for the presence of defects, and the rectum is examined for masses and the presence of impacted feces. The examination is completed by performing a proctosigmoidoscopy to exclude local organic pathology of the distal bowel and functional anatomical disorders (prolapsing hemorrhoids/rectal mucosa and rectocele). The finding of a solitary rectal ulcer may indicate the presence of an evacuatory disorder leading to secondary incontinence.

In the vast majority of cases, a comprehensive clinical history and examination will provide sufficient information to allow differentiation between patients with incontinence secondary to local organic pathology of the hindgut from those with functional disorders. However, in some cases, this may not be possible and additional consideration to more detailed radiological or endoscopic assessment of the hindgut is required. As alluded to above, most cases of fecal incontinence arise as a result of anorectal dysfunction. In such cases, elucidation of the underlying pathophysiological mechanisms requires formal physiological assessment of anorectal function.

Physiological Investigation in Patients with Fecal Incontinence

This section should be read in conjunction with the relevant parts in Section 1 of this book.

Indication

Rigorous laboratory assessment of colorectal/anorectal function is not required for all patients with fecal incontinence. However, those patients in whom empirical conservative measures have failed and coexisting disease has been excluded should be considered for further specialist investigation. As continence and the process of defecation depend upon multiple and complex physiological—and psychobehavioral—mechanisms, the pathophysiology of fecal incontinence may therefore be multifactorial. In order to systematically evaluate all aspects of anorectal function, it is our firm belief that patients should undergo a structured, comprehensive series of complementary tests that address:

1. anal sphincter and pelvic floor function,
2. anal sphincter morphology,
3. pudendal nerve function,
4. rectal "reservoir" function (sensation; compliance; capacity),
5. rectal evacuation,
6. gastrointestinal (primarily colonic) transit

For each individual, results of such tests hopefully will provide characterization of the sensory and motor disorders responsible for presenting symptoms, and thus promote evidence-based guidance of management strategy. Several studies have looked at the clinical impact of anorectal physiological investigation in patients with fecal incontinence and demonstrated that the information provided markedly improves diagnostic yield (67,68) and directly influences a change in management in a significant proportion of cases (67–71).

Anorectal physiological investigation also should be recommended in potential candidates for anorectal surgery no matter how "minor" the procedure (e.g., hemorrhoidectomy). This will provide the surgeon with objective prognostic information regarding anorectal function and the potential for developing postoperative incontinence, which obviously is crucial from a medico-legal standpoint. Following therapeutic intervention, data yielded from physiological investigation will allow an objective assessment of therapeutic efficacy.

Laboratory Investigations

A number of investigations exist for the assessment of anorectal function (Table 7.1-2); although many of these tests are now established in clinical practice, including anorectal manometry, endoanal ultrasound, etc., others (e.g., impedance planimetry, vectorvolume manometry) currently remain as research techniques limited to a few specialist centers.

Established Methodologies

Anorectal Manometry

This is the best established and most widely available tool. Anorectal manometric evaluation commonly encompasses a series of measurements designed to test for:

1. functional deficits in anal sphincter tone,
2. the presence or absence of rectoanal reflexes,
3. normal or abnormal rectal sensory function and compliance.

The biggest pitfall with anorectal manometry is the lack of uniformity regarding equipment and technique. Consequently, comparison of results between centers is problematic; therefore, each individual institution is encouraged to develop its own control values or, if using normative data from the literature, adopt similar methodology (72).

The apparatus required consists of four major components:

(a) an intraluminal pressure-sensing catheter (water-perfused, or with mounted solid-state microtransducers, air- or water-filled microballoon(s), or a sleeve sensor);
(b) pressure transducers;
(c) a balloon for inflation within the rectum (either integral to the catheter assembly or fixed to an independent catheter);
(d) the amplification/recording/display system.

For investigation of anal sphincter function, the objectives of assessment are to identify the functional anal canal length and to record the maximum resting anal canal pressure and voluntary anal squeeze pressure. A station

TABLE 7.1-2. Tests available for the assessment of anorectal and colorectal function in patients with fecal incontinence.

Test	Modality assessed	Pathophysiological information yielded	Clinical implications	Primary symptom
Mandatory investigations				
Anorectal manometry	(i) Anal sphincter function	Attenuated anal resting tone	Indicative of IAS dysfunction	Passive
		Attenuated anal squeeze pressures	Indicative of EAS dysfunction	Urge
	(ii) Rectal sensation	Altered sensory perception of rectal distension	Hypersensitivity associated with reduced reservoir capacity/ heightened perception	Urgency/urge
			Hyposensitivity associated with increased reservoir capacity/ blunted perception	Passive (overflow)/ post-defecation leakage
Endoanal ultrasound	Imaging of anal sphincters and associated structures	Anal sphincter defects	IAS defects	Passive
			EAS defects	Urge
Useful investigations				
Electrophysiology	Pudendal nerve terminal motor latencies (PNTML)	Prolonged latencies	Indicative of pudendal neuropathy—associated with attenuated EAS function	Urge
Anorectal manometry	Rectal compliance	Altered rectal biomechanical properties	Hypocompliance ("stiff" rectal wall) associated with reduced reservoir capacity	Urgency/urge
Prolonged anorectal/ rectosigmoid manometry	Anorectal/rectosigmoid motility	Disturbances of rectosigmoid contractile activity/motor patterns	Rectosigmoid dysmotility (hypercontractility: high-amplitude contractions/altered periodic motor activity)	Urgency/urge
	Coordination of rectal and anal motor events	Altered frequency and duration of transient IAS relaxations	Abnormal rectoanal motor/reflex coordination	Passive

TABLE 7.1-2. *Continued*

Test	Modality assessed	Pathophysiological information yielded	Clinical implications	Primary symptom
Evacuation proctography	Rectal evacuatory function	Disordered rectal evacuation secondary to mechanical or "functional" obstruction	Coexistent, possibly "occult" rectal evacuatory disorder	Passive (overflow)/post-defecation leakage
Transit studies	Gastrointestinal (primarily colonic) transit	Delayed transit	Coexistent colonic dysmotility—slow-transit constipation (±rectal evacuatory disorder)	Passive (overflow)/post-defecation leakage
		Rapid transit	Colonic/GI dysmotility—associated with loose stools	Urgency/urge
Investigations with limited value				
Anal mucosal electrosensitivity	Anal sensation	Altered sensory perception of anal electrostimulation	Blunted perception indicative of neuropathic process	Passive and urge
Anal manometry	Rectoanal inhibitory reflex (RAIR)	Attenuated reflex activity	Indicative of neuropathic process	Passive and urge
Non-established investigations				
Vectorvolume manometry	Anal sphincter function	Global or sector pressure deficits/pressure asymmetry	Indicative of IAS or EAS dysfunction or both	Passive and urge
3D endoanal ultrasound	Imaging of anal sphincters and associated structures	Anal sphincter defects	IAS or EAS defects	Passive and urge
Endoanal MRI	Imaging of anal sphincters and associated structures	Anal sphincter defects	IAS or EAS defects	Passive and urge
		Reduced EAS muscle bulk	EAS atrophy	Urge
Electronic barostat	(i) Rectal biomechanical properties	Altered rectal wall biomechanics	Attenuated reservoir function	Passive and urge
	(ii) visceral sensation	Altered sensory perception of rectal distension	Attenuated reservoir function	Urgency/urge
Impedance planimetry	Rectal biomechanical properties	Altered rectal wall biomechanics	Attenuated reservoir function	Passive and urge

pull-through (72,73), continuous pull-through (47,74), or stationary technique (75) is employed. The functional anal canal length usually is shorter in incontinent patients than normal control subjects (76). Symptoms of passive fecal incontinence correlate with low resting anal tone (65,77). This typically is due to internal anal sphincter (IAS) rupture (e.g., obstetric trauma, iatrogenic injury) (65), but also may be secondary to smooth muscle degeneration (20). Symptoms of urge or "stress" fecal incontinence often correlate with low anal squeeze pressures (65,77). In addition, squeeze duration is reduced (78) and squeeze "fatigue rate" is shortened significantly (79) in incontinent patients compared to controls. However, although low or poorly sustained voluntary anal squeeze pressures implies EAS weakness, standard manometry alone cannot differentiate between compromised muscle integrity or impaired innervation, or both, as a cause of that weakness. Anal squeeze pressure has been shown to be reasonably sensitive and specific for discrimination of patients with fecal incontinence (80,81); nevertheless, the correlation between anal canal pressures and incontinence is not perfect, given the range of normal values and the contribution of various other factors crucial to anorectal continence.

Relaxation of the caudal anus in response to rectal distension—the "rectoanal inhibitory reflex" (RAIR)—was first described by Gowers in 1877 (82), and it is believed to play an important role in the continence mechanism. Although differences in reflex parameters have been shown between incontinent patients and healthy subjects, the clinical significance of these findings is unclear. It has been shown that parametric assessment of the RAIR may correlate with fecal incontinence where a more rapid recovery of the inhibitory wave occurs in patients with demonstrable EAS atrophy (83). This would imply a more substantial role for IAS function in patients whose voluntary sphincter is already compromised.

Rectal sensory function is most commonly quantified using simple latex ("party") balloon distension. Two techniques are used for inflation: (1) ramp (continual) (84), or (2) intermittent, which can be either phasic (volumes injected and then withdrawn) (84) or stepwise (volumes are maintained between inflations) (85) in nature. Thresholds for first sensation, desire to defecate, and maximum toleration (86), as volunteered by the patient, are recorded. Both blunted (elevated thresholds; hyposensitivity) and hyperacute (lowered thresholds; hypersensitivity) rectal sensory function can be implied from this test. Both abnormalities have been reported in some patients with fecal incontinence. Those with rectal hypersensitivity typically complain of urgency/urge incontinence and increased frequency of defecation (40,48,50). Those with significant loss of the ability to sense distension may have passive (overflow) incontinence (49,51,87).

Compliance, which reflects rectal capacity and distensibility, may be measured in conjunction with the evaluation of rectal sensory thresholds. Intraballoon (intrarectal) pressure and the balloon volume must be monitored simultaneously; compliance is calculated as change in volume divided by change in pressure (ΔV/ΔP) over that part of the pressure–volume curve between first sensation and maximum toleration. This is somewhat simplistic, however, given that the pressure–volume relationship is nonlinear. In a proportion of patients with incontinence, the rectum has been shown to be poorly compliant (i.e., the rectal wall is "stiffer", primarily related to urgency) (38,39). Rectal compliance is most commonly measured using a catheter-mounted balloon and ramp inflation technique; this has been termed the proctometrogram (88). A more sophisticated evaluation of compliance and other properties of rectal sensorimotor function can be achieved using the electronic barostat (see below).

Other parameters or mechanisms of anorectal function that can be studied using manometric methods include: the rectoanal contractile reflex, anorectal pressures during coughing/straining maneuvers, rectal balloon expulsion, and the saline continence test. To date, these modalities have not found routine use in patients with fecal incontinence.

Anal Mucosal Electrosensitivity

Anal mucosal sensation can be quantified using a catheter-mounted bipolar ring electrode inserted into the anal canal. A current is passed through the electrode and steadily increased until sensation threshold is reported by the patient (89). Mucosal sensitivity is impaired in patients with fecal incontinence (89–92) and abnormal perineal descent (93), and this impairment may persist in the long-term following traumatic vaginal delivery (94). Although such findings have contributed to our understanding of the pathophysiology of fecal incontinence, the diagnostic value of this test and its influence on management are limited (92,95). Routine use is not recommended.

Electrophysiology

The pudendal nerve terminal motor latency (PNTML) is a measurement of the conduction time from stimulation of the pudendal nerve at the level of the ischial spine(s) to the evoked EAS contraction. This is achieved using a disposable glove-mounted stimulating and recording electrode (St. Mark's pudendal electrode) connected to a suitable recorder. Prolonged latencies are suggestive of pudendal neuropathy and have been demonstrated in incontinent patients who have suffered obstetric trauma (23–26), have excessive perineal descent (96,97), or a recognized neurological disorder (98). However, the value and, indeed, the validity of pudendal nerve latency testing has been increasingly questioned, given that most patients are now recognized as having identifiable muscle damage or degeneration (19,20). Although "grouped" data show that incontinent patients with bilaterally prolonged PNTMLs have reduced anal squeeze pressures compared to controls (37,99), thus supporting the concept that a neuropathic process impairs EAS function, the sensitivity and specificity of this test is poor; many patients with delayed latencies have squeeze pressures within the normal range and vice versa (37,100). This lack of agreement is likely to be due to methodological limitations:

1. PNTMLs increase with age, independent of continence status (101,102);
2. the PNTML reflects the function of the fastest conducting motor fibers, and thus normal latencies may be recorded in a damaged nerve as long as some fast-conducting fibers remain (101);
3. the test is operator-dependent and may be technically difficult to perform in some patients.

In conclusion, recording of PNTML may contribute little to the management of "individual" patients with fecal incontinence, and its routine use should now be questioned (37,95). Unilateral prolongation of PNTMLs is probably without clinical significance (102).

Other electrophysiological techniques exist for the evaluation of anal sphincter neuromuscular status in patients with fecal incontinence, including EAS electromyography (EMG) and motor- and somatosensory-evoked potentials. However, the clinical relevance of these techniques remains controversial, and the "gold-standard" has yet to be established. It recently has been suggested that the results of anal sphincter electromyography are more sensitive and more closely related to the anal functional status, as assessed on manometry, than measurement of PNTMLs (103).

Endoanal Ultrasonography

Endoanal ultrasound has superseded digital examination and needle EMG for the evaluation of sphincter integrity, and now provides the cornerstone for clinical investigation of patients with fecal incontinence. Accurate sonographic imaging of the sphincter muscles has revolutionized our understanding of the pathogenesis of incontinence and shown that structural damage rather than pudendal nerve damage is the underlying cause in most patients (32–35).

Given the predominantly cylindrical nature of the anal structures, imaging is best suited to a 360-degree axial view obtained at right angles to the lumen, and this is achieved using a 10-megahertz (MHz) transducer attached to a mechanically rotating endoprobe. Although operator-dependent, sensitivity and specificity approach 100% for the identification of anatomical defects if carried out by an experienced practitioner (104–106). Structural damage to either the internal or external anal sphincter can be identified clearly, as well as degenerative changes in the smooth muscle (20).

In incontinent patients, endoanal ultrasound has revealed that obstetric trauma followed by anal surgery are the major risk factors. Up to 90% of women in whom childbirth is the only apparent risk factor have ultrasonographic evidence of damage to one or both of the anal sphincters (32,34,35,57). In asymptomatic patients, "unsuspected" sphincter defects are also a common finding, as demonstrated by prospective studies of childbirth and various anal surgical procedures (32,53,57,107). The long-term effect of such occult damage is, as yet, unclear (60).

Of those physiological and imaging techniques available for the evaluation of patients with fecal incontinence, ultrasound is the test most likely to influence a change in management (70,71). Based on ultrasonographic findings (in conjunction with other test results), rational treatment can be planned, including the selection of patients who may benefit from surgery.

Ambulatory Manometry (See Chapter 2.6)

Prolonged assessment of anorectal or rectosigmoid motor activity may provide further invaluable information regarding the cause(s) of anorectal dysfunction in patients with fecal incontinence, and this technique is gaining increasing recognition as a clinical tool. A manometric catheter incorporating several solid-state pressure microtransducers is stationed intraluminally so that recording sites lie within the sigmoid, rectum, and anal canal. The catheter is connected to a portable, solid-state recording system, which allows monitoring of anorectal motility under "normal" physiological conditions over prolonged periods in ambulant subjects. This is particularly useful in patients in whom symptoms are intermittent.

In patients with incontinence, prolonged manometric studies have shown that transient IAS relaxation or "sampling" reflexes—equalization of rectal and anal canal pressures—occur more frequently than in control subjects, and that the duration of relaxation is longer (108–110). Symptoms of urgency or urge incontinence may be associated with high-amplitude contractions of the rectosigmoid (40,111) or altered periodic rectal motor activity (112), suggesting that rectal "hypercontractility" may contribute to the pathogenesis of this condition.

Evacuation Proctography

Passive (overflow) incontinence or post-defecation leakage may occur secondary to disorders of rectal evacuation. Evacuation proctography may be useful to exclude outlet obstruction due to an anatomical (e.g., large rectocele, intussusception, megarectum, etc.) (113,114) or a functional (e.g., pelvic floor dyssynergia, impaired rectal sensation, etc.) (51) cause. This simple, dynamic radiological technique involves fluoroscopic imaging of the process and assessment of the rate and completeness of rectal emptying following insertion of a barium paste (115).

In patients being considered for surgery, it has been shown that up to 40% may develop a "new" rectal evacuatory disorder following continence-restoring procedures (116). In such patients, either surgery has adversely affected the defecatory mechanism or an occult coexisting disorder of rectal evacuation has been "unmasked." Therefore, evacuation proctography should be considered in the preoperative work-up of patients with incontinence; any abnormalities revealed may be amenable to concurrent surgical correction or adjunctive postoperative conservative therapy (e.g., a bowel retraining program).

Evacuation proctography also can be used as a simple "continence test" and provides an objective means by which treatment can be assessed. Additionally, it may be used as an interim procedure to evaluate the efficacy of some surgical procedures, therefore, prior to stoma reversal.

Transit Studies

In patients in whom "constipation" and incontinence coexist, transit studies provide objective confirmation of a subjective complaint of infrequent defecation. A simple radiopaque marker study with plain abdominal film(s) taken three to five days later is adequate for detecting transit abnormalities (117–119). However, for accurate assessment of segmental colonic transit, radionuclide scintigraphy is required (120,121). If a delay in colonic transit is identified, management strategy can be altered accordingly.

Conversely, rapid gastrointestinal transit may result in diarrhea and underlie symptoms of urgency and frequency of defecation in patients with incontinence. Evaluation of accelerated transit is feasible using scintigraphy (122,123), but methodologies need to be refined and more robust normative data need to be acquired.

Non Established (Research) Methodologies

Several other techniques available for the investigation of anorectal function have yet to find a universally accepted role in the evaluation of patients with incontinence, and have thus far been limited to specialist research centers. These include vectorvolume manometry, three-dimensional (3D) endoanal ultrasonography, endoanal magnetic resonance imaging (MRI), use of the electronic barostat, and impedance planimetry. Many of these modalities are described in detail elsewhere in this volume.

Vectorvolume manometry utilizes multichannel manometric catheters with radially orientated side holes (typically eight orifices set 45 degrees apart), which allow a computer-derived 3D pressure profile of the anal canal to be obtained. Cross-sectional analysis permits accurate localization of pressure defects and allows differentiation between global and sector pressure deficits in patients with incontinence (124,125). Sphincter asymmetry may be a useful parameter for assessing the competence of anal sphincter function (126,127).

In terms of imaging techniques, 3D reconstruction of two-dimensional (2D) ultrasound images using dedicated computer software has contributed significantly to our understanding of normal anal canal anatomy (128, 129). However, the potential benefits of 3D endoanal ultrasound in the investigation of patients with fecal incontinence have yet to be ascertained (130). With regard to visualization of the EAS, endoanal MRI may be superior to ultrasonography, as there is a large contrast difference between the EAS and surrounding fat (131–133). Reduction in EAS muscle bulk, or atrophy, has been demonstrated in some patients with incontinence (131,134,135).

Assessment of rectal function can be performed more elaborately using the electronic barostat. This has the advantages that:

1. an infinitely compliant bag is used for inflation, which negates the problems faced when using traditional latex balloons, which have their own intrinsic elasticity;
2. the bag is attached at both ends to the catheter, which reduces the extent of its axial migration toward the sigmoid;
3. the procedure is computerized, which improves reproducibility and removes some observer bias.

In simple terms, the barostat rapidly aspirates air from the bag when the rectum contracts and injects air when the rectum relaxes. The volume of air aspirated/injected is proportional to the magnitude of contraction/relaxation. Various aspects of rectal sensorimotor function can be evaluated using this technique, including parameters of visceral perception, reflexes, tone, compliance, wall tension, and capacity (136,137). Use in patients with fecal incontinence has been limited thus far (39,49). An alternative methodology for studying biomechanical properties of the rectal wall is impedance planimetry, which combines rectal balloon inflation with measurement of intrabag (i.e., intraluminal) impedance (138,139) and may give a better appreciation of capacity (cross-sectional area) and tension–strain relationships in comparison to studies utilizing the barostat.

Treatment

Non Surgical Therapies

Most patients with mild to moderate symptoms (i.e., those seen at primary care level) will respond successfully to conservative management, and this must be considered as first-line therapy. Therapeutic strategies comprise pharmacological, behavioral, and physical modalities. Only patients who fail to respond to such measures (i.e., those with severe symptoms/major incontinence) should be referred to a specialist tertiary center for further investigation; however, it is remarkable how many patients who reach this stage have not, for example, undergone a simple trial of anti-diarrheal medication. Any underlying or coexistent gastrointestinal pathology needs to be identified and treated concomitantly, notably those conditions characterized by chronic diarrhea (140), which will exacerbate the symptoms of incontinence (e.g., diarrhea-predominant IBS, post-cholecystectomy diarrhea, pancreatic exocrine insufficiency, etc.). It should be remembered that conservative therapies may be used in combination and can be used successfully as an adjunct to surgery.

Dietary Manipulation

Modification of dietary intake may provide symptomatic benefit, although there are few "scientific" data available to support the efficacy of such an approach. Three separate factors need to be considered:

1. reduction/exclusion of diarrhea-inducing foods, e.g., caffeine, alcohol, dairy products, some vegetables (141);
2. identification/exclusion of sources of food intolerance (e.g., lactose, gluten);
3. addition or subtraction of stool-bulking agents.

Although there is a long-held belief that increasing dietary fiber to increase stool bulk is beneficial (142), some argue that greater volumes of softer stool will further challenge an incompetent continence mechanism and exacerbate symptoms (143,144). Indeed, the incompetent anal sphincters/rectal reservoir may be able to cope better with the smaller and firmer stool produced by reducing fiber intake (144).

Drug Treatment

Pharmacological therapy, although often empirical (first-line treatment), may be rationalized in view of clinical evaluation and the results of appropriate investigation, including tests of anorectal physiological function. Drug treatment is used primarily to solidify soft stool and prolong gastrointestinal transit (e.g., anti-diarrheals). However, improved understanding of the complex and multifactorial mechanisms governing both continence and defecation has led to the use of agents aimed at addressing specific aspects of those processes, therefore, enhancement of IAS tone in patients with passive fecal leakage, suppression of rectal "irritability" in patients with fecal urgency/urge incontinence, etc.

Drug classes currently available are listed below.

Constipating Agents

These drugs can benefit those with either passive fecal leakage or urge incontinence by reducing stool weight, frequency of defecation, and fecal urgency. Adsorbents act by absorbing excess fluid in stool, whereas opiate derivatives—loperamide (Imodium), codeine phosphate, and diphenoxylate hydrochloride (Lomotil)—may have multiple actions including:

1. slowing of gut transit, secondary to an effect on upper and lower gastrointestinal (GI) motility;
2. increasing fluid absorption;
3. inhibition of mucus secretion;
4. increasing anal sphincter pressures (145,146).

Loperamide is most commonly used due to its low side-effect profile (147); syrup may be more practical than capsule preparations, as the dose can be individually titrated to provide an effective balance between symptom response and avoidance of "constipation" (144).

Bile salt resins such as cholestyramine are not strictly anti-diarrheal, but may benefit patients with post-cholecystectomy diarrhea or those with altered small bowel re-absorption of bile salts. These agents act by binding bile salts in the small intestine and altering the absorption of fat-soluble vitamins (141,143).

Evacuation Aids

In adults, the major cause of fecal soiling is either incomplete rectal emptying (post-defecation leakage) or fecal impaction (overflow; notably in the geriatric population) (18,144). For overflow incontinence, disimpaction is the first step, either manually (sometimes under general anesthetic) or with enemas, followed by use of a cathartic, such as polyethylene glycol (PEG); recurrence is prevented by combining a daily osmotic laxative with a bowel habit training regimen aimed at getting the patient to attempt defecation at scheduled times each day [e.g., after meal(s)]. Defecation may be aided with suppositories with or without enemas (18,141). In patients with passive fecal leakage secondary to rectal evacuatory dysfunction, measures aimed at promoting efficient and complete rectal emptying should be employed, such as use of suppositories (glycerine, Bisacodyl), and/or retrograde rectal washouts (tap water, phosphate) (144).

Others

In patients with decreased anal resting tone and passive fecal soiling, the use of topical agents to stimulate smooth muscle function is currently being explored. The α-adrenoreceptor agonist phenylephrine has been shown to increase resting anal pressures in a dose-dependent manner in subjects with passive fecal incontinence (148), although a consistent clinical improvement has not been demonstrated (148,149).

Other agents that may be useful in ameliorating symptoms of fecal incontinence include: estrogen replacement therapy, which has been shown to significantly increase anal resting pressures and voluntary squeeze increments in postmenopausal women (150), and low-dose amitriptyline, which has been reported to modulate rectal (hyper)contractility in patients with urge fecal incontinence (112).

Physical Treatments

In nursing homes, pads may be the mainstay for management of fecal or urinary incontinence. Anal plugs may have a use in the medical management of patients with incontinence not amenable to surgery. This device expands after insertion into the anal canal to produce a watertight seal. Data are lacking as to their effectiveness, although results appear to be reasonable in those who can tolerate regular use (~50%). Patients with blunted anal canal sensation or neurological disorders are more likely to succeed with these devices (143,144).

Bowel Retraining ("Biofeedback")

If medication and dietary alterations alone are unsuccessful in treating the incontinence, a bowel retraining or bowel-directed behavioral management program should be considered as the next line of therapy. Such a program often is referred to as "biofeedback"; strictly speaking, however, biofeedback refers to a specific technique based on operant conditioning (151) that, in practice, forms only one part of a complex package of care. Elements of the care program include structured assessment of the problem (bowel diary, symptom and quality of life questionnaires), patient education (e.g., dietary and lifestyle advice, toilet behavior), emotional support, practical management of fecal incontinence (e.g., careful titration of anti-diarrheal drugs), and "retraining" measures aimed at enhancing selected aspects of anorectal function (e.g., anal sphincter strength, rectal sensory discrimination), involving the use of biofeedback (144).

In principle, biofeedback techniques aim to enable the patient (the "operator" being conditioned) to consciously manipulate a physiological measurement (e.g., the pressure generated by EAS contraction) via a visual and/or auditory representation of that parameter (i.e., "feedback"). Biofeedback as a treatment option for fecal incontinence was first described by Engel et al. in 1974 (151). Unfortunately, no standardized procedure exists for biofeedback therapy; many varying treatment protocols have been described in combination with many adjunctive measures (152). However, three main modalities are commonly employed (18,152).

1. Anal sphincter exercises. Anal sphincter function is recorded via an intra-anal manometric probe or EMG sensor or perianal EMG electrode. The patient is taught correct isolation of anal squeeze maneuvers (i.e., avoidance of contracting the abdominal wall), and then to "train" the striated musculature using pelvic floor or "Kegel" exercises to enhance both the strength and endurance of muscle contraction. Such exercises can be carried out at home and the biofeedback session used to monitor progress (see Chapter 6.5).
2. Anal sphincter exercises in response to rectal distension. External anal sphincter function is recorded via intra-anal pressure sensors (as above) and

rectal sensation is elicited by distension of a balloon positioned in the mid rectum. Commonly, the recording sensors and balloon are mounted on the same catheter. The patient is taught to correctly identify the sensation of rectal distension (i.e., urge to defecate), and then, without delay, to contract their EAS in response to this stimulus.

3. Rectal sensory discrimination. A rectal balloon is used to retrain rectal sensory (usually urge) thresholds. With visual feedback of intraballoon (rectal) pressure or volume, the patient is taught to discriminate, and thus respond to smaller rectal volumes. Conversely, rectal hypersensitivity—reduced sensory thresholds—is associated with symptoms of fecal urgency and frequency of defecation in some patients with urge fecal incontinence (40,81), and thus a protocol involving tolerance of progressively larger rectal volumes in an attempt to train the patient to resist urge is favored.

In terms of outcome, most studies report an improvement in approximately 75% of patients with mild to moderate fecal incontinence, with complete resolution of symptoms in nearly half (18,152). Only one study has reported no benefit at all (153). The precise mechanism by which biofeedback works is unclear; indeed, biofeedback may not be the most important element of the care package as a whole. However, studies in which rectal sensory retraining is synchronized with enhanced—and appropriate—anal sphincter contraction appear to be amongst the most successful (18,154). There is certainly consensus agreement regarding the need for careful selection of highly motivated patients, as well as the crucial interaction between an enthusiastic and dedicated therapist and the patient (154).

Evidence is contradictory as to which patients are most likely to benefit from a biofeedback program, and there are no clear predictors of success or failure (18,152). Improvement in anal sphincter function alone may not mirror symptomatic improvement and vice versa (152). Successful treatment has been reported in patients with or without structural damage to the anal sphincters and in those with normal or abnormal pudendal nerve function. Perhaps the only consistent finding is that patients with intact rectal sensation may be expected to have a more favorable response than those with rectal insensitivity. In addition, patients with urge incontinence tend to fare better than do those with passive incontinence (152). However, a recent Cochrane review has concluded that "there is not enough evidence from trials to judge . . . which aspects of the treatment are the most helpful and which patients are the most likely to be helped" (154). Nevertheless, biofeedback therapy does appear to have a clinical effect; it is safe, painless, inexpensive, and it does not preclude other treatments. Further long-term studies are required in line with standardization of therapeutic protocols.

Surgical Management of Patients with Fecal Incontinence

Principles of Management

The surgical management of fecal incontinence is often complex, and in common with any surgical procedure, it has its own inherent risks and complications. Therefore, it should be reserved for patients with intractable incontinence with impaired quality of life who have failed or who are deemed unsuitable for non-surgical management. The modern management of patients with fecal incontinence in a specialist surgical unit involves a multidisciplinary team of professionals, reflecting the multifaceted approach to the different aspects of patient assessment, education, support, and treatment.

The importance of a thorough and comprehensive assessment has been highlighted above, but this cannot be stressed strongly enough when considering surgery, as patient selection is crucial for a successful outcome. In addition to clinical assessment prior to surgery, due consideration also should be given to the evaluation of the cognitive and psychological status of potential candidates for surgery. Currently, no form of surgical intervention offers a 100% cure rate for incontinence, and thus preoperative counseling before surgery is obligatory so that patients can understand that surgery will frequently only improve rather than cure symptoms. Postoperatively, continued patient education and support, frequently provided by highly skilled nurses, are essential to successful recovery and rehabilitation.

The selection of patients for surgery, and the selection of an appropriate surgical procedure for individual patients, is a complex process. Consequently, the following description represents an over simplification of this process and concentrates specifically on the choice of surgical procedure appropriate to the underlying pathophysiology of the incontinence.

Surgical Correction of Underlying Organic Pathology

As discussed above, fecal incontinence will be secondary to underlying organic pathology of the anorectum (e.g., inflammatory bowel disease, neoplasia, stricture, fistulae, hemorrhoids, prolapse, etc.) in a proportion of patients. In such cases, appropriate surgical correction should relieve the symptoms of incontinence in the vast majority. A detailed discussion of the individual procedures available to address such pathology is beyond the scope of this chapter.

Simple Sphincter Defects

Isolated EAS Defects

Sphincteroplasty

Direct repair is appropriate in patients with isolated defects affecting one-third or less of the circumference of the EAS on endosonography. Anterior sphincter defects usually follow obstetric trauma and thus may be repaired immediately if identified at the time of injury (155). However, delayed repair is performed more frequently because of unrecognized injury or failure of primary repair.

Previously, sphincter repair was performed by apposition of the separated edges of the external sphincter. However, superior results are achieved using an overlapping repair, which is now considered the operation of choice for definable sphincter defects. The results of numerous studies of functional outcome following overlapping sphincteroplasty have been published in the literature (Table 7.1-3), with most reporting early success rates of 70% to 90%.

Certain factors, such as patient age and pudendal nerve function, may be important in predicting outcome following surgery, although the literature is largely contradictory in this regard. Sitzler and Thomson (156) reported a higher mean age in patients with failed repairs. Similarly, patient age

TABLE 7.1-3. The outcome of overlapping sphincteroplasty.

Study	Reference	Year	Number	% Continent (solid and liquid)
Browning	(228)	1984	97	74
Fang	(229)	1984	79	89
Pezim	(230)	1987	40	85
Laurberg	(231)	1988	19	47
Ctercteko	(232)	1988	58	64
Yoshioka	(233)	1989	27	74
Wexner	(234)	1991	16	76
Fleshman	(235)	1991	28	75
Engel	(236)	1994	52	69
Engel	(237)	1994	53	79
Sitzler	(156)	1996	31	74
Nickiteas	(157)	1996	42	67
Oliveira	(158)	1996	55	71
Engel	(238)	1997	20	65
Ternent	(239)	1997	16	62
Young	(240)	1998	56	87
Gilliland	(162)	1998	77	56
Hool	(241)	1999	51	80
Karoui	(242)	2000	86	81
Buie	(165)	2001	158	62

Median (range) = 74 (47–89).

greater than 50 years (157) has been identified as a predictor of failure. In contrast, Oliveira et al. (158) and Simmang et al. (159) found no influence of age on functional outcome. Indeed, Ha et al. (160) reported a superior functional outcome in patients older than 50 years when compared with their younger counterparts. Controversy also exists relating to pudendal nerve function. Several studies have implicated pudendal neuropathy as a predictor of failure following sphincteroplasty (161,162); indeed, it has been reported that even unilateral neuropathy is related to inferior postoperative outcome (163). However, other studies have failed to identify any relationship (157,164,165) and concluded that repair of anatomical sphincter defects should still be considered in the presence of pudendal neuropathy (166).

The majority of studies addressing the outcome of sphincteroplasty are restricted to short-term follow-up. Reported success rates appear lower in studies that have a longer period of follow-up. Londono-Schimmer et al. (161) evaluated 128 patients five years after surgery and found that only 50% had satisfactory results. More recently, Malouf et al. (116) and Halverson and Hull (167) also reported that only half of patients were continent to stool at five years following surgery. Furthermore, not only will many patients have residual symptoms following surgery, but some also may develop new evacuation disorders (116), and this should be taken into consideration when counseling patients preoperatively.

Surgery Following Failed Sphincteroplasty

Given the 70% to 90% short-term and 50% long-term success rates of overlapping sphincteroplasty, it is clear that some patients will have persistent fecal incontinence after surgery. It has been shown that many of these patients have residual anterior sphincter defects (168). Consequently, one surgical option is to perform a repeat overlapping sphincter repair. The outcome of repeat sphincter repair does not appear to be affected by previous surgery (162) and is associated with significant improvements in patient continence scores (169,170). Procedures that augment or replace the anal sphincter (see below) usually are reserved for defects that are irreparable.

Isolated IAS Defects

Surgical repair of isolated internal sphincter defects has been attempted, but has not proved successful in patients with passive fecal soiling (171,172). Consequently, alternative methods are required to address this problem.

Perianal Injection of Biomaterials

Various biomaterials have been injected perianally in an attempt to augment the internal sphincter. The materials used include: polytetrafluoroethylene (PTFE) paste (144,173), autologous fat (174), gluteraldehyde cross-linked collagen (175), silicone micro-implants (176), and pyrolytic carbon-coated beads suspended in a water-based carrier gel (177). Although these studies have shown some improvement in symptoms in approximately two-thirds of patients in the short term, whether such improvement is maintained at long-term follow-up has yet to be established.

Radiofrequency Energy Delivery to the Anal Canal

More recently, radiofrequency energy has been delivered deep to the mucosa of the anal canal via multiple needle electrodes during proctoscopy in ten female patients with fecal incontinence (178). Initially, eight patients responded to the treatment, and the modality was found to be safe and associated with improved continence and quality of life scores (178). Extended follow-up (two years) has suggested that symptomatic improvement is sustained (179). The proposed mechanism of action is heat-induced tissue contraction and remodeling of the anal canal and distal rectum (179). Clearly, further studies of greater numbers of patients are required before its widespread use can be recommended.

Dysfunctional Intact Sphincters

In a proportion of patients, physiological assessment of the anorectum reveals the presence of attenuated function of the internal or external anal sphincter in the absence of identifiable structural defects on endosonography. Such patients usually are managed with conservative therapies such as dietary manipulation, anti-diarrheal agents, topical phenylephrine, and biofeedback (see above). However, such measures are not always successful and surgical management may be indicated.

Pelvic Floor Procedures

Traditionally, pelvic floor procedures—postanal repair, anterior levatorplasty, total pelvic floor repair—have been performed for patients without a specific sphincter defect who suffer with idiopathic or neurogenic incontinence. The postanal repair was described by Sir Alan Parks in 1975 (180) and involves plication of the levator ani, puborectalis, and the EAS in an attempt to reconstitute the anorectal angle and lengthen the anal canal. Follow-up studies of the results of postanal repair have been disappointing and have not replicated the successful outcomes of the original reports, with typically only one-third to one-half of patients having improved continence (181–183). Consequently, although once popular in the United Kingdom and Europe, it has been performed less frequently in recent years (184); however, some surgeons still believe that it provides an alternative to more complicated procedures or a stoma (185).

Anterior levator ani plication (or anterior levatorplasty) is an alternative to postanal repair in patients with idiopathic or neurogenic incontinence, although it is more commonly performed in combination with direct sphincter repair (sphincteroplasty) in patients with traumatic EAS defects. Reports have suggested that the outcome of anterior levatorplasty is no different to that of postanal repair (186), with only 45% to 62% of patients with idiopathic incontinence benefiting from surgery (187–189).

Total pelvic floor repair involves a combination of a postanal repair with an anterior levatorplasty and sphincter plication. Early results demonstrated that approximately 60% were continent to solid and liquid stool (190), and longer-term follow-up revealed improved continence and quality of life in approximately half of all patients (191). Total pelvic floor repair was associated with significantly better results than postanal repair or anterior levatorplasty alone in a randomized trial performed by Deen et al. (192), with two-thirds of patients achieving restored continence compared to only approximately one-third of patients undergoing the other procedures. However, in the only other randomized trial comparing pelvic floor procedures performed to date (total pelvic floor repair vs. postanal repair), less than half of patients in each group benefited from surgery (193).

Sacral Nerve Stimulation (See Chapter 7.4)

The lack of simple surgical procedures that are effective in patients with intact, but functionally weak anal sphincters indicate that alternative treatments are required. Direct electrical stimulation of the sacral nerve roots was initially used in patients with urinary urge incontinence and was extended for use in the treatment of fecal incontinence by Matzel et al. in 1995 (194); however, its mechanism of action remains unclear. The nerve roots responsible for innervation of the anal sphincters and pelvic floor are S2, S3, and S4. Initially, patients undergo a short trial of percutaneous stimulation of the sacral nerve root that produces the maximal anal response to stimulation (usually S3) for a period of one to three weeks using an external stimulator. If this trial is associated with symptomatic improvement, the patient progresses to insertion of a permanent electrode connected to a stimulator inserted into the anterior abdominal wall or buttock.

In their original series, Matzel et al. (194) reported a marked improvement in fecal incontinence and EAS pressures in three patients. Subsequently, similar studies have shown successful short-term results in small numbers of patients, with marked improvements in clinical symptoms and quality of life associated with improvement of physiological parameters such as anal canal pressures and rectal sensory function (195–197). The results of a double-blind crossover study of sacral nerve stimulation also support these findings, with a marked, unequivocal improvement in fecal incontinence and patient quality of life (198). More recently, sustained medium-term benefit has been demonstrated in 15 patients after a median follow-up of 24 months, with 11 patients being fully continent (199). Similarly, Rosen et al. (200) reported significant improvement in clinical, quality of life, and physiological parameters in 16 patients at a median of 15 months follow-up. Early results appear very encouraging and sacral nerve stimulation appears to be a promising new modality for patients with dysfunctional, intact anal sphincters, although larger studies are required to confirm these initial results.

Irreparable Anal Sphincters

In certain patients, the anal sphincter muscles are irreparable. This includes those with disrupted anal sphincters that are unsuitable for—or have already failed—the procedures discussed above, together with those that have isolated internal sphincter defects resulting in severe passive leakage, refractory to all other treatments, and patients with congenital abnormalities of the anorectum. In such cases, sphincter reconstruction is performed using either native skeletal muscle or an artificial anal sphincter.

Electrically Stimulated (Dynamic) Graciloplasty (See Chapter 10.2)

Encirclement procedures involving transposition of skeletal muscle around the anus to augment or replace the anal sphincters have been performed for many years, and during that time, the gluteus maximus (201) and adductor longus and obturator internus (202) muscles have all been used. However, it is the gracilis muscle that is the favored option, being the most superficial medial adductor muscle with a sufficiently plastic neurovascular supply. Graciloplasty was first described by Pickrell et al. in 1952 (203). However, in contrast to the EAS, which is fatigue-resistant and comprised predominantly of slow-twitch fibers, the gracilis muscle largely consists of type II fast-twitch fibers that are unable to maintain a sustained contraction. Consequently, improvements in continence at that time were dependent on causing a degree of anal canal obstruction; thus, the results were generally poor (204,205).

Dynamic graciloplasty, as described by Williams (Figure 7.1.1) (206) and Baeten (207), involves the application of chronic low-frequency electrical stimulation to the gracilis muscle via a subcutaneously placed generator, transforming it to a slow-twitch non-fatigable muscle capable of a tonic state of contraction. Since its inception, the dynamic graciloplasty has been the subject of rigorous evaluation. In prospective multicenter trials, between 56% and 72% (208–210) of patients have achieved and maintained a successful outcome, with the best outcomes observed in those with traumatic incontinence. More recently, a systematic review revealed that dynamic graciloplasty was successful at restoring continence in 42% to 85% of patients (211). In the largest published series to date from a single center, 145 of 200 patients (72%) were continent to at least solid and liquid stool after a median follow-up of five years (212). Our own success rates for this procedure have been markedly influenced following the establishment of a specialist, dedicated, multidisciplinary team (Colorectal Development

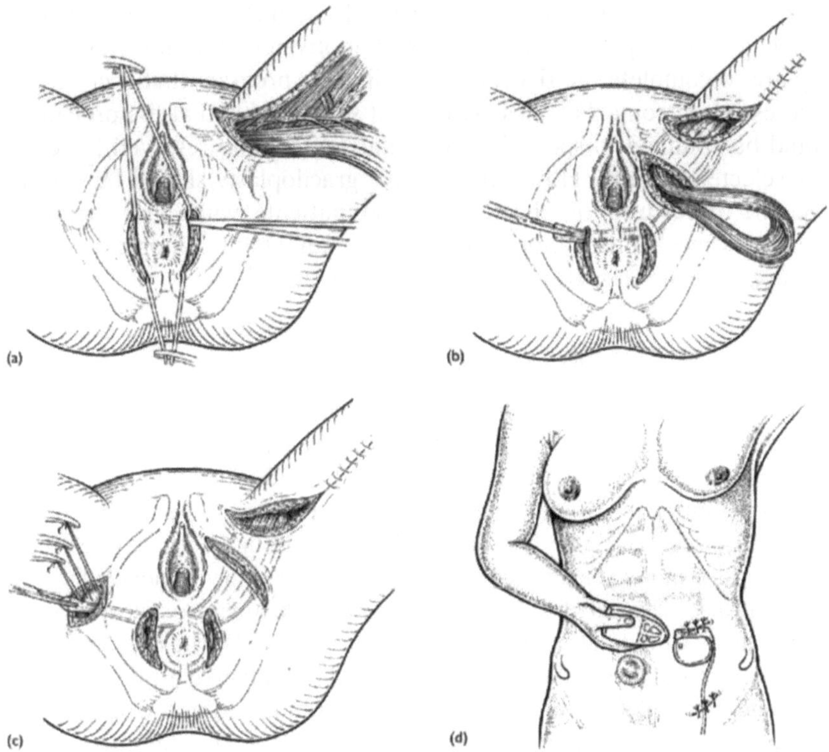

FIGURE 7.1.1. (a) A circumferential subcutaneous tunnel is developed around the anus through two lateral incisions. (b) The tendon of the gracilis is routed around the anus. (c) The tendon is then sutured to the opposite ischial tuberosity through a separate incision. (d) The stimulator is turned on with a hand-held telemetry device. (Reprinted with permission from Keighley MRB, Williams NS, editors. Surgery of the anus, rectum and colon. Second Edition. London: WB Saunders; 1999. p. 677.)

Unit), funded and independently assessed by a national government commissioning body. Since the Colorectal Development Unit was founded in 1997, 33 of 47 patients (70%) have had a good functional outcome (unpublished data).

Dynamic graciloplasty operations are technically demanding and may be associated with high morbidity. Infection may occur in up to one-third of cases (209), but is usually controlled with antibiotics if treatment is prompt and aggressive. Before the introduction of purpose-designed equipment, technical failure was problematic. However, it is the occurrence of postoperative evacuatory disorders, present in up to one-quarter of patients

(208), that are more difficult to resolve. Finally, it must be remembered that following surgery, patients must be highly motivated and fully educated if they are to complete the rigorous rehabilitation program that is crucial to a successful outcome. For these reasons, it seems likely that the procedure should be confined to specialist colorectal centers and reserved for carefully selected patients. However, dynamic graciloplasty should be considered the procedure of choice in those patients with an irreparable sphincteric mechanism, anorectal atresia, or undergoing anorectal reconstruction who are desperate to avoid a stoma.

Artificial Bowel Sphincter (See Chapter 10.3)

An alternative to the use of transposed skeletal muscle is to use a synthetic sphincter device. Indeed, the indications for their use are the same as for graciloplasty as discussed above. However, they additionally may be used in fecal incontinence of neuromuscular origin (e.g., myasthenia gravis and neuropathy secondary to diabetes mellitus). Although such devices have been used for many years in the treatment of urinary incontinence, the first successful use of an artificial sphincter for the treatment of fecal incontinence was by Christiansen and Lorentzen in 1987 (213). The contemporary device consists of an inflatable silicon cuff that is implanted around the anal canal and controlled by the patient via a pump located in the scrotum or labium majus. Activation of the pump forces fluid from the cuff into a reservoir implanted suprapubically in the space of Retzius, deflating the cuff and allowing defecation. Subsequently, the cuff automatically re-inflates slowly to maintain continence until the next evacuation.

Since its first use in 1987, several groups have reported their experiences with the artificial bowel sphincter (ABS) (Table 7.1-4). Overall improvements in continence are reported in approximately one-half to three-quarters of patients. Experience with the ABS remains limited and studies are restricted to small numbers of patients [with the exception of Devesa et al. (214)]. Long-term outcome appears less encouraging, with two studies with a median follow-up of approximately seven years documenting success rates of less than 50% and explantation rates as high as 41% and 49% respectively (215,216). Infection rates are also reported in up to one-third of cases (216,217).

Therefore, an artificial sphincter may be of benefit in selected patients with refractory incontinence, but the morbidity related to infection and erosion of the device, necessitating explantation, is high. Furthermore, as with graciloplasty, there appears to be a high incidence of postoperative evacuatory difficulties, which are present in up to one-half of patients (218,219). Long-term results suggest that the ABS is a less successful treatment option to dynamic graciloplasty, but it does provide a further alternative to a stoma, particularly for patients with a neuromuscular disease in whom graciloplasty is contraindicated.

TABLE 7.1-4. The results of artificial bowel sphincter implantation.

Study	Reference	Year	Number	Successful Outcome (%)	Infection (%)	Removal (%)
Single institution						
Christiansen	(243)	1992	12	50	25	17
Lehur	(244)	1996	13	69	15	31
Vaizey	(217)	1998	6	83	33	17
Christiansen*	(215)	1999	17	47	18	41
Lehur	(245)	2000	24	75	12	29
O'Brien	(246)	2000	13	77	15	23
Dodi	(247)	2000	8	75	25	25
Ortiz	(248)	2002	22	64	14	32
Devesa	(214)	2002	53	65	13	19
Parker*	(216)	2003	45	47	34	49
Multicenter						
Altomare	(218)	2002	28	75	18	25
Wong	(219)	2002	112	53	25	29

* Long-term follow-up median (range) = 67 (47–83) 18 (12–34) 27 (17–49).

Dysfunction Rectal Reservoir (See Chapter 9.1)

In addition to occurring secondary to anal sphincter dysfunction, fecal incontinence also may result from dysfunction of the rectal reservoir, which may manifest as either an impaired ability to store or evacuate feces. Reservoir dysfunction may occur in isolation or combination with other pathophysiological abnormalities, and it may complicate surgical procedures designed to improve continence (116).

Storage Dysfunction

Rectal Augmentation. Even in the absence of anal sphincter dysfunction, patients still may suffer with severe urgency of defecation and urge incontinence secondary to derangements of rectal sensorimotor function, manifesting as reduced wall compliance, hypersensitivity to distension, and hypercontractility on prolonged manometric investigation (40). We sought to address these physiological abnormalities by surgically increasing the capacity of the rectum in carefully selected patients. Consequently, we have developed the procedure of rectal augmentation (Figure 7.1.2), or ileorectoplasty, that involves incorporating a 10-centimeter patch of ileum on its vascular pedicle into the anterior rectal wall to increase its capacity (40). Our initial experience in 11 patients (seven with combined augmentation/dynamic graciloplasty) has suggested that there is a sustained increase in rectal capacity, as demonstrated by restoration of sensory threshold volumes and rectal compliance to normal in all (unpublished data), associated with a concomitant improvement in clinical symptoms (increased ability to defer defecation, reduced frequency of episodes of incontinence) and quality of life (220).

Evacuatory Dysfunction

Antegrade Continence Enema. In patients with fecal incontinence resulting from disordered evacuation, rectal enemas may be used to improve symptoms. An alternative is to maintain efficient emptying of the lower bowel through regular irrigation of water/saline, with or without aperients, via a catheter inserted into the proximal colon. In 1990, Malone et al. (221) described their experience with administration of antegrade colonic enemas via an appendicostomy fashioned in the right iliac fossa. This procedure has been used in patients with fecal incontinence resulting from congenital abnormalities, neurological disease, and chronic constipation, and is associated with success rates as high as 79% in pediatric patients (222). However, success is more limited when used in adult patients with fecal incontinence to achieve colonic emptying (223). Furthermore, long-term problems include appendiceal stenosis and reflux of colonic contents and irrigation fluid into the ileum.

Continent Colonic Conduit. The complications of the antegrade continence enema, coupled with the fact that the appendix may have been removed or be of too narrow a caliber to allow antegrade irrigation in adults, led us to develop the continent colonic conduit (224). The continent colonic conduit enables colonic irrigation to be performed by passing a catheter through a channel leading from the skin to the colonic lumen that incorporates an intussuscepted valve to prevent reflux. It has been most successful in patients with incontinence related to evacuation disorders (225). The conduit is best constructed in the transverse colon and permits the use of a larger catheter, allowing more rapid irrigation (226).

End Stage/Refractory Fecal Incontinence

Fecal Diversion

The distortion of body image associated with a stoma makes it an unacceptable option for most patients with fecal incontinence. Therefore, an end colostomy usually is reserved for intractable incontinence when other treatments have failed or are impractical. Stoma complications may occur in up to 40% of patients (227), and it is important to appreciate that patients still may experience troublesome incontinence of mucus produced in the rectum.

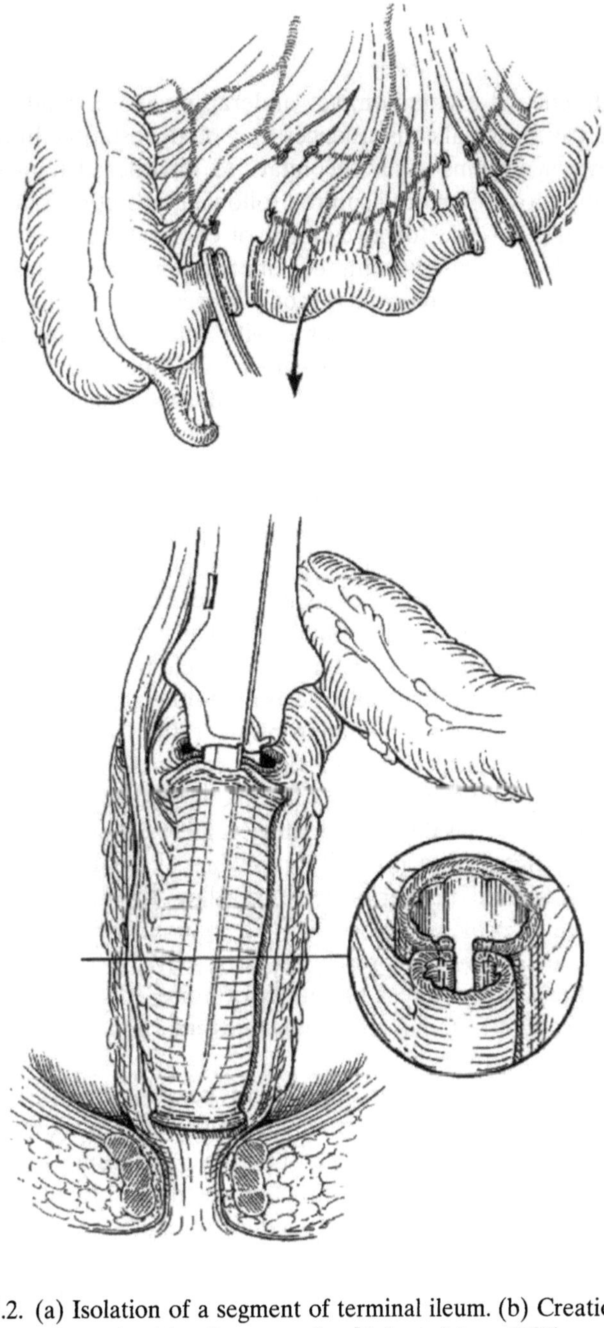

a

b

FIGURE 7.1.2. (a) Isolation of a segment of terminal ileum. (b) Creation of a side-to-side ileorectal pouch with a linear stapler. [Adapted from Williams et al. (40).]

Summary

Fecal incontinence is a common, yet underappreciated, condition whose physical and psychosocial consequences may be devastating. In the majority of patients, symptoms occur secondary to disordered function of the anorectum and most often are acquired following obstetric trauma or anal surgery. Specialist referral for assessment of colorectal/anorectal function is not required for all patients with fecal incontinence, as the majority with mild to moderate symptoms will respond successfully to simple medical management. However, those patients with intractable and sufficiently severe symptoms, in whom such measures have failed, warrant rigorous clinical evaluation at a tertiary centre. The modern management of patients with fecal incontinence should involve a multidisciplinary team of professionals, reflecting the multifaceted approach to the different aspects of patient assessment, education, support, and treatment.

In recent years, with the advent of anorectal physiological investigations, a more detailed understanding of the pathophysiological mechanisms underlying fecal incontinence is evolving. As several physiological abnormalities may be present, it is recommended that patients with intractable symptoms should undergo a structured, comprehensive series of tests in order to systematically evaluate all aspects of anorectal function. The results of these tests will help to suggest appropriate, rather than empirical management, both nonsurgical and, in particular, surgical. Currently, anorectal manometry (anal sphincter function and rectal sensation) and endoanal ultrasound should be considered mandatory in all cases, whereas other complementary investigations (e.g., rectal compliance, evacuation proctography, transit studies) should be performed according to the clinical picture. Certain tests (e.g., prolonged rectosigmoid manometry, endoanal MRI), which may be considered at present to be research investigations, offer future clinical promise, whereas the utility of more established techniques (e.g., pudendal nerve terminal motor latencies, anal sensation) are becoming increasingly controversial.

In those patients referred for surgical amelioration of their symptoms, the integration of the findings from clinical history, physical examination, and investigations enables the choice of suitable procedure to be tailored on an individual basis and to be directed specifically to the underlying abnormality or abnormalities. The procedure of choice for simple defects of the EAS appears to be direct repair, although success rates decrease in the long term. More complex operations have been devised in an attempt to avoid a permanent stoma in motivated patients with irreparable anal sphincters. Dynamic graciloplasty should be considered as the procedure of choice for such patients, as it is associated with better long-term results than the insertion of an ABS. Indeed, the continence rates following dynamic graciloplasty are equivalent, if not superior, to sphincteroplasty for simple sphincter defects at five-years follow-up. However, the complexity of such procedures and their relatively high morbidity suggest that they should currently be performed only in specialist colorectal centers.

Newer, less-invasive procedures, such as sacral nerve stimulation and delivery of biomaterials or radioenergy directly to the anal sphincter complex, offer hope to those patients with either dysfunctional intact sphincters or IAS defects and appear to be associated with encouraging early and medium-term benefit. Finally, the importance of addressing coexisting extrasphincteric physiological abnormalities should not be overlooked, and procedures such as rectal augmentation may be indicated in carefully selected cases.

In conclusion, the treatment of severe fecal incontinence remains challenging and the results of interventions, whether conservative or surgical, often may only improve rather than cure symptoms. Consequently, emphasis must be directed on the avoidance—whenever possible—of those risk factors known to be associated with the development of incontinence. Further understanding of the complex physiological and psychobehavioral factors contributing to bowel continence hopefully will lead to an improvement in outcomes following surgery. This is likely to be achieved only if the ultimate aim of surgery is the restoration of normal physiological function.

References

1. Lamah M and Kumar D. Fecal incontinence. Dig Dis Sci. 1999;44:2488–99.
2. Whitehead WE, Wald A, Diamant NE, Enck P, Pemberton JH, and Rao SS. Functional disorders of the anus and rectum. Gut. 1999;45 Suppl 2:II55–9.
3. Nelson R, Norton N, Cautley E, and Furner S. Community-based prevalence of anal incontinence. JAMA. 1995;274:559–61.
4. Perry S, Shaw C, McGrother C, Matthews RJ, Assassa RP, Dallosso H, Williams K, Brittain KR, Azam U, Clarke M, Jagger C, Mayne C, and Castleden CM. Prevalence of faecal incontinence in adults aged 40 years or more living in the community. Gut. 2002;50:480–4.
5. Kalantar JS, Howell S, and Talley NJ. Prevalence of faecal incontinence and associated risk factors; an underdiagnosed problem in the Australian community? Med J Aust. 2002;176:54–7.
6. Walter S, Hallbook O, Gotthard R, Bergmark M, and Sjodahl R. A population-based study on bowel habits in a Swedish community: prevalence of faecal incontinence and constipation. Scand J Gastroenterol. 2002;37:911–6.
7. Roberts RO, Jacobsen SJ, Reilly WT, Pemberton JH, Lieber MM, and Talley NJ. Prevalence of combined fecal and urinary incontinence: a community-based study. J Am Geriatr Soc. 1999;47:837–41.
8. Peet SM, Castleden CM, and McGrother CW. Prevalence of urinary and faecal incontinence in hospitals and residential and nursing homes for older people. BMJ. 1995;311:1063–4.
9. Nelson R, Furner S, and Jesudason V. Fecal incontinence in Wisconsin nursing homes: prevalence and associations. Dis Colon Rectum. 1998;41:1226–9.

10. Hinds JP, Eidelman BH, and Wald A. Prevalence of bowel dysfunction in multiple sclerosis. A population survey. Gastroenterology. 1990;98:1538–42.
11. Feldman M and Schiller LR. Disorders of gastrointestinal motility associated with diabetes mellitus. Ann Intern Med. 1983;98:378–84.
12. Drossman DA, Sandler RS, Broom CM, and McKee DC. Urgency and fecal soiling in people with bowel dysfunction. Dig Dis Sci. 1986;31:1221–5.
13. Rothbarth J, Bemelman WA, Meijerink WJ, Stiggelbout AM, Zwinderman AH, Buyze-Westerweel ME, and Delemarre JB. What is the impact of fecal incontinence on quality of life? Dis Colon Rectum. 2001;44:67–71.
14. Bharucha AE. Fecal incontinence. Gastroenterology. 2003;124:1672–85.
15. Malouf AJ, Chambers MG, and Kamm MA. Clinical and economic evaluation of surgical treatments for faecal incontinence. Br J Surg. 2001;88:1029–36.
16. Leigh RJ and Turnberg LA. Faecal incontinence: the unvoiced symptom. Lancet. 1982;1:1349–51.
17. Tobin GW and Brocklehurst JC. Faecal incontinence in residential homes for the elderly: prevalence, aetiology and management. Age Ageing. 1986;15:41–6.
18. Whitehead WE, Wald A, and Norton NJ. Treatment options for fecal incontinence. Dis Colon Rectum. 2001;44:131–44.
19. Kamm MA. Faecal incontinence. BMJ. 1998;316:528–32.
20. Vaizey CJ, Kamm MA, and Bartram CI. Primary degeneration of the internal anal sphincter as a cause of passive faecal incontinence. Lancet. 1997;349:612–5.
21. Engel AF, Kamm MA, and Talbot IC. Progressive systemic sclerosis of the internal anal sphincter leading to passive faecal incontinence. Gut. 1994;35:857–9.
22. Fernández-Fraga X, Azpiroz F, and Malagelada JR. Significance of pelvic floor muscles in anal incontinence. Gastroenterology. 2002;123:1441–50.
23. Snooks SJ, Swash M, Henry MM, and Setchell M. Risk factors in childbirth causing damage to the pelvic floor innervation. Int J Colorectal Dis. 1986;1:20–4.
24. Sultan AH, Kamm MA, and Hudson CN. Pudendal nerve damage during labour: prospective study before and after childbirth. Br J Obstet Gynaecol. 1994;101:22–8.
25. Tetzschner T, Sorensen M, Jonsson L, Lose G, and Christiansen J. Delivery and pudendal nerve function. Acta Obstet Gynecol Scand. 1997;76:324–31.
26. Rieger N and Wattchow D. The effect of vaginal delivery on anal function. Aust N Z J Surg. 1999;69:172–7.
27. Kiff ES, Barnes PR, and Swash M. Evidence of pudendal neuropathy in patients with perineal descent and chronic straining at stool. Gut. 1984;25:1279–82.
28. Snooks SJ, Barnes PR, Swash M, and Henry MM. Damage to the innervation of the pelvic floor musculature in chronic constipation. Gastroenterology. 1985;89:977–81.
29. Engel AF and Kamm MA. The acute effect of straining on pelvic floor neurological function. Int J Colorectal Dis. 1994;9:8–12.
30. Pfeifer J, Salanga VD, Agachan F, Weiss EG, and Wexner SD. Variation in pudendal nerve terminal motor latency according to disease. Dis Colon Rectum. 1997;40:79–83.

31. Kiff ES and Swash M. Slowed conduction in the pudendal nerves in idiopathic (neurogenic) faecal incontinence. Br J Surg. 1984;71:614–6.
32. Burnett SJ, Spence-Jones C, Speakman CT, Kamm MA, Hudson CN, and Bartram CI. Unsuspected sphincter damage following childbirth revealed by anal endosonography. Br J Radiol. 1991;64:225–7.
33. Law PJ, Kamm MA, and Bartram CI. Anal endosonography in the investigation of faecal incontinence. Br J Surg. 1991;78:312–4.
34. Deen KI, Kumar D, Williams JG, Olliff J, and Keighley MR. The prevalence of anal sphincter defects in faecal incontinence: a prospective endosonic study. Gut. 1993;34:685–8.
35. Nielsen MB, Hauge C, Pedersen JF, and Christiansen J. Endosonographic evaluation of patients with anal incontinence: findings and influence on surgical management. AJR Am J Roentgenol. 1993;160:771–5.
36. Vaizey CJ, Kamm MA, and Nicholls RJ. Recent advances in the surgical treatment of faecal incontinence. Br J Surg. 1998;85:596–603.
37. Hill J, Hosker G, and Kiff ES. Pudendal nerve terminal motor latency measurements: what they do and do not tell us. Br J Surg. 2002;89:1268–9.
38. Rasmussen O, Christensen B, Sorensen M, Tetzschner T, and Christiansen J. Rectal compliance in the assessment of patients with fecal incontinence. Dis Colon Rectum. 1990;33:650–3.
39. Salvioli B, Bharucha AE, Rath-Harvey D, Pemberton JH, and Phillips SF. Rectal compliance, capacity, and rectoanal sensation in fecal incontinence. Am J Gastroenterol. 2001;96:2158–68.
40. Williams NS, Ogunbiyi OA, Scott SM, Fajobi O, and Lunniss PJ. Rectal augmentation and stimulated gracilis anal neosphincter: a new approach in the management of fecal urgency and incontinence. Dis Colon Rectum. 2001;44: 192–8.
41. Denis P, Colin R, Galmiche JP, Geffroy Y, Hecketsweiler P, Lefrancois R, and Pasquis P. Elastic properties of the rectal wall in normal adults and in the patients with ulcerative colitis. Gastroenterology. 1979;77:45–8.
42. Varma JS, Smith AN, and Busuttil A. Correlation of clinical and manometric abnormalities of rectal function following chronic radiation injury. Br J Surg. 1985;72:875–8.
43. Carmona JA, Ortiz H, and Perez-Cabanas I. Alterations in anorectal function after anterior resection for cancer of the rectum. Int J Colorectal Dis. 1991;6: 108–10.
44. Quinn M. Reinnervation after chilbirth—a new paradigm for sensory bowel symptoms? Gut. 2001;49:597–8.
45. Chan CL, Facer P, Davis JB, Smith GD, Egerton J, Bountra C, Williams NS, and Anand P. Sensory fibres expressing capsaicin receptor TRPV1 in patients with rectal hypersensitivity and faecal urgency. Lancet. 2003;361: 385–91.
46. Lane RH and Parks AG. Function of the anal sphincters following colo-anal anastomosis. Br J Surg. 1977;64:596–9.
47. Rasmussen OØ. Anorectal function. Dis Colon Rectum. 1994;37:386–403.
48. Sun WM, Read NW, Miner PB. Relation between rectal sensation and anal function in normal subjects and patients with faecal incontinence. Gut. 1990;31: 1056–61.

49. Siproudhis L, Bellissant E, Pagenault M, Mendler MH, Allain H, Bretagne JF, and Gosselin M. Fecal incontinence with normal anal canal pressures: where is the pitfall? Am J Gastroenterol. 1999;94:1556–63.
50. Felt-Bersma RJ, Sloots CE, Poen AC, Cuesta MA, and Meuwissen SG. Rectal compliance as a routine measurement: extreme volumes have direct clinical impact and normal volumes exclude rectum as a problem. Dis Colon Rectum. 2000;43:1732–8.
51. Gladman MA, Scott SM, Chan CL, Williams NS, and Lunniss PJ. Rectal hyposensitivity: prevalence and clinical impact in patients with intractable constipation and fecal incontinence. Dis Colon Rectum. 2003;46:238–46.
52. Jorge JM and Wexner SD. Etiology and management of fecal incontinence. Dis Colon Rectum. 1993;36:77–97.
53. Felt-Bersma RJ, van Baren R, Koorevaar M, Strijers RL, and Cuesta MA. Unsuspected sphincter defects shown by anal endosonography after anorectal surgery. A prospective study. Dis Colon Rectum. 1995;38:249–53.
54. Ho YH, Low D, and Goh HS. Bowel function survey after segmental colorectal resections. Dis Colon Rectum. 1996;39:307–10.
55. Sood AK, Nygaard I, Shạhin MS, Sorosky JI, Lutgendorf SK, and Rao SS. Anorectal dysfunction after surgical treatment for cervical cancer. J Am Coll Surg. 2002;195:513–9.
56. Zbar AP, Beer-Gabel M, Chiappa AC, and Aslam M. Fecal incontinence after minor anorectal surgery. Dis Colon Rectum. 2001;44:1610–23.
57. Sultan AH, Kamm MA, Hudson CN, Thomas JM, and Bartram CI. Anal-sphincter disruption during vaginal delivery. N Engl J Med. 1993;329: 1905–11.
58. Chaliha C, Kalia V, Stanton SL, Monga A, and Sultan AH. Antenatal prediction of postpartum urinary and fecal incontinence. Obstet Gynecol. 1999;94: 689–94.
59. Fitzpatrick M and O'Herlihy C. The effects of labour and delivery on the pelvic floor. Best Pract Res Clin Obstet Gynaecol. 2001;15:63–79.
60. Sultan AH and Stanton SL. Occult obstetric trauma and anal incontinence. Eur J Gastroenterol Hepatol. 1997;9:423–7.
61. Jameson JS, Chia YW, Kamm MA, Speakman CT, Chye YH, and Henry MM. Effect of age, sex and parity on anorectal function. Br J Surg. 1994;81:1689–92.
62. Williams NS, Patel J, George BD, Hallan RI, and Watkins ES. Development of an electrically stimulated neoanal sphincter. Lancet. 1991;338:1166–9.
63. Pescatori M, Anastasio G, Bottini C, and Mentasti A. New grading and scoring for anal incontinence. Evaluation of 335 patients. Dis Colon Rectum. 1992;35: 482–7.
64. Vaizey CJ, Carapeti E, Cahill JA, and Kamm MA. Prospective comparison of faecal incontinence grading systems. Gut. 1999;44:77–80.
65. Engel AF, Kamm MA, Bartram CI, and Nicholls RJ. Relationship of symptoms in faecal incontinence to specific sphincter abnormalities. Int J Colorectal Dis. 1995;10:152–5.
66. Eckardt VF and Kanzler G. How reliable is digital examination for the evaluation of anal sphincter tone? Int J Colorectal Dis. 1993:8;95–7.
67. Keating JP, Stewart PJ, Eyers AA, Warner D, and Bokey EL. Are special investigations of value in the management of patients with fecal incontinence? Dis Colon Rectum. 1997;40:896–901.

68. Vaizey CJ and Kamm MA. Prospective assessment of the clinical value of anorectal investigations. Digestion. 2000;61:207–14.
69. Rao SS and Patel RS. How useful are manometric tests of anorectal function in the management of defecation disorders? Am J Gastroenterol. 1997;92:469–75.
70. Felt-Bersma RJ, Poen AC, Cuesta MA, and Meuwissen SG. Referral for anorectal function evaluation: therapeutic implications and reassurance. Eur J Gastroenterol Hepatol. 1999;11:289–94.
71. Liberman H, Faria J, Ternent CA, Blatchford GJ, Christensen MA, and Thorson AG. A prospective evaluation of the value of anorectal physiology in the management of fecal incontinence. Dis Colon Rectum. 2001;44:1567–74.
72. Rao SSC and Sun WM. Manometric assessment of anorectal function. Gastroenterol Clin North Am. 2001;30:15–32.
73. Jorge JMN and Wexner SD. Anorectal manometry: techniques and clinical applications. Southern Med J. 1993;86:924–31.
74. McHugh SM and Diamant NE. Anal canal pressure profile: a reappraisal as determined by rapid pullthrough technique. Gut. 1987;28:1234–41.
75. Rao SSC, Hatfield R, Soffer E, Rao S, Beaty J, and Conklin JL. Manometric tests of anorectal function in healthy adults. Am J Gastroenterol. 1999;94:773–83.
76. Nivatvongs S, Stern HS, and Fryd DS. The length of the anal canal. Dis Colon Rectum. 1981;24:600–1.
77. Enck P, Kuhlbusch R, Lubke H, Frieling T, and Erckenbrecht JF. Age and sex and anorectal manometry in incontinence. Dis Colon Rectum. 1989;32:1026–30.
78. Chiarioni G, Scattolini C, Bonfante F, and Vantini I. Liquid stool incontinence with severe urgency: anorectal function and effective biofeedback treatment. Gut. 1993;34:1576–80.
79. Marcello PW, Barrett RC, Coller JA, Schoetz DJ Jr, Roberts PL, Murray JJ, and Rusin LC. Fatigue rate index as a new measurement of external sphincter function. Dis Colon Rectum. 1998;41:336–43.
80. Felt-Bersma RJF, Klinkenberg-Knol EC, and Meuwissen SGM. Anorectal function investigations in incontinent and continent patients. Dis Colon Rectum. 1990;33:479–86.
81. Sun WM, Donnelly TC, and Read NW. Utility of a combined test of anorectal manometry, electromyography, and sensation in determining the mechanism of "idiopathic" faecal incontinence. Gut. 1992;33:807–13.
82. Gowers WR. The automatic action of the sphincter ani. Proc R Soc Lond. 1877;26:77–84.
83. Zbar AP, Aslam M, Gold DM, Gatzen C, Gosling A, and Kmiot WA. Parameters of the rectoanal inhibitory reflex in patients with idiopathic fecal incontinence and chronic constipation. Dis Colon Rectum. 1998;41:200–8.
84. Sun WM, Read NW, Prior A, Daly JA, Cheah SK, and Grundy D. Sensory and motor responses to rectal distention vary according to rate and pattern of balloon inflation. Gastroenterology. 1990;99:1008–15.
85. Whitehead WE and Schuster MM. Anorectal physiology and pathophysiology. Am J Gastroenterol. 1987;82:487–97.

86. Farthing MJG and Lennard-Jones JE. Sensibility of the rectum to distension and the anorectal distension reflex in ulcerative colitis. Gut. 1978;19:64–9.
87. Hoffmann BA, Timmcke AE, Gathright JB Jr, Hicks TC, Opelka FG, and Beck DE. Fecal seepage and soiling: a problem of rectal sensation. Dis Colon Rectum. 1995;38:746–8.
88. Varma JS and Smith AN. Reproducibility of the proctometrogram. Gut. 1986; 27:288–92.
89. Roe AM, Bartolo DC, and Mortensen NJ. New method for assessment of anal sensation in various anorectal disorders. Br J Surg. 1986;73:310–2.
90. Rogers J, Henry MM, and Misiewicz JJ. Combined sensory and motor deficit in primary neuropathic faecal incontinence. Gut. 1988;29:5–9.
91. Bielefeldt K, Enck P, and Erckenbrecht JF. Sensory and motor function in the maintenance of anal continence. Dis Colon Rectum. 1990;33:674–8.
92. Felt-Bersma RJ, Poen AC, Cuesta MA, and Meuwissen SG. Anal sensitivity test: what does it measure and do we need it? Cause or derivative of anorectal complaints. Dis Colon Rectum. 1997;40:811–6.
93. Gee AS, Mills A, and Durdey P. What is the relationship between perineal descent and anal mucosal electrosensitivity? Dis Colon Rectum. 1995;38:419–23.
94. Cornes H, Bartolo DC, and Stirrat GM. Changes in anal canal sensation after childbirth. Br J Surg. 1991;78:74–7.
95. Diamant NE, Kamm MA, Wald A, and Whitehead WE. American Gastroenterological Association medical position statement on anorectal testing techniques. Gastroenterology. 1999;116:732–60.
96. Jones PN, Lubowski DZ, Swash M, and Henry MM. Relation between perineal descent and pudendal nerve damage in idiopathic faecal incontinence. Int J Colorectal Dis. 1987;2:93–5.
97. Ho YH and Goh HS. The neurophysiological significance of perineal descent. Int J Colorectal Dis. 1995;10:107–11.
98. Pinna Pintor M, Zara GP, Falletto E, Monge L, Demattei M, Carta Q, and Masenti E. Pudendal neuropathy in diabetic patients with faecal incontinence. Int J Colorectal Dis. 1994;9:105–9.
99. Súilleabháin CB, Horgan AF, McEnroe L, Poon FW, Anderson JH, Finlay IG, and McKee RF. The relationship of pudendal nerve terminal motor latency to squeeze pressure in patients with idiopathic fecal incontinence. Dis Colon Rectum. 2001;44:666–71.
100. Wexner SD, Marchetti F, Salanga VD, Corredor C, and Jagelman DG. Neurophysiologic assessment of the anal sphincters. Dis Colon Rectum. 1991;34:606–12.
101. Cheong DM, Vaccaro CA, Salanga VD, Wexner SD, Phillips RC, Hanson MR, and Waxner SD. Electrodiagnostic evaluation of fecal incontinence. Muscle Nerve. 1995;18:612–9.
102. Rasmussen OO, Christiansen J, Tetzschner T, and Sorensen M. Pudendal nerve function in idiopathic fecal incontinence. Dis Colon Rectum. 2000;43:633–6.
103. Thomas C, Lefaucheur JP, Galula G, de Parades V, Bourguignon J, and Atienza P. Respective value of pudendal nerve terminal motor latency and anal sphincter electromyography in neurogenic fecal incontinence. Neurophysiol Clin. 2002;32:85–90.

104. Felt-Bersma RJ, Cuesta MA, Koorevaar M, Strijers RL, Meuwissen SG, Dercksen EJ, and Wesdorp RI. Anal endosonography: relationship with anal manometry and neurophysiologic tests. Dis Colon Rectum. 1992;35:944–9.
105. Sultan AH, Nicholls RJ, Kamm MA, Hudson CN, Beynon J, and Bartram CI. Anal endosonography and correlation with in vitro and in vivo anatomy. Br J Surg. 1993;80:508–11.
106. Sultan AH, Kamm MA, Talbot IC, Nicholls RJ, and Bartram CI. Anal endosonography for identifying external sphincter defects confirmed histologically. Br J Surg. 1994;81:463–5.
107. Willis S, Faridi A, Schelzig S, Hoelzl F, Kasperk R, Rath W, and Schumpelick V. Childbirth and incontinence: a prospective study on anal sphincter morphology and function before and early after vaginal delivery. Langenbecks Arch Surg. 2002;387:101–7.
108. Roberts JP and Williams NS. The role and technique of ambulatory anal manometry. Baillieres Clin Gastroenterol. 1992;6:163–78.
109. Farouk R, Duthie GS, Pryde A, McGregor AB, and Bartolo DC. Internal anal sphincter dysfunction in neurogenic faecal incontinence. Br J Surg. 1993;80: 259–61.
110. Mularczyk A and Basilisco G. Fecal incontinence induced by spontaneous internal anal sphincter relaxation: report of a case. Dis Colon Rectum. 2002;45:973–6.
111. Herbst F, Kamm MA, Morris GP, Britton K, Woloszko J, and Nicholls RJ. Gastrointestinal transit and prolonged ambulatory colonic motility in health and faecal incontinence. Gut. 1997;41:381–9.
112. Santoro GA, Eitan BZ, Pryde A, and Bartolo DC. Open study of low-dose amitriptyline in the treatment of patients with idiopathic fecal incontinence. Dis Colon Rectum. 2000;43:1676–81.
113. Felt-Bersma RJ. Clinical indications for anorectal function investigations. Scand J Gastroenterol. 1990;178 Suppl:1–6.
114. Rex DK and Lappas JC. Combined anorectal manometry and defecography in 50 consecutive adults with fecal incontinence. Dis Colon Rectum. 1992;35:1040–5.
115. Mahieu P, Pringot J, and Bodart P. Defecography: I. Description of a new procedure and results in normal patients. Gastrointest Radiol. 1984;9:247–51.
116. Malouf AJ, Norton CS, Engel AF, Nicholls RJ, and Kamm MA. Long-term results of overlapping anterior anal-sphincter repair for obstetric trauma. Lancet. 2000;355:260–5.
117. Hinton JM, Lennard-Jones JE, and Young AC. A new method for studying gut transit times using radioopaque markers. Gut. 1969;10:842–7.
118. Arhan P, Devroede G, Jehannin B, Lanza M, Faverdin C, Dornic C, Persoz B, Tetreault L, Perey B, and Pellerin D. Segmental colonic transit time. Dis Colon Rectum. 1981;24:625–9.
119. Metcalf AM, Phillips SF, Zinsmeister AR, MacCarty RL, Beart RW, and Wolff BG. Simplified assessment of segmental colonic transit. Gastroenterology. 1987;92:40–7.
120. Krevsky B, Malmud LS, D'Ercole F, Maurer AH, and Fisher RS. Colonic transit scintigraphy. A physiologic approach to the quantitative measurement of colonic transit in humans. Gastroenterology. 1986;91:1102–12.

121. Scott SM, Knowles CH, Lunniss PJ, Newell M, Garvie N, and Williams NS. Scintigraphic assessment of colonic transit in patients with slow transit constipation arising de novo (chronic idiopathic) and following pelvic surgery or childbirth. Br J Surg. 2001;88:405–11.
122. Charles F, Camilleri M, Phillips SF, Thomforde GM, and Forstrom LA. Scintigraphy of the whole gut: clinical evaluation of transit disorders. Mayo Clin Proc. 1995;70:113–8.
123. Bonapace ES, Maurer AH, Davidoff S, Krevsky B, Fisher RS, and Parkman HP. Whole gut transit scintigraphy in the clinical evaluation of patients with upper and lower gastrointestinal symptoms. Am J Gastroenterol. 2000;95: 2838–47.
124. Braun JC, Treutner KH, Dreuw B, Klimaszewski M, and Schumpelick V. Vectormanometry for differential diagnosis of fecal incontinence. Dis Colon Rectum. 1994;37:989–96.
125. Zbar AP, Aslam M, Hider A, Toomey P, and Kmiot WA. Comparison of vector volume manometry with conventional manometry in anorectal dysfunction. Tech Coloproctol. 1998;2:84–90.
126. Williams N, Barlow J, Hobson A, Scott N, and Irving M. Manometric asymmetry in the anal canal in controls and patients with fecal incontinence. Dis Colon Rectum. 1995;38:1275–80.
127. Jorge JM and Habr-Gama A. The value of sphincter asymmetry index in anal incontinence. Int J Colorectal Dis. 2000;15:303–10.
128. Williams AB, Cheetham MJ, Bartram CI, Halligan S, Kamm MA, Nicholls RJ, and Kmiot WA. Gender differences in the longitudinal pressure profile of the anal canal related to anatomical structure as demonstrated on three-dimensional anal endosonography. Br J Surg. 2000;87:1674–9.
129. Bollard RC, Gardiner A, Lindow S, Phillips K, and Duthie GS. Normal female anal sphincter: difficulties in interpretation explained. Dis Colon Rectum. 2002;45:171–5.
130. Gold DM, Bartram CI, Halligan S, Humphries KN, Kamm MA, and Kmiot WA. Three-dimensional endoanal sonography in assessing anal canal injury. Br J Surg. 1999;86:365–70.
131. de Souza NM, Puni R, Zbar A, Gilderdale DJ, Coutts GA, and Krausz T. MR imaging of the anal sphincter in multiparous women using an endoanal coil: correlation with in vitro anatomy and appearances in fecal incontinence. AJR Am J Roentgenol. 1996;167:1465–71.
132. Rociu E, Stoker J, Eijkemans MJ, Schouten WR, and Lameris JS. Fecal incontinence: endoanal US versus endoanal MR imaging. Radiology. 1999;212: 453–8.
133. Williams AB, Bartram CI, Halligan S, Marshall MM, Nicholls RJ, and Kmiot WA. Endosonographic anatomy of the normal anal canal compared with endocoil magnetic resonance imaging. Dis Colon Rectum. 2002;45:176–83.
134. Briel JW, Stoker J, Rociu E, Lameris JS, Hop WC, and Schouten WR. External anal sphincter atrophy on endoanal magnetic resonance imaging adversely affects continence after sphincteroplasty. Br J Surg. 1999;86:1322–7.
135. Williams AB, Malouf AJ, Bartram CI, Halligan S, Kamm MA, and Kmiot WA. Assessment of external anal sphincter morphology in idiopathic fecal incontinence with endocoil magnetic resonance imaging. Dig Dis Sci. 2001;46:1466–71.

136. Whitehead WE, Delvaux M; The Working Team. Standardization of barostat procedures for testing smooth muscle tone and sensory thresholds in the gastrointestinal tract. Dig Dis Sci. 1997;42:223–41.
137. van der Schaar PJ, Lamers CBHW, and Masclee AAM. The role of the barostat in human research and clinical practice. Scand J Gastroenterol. 1999;34 (Suppl 230):52–63.
138. Dall FH, Jorgensen CS, Houe D, Gregersen H, and Djurhuus JC. Biomechanical wall properties of the human rectum. A study with impedance planimetry. Gut. 1993;34:1581–6.
139. Krogh K, Mosdal C, Gregersen H, and Laurberg S. Rectal wall properties in patients with acute and chronic spinal cord lesions. Dis Colon Rectum. 2002;45:641–9.
140. Thomas PD, Forbes A, Green J, Howdle P, Long R, Playford R, Sheridan M, Stevens R, Valori R, Walters J, Addison GM, Hill P, and Brydon G. Guidelines for the investigation of chronic diarrhoea, 2nd edition. Gut. 2003;52 (Suppl 5):v1–15.
141. Parker SC and Thorsen A. Fecal incontinence. Surg Clin N Am. 2002;82: 1273–90.
142. Bliss DZ, Jung HJ, Savik K, Lowry A, LeMoine M, Jensen L, Werner C, and Schaffer K. Supplementation with dietary fiber improves fecal incontinence. Nurs Res. 2001;50:203–13.
143. Eccersley AJ and Williams NS. Fecal incontinence—pathophysiology and management. In: Pemberton JH, Swash M, and Henry MM, editors. The pelvic floor. Its function and disorders. London: WB Saunders; 2002. p. 341–57.
144. Cheetham MJ, Kenefick NJ, and Kamm MA. Non-surgical management of faecal incontinence. Hosp Med. 2001;62:538–41.
145. Ruppin H. Review: loperamide—a potent antidiarrhoeal drug with actions along the alimentary tract. Aliment Pharmacol Ther. 1987;1:179–90.
146. Sun WM, Read NW, and Verlinden M. Effects of loperamide oxide on gastrointestinal transit time and anorectal function in patients with chronic diarrhoea and faecal incontinence. Scand J Gastroenterol. 1997;32:34–8.
147. Gattuso JM and Kamm MA. Adverse effects of drugs used in the management of constipation and diarrhoea. Drug Saf. 1994;10:47–65.
148. Cheetham MJ, Kamm MA, and Phillips RK. Topical phenylephrine increases anal canal resting pressure in patients with faecal incontinence. Gut. 2001;48: 356–9.
149. Carapeti EA, Kamm MA, and Phillips RK. Randomized controlled trial of topical phenylephrine in the treatment of faecal incontinence. Br J Surg. 2000; 87:38–42.
150. Donnelly V, O'Connell PR, and O'Herlihy C. The influence of oestrogen replacement on faecal incontinence in postmenopausal women. Br J Obstet Gynaecol. 1997;104:311–5.
151. Engel BT, Nikoomanesh P, and Scuster MM. Operant conditioning of rectosphincteric responses in the treatment of faecal incontinence. N Engl J Med. 1974;290:646–9.
152. Norton C and Kamm MA. Anal sphincter biofeedback and pelvic floor exercises for faecal incontinence in adults—a systematic review. Aliment Pharmacol Ther. 2001;15:1147–54.

153. van Tets WF, Kuijpers JH, and Bleijenberg G. Biofeedback treatment is ineffective in neurogenic fecal incontinence. Dis Colon Rectum. 1996;39:992–4.
154. Norton C, Hosker G, and Brazzelli M. Biofeedback and/or sphincter exercises for the treatment of faecal incontinence in adults. Cochrane Database Syst Rev. 2000;2:CD002111.
155. Sultan AH, Monga AK, Kumar D, and Stanton SL. Primary repair of obstetric anal sphincter rupture using the overlap technique. Br J Obstet Gynaecol. 1999;106:318–23.
156. Sitzler PJ and Thomson JP. Overlap repair of damaged anal sphincter. A single surgeon's series. Dis Colon Rectum. 1996;39:1356–60.
157. Nikiteas N, Korsgen S, Kumar D, and Keighley MR. Audit of sphincter repair. Factors associated with poor outcome. Dis Colon Rectum. 1996;39:1164–70.
158. Oliveira L, Pfeifer J, and Wexner SD. Physiological and clinical outcome of anterior sphincteroplasty. Br J Surg. 1996;83:502–5.
159. Simmang C, Birnbaum EH, Kodner IJ, Fry RD, and Fleshman JW. Anal sphincter reconstruction in the elderly: does advancing age affect outcome? Dis Colon Rectum. 1994;37:1065–9.
160. Ha HT, Fleshman JW, Smith M, Read TE, Kodner IJ, and Birnbaum EH. Manometric squeeze pressure difference parallels functional outcome after overlapping sphincter reconstruction. Dis Colon Rectum. 2001;44:655–60.
161. Londono-Schimmer EE, Garcia-Duperly R, Nicholls RJ, Ritchie JK, Hawley PR, and Thomson JP. Overlapping anal sphincter repair for faecal incontinence due to sphincter trauma: five year follow-up functional results. Int J Colorectal Dis. 1994;9:110–3.
162. Gilliland R, Altomare DF, Moreira H Jr, Oliveira L, Gilliland JE, and Wexner SD. Pudendal neuropathy is predictive of failure following anterior overlapping sphincteroplasty. Dis Colon Rectum. 1998;41:1516–22.
163. Sangwan YP, Coller JA, Barrett MS, Murray JJ, Roberts PL, and Schoetz DJ Jr. Unilateral pudendal neuropathy. Significance and implications. Dis Colon Rectum. 1996;39:249–51.
164. Rasmussen OO, Colstrup H, Lose G, and Christiansen J.A technique for the dynamic assessment of anal sphincter function. Int J Colorectal Dis. 1990;5: 135–41.
165. Buie WD, Lowry AC, Rothenberger DA, and Madoff RD. Clinical rather than laboratory assessment predicts continence after anterior sphincteroplasty. Dis Colon Rectum. 2001;44:1255–60.
166. Chen AS, Luchtefeld MA, Senagore AJ, Mackeigan JM, and Hoyt C. Pudendal nerve latency. Does it predict outcome of anal sphincter repair? Dis Colon Rectum. 1998;41:1005–9.
167. Halverson AL and Hull TL. Long-term outcome of overlapping anal sphincter repair. Dis Colon Rectum. 2002;45:345–8.
168. Engel AF, Kamm MA, Sultan AH, Bartram CI, and Nicholls RJ. Anterior anal sphincter repair in patients with obstetric trauma. Br J Surg. 1994;81:1231–4.
169. Giordano P, Renzi A, Efron J, Gervaz P, Weiss EG, Nogueras JJ, and Wexner SD. Previous sphincter repair does not affect the outcome of repeat repair. Dis Colon Rectum. 2002;45:635–40.
170. Pinedo G, Vaizey CJ, Nicholls RJ, Roach R, Halligan S, and Kamm MA. Results of repeat anal sphincter repair. Br J Surg. 1999;86:66–9.

171. Leroi AM, Kamm MA, Weber J, Denis P, and Hawley PR. Internal anal sphincter repair. Int J Colorectal Dis. 1997;12:243–5.
172. Morgan R, Patel B, Beynon J, and Carr ND. Surgical management of anorectal incontinence due to internal anal sphincter deficiency. Br J Surg. 1997;84:226–30.
173. Shafik A. Polytetrafluoroethylene injection for the treatment of partial fecal incontinence. Int Surg. 1993;78:159–61.
174. Shafik A. Perianal injection of autologous fat for treatment of sphincteric incontinence. Dis Colon Rectum. 1995;38:583–7.
175. Kumar D, Benson MJ, and Bland JE. Glutaraldehyde cross-linked collagen in the treatment of faecal incontinence. Br J Surg. 1998;85:978–9.
176. Kenefick NJ, Vaizey CJ, Malouf AJ, Norton CS, Marshall M, and Kamm MA. Injectable silicone biomaterial for faecal incontinence due to internal anal sphincter dysfunction. Gut. 2002;51:225–8.
177. Davis K, Kumar D, and Poloniecki J. Preliminary evaluation of an injectable anal sphincter bulking agent (Durasphere) in the management of faecal incontinence. Aliment Pharmacol Ther. 2003;18:237–43.
178. Takahashi T, Garcia-Osogobio S, Valdovinos MA, Mass W, Jimenez R, Jauregui LA, Bobadilla J, Belmonte C, Edelstein PS, and Utley DS. Radio-frequency energy delivery to the anal canal for the treatment of fecal incontinence. Dis Colon Rectum. 2002;45:915–22.
179. Takahashi T, Garcia-Osogobio S, Valdovinos MA, Belmonte C, Barreto C, and Velasco L. Extended two-year results of radio-frequency energy delivery for the treatment of fecal incontinence (the Secca procedure). Dis Colon Rectum. 2003;46:711–5.
180. Parks AG. President's Address. Anorectal incontinence. Proc R Soc Med. 1975;68:681–90.
181. Matsuoka H, Mavrantonis C, Wexner SD, Oliveira L, Gilliland R, and Pikarsky A. Postanal repair for fecal incontinence—is it worthwhile? Dis Colon Rectum. 2000;43:1561–7.
182. Jameson JS, Speakman CT, Darzi A, Chia YW, and Henry MM. Audit of postanal repair in the treatment of fecal incontinence. Dis Colon Rectum. 1994;37:369–72.
183. Scott AD, Henry MM, and Phillips RK. Clinical assessment and anorectal manometry before postanal repair: failure to predict outcome. Br J Surg. 1990;77:628–9.
184. Varma JS, Binnie NR, Kawimbe B, Papachrysostomou M, and Smith AN. A regional audit of the investigation and treatment of colorectal and pelvic floor disorders (1984–1991). Int J Colorectal Dis. 1993;8:66–70.
185. Rieger NA, Sarre RG, Saccone GT, Hunter A, and Toouli J. Postanal repair for faecal incontinence: long-term follow-up. Aust N Z J Surg. 1997;67:566–70.
186. Orrom WJ, Miller R, Cornes H, Duthie G, Mortensen NJ, and Bartolo DC. Comparison of anterior sphincteroplasty and postanal repair in the treatment of idiopathic fecal incontinence. Dis Colon Rectum. 1991;34:305–10.
187. Miller R, Orrom WJ, Cornes H, Duthie G, and Bartolo DC. Anterior sphincter plication and levatorplasty in the treatment of faecal incontinence. Br J Surg. 1989;76:1058–60.

188. Osterberg A, Graf W, Holmberg A, Pahlman L, Ljung A, and Hakelius L. Long-term results of anterior levatorplasty for fecal incontinence. A retrospective study. Dis Colon Rectum. 1996;39:671–4.
189. Osterberg A, Edebol Eeg-Olofsson K, and Graf W. Results of surgical treatment for faecal incontinence. Br J Surg. 2000;87:1546–52.
190. Pinho M, Ortiz J, Oya M, Panagamuwa B, Asperer J, and Keighley MR. Total pelvic floor repair for the treatment of neuropathic fecal incontinence. Am J Surg. 1992;163:340–3.
191. Korsgen S, Deen KI, and Keighley MR. Long-term results of total pelvic floor repair for postobstetric fecal incontinence. Dis Colon Rectum. 1997;40:835–9.
192. Deen KI, Oya M, Ortiz J, and Keighley MR. Randomized trial comparing three forms of pelvic floor repair for neuropathic faecal incontinence. Br J Surg. 1993;80:794–8.
193. van Tets WF and Kuijpers JH. Pelvic floor procedures produce no consistent changes in anatomy or physiology. Dis Colon Rectum. 1998;41:365–9.
194. Matzel KE, Stadelmaier U, Hohenfellner M, and Gall FP. Electrical stimulation of sacral spinal nerves for treatment of faecal incontinence. Lancet. 1995;346:1124–7.
195. Malouf AJ, Vaizey CJ, Nicholls RJ, and Kamm MA. Permanent sacral nerve stimulation for fecal incontinence. Ann Surg. 2000;232:143–8.
196. Ganio E, Masin A, Ratto C, Altomare DF, Ripetti V, Clerico G, Lise M, Doglietto GB, Memeo V, Landolfi V, Del Genio A, Arullani A, Giardiello G, and de Seta F. Short-term sacral nerve stimulation for functional anorectal and urinary disturbances: results in 40 patients: evaluation of a new option for anorectal functional disorders. Dis Colon Rectum. 2001;44:1261–7.
197. Leroi AM, Michot F, Grise P, and Denis P. Effect of sacral nerve stimulation in patients with fecal and urinary incontinence. Dis Colon Rectum. 2001;44:779–89.
198. Vaizey CJ, Kamm MA, Roy AJ, and Nicholls RJ. Double-blind crossover study of sacral nerve stimulation for fecal incontinence. Dis Colon Rectum. 2000; 43:298–302.
199. Kenefick NJ, Vaizey CJ, Cohen RC, Nicholls RJ, and Kamm MA. Medium-term results of permanent sacral nerve stimulation for faecal incontinence. Br J Surg. 2002;89:896–901.
200. Rosen HR, Urbarz C, Holzer B, Novi G, and Schiessel R. Sacral nerve stimulation as a treatment for fecal incontinence. Gastroenterology. 2001;121:536–41.
201. Pearl RK, Prasad ML, Nelson RL, Orsay CP, and Abcarian H. Bilateral gluteus maximus transposition for anal incontinence. Dis Colon Rectum. 1991;34:478–81.
202. Skacel V and Laichman S. An anal neosphincter from the internal obturator muscle. Rozhl Chir. 1987;66:394–9.
203. Pickrell KL, Broadbent IR, Masters FW, and Metzger JT. Construction of a rectal sphincter and restoration of anal continence by transplanting the gracilis muscle. A report of four cases in children. Ann Surg. 1952;135:853–62.
204. Faucheron JL, Hannoun L, Thome C, and Parc R. Is fecal continence improved by nonstimulated gracilis muscle transposition? Dis Colon Rectum. 1994;37: 979–83.

205. Corman ML. Gracilis muscle transposition for anal incontinence: late results. Br J Surg. 1985;72 Suppl:S21–2.
206. Williams NS, Hallan RI, Koeze TH, and Watkins ES. Construction of a neorectum and neoanal sphincter following previous proctocolectomy. Br J Surg. 1989;76:1191–4.
207. Baeten C, Spaans F, and Fluks A. An implanted neuromuscular stimulator for fecal continence following previously implanted gracilis muscle. Report of a case. Dis Colon Rectum. 1988;31:134–7.
208. Mander BJ, Wexner SD, Williams NS, Bartolo DC, Lubowski DZ, Oresland T, Romano G, and Keighley MR. Preliminary results of a multicentre trial of the electrically stimulated gracilis neoanal sphincter. Br J Surg. 1999;86:1543–8.
209. Madoff RD, Rosen HR, Baeten CG, LaFontaine LJ, Cavina E, Devesa M, Rouanet P, Christiansen J, Faucheron JL, Isbister W, Kohler L, Guelinckx PJ, and Pahlman L. Safety and efficacy of dynamic muscle plasty for anal incontinence: lessons from a prospective, multicenter trial. Gastroenterology. 1999; 116:549–56.
210. Wexner SD, Baeten C, Bailey R, Bakka A, Belin B, Belliveau P, Berg E, Buie WD, Burnstein M, Christiansen J, Coller J, Galandiuk S, Lange J, Madoff R, Matzel KE, Pahlman L, Parc R, Reilly J, Seccia M, Thorson AG, and Vernava AM 3rd. Long-term efficacy of dynamic graciloplasty for fecal incontinence. Dis Colon Rectum. 2002;45:809–18.
211. Chapman AE, Geerdes B, Hewett P, Young J, Eyers T, Kiroff G, and Maddern GJ. Systematic review of dynamic graciloplasty in the treatment of faecal incontinence. Br J Surg. 2002;89:138–53.
212. Rongen MJ, Uludag O, El Naggar K, Geerdes BP, Konsten J, and Baeten CG. Long-term follow-up of dynamic graciloplasty for fecal incontinence. Dis Colon Rectum. 2003;46:716–21.
213. Christiansen J and Lorentzen M. Implantation of artificial sphincter for anal incontinence. Lancet. 1987;2:244–5.
214. Devesa JM, Rey A, Hervas PL, Halawa KS, Larranaga I, Svidler L, Abraira V, and Muriel A. Artificial anal sphincter: complications and functional results of a large personal series. Dis Colon Rectum. 2002;45:1154–63.
215. Christiansen J, Rasmussen OO, and Lindorff-Larsen K. Long-term results of artificial anal sphincter implantation for severe anal incontinence. Ann Surg. 1999;230:45–8.
216. Parker SC, Spencer MP, Madoff RD, Jensen LL, Wong WD, and Rothenberger DA. Artificial bowel sphincter: long-term experience at a single institution. Dis Colon Rectum. 2003;46:722–9.
217. Vaizey CJ, Kamm MA, Gold DM, Bartram CI, Halligan S, and Nicholls RJ. Clinical, physiological, and radiological study of a new purpose-designed artificial bowel sphincter. Lancet. 1998;352:105–9.
218. Altomare DF, Dodi G, La Torre F, Romano G, Melega E, and Rinaldi M. Multicentre retrospective analysis of the outcome of artificial anal sphincter implantation for severe faecal incontinence. Br J Surg. 2001;88:1481–6.
219. Wong WD, Congliosi SM, Spencer MP, Corman ML, Tan P, Opelka FG, Burnstein M, Nogueras JJ, Bailey HR, Devesa JM, Fry RD, Cagir B, Birnbaum E, Fleshman JW, Lawrence MA, Buie WD, Heine J, Edelstein PS, Gregorcyk S, Lehur PA, Michot F, Phang PT, Schoetz DJ, Potenti F, and Tsai JY. The safety

and efficacy of the artificial bowel sphincter for fecal incontinence: results from a multicenter cohort study. Dis Colon Rectum. 2002;45:1139–53.
220. Chan C, Williams N, Tillin T, Scott M, and Lunniss P. Rectal augmentation: evaluation of a novel surgical procedure for the management of severe faecal urgency [abstract]. Dis Colon Rectum. 2002;45(12):A35.
221. Malone PS, Ransley PG, and Kiely EM. Preliminary report: the antegrade continence enema. Lancet. 1990;336:1217–8.
222. Curry JI, Osborne A, and Malone PS. The MACE procedure: experience in the United Kingdom. J Pediatr Surg. 1999;34:338–40.
223. Gerharz EW, Vik V, Webb G, Leaver R, Shah PJ, and Woodhouse CR. The value of the MACE (Malone antegrade colonic enema) procedure in adult patients. J Am Coll Surg. 1997;185:544–7.
224. Williams NS, Hughes SF, and Stuchfield B. Continent colonic conduit for rectal evacuation in severe constipation. Lancet. 1994;343:1321–4.
225. Hughes SF and Williams NS. Continent colonic conduit for the treatment of faecal incontinence associated with disordered evacuation. Br J Surg. 1995;82: 1318–20.
226. Hughes SF and Williams NS. Antegrade enemas for the treatment of severe idiopathic constipation. Br J Surg. 1995;82:567.
227. Pearl RK, Prasad ML, Orsay CP, Abcarian H, Tan AB, and Melzl MT. Early local complications from intestinal stomas. Arch Surg. 1985;120:1145–7.
228. Browning GG and Motson RW. Anal sphincter injury. Management and results of Parks sphincter repair. Ann Surg. 1984;199:351–7.
229. Fang DT, Nivatvongs S, Vermeulen FD, Herman FN, Goldberg SM, and Rothenberger DA. Overlapping sphincteroplasty for acquired anal incontinence. Dis Colon Rectum. 1984;27:720–2.
230. Pezim ME, Spencer RJ, Stanhope CR, Beart RW Jr, Ready RL, and Ilstrup DM. Sphincter repair for fecal incontinence after obstetrical or iatrogenic injury. Dis Colon Rectum. 1987;30:521–5.
231. Laurberg S, Swash M, and Henry MM. Delayed external sphincter repair for obstetric tear. Br J Surg. 1988;75:786–8.
232. Ctercteko GC, Fazio VW, Jagelman DG, Lavery IC, Weakley FL, and Melia M. Anal sphincter repair: a report of 60 cases and review of the literature. Aust N Z J Surg. 1988;58:703–10.
233. Yoshioka K and Keighley MR. Sphincter repair for fecal incontinence. Dis Colon Rectum. 1989;32:39–42.
234. Wexner SD, Marchetti F, and Jagelman DG. The role of sphincteroplasty for fecal incontinence reevaluated: a prospective physiologic and functional review. Dis Colon Rectum. 1991;34:22–30.
235. Fleshman JW, Dreznik Z, Fry RD, and Kodner IJ. Anal sphincter repair for obstetric injury: manometric evaluation of functional results. Dis Colon Rectum. 1991;34:1061–7.
236. Engel AF, Kamm MA, and Hawley PR. Civilian and war injuries of the perineum and anal sphincters. Br J Surg. 1994;81:1069–73.
237. Engel AF, Kamm MA, Sultan AH, Bartram CI, and Nicholls RJ. Anterior anal sphincter repair in patients with obstetric trauma. Br J Surg. 1994;81:1231–4.
238. Engel AF, Lunniss PJ, Kamm MA, and Phillips RK. Sphincteroplasty for incontinence after surgery for idiopathic fistula in ano. Int J Colorectal Dis. 1997; 12:323–5.

239. Ternent CA, Shashidharan M, Blatchford GJ, Christensen MA, Thorson AG, and Sentovich SM. Transanal ultrasound and anorectal physiology findings affecting continence after sphincteroplasty. Dis Colon Rectum. 1997;40:462–7.
240. Young CJ, Mathur MN, Eyers AA, and Solomon MJ. Successful overlapping anal sphincter repair: relationship to patient age, neuropathy, and colostomy formation. Dis Colon Rectum. 1998;41:344–9.
241. Hool GR, Lieber ML, and Church JM. Postoperative anal canal length predicts outcome in patients having sphincter repair for fecal incontinence. Dis Colon Rectum. 1999;42:313–8.
242. Karoui S, Leroi AM, Koning E, Menard JF, Michot F, and Denis P. Results of sphincteroplasty in 86 patients with anal incontinence. Dis Colon Rectum. 2000;43:813–20.
243. Christiansen J and Sparso B. Treatment of anal incontinence by an implantable prosthetic anal sphincter. Ann Surg. 1992;215:383–6.
244. Lehur PA, Michot F, Denis P, Grise P, Leborgne J, Teniere P, and Buzelin JM. Results of artificial sphincter in severe anal incontinence. Report of 14 consecutive implantations. Dis Colon Rectum. 1996;39:1352–5.
245. Lehur PA, Roig JV, and Duinslaeger M. Artificial anal sphincter: prospective clinical and manometric evaluation. Dis Colon Rectum. 2000;43:1100–6.
246. O'Brien PE and Skinner S. Restoring control: the Acticon Neosphincter artificial bowel sphincter in the treatment of anal incontinence. Dis Colon Rectum. 2000;43:1213–6.
247. Dodi G, Melega E, Masin A, Infantino A, Cavallari F, and Lise M. Artificial bowel sphincter (ABS) for severe faecal incontinence: a clinical and manometric study. Colorectal Dis. 2000;2:207–11.
248. Ortiz H, Armendariz P, DeMiguel M, Ruiz MD, Alos R, and Roig JV. Complications and functional outcome following artificial anal sphincter implantation. Br J Surg. 2002;89:877–81.

Editorial Commentary

The severity of fecal incontinence (FI) depends on the type and frequency of symptoms and may entail the inability to retain gas, both gas and liquid faeces, or only solid feces. Severe FI is likely to require surgery, whereas mild or moderate FI is better managed conservatively. Establishment of a correlation between the severity of symptoms and the cause of the disease would help in selecting the proper treatment for individual patients. Classifications should take into account both the severity and the frequency of symptoms where patients with incontinence due to congenital and traumatic causes have a higher mean score than other groups. Patients who require an operation more frequently are those whose incontinence is due to congenital or traumatic factors and patients with FI associated with rectal prolapse. There are a legion of new operative procedures for FI although these are specialized techniques which need to be prospectively conducted and assessed in tertiary coloproctological facilities. The predictive benefits of biofeedback and neuromodulatory procedures are still being defined.

Different outcomes are reported to the literature following pelvic floor rehabilitation for faecal incontinence, possibly due to the types of procedures employed, whether biofeedback or physiotherapy or electrostimulation. We analyzed the results achieved in a group of patients treated with a combination of three procedures. Thirty-two patients (24 females) with fecal incontinence underwent a course of combined rehabilitation (CR) in our unit. Patients were taught perineal exercises and biofeedback was either sensory or electromyographic with electrostimulation being performed with a 10–20 MHz endoanal probe. Twenty-seven patients were available for follow-up. The mean incontinence scores improved from 4.0 ± 0.8 to 2.1 ± 1.7 (mean ± sd) ($p > 0.001$); where19 patients (70%) were satisfied after CR and 11 (44%) became fully continent. Rectal sensation thresholds improved in 55% of the cases and 86% of them had a corresponding positive clinical outcome. Although the exact mechanisms behind successful conservative therapies is unclear, pelvic floor rehabilitation seems to be effective for the management of fecal incontinence when carried out combining different types of procedures. An increase of rectal sensation may be responsible for some of the clinical improvement.

MP

Chapter 7.2
Quality of Life Issues

Lucia Oliveira

Fecal incontinence is an important condition that has received more prominent attention in the last several years. It is a complex and usually multifactorial condition that merits adequate management due to its tremendous socioeconomic impact and, more importantly, its impact on the patient's quality of life.

Fecal incontinence can be a devastating condition, causing disability and compromising the patient's dignity with significant impairment in quality of life, well-being, and social/economic relations. It is one of the most debilitating conditions in an otherwise healthy individual that can lead to social isolation, loss of self-esteem, and a variety of psychological states including depression.

The economic impact of fecal incontinence is great, with costs averaging more than $4 million dollars per year in the United States for incontinence supplies and diapers (1). Furthermore, the estimated long-term cost of treating fecal incontinence secondary to obstetric injury alone is in the range of $17 166.00 per patient (2).

In the elderly population, fecal incontinence is the second leading cause of hospitalization, contributing to the increased number of urinary tract infections and other disabilities that constitute an important public health problem. Although the exact incidence of fecal incontinence is still unknown, the reported incidence in the literature varies from 1% to 5% in the general population (3–5). In a recent survey that included 15 904 adults aged 40 years or more and excluding residents of nursing and residential homes, 1.4% reported major fecal incontinence and 0.7% reported major fecal incontinence with bowel symptoms that impaired quality of life (6).

Assessment

The assessment of an incontinent patient begins with a detailed clinical history and physical examination that will provide an indication of the best treatment approach for these patients (7). In addition, the clinical examination can provide important information about the severity of the problem and the objective impairment in quality of life. With this purpose, a number of incontinence scales and quality of life instruments have been developed in the last decades with some specific applications. These scales provide important information about the frequency and severity of the problem and can facilitate the more objective statistical comparison of results between various institutions.

The practical application of an incontinence severity index is to guide treatment options wherein an 85-year-old female patient who has leakage to liquid stool once per week may benefit significantly from simple clinical measures such as the introduction of bulking agents or constipating medications. Conversely, a 35-year-old active female patient who remains incontinent following a third vaginal delivery will most likely benefit from a more intensive investigation in order to select adequate surgical treatment and to predict for likely surgical success.

The impact of any medical condition on quality of life has recently gained more interest. The importance of more objective assessment of the impact of fecal incontinence on the patient's quality of life is to selectively tailor more ideal treatment options for each patient depending on the severity of the problem. As fecal incontinence can be a subjective complaint, it is important to have an instrument that can quantify more objectively the degree of that incontinence. Initial incontinence scales aimed at quantifying the degree of the incontinence, but they usually did not assess the impact of that condition on the patient's quality of life. Here, there has been a plea for the inclusion within scoring systems of aspects pertaining to fecal urgency and the effect of anti-diarrheal medication. Patients may avoid incontinence by close proximity to a toilet, and consistent use of anti-diarrheals may mask the underlying condition (8). In addition, there was no uniformity amongst various scale users relative to interpretation of the different scales; therefore, comparisons of the results in the literature were conflicting and occasionally inaccurate (Table 7.2-1) (9–20).

In these comparative analyses, whereas Parks (10) considered a score of one as normal continence and a score of four as total incontinence to solid stool, other authors such as Holschneider (13) included in his classification manometric results for patient categorization. Keighley and Fielding (14) considered fecal incontinence as minor, moderate, or severe, whereas Corman (15) utilized an excellent to poor scale for his patients, showing that it is effectively impossible to compare results of these various classifications. In addition, most of these classifications do not mention the frequency of episodes of incontinence that, from the patient's perspective, can profoundly compromise the patient's quality of life.

In 1992, Pescatori and colleagues (21) published one of the first attempts in the development of a new incontinence grading system to evaluate both the degree and frequency of symptoms. Subsequently, the following year, Jorge and Wexner (22) introduced the Cleveland Clinic Florida

TABLE 7.2-1. Different classification or scoring systems for fecal incontinence in the literature.

Author	Scoring system
Kelly (8)	Points: 0–2 = poor; 2–4 = fair; 5–6 = good
	0 = 50% accidents, always soiling, absent sphincters
	1 = occasional acdcidents, occasional soiling, weak sphincters
Parks (10)	1 = normal
	2 = difficult control of flatus and diarrhea
	3 = no control of diarrhea
	4 = no control of solid stool
Lane (11)	True incontinence = loss of feces without knowledge or control
	Partial incontinence = passage of flatus por mucus under same conditions
	Overflow incontinence = result of rectal distension without sphincter relaxation
Rudd (12)	1 = continence
	2 = minor leak
	3 = acceptable leak
	4 = unsatisfactory major leak
	5 = total failure
Holschneider (13)	Continence [resting tone at manometry (rt) > 16 mmHg]
	Partial continence (rt = 9–15)
	Incontinence (rt < 8)
Keighley and Fielding (14)	Minor = fecal leakage once a month or less, to diarrhea
	Moderate = incontinence once a week to solid stool
	Severe = incontinence in most days, perineal pad
Corman (15)	Excellent = continent all time
	Good = continent, but may require enemas
	Fair = incontinent for liquid stool
	Poor = incontinent for solid stool
Hiltunen (16)	Continent, partially continent, totally incontinent
Broden (17)	1 = none
	2 = medium
	3 = severe incontinence
Womack (18)	A = continence
	B = incontinence for liquid stool
	C = incontinence to flatus and diarrhea
	D = totally incontinent
Rainey (19)	A = continence
	B = incontinence to liquid stool
	C = incontinence to solid stool
Miller (20)	Grade I = incontinence less frequent than once a month
	Grade II = between once a month and once a week
	Grade III = more than once a week
	Score = flatus 1–3, fluid 4–6, solid 7–9
Pescatori (21)	Incontinence for A = flatus/mucus; B = diarrhea; C = solid stool
	1 = occasionally
	2 = weekly
	3 = daily
	Score = from 0 (continent) to 6 (severe totally incontinent)

Incontinence Scoring System based on modifications of the existing scoring systems (Table 7.2-2). These authors stratified the frequency of incontinent episodes to gas, liquid, or solid stool with any alterations in lifestyle, where perfect continence was recorded as zero and total incontinence was maximally scored as 20. This proposed scoring system was a simple and relatively easy method for objectively evaluating fecal incontinence and has since become very popular. In fact, it recently has undergone a validation process by Rothbarth and colleagues (23). Despite the limited number of patients, the authors of this study demonstrated that there was a correlation between the Wexner incontinence score and the patient's quality of life, where a Wexner incontinence score higher than nine was associated with a significant decrease in quality of life and where almost all patients with scores higher than nine were incontinent to solid stool more than once per week, necessitating the use of pads on a daily basis.

Based on these initial fecal incontinence scoring systems—in particular the Wexner/Jorge index—a scoring severity index was proposed by Rockwood in 1999 that subsequently has gained popularity (24). Based on the type and frequency of incontinence, they assessed the patients' scores relative to incontinence to gas, mucus, liquid, and solid stool (Table 7.2-3), where it was demonstrated that, overall, the surgeon and patient ratings were similar and that only minor differences between grades were associated with accidental loss of solid stool.

As the impact of fecal incontinence on quality of life has been gaining more widespread interest, evaluation of the patient with fecal incontinence involves a wider and more complex process. Specifically, defining the patient's quality of life is a multifaceted aspect of the assessment and usually is related to a combination of physical, psychological, and social factors of well-being. In addition, quality of life needs to be assessed subjectively from the patient's point of view, rendering this process significantly more complex.

Subsequent to their initial publication, Rockwood et al. published a Fecal Incontinence Quality of Life (FIQOL) Scale in 2000 that represented one of the first attempts in the development of a psychometric evaluation of a

TABLE 7.2-2. Cleveland Clinic Florida Scoring System.

Type of incontinence	Never	Rarely	Sometimes	Usually	Always
Solid	0	1	2	3	4
Liquid	0	1	2	3	4
Gas	0	1	2	3	4
Wears Pad	0	1	2	3	4
Lifestyle Alteration	0	1	2	3	4

never, 0 (never); rarely (<1/month); sometimes (<1/week >1/month); usually (<1/day >1/week); always (>1/day).
0 = perfect continence; 20 = complete incontinence.

TABLE 7.2-3. Fecal Incontinence Severity Index.

A	2 or more time/day	Once a day	2 or more times/week	Once a week	1–3 times a month
Gas					
Mucus					
Liquid					
Solid					

B	2 or more times/week	Once a day	2 or more times/week	Once a week	1–3 times a month	Never
Gas		?	?	?	?	
Mucus	?	?	?	?	?	
Liquid	?	?	?	?	?	
Solid	?	?	?	?	?	

A. Fecal Incontinence Severity Index Event × frequency matrix presented to surgeons and patients to develop weightings and overall severity score. Participants were instructed to rank the importance of each cell by placing a "1" in the most severe cell and a "20" in the least severe cell.
B. Fecal Incontinence Severity Index Questionnaire. Presented to the fecal incontinence study population, the question asked, "For each of the following, please indicate on average how often in the past month you experienced any amount of accidental bowel leakage (check only one box per row)."

quality of life measure designed to assess the impact of specific treatment for fecal incontinence (25). They based this FIQOL scale on the SF-36 general health survey (26) in order to establish the validity of the new condition-specific measures. The scale is composed of 29 items forming four scales or domains:

1. Lifestyle (10 items);
2. Coping/Behavior (9 items);
3. Depression/Self-perception (7 items); and
4. Embarrassment (3 items) (Table 7.2-4).

A panel of experts was enrolled to identify the quality of life-related domains adversely affected by fecal incontinence in two distinct populations; namely, patients with fecal incontinence and an age-matched control group without incontinence symptoms. The authors demonstrated that the scales were both reliable and valid, with each demonstrating stability over time and an acceptable internal reliability. However, this study had some drawbacks in that the scales contain redundant items that could very readily be removed without affecting statistical validity. Furthermore, it would be important to apply the scales to patients with varying degrees of incontinence in an effort to completely validate this measurement instrument. Another point of interest would be to correlate the results of this instrument with objective physiological testing such as anal manometry.

TABLE 7.2-4. Fecal Incontinence Quality of Life Scale composition.

Scale 1: Lifestyle
I cannot do many of things I want to do
I am afraid to go out
It is important to plan my schedule (daily activities) around my bowel pattern
I cut down on how much I eat before I go out
It is difficult for me to get out and do things like going to a movie or to church
I avoid traveling by plane or train
I avoid visiting friends
I avoid going out to eat
I avoid staying overnight away from home

Scale 2: Coping/behavior
I have sex less often than I would like to
The possibility of bowel accidents is always on my mind
I feel I have no control over my bowels
Whenever I go someplace new, I specifically locate where the bathrooms are
I worry about not being able to get to the toilet in time
I worry about bowel accidents
I try to prevent bowel accidents by staying very near a bathroom
I can't hold my bowel movement long enough to get to the bathroom
Whenever I am away from home, I try to stay near a restroom as much as possible

Scale 3: Depression/Self-perception
In general, would you say your health is
I am afraid to have sex
I feel different from other people
I enjoy life less
I feel like I am not a healthy person
I feel depressed
During the past month, have you felt so sad, discouraged, hopeless, or had so many problems that you wondered if anything was worthwhile

Scale 4: Embarrassment
I leak stool without even knowing it
I worry about others smelling stool on me
I feel ashamed

Quality of Life Scale for fecal Incontinence
Q1: In general, would you say your health is:
1 Excellent
2 Very Good
3 Fair
4 Poor

Q2: For each of the items, please indicate how much of the time the issue is a concern for you due to accidental bowel leakage. [If it is a concern for you for reasons other than accidental bowel leakage, then check the box under Not Apply (N/A)]

Q2 Due to accidental bowel leakage: N/A	Most of the time	Some of the time	A little of the time	None of the time
a. I am afraid to go out				
b. I avoid visiting friends				
c. I avoid staying overnight away from home				
d. It is difficult for me to get out and do things like going to a movie or to church				

TABLE 7.2-4. *Continued*

e. I cut down on how much I eat before I go out
f. Whenever I am away from home, I try stay near a restroom as much as possible
g. It is important to plan my schedule (daily activities) around my bowel pattern
h. I avoid traveling
i. I worry about not being able to get to the toilet in time
j. I feel I have no control over my bowels
k. I can't hold my bowel movement long enough to get to the bathroom
l. I leak stool without even knowing it
m. I try to prevent bowel accidents by staying very near a bathroom

Q3: Due to accidental bowel leakage, indicate the extent to which you agree or disagree with each of the following items. [If it is a concern for you for reasons other than accidental bowel leakage, then check the box under Not Apply (N/A).]

Q3 Due to accidental bowel leakage	Strongly agree	Somewhat agree	Somewhat disagree	Strongly disagree
a. I feel ashamed	1	2	3	4
b. I cannot do many of things I want to do	1	2	3	4
c. I worry about bowel accidents	1	2	3	4
d. I feel depressed	1	2	3	4
e. I worry about others smelling stool on me	1	2	3	4
f. I feel like I am not a healthy person	1	2	3	4
g. I enjoy life less	1	2	3	4
h. I have sex less often than I would like to	1	2	3	4
i. I feel different from other people	1	2	3	4
j. The possibility of bowel accidents is always on my mind	1	2	3	4
k. I am afraid to have sex	1	2	3	4
l. I avoid traveling by place or train	1	2	3	4
m. I avoid going out to eat	1	2	3	4
n. Whenever I go someplace new, I especially locate where the bathrooms are	1	2	3	4

Q4: During the past month, have you felt so sad, discouraged, hopeless, or had so many problems that you wondered if anything was worthwhile?
1 extremely so—to the point that I have just about given up
2 very much so
3 quite a bit
4 some—enough to bother me
5 a little bit
6 not at all

The evaluation of quality of life in patients with anal incontinence is therefore complicated and difficult and is somewhat dependent on the examiner's perspective, with varying (and at times contradictory) results and distinct weightings attributable to the various items evaluated. From the surgeon's point of view, objective data such as the type of incontinence and the frequency of incontinent episodes seem to be the most relevant aspects from which a surgical or non-surgical treatment option is proposed and evaluated. However, from the patient's perspective—which, in fact, should be more important and relevant in our evaluation—information related to the effect of hygiene, impact of continence on social activities, and normal daily activities, as well as the occurrence and timing of episodes of leakage, are often the most worrisome specific personal issues. One recent publication aimed to assess qualitatively the impact of fecal incontinence and treatment on the patient's quality of life using some of these parameters (27). Here, the authors interviewed 118 patients with varying degrees of neuropathic fecal incontinence prior to randomization to biofeedback therapy. They utilized a Direct Questioning of Objectives Quality of Life measure that was used previously in the evaluation of patients who underwent surgical treatment for ulcerative colitis (28). The patients were asked to list one to four important aspects related to their incontinence that they hoped would improve with treatment and to rate each aspect according to its importance on a scale from 0 to 10. After treatment, patients were asked to rate their current ability to perform each previously listed objective on a similar scale of 0 to 10. The combined list of objectives was then categorized into 18 groups for analysis; these then were condensed further into eight major categories for statistical assessment (Table 7.2-5). In this interesting trial, the authors demonstrated that, in this particular group of patients with neurogenic incontinence, the most frequent and important aspect of quality of life affected related to the ability to participate in such social activities as shopping and traveling without the concern of having a toilet nearby. Their results demonstrated that further studies in fecal incontinence and its impact on quality of life issues will require the development of more complete incontinence measurement instruments.

The importance of quality of life in various disorders where fecal incontinence may be significantly involved also has been demonstrated in different studies. In 1995, O'Keefe and colleagues (29) sampled 704 Minnesota residents 65 years of age and older, showing that functional bowel disorders interfere with daily living and quality of life. In a group of 892 diabetic patients, Talley and colleagues evaluated the impact of gastrointestinal symptoms related to quality of life using the SF-36 general health survey (30), where they observed a significant decrease in quality of life scores in diabetics, specifically those with type 2 diabetes. In another group of patients with Parkinson's disease, a questionnaire-based assessment of pelvic organ dysfunction was applied to 115 patients (31). Here, the authors

TABLE 7.2-5. Major categories derived from objectives.

Category	Frequency	Importance	Ability	Improvement	No. of Patients who nominated an objective in this category (%)
1. Getting out of house, socializing and shopping (objectives 1, 2, 3, 4)	123	8.2 (2)	4.4 (2.4)	2 (2.4)	85 (72)
2. Personal and psychological (objectives 5, 6, 7)	55	8.4 (1.8)	4.2 (2.3)	2.5 (2.3)	36 (30)
3. Hygiene and groming (objectives 8, 9, 10)	41	8.7 (1.6)	4.1 (2.1)	2.1 (2.7)	37 (31)
4. Travel—local or overseas (objectives 11, 12)	40	8.1 (1.9)	4.2 (2)	1.8 (3)	34 (29)
5. Exercise and walking (objectives 13, 14)	33	7.8 (1.7)	4.9 (2.9)	2.0 (3.4)	30 (25)
6. Family and relationships (objectives 15, 16)	30	9.0 (1.1)	5 (3.2)	2.4 (2.5)	26 (22)
7. Home duties (objective 17)	25	8.2 (1.7)	5.6 (3.4)	2.2 (2.7)	23 (19)
8. Job and work (objective 18)	17	8.9 (1.5)	4.7 (2.7)	1.7 (2)	16 (13)

demonstrated that fecal incontinence was commonly associated with urinary incontinence and that both significantly affected the patients' reported quality of life independent of their neurological condition (see Chapter 7.3).

In summary, the assessment of quality of life issues in patients with fecal incontinence plays an important role in the evaluation process and can help surgeons and general practitioners in selecting the most suitable treatment option. In addition, the validation of a universal quality of life instrument for fecal incontinence can help maintain uniformity in order to effectively compare the results of operative and biofeedback therapies between different institutions.

At this point, the fecal incontinence quality of life scales as proffered by Rockwood and colleagues represent an initial step forward for colorectal surgeons to objectively rate their results and to evaluate patients with fecal incontinence in a more humanistic and complete manner.

References

1. Clarke N, Hughes AP, and Dodd KJ. The elderly in residential care: patterns of disability. Health Trends. 1979;11:17–21.
2. Mellgren A, Jensen LL, Zetterstrom JP, Wong WD, Hofmeister JH, and Lowry AC. Long-term cost of fecal incontinence secondary to obstetric injuries. Dis Colon Rectum. 1999;42(7):857–65; discussion, 865–7.
3. Thomas TM, Egan M, Walgrave A, and Meade TW. The prevalence of faecal and double incontinence. Community Med. 1984;6:216–20.

4. Enck P, Bielefeldt K, Rathmann W, Purrmann J, Tschope D, and Erckenbrecht JF. Epidemiology of fecal incontinence in selected patients groups. Int J Colorectal Dis. 1991;6:143–6.
5. Johanson JF and Lafferty J. Epidemiology of fecal incontinence: the silent affliction. Am J Gastroenterol. 1996;91:33–6.
6. Perry S, Shaw C, McGrother C, Matthews RJ, et al. Prevalence of faecal incontinence in adults aged 40 years or more living in the community. Gut. 2002; 50(4):480–4.
7. Oliveira L and Wexner SD. In: Beck D and Wexner SD, editors. Fundamentals of anorectal surgery. 2nd ed. 1998. p. 115–52.
8. Vaizey CJ, Carapeti E, Cahill JA, and Kamm MA. Prospective comparison of faecal incontinence grading systems. Gut. 1999;44:77–80.
9. Kelly JH. Cinedefecography in anorectal malformations. J Pediatr Surg. 1969; 4:538–46.
10. Parks AG. Anorectal incontinence. J R Soc Med. 1975;68:21–30.
11. Lane RN. Clinical application of anorectal physiology. Proc Soc Med. 1975; 68:28–30.
12. Rudd WW. The transanal anastomosis: a sphincter-saving operation with improved continence. Dis Colon Rectum. 1979;22:102–5.
13. Holschneider AM. Treatment and functional results of anorectal continence in children with imperforate anus. Acta Chir Belg. 1983;3:191–204.
14. Keighley MR and Fielding WL. Management of faecal incontinence and results of surgical treatment. Br J Surg. 1983;70:463–8.
15. Corman M. Gracilis muscle transposition for anal incontinence. Late results. Br J Surg. 1985;72:S21–2.
16. Hiltunen KNM, Matikainen M, Auvinen O, and Hietanen P. Clinical and manometric evaluation of anal sphincter function in incontinent patients. Am J Surg. 1986;151:489–92.
17. Broden G, Dolk A, and Holmstroem B. Recovery of the internal anal sphincter following rectopexy:a possible explanation for continence improvement. Int J Colorectal Dis. 1988;3:23–8.
18. Womack NR, Morrison JF, and Williams NS. Prospective study of the effects of postanal repair in neurogenic fecal incontinence. Br J Surg. 1988;75:48–52.
19. Rainey JB, Donaldson DN, and Thomson JP. Postanal repair: which patients derive most benefit? J R Coll Surg Edinb. 1990;35:101–5.
20. Miller R, Bartolo DC, Lock-Edmunds JC, and Mortensen NJ. Prospective study of conservative and operative treatment for faecal incontinence. Br J Surg. 1988;75:101–5.
21. Pescatori M, Anastasio G, Bottini C, and Mentasti A. New grading and scoring for anal incontinence. Evaluation of 335 patients. Dis Colon Rectum. 1992; 35:482–487.
22. Jorge JMN and Wexner SD. Etiology and management of fecal incontinence. Dis Colon Rectum. 1993;36:77–97.
23. Rothbarth J, Bemelman WA, Meijerink WJHJ, Stiggelbout AM, Zwinderman AH, Buyze-Westerweel ME, and Delemarre JBVM. What is the impact of fecal incontinence on quality of life? Dis Colon Rectum. 2001;44:67–71.
24. Rockwood TH, Church J, Fleshman JW, Kane RL, Mavrantonis C, Thorson AG, Wexner SD, Bliss D, and Lowry AC. Patient and surgeon ranking of the sever-

ity of symptoms associated with fecal incontinence. The fecal incontinence severity index. Dis Colon Rectum. 1999;42:1525–32.
25. Rockwood TH, Church J, Fleshman JW, Kane RL, Mavrantonis C, Thorson AG, Wexner SD, Bliss D, and Lowry AC. Fecal Incontinence Quality of Life Scale. Quality of life instrument for patients with fecal incontinence. Dis Colon Rectum. 2000;43:9–17.
26. Ware L, Snow K, Kosinski M, and Gandek B. SF-36 health survey. Manual and interpretation guide. Boston: The Health Institute, New England Medical Center; 1993.
27. Byrne CM, Pager CK, Rex MA, Roberts R, and Solomon MJ. Assessment of quality of life in the treatment of patients with neuropathic fecal incontinence. Dis Colon Rectum. 2002;45:1431–6.
28. McLeod RS, Churchill DN, Lock AM, Vanderburgh S, and Cohen Z. Quality of life of patients with ulcerative colitis preoperatively and postoperatively. Gastroenterology. 1991;101:1307–13.
29. O'Keefe EA, Talley NJ, Zinsmeister AR, and Jacobsen SJ. Bowel disorders impair functional status and quality of life in the elderly:a population-based study. J Gerontol A Biol Sci Med Sci. 1995;50(4):M184–9.
30. Talley NJ, Young L, Bytzer P, Hammer J, Leemon M, Jones M, and Horowitz M. Impact of chronic gastrointestinal symptoms in diabetes mellitus on health-related quality of life. Am J Gastroenterol. 2001;96(1):71–6.
31. Sakakibara R, Shinotoh H, Uchiyama T, Sakuma M, Kashiwado M, Yoshiyama M, and Hattori T. Questionnaire-based assessment of pelvic organ dysfunction in Parkinson's disease. Auton Neurosci. 2001;92(1–2):76–85.

Editorial Commentary

Dr. Lucia Oliveira (an alumnus of the Department of Colorectal Surgery at Cleveland Clinic Florida) has developed significant expertise in anorectal physiology at her hospital in Rio De Janeiro, Brazil. One of her areas of special interest, quality of life assessment and fecal incontinence, has been clearly detailed within her chapter. The most salient feature is that the diligence of investigation should parallel the anticipated therapeutic offerings. For example, if there is little anticipation to offer the patient extensive therapy, then the cost and inconvenience of anorectal physiologic investigation may not be worthwhile to pursue. Conversely, if the patient may be a candidate for new interventions such as sacral nerve stimulation, artificial bowel sphincter, or stimulated graciloplasty, then by all means a detailed in-depth evaluation should be undertaken. Quality of life is probably the most important facet of determination of whether or not such physiologic assessment should be used as it is quality of life which is the ultimate endpoint and not a surrogate for the determination of success or failure of therapy. Dr. Oliveira has expertly and successfully addressed this topic.

SW

Chapter 7.3
Fecal and Urinary Incontinence: Epidemiology and Etiology

DANA R. SANDS and MINDA NEIMARK

As more is understood about the function of the pelvic floor, colorectal surgeons, urogynecologists, and urologists will find themselves working together to treat women with complex mixed forms of incontinence and pelvic organ prolapse. No longer should these issues be addressed in isolation. Several population-based studies have been conducted to ascertain the true incidence of isolated fecal and urinary incontinence. The incidence of dual incontinence is much less studied. The evolution of the concept of the pelvic floor as one functional unit with both anterior and posterior components has led physicians treating patients with isolated incontinence to search for evidence of dual incontinence. This has allowed us to provide more comprehensive medical care for our patients.

Fecal Incontinence

Epidemiology and Etiology

Fecal incontinence represents a significant public health concern. It is estimated that over 400 million dollars per year are spent on adult diapers in the United States (1). The prevalence of fecal incontinence is grossly underestimated due to the social stigma associated with the condition and the reluctance of both patient and physician to discuss these problems. The problem extends beyond geographic borders and stretches worldwide. Several studies from various countries have estimated the prevalence of fecal incontinence in the general population to be between 1.4% and 12.7% (Table 7.3-1). This range reported after meta-analysis of over 26000 people underscores the difficulty in fully assessing the magnitude of the problem.

The etiology of fecal incontinence can be classified into two groups: patients with normal pelvic floor function and those with abnormal pelvic floor function. Initially, it is important to rule out pseudoincontinence as the cause of the patient's symptoms. Pseudoincontinence results from perineal soiling that can be related to poor hygiene, prolapsing hemorrhoids, anal

TABLE 7.3-1. Prevalence of fecal incontinence in various countries.

Country	Year	Study Size (N)	Prevalence
United Kingdom (2)	2001	2818	3%
Nigeria (3)	2002	3963	6.96%
Australia (4)	2002	660	9%
United Kingdom (5)	2002	10116	1.40%
New Zealand (6)	2001	717	12.70%
United Arab Emirates (7)	2001	450	11.30%
Switzerland (8)	2001	984	4.40%
United States (9)	1995	6959	2.20%

fistula, or dermatologic conditions. Overflow incontinence is another cause for fecal incontinence. It often is seen in the elderly and is associated with fecal impaction. Fecal incontinence with normal pelvic floor function can result from persistent liquid stool, causing diarrhea and urgency, or may be related to systemic illnesses including diabetes, multiple sclerosis, scleroderma, or dementia. Acquired fecal incontinence related to pelvic floor dysfunction can be subdivided further into etiologies related to sphincter injury and those related to denervation injury. The most common cause of sphincter injury in otherwise healthy women is obstetric trauma. The true incidence of sphincter injury and subsequent fecal incontinence is difficult to assess because the symptom presentation often is delayed. Sangalli et al. (10) contacted over 200 women 13 years after obstetric related anal sphincter trauma. Fecal incontinence was noted in 11.5% and 25% of women with third- and fourth-degree lacerations, respectively. In the subgroup of women with fourth-degree lacerations, subsequent vaginal delivery was associated with a higher prevalence of severe incontinence. Ryhammer and colleagues (11) assessed the long-term effect of vaginal delivery on anorectal function in a group of normal perimenopausal women. Increasing parity correlated with increased perineal descent, decreased anal mucosa sensitivity, and prolonged pudendal nerve terminal motor latency (PNTML). They concluded that repeated vaginal deliveries had a long-term adverse effect on anorectal physiology and function.

Trauma to the anal sphincters is not limited to obstetric causes. Surgical treatment of anal fistulae fissures and hemorrhoids can all lead to varying degrees of incontinence (12). In a prospective study of 50 patients who underwent fistulectomy, hemorrhoidectomy, or sphincterotomy, Felt-Bersma and colleagues (13) found a 46% incidence of anal sphincter defects. Thirty percent of these patients had symptoms of fecal incontinence, whereas 70% had occult sphincter defects. The implications for future continence in the subgroup with occult injuries are unknown. The largely abandoned Lord technique for the treatment of hemorrhoidal disease, consisting of anal dilatation, has been reported to have associated incontinence rates as high as 52% in the long term (14). The presence of a rectal prolapse also can lead to incontinence secondary to the chronic dilatation of the anal sphincters and traction injury to the pudendal nerves, resulting in pudendal neuropathy, although the physiology here is complex with a mixture of sphincter damage, altered mucosal sensitivity, disabled anorectal sampling, and rectoanal incoordination, as well as fundamental alteration in the rectoanal inhibitory reflex (15). Neuropathic injury to the pelvic floor will be addressed further in this chapter. Female sex, previous anorectal surgery, and previous vaginal delivery are all risk factors for the development of fecal incontinence related to pelvic floor dysfunction.

Urinary Incontinence

Urinary incontinence (UI), defined as the involuntary loss of urine sufficient to be a social or hygiene problem, is a newly recognized health issue affecting millions of people worldwide (16). Urinary incontinence in the elderly is a major cause of disability and dependency, imposing a significant financial burden on both the patient and society as a whole. In 1995, the total estimated expense of UI was $26.3 billion, or $3565 per individual aged 65 and older with urinary incontinence (17).

Urinary incontinence, a generalized term, encompasses several etiologies of incontinence including stress incontinence, overactive bladder (OAB), mixed incontinence (stress and OAB), and overflow incontinence. Each condition of incontinence is characterized not only by distinct symptoms, but also by overlapping symptoms requiring investigative studies to define the etiology of the patient's UI. The following are etiologies of UI defined by International Continence Society (ICS) classification:

Stress Incontinence (SUI): urine loss coincident with an increase in intra-abdominal pressure in the absence of a detrusor contraction or overdistended bladder.

Overactive bladder (OAB): a term used to encompass a range of irritative bladder filling and storage symptoms. For this chapter, the term OAB will be used to define involuntary loss of urine associated with involuntary or uninhibited detrusor contractions documented by cystometry. Terms used to clinically define this condition are detrusor hyperreflexia or detrusor instability. Other terms that are used clinically, but have not been defined by the ICS, are motor urge incontinence and sensory urge incontinence.

Mixed incontinence is combined SUI and OAB.

Overflow Incontinence is defined as involuntary loss of urine associated with over distension of the bladder.

Epidemiology

The epidemiology of UI includes incidence, prevalence, types of incontinence, as well as associated risk factors such as age, gender, and medical illnesses (see Table 7.3-2). Although there recently has been an increased awareness of UI among physicians and the public, it still remains an underreported health condition due to the ongoing perception as a socially embarrassing condition. It has been estimated that almost 40% of women who experience urinary incontinence endure the condition for a year or more before consulting a doctor. In addition, although studies have been conducted in an attempt to determine the true prevalence of urinary incontinence, they have produced only estimates due to differences in methodology, as well as variations in the definitions of UI.

Urinary incontinence incidence is defined as the number of new cases over a certain period of time. The incidence of UI reported in the literature is limited due to factors such as dropouts by migration, noncompliance, and death. Elving (18) reported an increase in the incidence of urinary incontinence in women between the ages of 45 and 59 years.

Sex and Age

Urinary incontinence has been demonstrated to be more prevalent in women than in men, with prevalence ranging from 4.5% to 53% in women and 1.6% to 24% in men. This chapter will address only the epidemiology

TABLE 7.3-2. Risk factors associated with UI.

Age
Gender
Medical illness
Cerebrovascular events
Parkinson's
Multiple sclerosis
Pulmonary disease
Chronic bronchitis
Chronic obstructive pulmonary disease
Diabetes
Connective tissue disease
Congenital
Spina bifida
Medications
Thiazides
Oral estrogen
Body mass index
Previous pelvic surgery
Childbirth
Menopause
Smoking

of UI in the female patient. It is well documented that UI increases with age. The lifetime risk of undergoing a single operation for prolapse or incontinence by age 80 is 11.1% (19). A recent survey showed that 12.5% of women less than 80 years of age, 19% of women between 80 and 89 years of age, and 31.1% of women greater than 90 years of age reported daily UI (20). It has been demonstrated that functional urethral length—an important component of the continence mechanism—is affected by age and estrogen status. This is due to a decrease in both urethral vascularity and smooth and skeletal muscle, both of which are estrogen dependent. This has been made evident by studies demonstrating that the use of local estrogen improves incontinence symptoms.

Urinary incontinence is a very common condition in the nursing home setting, where it is the number one reason for admission to a nursing home, with an estimated prevalence as high as 70% (21).

Types of Incontinence

Stress incontinence—reportedly occurring in 49% of all women—is more predominant than OAB, which occurs in approximately 22% of women. Mixed incontinence is reported to occur in 47% of the female population. Reported symptoms have been shown to be a poor diagnostic tool for UI. Therefore, urodynamics should be performed prior to initiating treatment, especially when surgical treatment is considered (22).

Stress urinary incontinence results when there is loss of support to the bladder neck failing to maintain a watertight seal under conditions of increased intra-abdominal pressure. When the bladder neck can no longer maintain a seal at rest, the condition is called intrinsic sphincter deficiency (ISD)—a more severe form of stress incontinence.

Overactive bladder (OAB) has been popularized recently as a term for the condition encompassing a range of irritative bladder filling and storage symptoms. It includes urinary frequency, urgency, and urge incontinence, singly or in combination. Urgency is a strong desire to void accompanied by a fear of leakage. Frequency represents the need to urinate on an abnormally frequent basis—more than eight times per day or more than two times per night (nocturia). Urge incontinence refers to the symptom of urine loss preceded by a strong sense of urgency. Detrusor instability is the term used when loss of urine secondary to a spontaneous or provoked involuntary detrusor contraction is demonstrated during cystometry. If the uninhibited detrusor contractions are due to a neurologic etiology, such as multiple sclerosis or Parkinson's disease, then the term detrusor hyperreflexia is used. Complaints of bladder dysfunction may be the initial symptom of a neurologic lesion. In fact, 20% to 30% of patients with multiple sclerosis or Parkinson's disease will have bladder dysfunction complaints prior to a diagnosis of their primary neurological disease.

Race

The distribution of incontinence types differs between racial groups. It is theorized that these differences in distribution are due to genetic factors and lifestyle. In a recent study evaluating the prevalence of UI amongst first-degree relatives, there was a three-fold prevalence of UI amongst first-degree relatives of index female patients presenting with UI (23). It has been demonstrated that white postmenopausal women are more likely to report UI than black postmenopausal women (32% vs. 18%) (18). In a study of 200 women who had undergone multichannel urodynamic evaluation, white women were more likely to have a diagnosis of stress urinary incontinence than black women (61% vs. 27%). In addition, 56% of black women were more likely to have OAB, compared with 28% of white women (24). A recent study by Mattox and Bhatia (25) evaluated the prevalence of UI among white and Hispanic women with similar age, gravity, and parity. Hispanic women were more likely to have stress incontinence than white women (30% vs. 16%), and white women were more likely to have OAB than Hispanic women (44% vs. 27%).

Dual Incontinence

Epidemiology

After comparison of the etiology and relative risk factors for the development of isolated fecal and urinary incontinence, there is no surprise that these two afflictions frequently coexist. Dual incontinence is grossly underdiagnosed. In a population-based study from Minnesota, over 1500 people over the age of 50 responded to a questionnaire related to fecal and urinary incontinence (26). Here, 5.4% and 9.4% of men and women, respectively, suffered from combined fecal and urinary incontinence. Among people with fecal incontinence, the prevalence of concurrent urinary incontinence was 51.1% in men and 59.6% in women. In the younger age groups, the incidence of combined incontinence in women was twice as high as in men. These incidences are much higher than those previously reported by Nakanishi (27), who found the prevalence to be 53/1000 in a community-based review.

Lacima and colleagues (28) investigated the incidence of coexisting fecal incontinence in a subgroup of patients being treated in a urodynamic hospital unit. After interviewing 900 consecutive patients suffering from urinary incontinence, they found the incidence of dual incontinence to be 8.7%. The urodynamic evaluation of this group revealed stress incontinence in 42%, detrusor instability in 11%, mixed incontinence in 37%, voiding disorder in 3%, and no urodynamically detectable abnormality in 6%. A history of vaginal delivery and chronic straining was more frequent in the group of patients with dual incontinence. In a similar review, Meschia et al.

(29) investigated the prevalence of fecal incontinence in 881 women being treated for urinary incontinence or pelvic organ prolapse. Twenty percent of their patients suffered from fecal incontinence. Of the patients with urinary incontinence, 24% had coexistent fecal incontinence, and independently, the women with urinary incontinence were more likely to report their symptoms of fecal incontinence than those being treated for pelvic organ prolapse alone. Alnaif and Drutz (30) noted, however, that dual incontinence exists even in the nulliparous population of teenage girls in Canada. In a survey of 332 teenage girls, the prevalence of urinary incontinence symptoms was 17%, where 38% had minor symptoms of fecal incontinence (usually to gas), and 3% had major symptoms of fecal incontinence. Of interest, with the exception of the one woman who suffered from enuresis, none of the women with fecal or urinary incontinence symptoms had sought medical attention or felt that the symptoms were abnormal.

The experience at the Cleveland Clinic Florida again points to a high incidence of dual incontinence (31). In a group of patients who were treated surgically for fecal incontinence, the incidence of concomitant urinary incontinence was 54%, and 64% of patients treated surgically for rectal prolapse had associated urinary incontinence. These numbers are much higher than the general population, pointing to a common pathophysiology for urinary and fecal incontinence involving pelvic floor dysfunction.

Damage to the Pelvic Floor

Obstetrics

The pelvis traditionally has been separated into three compartments: the anterior containing the bladder, the middle compartment, which is occupied by the uterus and vagina, and the posterior compartment occupied by the rectum and anus. Because all three compartments share similar innervation and muscular support, it is logical to assume that damage to the nerves and muscles of the pelvic floor can lead to pelvic floor dysfunction and urinary and/or fecal incontinence. This concept of the pelvic floor as a single functional unit is gaining acceptance by physicians who address dysfunction of the pelvis resulting in incontinence, urinary or fecal. The pathophysiology behind fecal and urinary incontinence is thought to be the result of a combination of factors including childbirth, connective tissue disorders, pelvic neuropathies, congenital factors, pelvic surgery, and miscellaneous factors such as obesity, respiratory disorders, occupational and recreational stress, and hypoestrogenism. This is important for a physician to understand because it is traditionally thought that most of the damage that occurs to the pelvis is iatrogenic.

As stated previously, there are many factors contributing to damage of the pelvic floor. Obstetrical injury is thought to be the principal factor contributing to the development of incontinence. It has been well established that a vaginal delivery—notably the first—is associated strongly with the future development of urinary and fecal incontinence. Approximately 40% of women who undergo a vaginal delivery will at some point develop urinary and/or fecal incontinence. It also has been shown that women who undergo elective cesarean section without previous labor have fewer complaints of these symptoms. This would indicate there has been little to no damage sustained by that mode of delivery. Instrumental vaginal deliveries with forceps have been shown to be responsible for a greater decrease in intra-anal pressure and a greater incidence of weak pelvic floor musculature compared with vaginal delivery without forceps. This determination was based on objective data including physical examination and urodynamics (32).

Pelvic floor dysfunction caused by obstetrical injury is related to damage of the anatomical support or denervation injury of the pudendal nerve. The event of a vaginal delivery results in dilation and stretching of the pelvic floor, connective tissue supports including the perineal body, and the muscles of the anal sphincter. Episiotomy and occult damage to the external anal sphincter (EAS) as evidenced by endoanal ultrasound reveals many unsuspected defects of both the internal and external anal sphincters following vaginal delivery. Sultan et al. (33) used endoanal ultrasonography to evaluate the sphincter morphology in 202 women before and after delivery and six weeks postpartum. Thirty-five percent of the primiparous and 44% of the multiparous patients had anal sphincter disruptions after delivery.

There are multiple studies that have found childbirth, particularly with a vaginal delivery, to be associated with the development of pelvic neuropathies either by direct compression or stretching of the nerve. The pudendal nerve innervates the pelvic floor muscles, as well as the anal and the external striated urethral sphincter, as the nerve travels along the pelvic sidewall. Specifically, the inferior hemorrhoidal branches innervate the EAS and the perineal branches of the pudendal nerve innervate the periurethral sphincter. The site of damage to the pudendal nerve determines the extent of dysfunction to the various muscles it innervates (34,35).

Snooks et al. (36) demonstrated slowed conduction of the perineal nerve in those patients with stress urinary incontinence. The type of obstetrical event that results in a neuropathy has been evaluated in studies assessing pudendal nerve function. Tetzschner and colleagues (37) demonstrated an increase in terminal motor latency of the pudendal nerve (PTML) in women who underwent a vaginal delivery. In a recent study, PTML recordings were compared in women beyond 34 weeks gestation who either delivered vaginally or by elective Caesarean section. Terminal motor latency of the pudendal nerve values were significantly more prolonged in those women who had a vaginal delivery when compared with women who had an elective Caesarean section, either in primipara or multipara, and women who had a Caesarean section after the onset of labor also had prolongation of PTML (38,39).

Pelvic Surgery

Pelvic surgery—especially radical pelvic surgery with extensive dissection—can lead to pelvic floor dysfunction. Several studies have shown that a major cause of pelvic morbidity after radical surgery for gynecologic cancer is damage to the pelvic nerve plexus. Bladder dysfunction after pelvic surgery from either blunt or sharp dissection has been attributed to damage to the autonomic nerves: the sacral splanchnic (parasympathetic), hypogastric (sympathetic), and the pelvic autonomic nerve plexus.

Surgical repair of pelvic organ prolapse when performed through the vaginal route has been shown to result in damage to the pudendal nerve and its perineal branch because the perineal branch supplies the anterior vaginal wall. Women evaluated up to 32 months postoperatively who underwent vaginal reconstruction and had a suboptimal outcome of their prolapse determined by physical examination demonstrated a neuropathy documented by an increase in the PTML of the perineal branch of the pudendal nerve (40). It also has been demonstrated that vaginal dissection can worsen preexisting perineal neuropathy in patients with pelvic relaxation and stress incontinence. Benson and McClellan (41) found that pelvic floor surgery involving vaginal dissection with or without needle urethropexy in patients with pelvic floor relaxation or urinary incontinence resulted in further deterioration of nerve function based on terminal motor latency studies of both the perineal and inferior rectal branches of the pudendal nerve six weeks following surgery.

Menopause

Epidemiologic studies have demonstrated a higher prevalence of UI in postmenopausal women. This most likely is due to a combination of lower urinary tract changes that occur in the postmenopausal woman, as well as the higher incidence of medical illnesses that have been associated with UI. Urethral function is affected by age. Maximal urethral pressure and functional urethral length increase from infancy to early adulthood, and then decrease with advancing age. It also has been shown that the pelvic floor, bladder, and vagina are estrogen-dependent. Because normal urethral function is dependent on estrogen, further decrease in functional length occurs after menopause because of estrogen deficiency, contributing to the development of UI.

Surgical Outcome for Combined Fecal and Urinary Incontinence

There are limited data available on combined surgery for urinary and fecal incontinence. Advantages to performing a combined procedure as compared with several surgeries include lower cost, fewer in-hospital days, and only one exposure to general anesthesia. In addition, a single combined surgery would ideally decrease the amount of trauma to the pelvic floor, thus decreasing the potential for neuropathy. Halverson and colleagues (42) reported surgical outcomes in patients who underwent sphincteroplasty alone versus sphincteroplasty and urogynecologic surgery, including transvaginal hysterectomy, vaginal prolapse repair, and urethropexy. There were no significant differences in terms of surgical success, morbidity, or mortality between the two groups. There was also no significant difference in limitation—physically, socially, or sexually—between the two groups. In addition, 92% of the patients were satisfied that their double incontinence was repaired at the same time. Silvis and colleagues (43) evaluated the overall benefit of performing a rectovaginovesicopexy for 25 women with combined fecal and urinary incontinence. In this small series, constipation was improved in 78%, fecal incontinence in 69%, and urinary incontinence in 50%, based on defecography, physical examination, and mailed response questionnaires.

Ross (44) evaluated 46 women who had UI and fecal incontinence treated surgically by laparoscopic Burch colposuspension and overlapping sphincteroplasty. At one year postoperatively, 89% were objectively dry and 82% had no reported fecal incontinence. Sacral nerve stimulation has been shown to be successful for UI, urge incontinence, and detrusor instability (see Chapter 7.4). New data regarding sacral nerve stimulation for combined treatment of fecal and urinary incontinence are now being analyzed and are awaited. Perhaps the most convincing evidence for a similar neuropathic etiology for fecal and urinary incontinence has been the success associated with sacral nerve stimulation. Initially used for the treatment of urinary incontinence, patients with concomitant fecal incontinence soon noted improvement in both symptoms. Early and mid-term results have shown sacral nerve stimulation to be beneficial in the treatment of complex forms of incontinence (45,46).

Conclusions

The true epidemiology of combined urinary and fecal incontinence is difficult to assess. The social stigma associated with these conditions has made it difficult for physicians to adequately identify affected patients. As we learn more about the function of the pelvic floor and recognize the common etiology of both anterior and posterior compartment dysfunction, we will offer better and more comprehensive care to our patients.

References

1. Johanson JF and Lafferty J. Epidemiology of fecal incontinence: The silent affliction. Am J Gastroenterol. 1996;91:33–6.
2. Edwards NI and Jones D. The prevalence of fecal incontinence in older people living at home. Age Ageing. 2001;30:503–7.
3. Okonkwo JE, Obionu CN, Okonkwo CV, and Obiechina NJ. Anal incontinence among Igbo (Nigerian) women. Int J Clin Prac. 2002;56:178–80.
4. Kalantar JS, Howell S, and Talley NJ. Prevalence of fecal incontinence and associated risk factors; an underdiagnosed problem in the Australian community? Med J Aust. 2002;176:47–8.
5. Shaw P, McGrother C, Matthews RJ, et al. Prevalence of faecal incontinence in adults aged 40 years or more living in the community. Gut. 2002;50:480–4.
6. Lynch AC, Dobbs BR, Keating J, and Frizelle FA. The prevalence of faecal incontinence and constipation in a general New Zealand population; a postal survey. N Z Med J. 2001;114:474–7.
7. Rizk DE, Hassan MY, Shaheen H, Cherian JV, Micaleff R, and Dunn E. The prevalence and determinants of health care seeking behavior for fecal incontinence in multiparous United Arab Emirates females. Dis Colon Rectum. 2001;44:1850–6.
8. Faltin DL, Sangalli MR, Curtin F, Morabia A, and Weil A. Prevalence of anal incontinence and other anorectal symptoms in women. Int Urogynecol J Pelvic Floor Dysfunct. 2001;12:117–21.
9. Nelson R. Community-based prevalence of anal incontinence. JAMA. 1995; 274:559–61.
10. Sangalli MR, Floris L, Faltin D, and Weil A. Anal incontinence in women with third or fourth degree perineal tears and subsequent vaginal deliveries. Aust N Z Obstet Gynaecol. 2000;40:244–8.
11. Ryhammer AM, Laurberg S, and Hermann AP. Long-term effect of vaginal delivery on anorectal function in normal perimenopausal women. Dis Col Rectum. 1996;39:852–9.
12. Zbar AP, Beer-Gabel M, Chiappa AC, and Aslam M. Fecal incontinence after minor anorectal surgery. Dis Colon Rectum. 2001;44:1610–23.
13. Felt-Bersma RJ, van Baren R, Koorevaar M, Strijers RL, and Cuesta MA. Unsuspected sphincter defects shown by anal ultrasonography after anorectal surgery. A prospective study. Dis Col Rectum. 1995;38:249–53.
14. Konsten J and Baeten CG. Hemorrhoidectomy vs. Lord's method: 17 year follow up of a prospective randomized trial. Dis Col Rectum. 2000;43:503–6.
15. Zbar AP, Takashima S, Hasegawa T, and Kitabayashi K. Perineal rectosigmoidectomy (Altemeier's procedure): a review of physiology, technique and outcome. Tech Coloproctol. 2002;6:109–16.
16. Fantl JA, Newman DK, Collong J, et al. Urinary incontinence in adults: acute and chronic management. Clinical practice guideline, No. 2, 1996 update. Rockville, MD: U.S. Department of Health and Human Services, Public Health Service, Agency for Health and Human Services. Public Health Service, Agency

for Health Care Policy and Research. AHCPR Publication No. 9-0682; March 1996.
17. Wagner TH and Hu T. Economic costs of urinary incontinence. Int Urogynecol J. 1998;9:127–8.
18. Elving LB, Foldspang A, Lam OW, and Mommsen S. Descriptive epidemiology of urinary incontinence in 3100 women age 30–59. Scand J Urol Nephrol. 1989;125(Suppl):37–43.
19. Olsen AL, Smith VJ, Bergstrom JO, Colling JC, and Clark AL. Epidemiology of surgically managed pelvic organ prolapse and urinary incontinence. Obstet Gynecol. 1997;89:501–6.
20. Brown JS, Seeley DG, Fong J, Black D, Ensurd KE, and Grady D. Urinary incontinence in older women: Who is at risk? Obstet Gynecol. 1996;87:715–21.
21. Ouslander JG and Schnelle JF. Incontinence in the nursing home. J Am Geriatr Soc. 1990;38:289–91.
22. Jensen JK, Nielsen FR Jr, and Ostergard DR. The role of patient history in the diagnosis of urinary incontinence. Obstet Gynecol. 1994;83:904–10.
23. Mushkat Y, Bulovsky I, and Langer R. Female urinary stress incontinence—does it have familial prevalence? Am J Obstet Gynecol. 1996;174:617–19.
24. Bump RC. Racial comparisons and contrasts in urinary incontinence and pelvic organ prolapse. Obstet Gynecol. 1993;81:421–5.
25. Mattox TF and Bhatia N. The prevalence of urinary incontinence or prolapse among white and Hispanic women. Am J Obstet Gynecol. 1996;174:646–8.
26. Roberts RO, Jacobsen SJ, Reilly WT, Pemberton JH, Lieber MM, and Talley NJ. Prevalence of combined fecal and urinary incontinence: A community based study. J Am Geriatr Soc. 1999;47:837–42.
27. Nakanishi N, Tatara K, Nakajima K, Takabayashi H, Takahashi S, Naramura H, and Ikeda K. Urinary and fecal incontinence in a community residing older population in Japan. J Am Geriatr Soc. 1997;45:215–19.
28. Lacima G, Espuna M, Pera M, Puig-Clota M, Quinto L, and Garcia-Valdecasas JC. Clinical, urodynamic and manometric findings in women with combined fecal and urinary incontinence. Neurourol Urodyn. 2002;21:464–9.
29. Meschia M, Buonaguidi A, Pifarotti P, Somigliana E, Spenacchio M, and Amicarelli F. Prevalence of anal incontinence in women with symptoms of urinary incontinence and genital prolapse. Obstet Gynecol. 2002;100:719–23.
30. Alnaif B and Drutz HP. The prevalence of urinary and fecal incontinence in Canadian secondary school teenage girls: Questionnaire study and review of the literature. Int Urogynecol J. 2001;12:134–8.
31. Gonzalez-Argente FX, Jain A, Nogueras JJ, Davila GW, Weiss EG, and Wexner SD. Prevalence and severity of urinary incontinence and pelvic genital prolapse in females with anal incontinence or rectal prolapse. Dis Colon Rectum. 2001;44:920–6.
32. Meyer A, Hohfeld P, Actari C, Russolo A, and De Grandi P. Birth trauma: Short and long term effects of forceps delivery compared with spontaneous delivery on various pelvic floor parameters. Brit J Obstet Gynecol. 2000;107:1360–5.
33. Sultan AH, Kamm MA, Hudson CN, Thomas JM, and Bartram CI. Anal sphincter disruptions during vaginal delivery. N Eng J Med. 1993;329:1905–11.
34. Pregazzi R, Sartore A, Bortoli P, Grimaldi E, Ricci G, and Guaschino S. Immediate postpartum perineal examination as a predictor of puerperal pelvic floor dysfunction. Obstet Gynecol. 2002;99:581–4.

35. Smith ARB, Hosker GL, and Warrell DW. The role of pudendal nerve damage in the etiology of genuine stress incontinence in women. Brit J Obstet Gynecol. 1989;96:29–32.
36. Snooks SJ, Badenoch DF, Tiptaft RC, and Swash M. Perineal nerve damage in genuine stress incontinence. Brit J Urol. 1985;57:422–6.
37. Tetzschner T, Sorensen M, Johnson L, Lose G, and Christiansen J. Delivery and pudendal nerve function. Acta Obstet Gynecol Scand. 1997;76:324–31.
38. Sultan AH, Kamm MA, and Hudson CN. Pudendal nerve damage during labor: prospective study before and after childbirth. Br J Obstet Gynaecol. 1994; 101:22–8.
39. Fynes M, Donnelly VS, O'Connell PR, and O'Herlihy C. Caesarean delivery and anal sphincter injury. Obstet Gynecol. 1998;92(4 Pt 1):496–500.
40. Welgoss JA, Vogt VY, McClellan EJ, and Benson JT. Relationship between surgically induced neuropathy and outcome of pelvic organ prolapse surgery. Int Urogynecol J. 1999;10:11–14.
41. Benson JT and McClellan E. The effect of vaginal dissection on the pudendal nerve. Obstet Gynecol. 1993;82:387–9.
42. Halverson AL, Hull TL, Paraiso MF, and Floruta C. Outcome of sphincteroplasty combined with surgery for urinary incontinence and pelvic organ prolapse. Dis Colon Rectum. 2001;44:1421–6.
43. Silvis R, Gooszen HG, Kahraman T, Groenendijk AG, Lock MT, Itiliaander MV, and Janssen LW. Novel approach to combined defecation and micturition disorders with rectovaginovesicopexy. Brit J Surgery. 1998;85:813–17.
44. Ross JW. Laparoscopic burch colposuspension and overlapping sphincteroplasty for double incontinence. JSLS. 2001;5:203–9.
45. Kenefick NJ, Vaizey CJ, Cohen CG, Nicholls RJ, and Kamm MA. Medium-term results of permanent sacral nerve stimulation for fecal incontinence. Br J Surg. 2002;89:896–901.
46. Ganio E, Masin A, Ratto C, Altomare DF, Ripetti V, Clerico G, Lise M, Doglietto GB, Memeo V, Landolfi V, Del Genio A, Arullani A, Giardiello G, and De Seta F. Short-term sacral nerve stimulation for functional anorectal and urinary disturbances: Results in forty patients. Dis Colon Rectum. 2001;44: 1261–7.

Editorial Commentary

Dr. Dana Sands (an alumnus in the Department of Colorectal Surgery at Cleveland Clinic Florida) and Dr. Minda Neimark (an alumnus of the Section of Urogynecology at Cleveland Clinic Florida) work closely together on a routine basis to address mixed fecal and urinary incontinence. They have brought to this book their collective wisdom and have helped us to recognize a fact often overlooked by colorectal surgeons, specifically that urinary incontinence may well coexist with fecal incontinence and that the treatment of one condition may exacerbate the other. Their work together has highlighted the fact that prior to any intervention for one type of incontinence the other type of incontinence should be assessed with whatever tests are appropriate and if appropriate, simultaneously treated to prevent such exacerbation. I think that the very high incidence of dual incontinence may be striking to many readers along with the fact that both etiologies can often be successfully simultaneously addressed. Their contribution represents the future of pelvic floor physiologic evaluation and treatment. It is important for coloproctologists to understand that we should work as a team with our urogynecology colleagues to ensure proper evaluation and treatment in these patients.

SW

Chapter 7.4
Sacral Neuromodulation

Ezio Ganio

Introduction

Until recently, the treatment of fecal incontinence had focused solely on the anal sphincters. However, if incontinence is a result of a sphincteric functional deficit or of a rectal pressure that exceeds anal pressure for rectal hypersensitivity and hypertonia in a patient with an intact anal sphincter mechanism, this approach is unsatisfactory. Sacral neuromodulation (SNM) has now proven to be a valid approach for some of these patients with functional fecal incontinence. Urologists first began to study the possibilities of an electrical stimulation to control bladder dysfunction in the 1950s. Initial attempts to provoke artificial micturition involved direct stimulation of the spinal cord (1,2), the detrusor muscle (1,3,4), and the striated sphincter (4,5). None of these methods produced satisfactory bladder emptying. Research then was focused on electrical stimulation of the sacral nerve roots in order to treat serious bladder emptying dysfunction (4,6,7). Tanagho and Schmidt (8) of the University of California in San Francisco applied the principles of sacral nerve stimulation to patients affected by voiding dysfunction or incontinence due to bladder instability. In 1981, they performed the first sacral nerve stimulation implant. Currently, stimulation of the sacral nerve roots has been used successfully to control voiding difficulties and urinary incontinence.

The first report on the possible use of sacral neuromodulation in the treatment of fecal incontinence was published in 1995 (9). Although the mechanism of sacral stimulation is today still far from understood, it is likely that the effects are multifactorial. The stimulated target is a mixed nerve carrying efferent (somatomotor) and afferent (sensory) nerves, as well as autonomic nerves (10), and the interaction between the autonomic and somatic nervous system is an integral part of the nerve control of the mechanisms of defecation. Sacral nerve stimulation seems to have an effect on rectal motility, which could be of clinical importance (11). The improvement in continence could be related to a change of rectal sensibility leading to a better coordination between the rectum and the anorectal sphincter. Blockade of C-afferent fibers is one of the suggested mechanisms of action of sacral neuromodulation (12), with a modulation/inhibition of sacral reflex arcs regulating rectal tone and contractility. Additionally, SNM offers the possibility of predicting the beneficial effects through temporary percutaneous stimulation.

Technique of Sacral Neuromodulation

Sacral nerve stimulation therapy consists of two stages: peripheral nerve evaluation—the diagnostic stage—and permanent implant—the therapeutic stage. Each step follows specific principles and has specific goals.

Percutaneous Nerve Evaluation

Percutaneous nerve evaluation (PNE) of the sacral roots (S2, S3, and S4) is divided into two phases: an acute phase to test the functional relevance and integrity of each sacral spinal nerve to striated anal sphincter function (9), and a chronic phase of 10 to 14 days to assess the therapeutic potential of sacral spinal nerve stimulation in individual patients.

Percutaneous Nerve Evaluation Procedure

With the patient in the prone position, the three sacral foramina S2, S3, and S4 are located using bony landmarks (Figures 7.4.1 and 7.4.2). The sacral foramen S2 is typically found just under the projection of the posterior

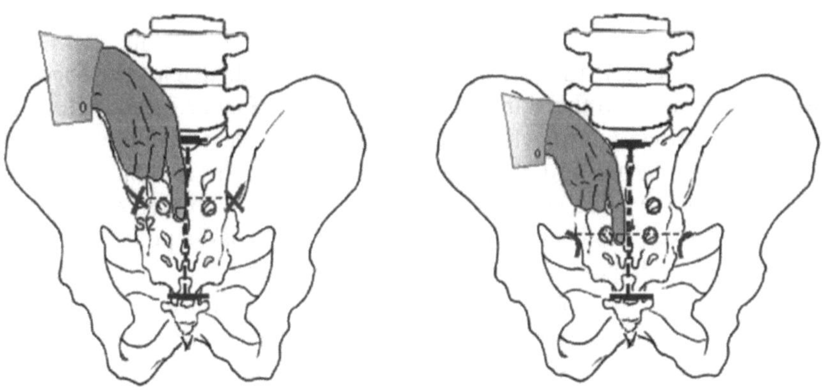

FIGURE 7.4.1. Bony landmarks.The dorsal sacral foramina are positioned approximately two centimeters laterally to the sacral crest. S2 is about one centimeter medially and one centimeter below the posterior superior iliac spine; S3 is positioned on a level with the upper border of the sciatic notch.

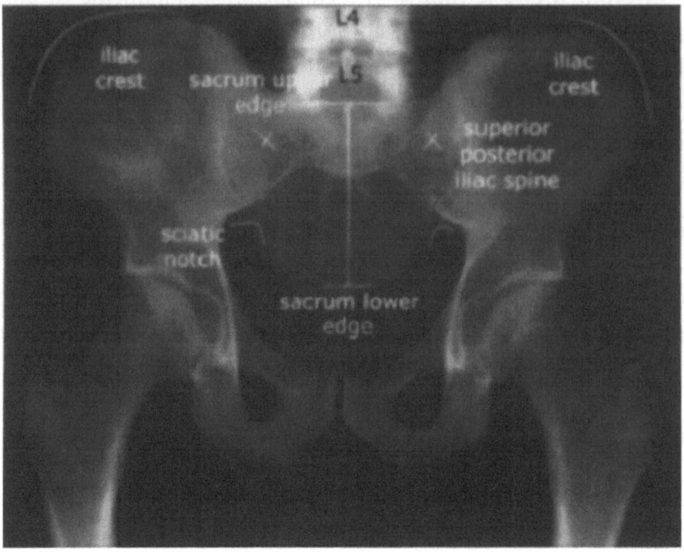

FIGURE 7.4.2. Antero-posterior X-ray. Schematic representation on a pelvis X-ray of the bony landmarks for sacral foramina location.

superior iliac spines and about one finger breadth lateral to the mid-line. The sciatic notches, which correspond to level S3, are identified with the S4 foramen about two centimeters under the S3 foramen. Foramina S3 and S4 also are positioned about one finger breadth from the mid-line.

The acute phase test is performed under local anesthesia using a 20-gauge insulated spinal needle (Medtronic™ #041828-004) and an external neurostimulator (Medtronic™ Model 3625 Screener or Medtronic™ Model 3628 Dual Screener). The needle is inserted perpendicular to the sacrum, with an inclination to the skin of 60 to 80 degrees (Figure 7.4.3). After the needle is positioned in the chosen foramen, it is connected to the external neurostimulator. The stimulation parameters used in the acute phase are a pulse width (PW) of 210 microseconds, a frequency of 25 Hertz (Hz), and an amplitude that results in an increased contraction of the pelvic floor and a deepening and flattening of the buttock muscle. This usually occurs between one and six volts. Stimulation of specific sacral nerves typically results in specific movements of the perineum, anal sphincter, and ipsilateral lower extremity. This ensures correct lead placement. Stimulation of S2 causes some movement of the perineum and the external sphincter along with a lateral rotation of the leg and contraction of the toes and foot. Stimulation of S3 causes a contraction of the pelvic floor and the external anal sphincter (EAS), the "bellows" contraction, and a plantar flexion of the big toe. Stimulation of S4 causes a contraction of the anus with a clamp-like perineal movement with no leg or foot movement. Vesical, vaginal (or scrotal), and rectal paraesthesia may be perceived by the patient during sacral nerve stimulation.

Temporary Sacral Nerve Stimulation

Once an adequate muscular response is obtained, a temporary stimulator lead (Model 3065U Medtronic™, Minneapolis MN, USA, or Model 3057-1, Minneapolis MN, USA) is inserted through the needle, following which, the needle is removed. The lead is connected to an external stimulator (Screener Model 3625, Minneapolis MN, USA) to allow evaluation of the functional responses to the test, both subjectively with regard to continence and objectively using rectoanal manometry (Figure 7.4.4). Ten to fourteen days of stimulation is the minimum period accepted for this test. To evaluate the functional results of PNE, patients complete a clinical diary of fecal incontinence and bowel movement episodes in the two weeks preceding, during, and in the two weeks following the PNE test.

Surgical Technique for Permanent Implant

The surgical technique recently has evolved from a classically open to a minimally invasive implant approach. Both methods are explained below.

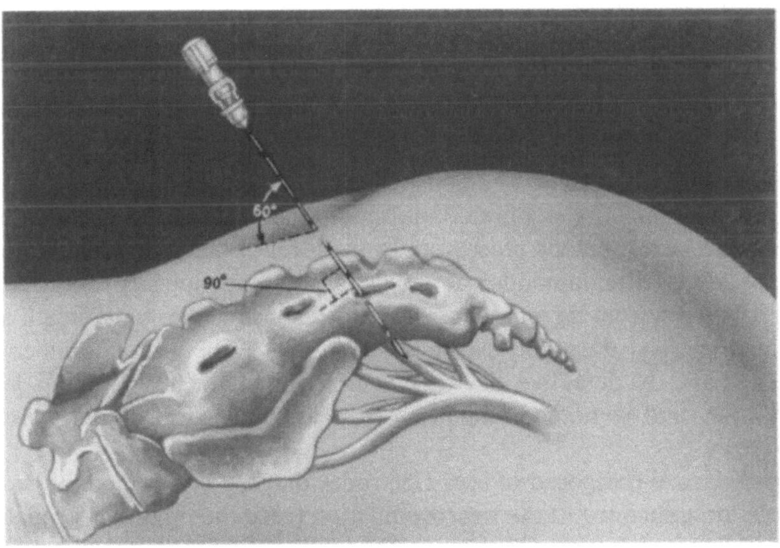

FIGURE 7.4.3. Needle puncture. The needle is inserted parallel to the foraminal axes with an inclination to the skin of 60 to 80 degrees.

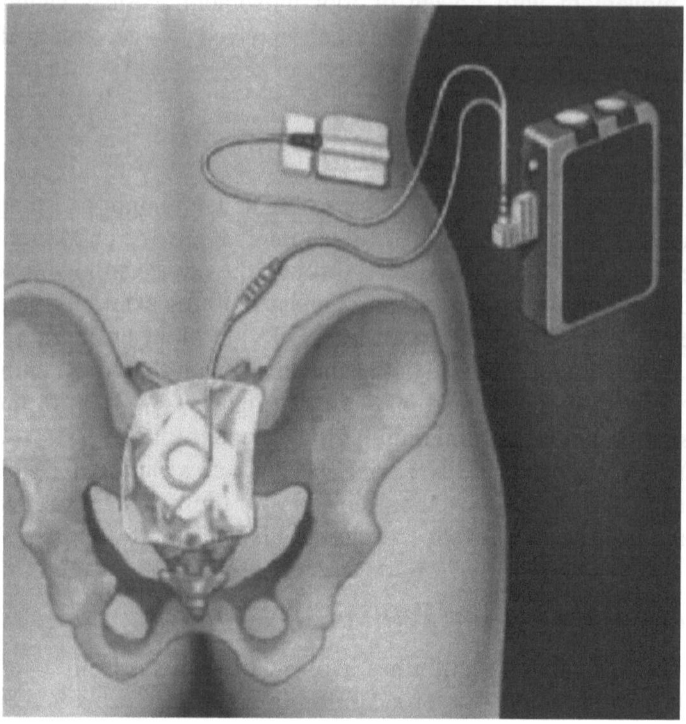

FIGURE 7.4.4. Percutaneous nerve evaluation—chronic phase. A temporary lead is connected to an external stimulator to evaluate the functional responses with regards to continence.

Classical Open Surgical Technique

Before incision, the sacral foramen is checked with an isolated needle. Once the sacral foramen is confirmed, an incision is made along the mid-line above the sacral spinous process up to the level of the underlying lumbo-dorsal fascia. The lumbodorsal fascia is cut longitudinally, about one finger breadth from the mid-line. The paraspinous muscles underneath are divided sharply along the length of their fibers. The sacral foramen is checked and the definitive electrode is inserted (Model 3080, Minneapolis MN, USA) and anchored to the periosteum using non-reabsorbable thread or screws.

Each lead is composed of four electrodes that can be selected individually by programming of the neurostimulator. Once the tip is anchored, the rest of the lead is tunneled through the layer of subcutaneous tissue to a small incision made on the patient's side. The patient is turned on their side and a subcutaneous pocket is prepared in the lower quadrant of the abdomen. An extension is used to connect the electrode to the neurostimulator (Interstim 3023, Minneapolis MN, USA).

The stimulator [implantable pulse generator (IPG)] can be activated the day after surgical implantation using a control unit (Model 7432, Minneapolis MN, USA) that allows all parameters to be set percutaneously via a radiofrequency (RF) signal. Each stimulator is programmed in the most effective way to suit that individual patient. This classical open surgical procedure requires a long operation time (40–70 minutes), and for the IPG abdominal position, some patients complain of displacement or pain at the IPG site postoperatively. A new modality of buttock placement of the IPG was proposed in 2001 to shorten the operating time and to reduce complications (13).

To simplify the technique of implant, a less-invasive surgical approach using a small paramedian incision was proposed by Mamo. Here, fluoroscopy is used to localize the sacral foramen and the insulated needle used for the PNE test, and a 14-gauge angiocath is used to direct the permanent lead into the selected sacral foramen without dissection. The lead then is anchored to the lumbodorsal fascia (superficial to the sacral periosteum) using a moveable lead anchor system (14).

Minimally Invasive Technique

A new tined lead, required for percutaneous implant, is available. After insertion of the needle in the selected sacral foramen and testing for nerve responses, a metal stylet (directional guide) is inserted through the needle. The needle is removed and two small incisions are made on either side of the guide with two dilators inserted along the directional guide and advanced into the sacral foramen. Leaving the introducer sheath in place, the chronic tined lead is inserted and advanced under fluoroscopic control (Figure 7.4.5). Once the responses of the various electrodes are confirmed, the introducer sheath is removed, thereby deploying the tines and anchoring the lead (15).

Finally, the classical one-stage permanent implant could be replaced by a two-stage procedure. Once the permanent lead is implanted, a percutaneous extension is used to connect it to a temporary external stimulator (Figure 7.4.6), allowing a long period of evaluation (1–2 months) of the effectiveness of sacral neuromodulation. If the response is confirmed, the percutaneous extension will be replaced by an implantable extension and connected to the IPG. Following the introduction of the minimally invasive technique, the two-stage modality recently has been proposed as an alternative to the PNE itself.

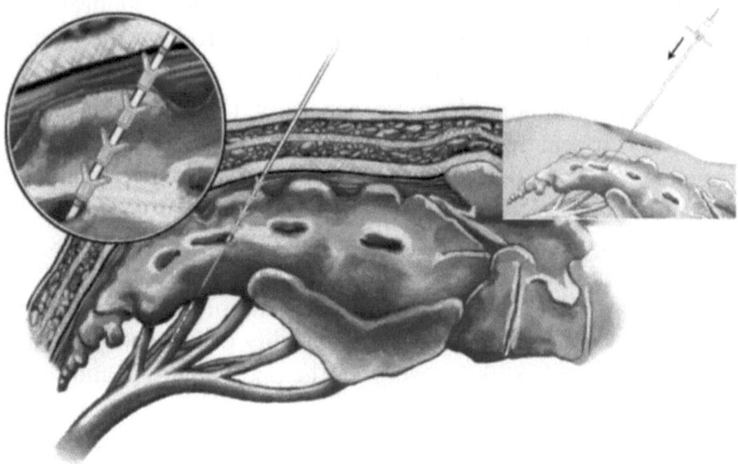

FIGURE 7.4.5. Minimally invasive implant procedure. Under local anesthesia, the permanent lead is inserted using an introducer sheath on the guide of a foramen needle (right panel). While holding the lead in place, the introducer sheath is removed, which deploys the tines and anchors the lead in place (left panel).

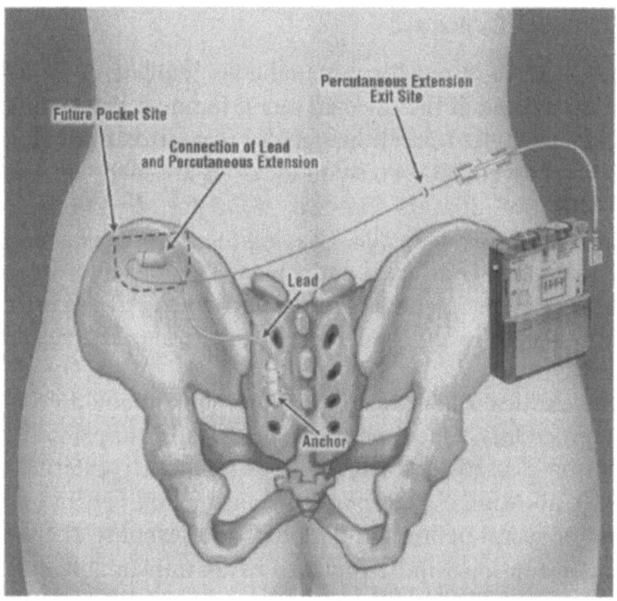

FIGURE 7.4.6. Two-stage procedure. In the first stage, the permanent lead is connected through a percutaneous extension to a temporary external stimulator. This allows a long evaluation period (1–2 months). If the response is confirmed, the percutaneous extension will be replaced in the second stage by an implantable extension and connected to the IPG.

Indications and Patient Evaluation

The lack of knowledge of the mechanism of action of neurostimulation makes it difficult to give precise indications for potentially eligible patients. Two recommendations are proposed; namely, clinical and anatomical.

It is a shared belief that the indication for neuromodulation is severe incontinence not amenable to standard drugs or biofeedback therapy or failed conventional surgical management. Incontinence to solid or liquid feces at least once a week during the last two months, as reflected in a defecation diary kept by the patient, is a good practical guide. Patients with only gas incontinence or minor staining are not good candidates for this procedure at this time. If the type of incontinence is considered, patients with urge incontinence—fecal loss at the first signs of the urge to defecate—show a better improvement when compared with passively incontinent patients (inadvertent and unpredictable fecal loss) (16).

Among anatomical considerations, both the sphincteric muscular integrity and the integrity of the nervous supply must be considered. As regards the muscular integrity, these patients can still be included if they have small defects so limited that they could not be considered as a potential cause of incontinence, as can patients with persistent severe incontinence after failed sphincter repair (17). Patients with complete spinal cord lesions or peripheral nervous lesions such as spina bifida or iatrogenic nerve lesions generally are not candidates for sacral neuromodulation (16,17).

Initial assessment includes a complete clinical history and physical examination. Before applying the stimulator, patients undergo anorectal physiological evaluation and an anal ultrasound to exclude sphincteric lesions. This evaluation includes rectoanal manovolumetry (16) and pudendal nerve terminal motor latency (PNTML) measurements. Rectoanal manovolumetric evaluation includes the sphincter parameters of maximum resting pressure and maximum squeeze pressure, rectoanal inhibitory reflex (RAIR) threshold, urge to defecate expressed as volume and distension pressure, maximum rectal volume at one minute of distention with 40 centimeters of H_2O, the contraction rectal response to a rapid distension of 30 centimeters of H_2O, and rectal compliance (Δ volume/Δ pressure). Manometric evaluation is performed before stimulation, during the acute stimulation phase, and on the last day of PNE testing. It is repeated again at one- and four-month follow-up visits in patients with permanent implants; however, anal manometry is not a specific examination for the selection of eligible patients, although it may help in better understanding the mechanisms of sacral stimulation.

In contrast, PNTML evaluation is a useful parameter, where an immeasurable latency is a sign of a complete peripheral nervous lesion and represents a relative contraindication to sacral neuromodulation. To establish baseline function, patients complete a 14-day fecal incontinence diary of episodes of fecal incontinence and bowel movements prior to PNE. The same diary is used during the PNE and in the two weeks following PNE. The evaluation of the clinical diary is the only parameter that currently allows selection of patients for a definitive implant. Usually, a PNE test is considered positive if there is a complete cessation or reduction of more than 50% to 80% in leakage episodes for liquid or solid stool during the test period and a rapid return to pre-PNE conditions when stimulation is turned off. After permanent sacral implant, patients are evaluated for functional disorders with clinical examination and anorectal manometry. Additionally, all patients complete a 14-day continence diary prior to each scheduled follow-up visit at three and six months after implant, and then every 6 months thereafter.

Clinical Trial Results

In 1995, at a follow-up of six months, Matzel and colleagues (9) reported a complete recovery of continence in two cases, soiling in one patient with definitive implant of a sacral electrode and an improvement of resting and squeezing anal pressure. In July 2000, Malouf et al. (18) reported an improvement in the Wexner incontinence scale from 16 to 20 to three to six in five patients followed for at least 16 months after definitive implant of a sacral electrode. The resting anal tone showed consistent improvement, but no variation was observed in the squeeze anal pressure. In September 2001, Rosen et al. (19) published the results of 16 permanent implants selected out of 20 (80%) incontinent patients tested over a period of 10 to 14 days with PNE. Three patients had their electrodes removed because of infection. The remaining 13 (81.2%) had functioning implants with a significant improvement in fecal continence. Resting and squeeze anal pressures improved significantly only in patients with neurologic incontinence, but not in those with idiopathic incontinence. For the first time, a dedicated Quality of Life questionnaire was used, showing clear improvement in all four items investigated—lifestyle, coping behavior, depression, and embarrassment.

In our experience (16) with five patients implanted out of 23 PNE tests (22%), definitive electrical stimulation of sacral roots was associated with an improvement in fecal continence from a mean of 4.8 episodes per week to a complete cessation at a median follow-up of 19.2 months (range 5 to 37). A significant increase of the resting anal pressure, but not squeeze anal pressure, was observed, and an earlier rectal sensation to balloon distension was recorded in this first series of patients. Using isobaric rectal distension, the pressure applied for the first sensation threshold decreased significantly ($p = 0.012$), as did the pressure for the urge threshold ($p = 0.008$). The distension pressure decrease for the first sensation and urge threshold is considered important because it indicates a better sensibility or a facilitation of the rectal receptors.

In the same year, Anne-Marie Leroi (20) reported the results of SNM in six patients simultaneously affected by fecal and urinary incontinence. All these patients improved their urinary and fecal symptoms significantly, but no changes were documented in resting and squeeze anal pressures. On the contrary, the volume required to induce early and urge rectal sensation was significantly lower than before SNM. In 2001, the first report of the multicentric Italian experience of GINS (Italian group for sacral neuromodulation) (21) showed results of SNM in 16 incontinent patients after a mean follow-up of 15.5 (range 3–45) months. Fecal incontinence improved significantly in all patients, and the number of incontinence accidents for liquid or solid stool in 14 days decreased from 11.5 ± 4.8 (range 2–20) pre-implant to 0.6 ± 0.9 (range 0–2) at the last follow-up. Resting anal pressure, but not squeeze pressure, increased significantly after SNM. The rectal volume for the urge threshold decreased significantly ($p = 0.04$) with chronic sacral stimulation. Eleven of these patients also suffered from urinary dysfunction (incontinence or retention), and all had a marked improvement of their urinary symptoms.

The first medium-term results of SNM for fecal incontinence have been published by Kenefick and colleagues (22) in July 2002, reporting good results in 15 incontinent patients followed up for a mean of 24 months, with 11 patients becoming fully continent. Episodes of fecal incontinence decreased from 11 (2–30) per week before stimulation to 0 (0–4) per week after permanent stimulation ($P < 0.001$). Urgency and ability to defer defecation improved in all patients. Resting and squeeze anal pressures significantly increased and the volume required for rectal sensitivity to initial distension was significantly lower ($P < 0.05$) than before SNM. There were no major complications. In this group of patients, the quality of life questionnaire [36-item Short Form Healthy Survey (SF36)] was performed before and after stimulation, where “social function” and “role—physical” subscales of the SF36 improved significantly.

Medium-term results of a substantial series were presented by the GINS (23) group in the spring of 2002. Thirty-one patients had a permanent implant out of 116 (27%) PNE tests, and PNE results were reproduced in all patients at a mean follow-up of 25.6 (range 1–56) months. The mean number of incontinence episodes for solid or liquid stools (per 14 days) decreased from 15 (range 2–22) at baseline to 3.2 (range 0–10) at three months follow-up ($p = 0.02$), to 2.9 (range 0–13) at six months, and to 0.3 (range 0–4) at 12 months follow-up. Again, anorectal manometry shows a positive trend in increasing sphincter pressure and rectal sensitivity. With regard to adverse events, one patient complained of pain at the implant site when the IPG case was used as an anode (unipolar impulse), and another necessitated electrode repositioning for displacement after three months. In one patient, interruption of the electrode caused decreased effectiveness at 11 months post implant, where the lead was changed and the patient recovered continence. No local sepsis occurred. The SF36 was used in 18 of these patients before and after SNM. Improvement of continence had a positive impact on the health state, particularly in the reduction of physical limitations or disabilities. An overall analysis showed a significant improvement in patients' physical ($p < 0.05$) and mental health ($p < 0.05$) following implant.

An update of the experiences of the various groups confirmed a substantial improvement of continence with SNM. In October 2002, Leroi (24) reported a significant improvement of continence—episodes of fecal incontinence, urgent need to defecate, and delay to postpone defecation—in 12 implanted patients. Nevertheless, two patients did not have the same results as during temporary stimulation. One patient necessitated electrode reimplantation for lead displacement, and afterwards the patient complained of pain at the electrode site, which necessitated removal of the stimulator. Two patients were explanted, one for pain and one for severe infection, resulting in removal of the stimulator in 25% of cases.

Long-term results have been reported recently by Matzel et al. (25), and functional improvement was achieved in 94% of 16 patients. At a median follow-up of 32.5 months (3–99), treatment was successful in 81% of cases. Two of the electrodes were removed after five and 45 months, respectively, for intractable pain. The mean squeeze pressure increased, but maximum squeeze pressures improved in only three patients. Resting pressure, perception, urge threshold, and maximum tolerable volume were not significantly changed. Using the disease-specific quality of life instrument (FIQL-ASCRS) before and during stimulation, the quality of life index was improved in all cases.

In our experience, the results of the PNE test has been reproduced in all 14 patients we have implanted. With a follow-up of 32.2 months (2–84), treatment was effective in 84.6% of cases. Two patients have been explanted after 11 and 24 months, respectively. In the first patient, an electrode displacement occurred as a consequence of sacral trauma, and after reimplantation, the positive effects of SNM were not reproduced, whereas in the second patient, the stimulator was removed for loss of effectiveness despite the device functioning normally.

Proposed Mechanism of Action

Debate as to the mechanism of action for sacral stimulation in patients with fecal incontinence is still ongoing. Action on the striated sphincters and a facilitation of voluntary contraction have been suggested and attributed to direct alpha motor fiber stimulation (10). Several studies have tried to show an improvement of the EAS during neuromodulation, but results are controversial. However, according to observations by Fowler et al. (26), studies on the latencies of the pelvic floor contraction during peripheral nerve evaluation showed that the muscle response is reflexively mediated, with a minimum latency ranging from 50 to 57 milliseconds instead of the four to five milliseconds observed with sacral root magnetic depolarization (11).

The trend towards an improvement in rectal sensitivity with a reduction in the threshold of perception of rectal distension is of particular interest, and an effect at the level of the central nervous system by afferent stimulation has been hypothesized. Vaizey et al. (11) recorded rectal and anal pressures in one patient for several hours before and during neuromodulation. The baseline spontaneous contractile rectal activity and inappropriate relaxations of the internal anal sphincter (IAS) recorded disappeared during neuromodulation. The IAS relaxations were replaced by a spontaneous activity of ultra-slow waves.

The contractile response of the ampulla recti evoked with rapid rectal distension at a pressure of 30 centimeters of H_2O (manovolumetrically measured) decreases during SNM (16). This rectal reflex motor activity is smaller if compared with the sigmoid contractions observed during balloon sigmoid distension. This rectal response is considered characteristic of a reservoir organ and is believed to be mediated by an inhibitory spinal reflex (27), where a reduction in activity could be an inhibiting mechanism. These observations imply a special effect on afferent fiber stimulation and medulla synaptic integrity, both for the sensitive and rectal (or sphincteric) motility during chronic sacral neuromodulation, and confirm the canine animal experiments of Tanagho and Schmidt (28), in which stimulation of the intact dorsal component (afferent) of S2 produced responses in the bladder and the anal sphincter that were similar to those induced by stimulation of the intact nerve.

Three types of fibers generally are recognized in the sensory subclass of nerve fibers: A-beta fibers (the largest fibers, mediating the sensations of touch and mild pressure, as well as the sensation of position of joints and vibration), A-delta fibers (smaller than A-beta fibers mediating the sensation of cold and the first components of the sensation of pain), and C-fibers (the slowest and smallest fibers mediating the sensation of warmth and the main component of the sensation of pain). In addition, C fibers subserve most of the autonomic peripheral nerve functions. Some experimental animal studies seem to confirm the hypothesis that neuromodulation has an effect on the central nervous system via afferent sensory fibers. A double-blind randomized study with spinally transected rats has evaluated the role of neuromodulation on C-afferent fibers that form the afferent arc of the pathological reflex responsible for bladder hyperreflexia after spinal cord trauma. T10 spinal transection results in bladder hyperreflexia after three weeks and is associated with an increase in the neuropeptide content—substance P, neurokinin A, and calcitonin gene-related peptide (CGRP)—in L6 dorsal root ganglia. The electric stimulation of S1 reduces the increase in neuropeptide concentration at L6 and abolishes bladder hyperreflexia, suggesting that the blockade of C-afferent fibers is one of the mechanisms of action of sacral neuromodulation (29).

Recently, Chan et al. (30) have shown an increase of nerve fibers immunoreactive to vanilloid receptor subtype 1 (VR1) in the mucosal, submucosal, and muscle layers of patients with rectal hypersensitivity and fecal urgency. The VR1, present in A-delta and C-fibers and postsynaptic sites within the spinal cord dorsal horn, is known as an integrator of noxious stimuli. Vanilloid receptor subtype 1 is activated by heat, protons, and capsaicin—an alkaloid extractable from red pepper—and induces a flow of cations, especially Ca+ and Na+). Intravenous injection of capsaicin has produced dose-dependent sensations in the rectum of healthy people, indicating a high density of functional VR1 in this organ (31). An increased density of VR1 fibers could lead to hyperexcitability of the dorsal spinal cord, which results in a deregulation of the sacral reflexes. These efferent reflexes include neurogenic inflammation and an increase in the sympathetic tone resulting in vasospasm and reflexive striated muscular spasticity (32). Further work on local neuromodulators that are likely to reflexively stimulate the anorectal sphincter is now required.

In our experience, only patients with urge incontinence showed benefit from sacral neurostimulation (16). Although animal experiments are not directly applicable, if an increase of VR1 receptors is at the heart of urge incontinence, the effect of SNM in humans could be attributed to the inhibition of C-fibers. An interesting contribution to the comprehension of the mechanism of action of the SNM comes from Hamdy and colleagues (33), who showed that anal sphincter contraction induced by magnetic cortical stimulation was facilitated when this stimulation was preceded by repetitive stimulation of the pudendal or sacral nerve, suggesting that repetitive stimulation of a sacral nerve could cause sensory–motor interactions with better control of sphincter function.

Conclusions

Sacral neuromodulation represents a promising therapy for patients with fecal incontinence. Overall, the published series demonstrate a high effectiveness, with a median of 90.8% success rates with minimal morbidity. The possibility of selecting patients on the basis of a preliminary peripheral nerve evaluation allows sacral neuromodulation a unique place in the spectrum of possible treatments for patients with fecal incontinence. The mechanism of action appears complex, with alterations in neuromodulatory reflex arcs and local neuropeptide expression. An improved understanding of these mechanisms will permit classification of the indications for this technique, which is likely to result in greater success.

References

1. Bradley WE, Timm GW, and Chou SN. A decade of experience with electronic stimulation of the micturition reflex. Urol Int. 1971;26:283–302.

2. Held T, Agrawal G, and Kantrowitz A. Studies in stimulation of the bladder and its motor nerves. Surgery. 1966;60:848–56.
3. Jonas U, Jones LW, and Tanagho EA. Spinal cord versus detrusor stimulation. A comparative study in six acute dogs. Invest Urol. 1975;13:171–4.
4. Ingersoll EH, Jones LL, and Hegre ES. Effect on urinary bladder of unilateral stimulation of pelvic nerves in the dog. Amer J Physiol. 1957;189:167–71.
5. Holmquist B. Electromicturition by pelvic nerve stimulation in dogs. Scand J Urol Nephrol. 1968;2 (suppl):1–27.
6. Heine JP, Schmidt RA, and Tanagho EA. Intraspinal sacral root stimulation for controlled micturition. Invest Urol. 1977;15(1):78–82.
7. Schmidt RA, Bruschini H, and Tanagho EA. Urinary bladder and sphincter responses to stimulation of dorsal and ventral sacral roots. Invest Urol. 1979; 16:300–4.
8. Tanagho EA AND Schmidt RA. Bladder pacemaker: Scientific basis and clinical future. Urology. 1982;20:614–19.
9. Matzel KE, Stadelmaier U, Hohenfellner M, and Gall FP. Electrical stimulation of sacral spinal nerves for treatment of faecal incontinence. Lancet. 1995; 346:1124–7.
10. Matzel KE. Sacral neurostimulation: principles and its role in the treatment of feacal incontinence. Proceeding of the 6th Biennial International Meeting of Coloproctology, 2000 Apr; 101–3.
11. Vaizey CJ, Kamm MA, Turner IC, Nicholls RJ, and Woloszko J. Effects of short-term sacral nerve stimulation on anal and rectal function in patients with anal incontinence. Gut. 1999;44:407–12.
12. Shaker H, Wang Y, Loung D, Balbaa L, Fehlings MG, and Hassouna MM. Role of C-afferent fibres in the mechanism of action of sacral nerve root neuromodulation in chronic spinal cord injury. BJU Int. 2000;85(7):905–10.
13. Scheepens WA, Weil EH, van Koeveringe GA, Rohrmann D, Hedlund HE, Schurch B, Ostardo E, Pastorello M, Ratto C, Nordling J, and van Kerrebroeck PE. Buttock placement of the implantable pulse generator: a new implantation technique for sacral neuromodulation—a multicenter study. Eur Urol. 2001; 40(4):434–8.
14. Chai TC and Mamo GJ. Modified techniques of S3 foramen localization and lead implantation in S3 neuromodulation. Urology. 2001;58(5):786–90.
15. Spinelli M, Giardiello G, Arduini A, and van den Hombergh U. New percutaneous technique of sacral nerve stimulation has high initial success rate: preliminary results. Eur Urol. 2003;43(1):70–4.
16. Ganio E, Luc AR, Clerico G, and Trompetto M. Sacral nerve stimulation for treatment of fecal incontinence: a novel approach for intractable fecal incontinence. Dis Colon Rectum. 2001;44(5):619–29.
17. Michot F, Leroi AM, Grise P, and Denis P. Effect of sacral nerve stimulation on pelvic floor function in patients with faecal incontinence. Acts from 6th Biennial Course—International Meeting of Coloproctology" Saint Vincent 5–7/4/2000. p. 135–7.
18. Malouf AJ, Vaizey CJ, Nicholls RJ, and Kamm MA. Permanent sacral nerve stimulation for fecal incontinence. Ann Surg. 2000;232:143–8.
19. Rosen HR, Urbarz C, Holzer B, Novi G, and Schiessel R. Sacral nerve stimulation as a treatment for fecal incontinence. Gastroenterology. 2001;121:536–41.
20. Leroi AM, Michot F, Grise P, and Denis P. Effect of sacral nerve stimulation in patients with fecal and urinary incontinence. Dis Colon Rectum. 2001;44:779–89.

21. Ganio E, Ratto C, Masin A, Luc AR, Doglietto GB, Dodi G, Ripetti V, Arullani A, Frascio M, BertiRiboli E, Landolfi V, Del Genio A, Altomare DF, Memeo V, Bertapelle P, Carone R, Spinelli M, Zanollo A, Spreafico L, Giardiello G, and de Seta F. Neuromodulation for fecal incontinence: outcome in 16 patients with definitive implant. The initial Italian Sacral Neurostimulation Group (GINS) experience. Dis Colon Rectum. 2001;44:965–70.
22. Kenefick NJ, Vaizey CJ, Cohen RC, Nicholls RJ, and Kamm MA. Medium-term results of permanent sacral nerve stimulation for faecal incontinence. Br J Surg. 2002;89:896–901.
23. Ganio E, Realis LA, Ratto C, Doglietto GB, Masin A, Dodi G, Altomare DF, Memeo V, Ripetti V, Arullani A, Falletto E, Gaetini A, Scarpino O, Saba V, Infantino A, La Manna S, Ferulano, and Villani R. Sacral Nerve Modulation for fecal incontinence. Functional results and assessment of the Quality of Life. Acts from 13th Annual Colorectal Disease; 2002 Feb 14–16; Fort Lauderdale, Florida.
24. Leroi AM. Sacral Nerve Modulation for fecal incontinence. Running clinical studies update. Acts from 7th Biennal Course—International Meeting of coloproctology" Saint Vincent; 2002 Sept.
25. Matzel KE, Bittorf B, Stadelmaier U, and Hohenberger W. Sacral nerve stimulation in the treatment of faecal incontinence. Chirurg. 2003;74(1):26–32.
26. Fowler CJ, Swinn MJ, Goodwin RJ, Oliver S, and Craggs M. Studies of the latency of pelvic floor contraction during peripheral nerve evaluation show the muscle response is reflexly mediated. J Urol. 2000;163(3):881–3.
27. Åkerval S, Fasth S, Nordgres S, Òlresland T, and Hultén L. Manovolumetry: a new method for investigation of anorectal function. Gut. 1988;29:614–23.
28. Tanagho EA and Schmidt RA. Electrical stimulation in the clinical management of the neurogenic bladder. J Urol. 1988;140:1331–9.
29. Chan CLH, Facer P, Davis JB, Smith GD, Egerton J, Bountra C, Williams NS, and Anand P. Sensory fibres expressing capsaicin receptor TRPV1 in patients with rectal hypersensitivity and faecal urgency. The Lancet. 2003;361:385–91.
30. Shaker H, Wang Y, Loung D, Balbaa L, Fehlings MG, and Hassouna MM. Role of C-afferent fibres in the mechanism of action of sacral nerve root neuromodulation in chronic spinal cord injury. BJU Int. 2000;85(7):905–10.
31. Winning AJ, Hamilton RD, Shea SA, and Guz A. Respiratory and cardiovascular effects of central and peripheral intravenous injections of capsaicin in man: evidence for pulmonary chemosensitivity. Clin Sci (Lond). 1986;71:519–26.
32. Black PH. Stress and the inflammatory response: A review of neurogenic inflammation. Brain Behav Immun. 2002;16(6):622–53.
33. Hamdy S, Enck P, Aziz Q, Rothwell JC, Uengoergil S, Hobson A, and Thompson D. Spinal and pudendal nerve modulation of human corticoanal motor pathways. Am J Physiol. 1998;G419–23.

Editorial Commentary

Since the first report in 1982 showing that spinal stimulation effectively treated two constipated patients by increasing large bowel peristalsis and decreasing intestinal transit times, the technique of neuromodulation (NM) has become more sophisticated and permitted successful managent of various pelvic floor and colonic motility dysfunctions, among them fecal incontinence. Sacral NM achieves a success rate of 85% in patients treated by Dr. Ganio's group and followed up for a median of 32 months. Such outcomes compare favorably with all the other techniques currently used to manage fecal incontinence providing a better selection of patients by the utlization of temporary stimulation protocols. The undoubted high cost seems adequately balanced by this high success rate, even if at the present time long-term results are still lacking. According to the author, the presence of anatomically interrupted anal sphincters is a contraindication to sacral NM. Nevertheless 25% of patients "cured" with sacral NM, in recently published small series, had some degree of demonstrable sphincter division prior to treatment. The procedure is minimally invasive, may be carried out under local anesthesia and is much less traumatic when compared with other techniques such as graciloplasty or the artificial bowel sphincter; both of which may require a temporary diverting stoma. Moreover sacral NM appears relatively effective in cases of pudendal neuropathy; a finding which may negate the utilization of external anal sphincteroplasty.

MP

Chapter 8
Urogynecological Assessment and Perspective in Patients Presenting with Evacuatory Dysfunction

Jennifer T. Pollak and G. Willy Davila

Background

Enteroceles and rectoceles represent a herniation of the rectum or upper posterior vaginal wall and its underlying intraperitoneal contents into the vaginal canal resulting in a vaginal bulge. Women typically complain of perineal and vaginal pressure, obstructive defecation, or constipation, and many splint or digitally reduce the vagina in order to effectuate a bowel movement. These anatomic defects arise from either a tear or stretching of the rectovaginal fascia analogous to an abdominal wall ventral hernia. Although anatomic cure rates are high, there are conflicting reports with regard to functional outcome, postoperative defecatory symptoms, and sexual dysfunction, including dyspareunia. Marked differences exist between management approaches followed by urogynecologists and colorectal surgeons. This chapter should be read in conjunction with Chapter 6.3 concerning rectocele/enterocele pathogenesis and management. A gynecologist's perspective of evacuatory dysfunction and the standard nature of gynecological assessment of these patients is highlighted here.

Introduction

With the growth of the sub-specialty of urogynecology and its related research, a growing number of clinicians are recognizing the concept of the female pelvic floor. The pelvic floor is a single functional unit composed of three compartments. The anterior compartment consists of the bladder and urethra, the middle compartment consists of the vagina and uterus, and the posterior compartment is comprised of the rectum and anus. Traditionally, dysfunction of the different compartments is cared for by different clinicians, and thus, coexistent problems of the other organs often go unrecognized. In addition, dysfunction in one compartment may be managed very differently by those specialists who care for that specific compartment. This lack of consensus is exemplified in the management of rectovaginal septum weakness by gynecologists and colorectal surgeons.

The coexistence of pelvic floor dysfunction in a single patient is extremely common. In a questionnaire study, 53% of patients with fecal incontinence also had urinary incontinence and 18% of them had genital prolapse (1). In the same study, 66% of patients with rectal prolapse had urinary incontinence and 34% had genital prolapse. In another series, 31% of women surveyed with urinary incontinence also had fecal incontinence and 7% of women with genital prolapse had fecal incontinence (2). In a large series of over 800 women with urinary incontinence and/or genital prolapse, 20% of patients had anal incontinence (3).

Both gynecologists and colorectal surgeons treat rectoceles and enteroceles, and rectocele repair represents one of the most commonly performed gynecologic pelvic reconstructive procedures in women. In fact, 100% of gynecologists surveyed manage rectoceles, whereas 68% of colorectal surgeons manage this disorder (4–6). Gynecologic surgeons frequently perform rectocele repairs as isolated procedures or in conjunction with other reconstructive procedures. The restoration of normal anatomy to the posterior vaginal wall is referred to as an enterocele repair if it involves a peritoneal bulge into the upper posterior vaginal wall. If the lower wall is involved, it is termed a posterior repair or posterior colporrhaphy. Although sometimes used interchangeably with the term rectocele repair, these two operations may have varying treatment goals. A rectocele repair focuses on correcting a hernia of the anterior rectal wall into the vaginal canal secondary to a weakened or torn rectovaginal septum, whereas a posterior colporrhaphy corrects a rectal bulge and normalizes vaginal caliber by restoring structural integrity to the posterior vaginal wall and introitus.

Unlike other reconstructive procedures, such as surgery to treat urinary stress incontinence, the gynecologic preoperative evaluation of a symptomatic posterior vaginal bulge typically includes only a history and physical examination. Gynecologists generally have not adopted the performance of defecography or other evaluation techniques for the evaluation of this anatomic defect. While 80% of colorectal surgeons use defecography, only 6% of surveyed gynecologists use this investigation (4–6). In addition, differentiation between enterocele and rectocele components of posterior vaginal wall prolapse typically is performed on a clinical and intraoperative basis. It is unclear at this time whether surgical therapy outcomes are impacted negatively by the lack of preoperative evaluation beyond this history and physical examination. By far, gynecologists consider repair of the rectocele a commonly necessary procedure with low morbidity for their patients.

This chapter will cover various aspects of the gynecologic approach to rectocele and enterocele repair, including physical examination and anatomy, symptoms, indications for repair, surgical techniques, and treatment outcomes.

Physical Examination

The typical physical finding in a woman with a symptomatic enterocele or rectocele is a lower posterior vaginal wall bulge. An enterocele is identified as a bulge of the superior posterior vaginal wall between the vaginal apex and the levator plate. It may extend superiorly to weaken the support of the vaginal apex, leading to vaginal vault prolapse. In an isolated rectocele, the bulge extends from the edge of the levator plate to the perineal body (Figure 8.1). As a rectocele enlarges, the perineal body may distend further and loose its bulk, leading to an evident perineocele. Enteroceles and rectoceles frequently coexist. The physical examination should include not only a vaginal examination, but also a rectal examination, as a perineocele may not be evident on vaginal examination. At times, it can be identified only upon digital rectal examination, where an absence of fibromuscular tissue in the perineal body is confirmed.

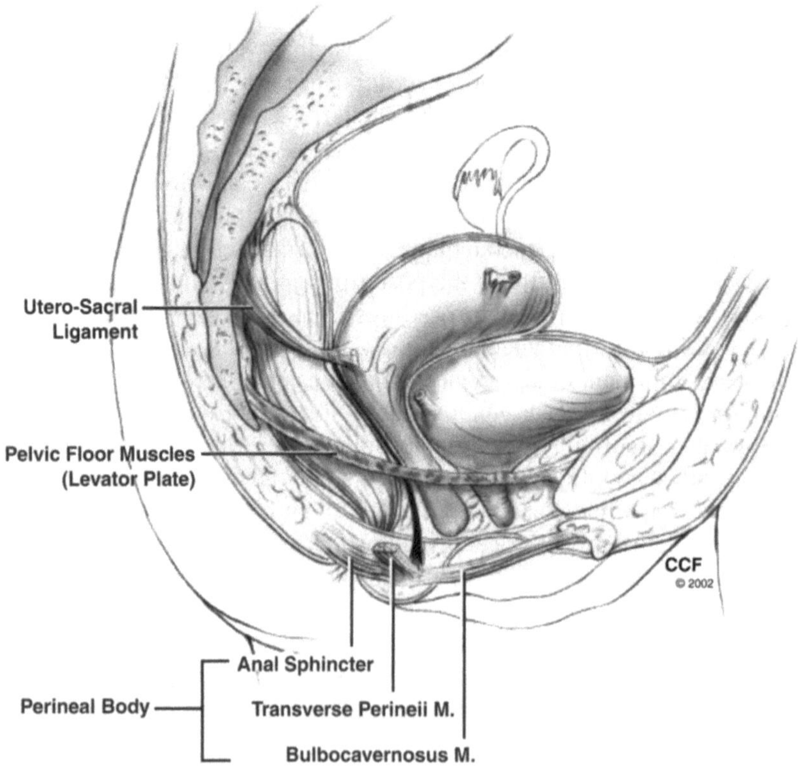

FIGURE 8.1. Lateral view of pelvis. Rectoceles typically develop between the levator plate and the perineal body due to weakness of the rectovaginal septum endopelvic fascia.

Various classification schemes describe enterocele and rectocele severity. In the traditional Baden–Walker system, which uses the mid-vaginal plane as a landmark, anatomic defects are graded from 0 to 4. Grade 0 is normal, whereas a grade 4 extends beyond the hymen. In the pelvic organ prolapse quantification (POPQ) system, two points along the posterior vaginal wall are identified (Ap, 3 cm proximal to the hymen; Bp, the most dependent part) and their distances from the hymenal ring are measured in centimeters with maximum Valsalva effort. In the POPQ system, discrete points and their displacement are measured rather than the underlying prolapsing organ. The more traditional approach has a surgical focus, whereas the newer POPQ simply identifies specific vaginal site prolapse (7).

Additional factors that should be evaluated during the physical examination include associated pelvic support defects such as vaginal vault prolapse or cystocele, pelvic neuromuscular function, and vaginal mucosal thickness and estrogenation. All pelvic floor anatomic defects should be repaired during a reconstructive surgical procedure because untreated small anatomical defects of the anterior and apical vagina may enlarge after repair of the posterior vaginal wall. Thus, preoperative identification of specific individual defects is crucial. Levator contraction strength and tone are important factors in enhancing the long-term success rate of pelvic reconstructive surgery. Regular Kegel exercises should be recommended following pelvic reconstructive procedures. Biofeedback therapy may be necessary to instruct patients how to adequately isolate and contract their pelvic floor muscles. Poorly estrogenized thin vaginal mucosa should be treated with local estrogen prior to surgical therapy.

Anatomy

Enterocele and rectocele result from defects in the integrity of the posterior vaginal wall and rectovaginal septum and herniation of the posterior wall into the vaginal lumen through these defects. The normal posterior vagina is lined by squamous epithelium that overlies the lamina propria, a layer of loose connective tissue. A fibromuscular layer of tissue composed of smooth muscle, collagen, and elastin underlies this lamina propria and is referred to as the rectovaginal fascia. This is an extension of the endopelvic fascia that surrounds and supports the pelvic organs and contains blood vessels, lymphatics, and nerves that supply and innervate the pelvic organs.

Denonvilliers originally described a dense tissue layer in men between the bladder and the rectum and named it the rectovesical septum (8). Many clinicians refer to this layer as Denonvilliers' fascia. The layer of tissue between the vagina and the rectum was felt to be analogous to the rectovesical septum and became known as Denonvilliers' fascia in the female, or the rectovaginal septum (8). Others described the rectovaginal septum, or rectovaginal fascia, as a support mechanism of the pelvic organs, and they were successful in identifying this layer during surgical and autopsy dissections (8–11).

The normal vagina is stabilized and supported at three levels. Superiorly, the vaginal apical endopelvic fascia is attached to the cardinal uterosacral ligament complex (Level I). Laterally, the endopelvic fascia is connected to the arcus tendineus fasciae pelvis (Level II), with the lateral posterior vagina attaching to the fascia overlying the levator ani muscles. Inferiorly, the lower posterior vagina connects to the perineal body (Level III) (12). The cervix—or vaginal cuff in the hysterectomized woman—is considered to be the superior attachment site or "central tendon," and the perineal body the inferior attachment site or "central tendon." The endopelvic fascia extends between these two "tendons," comprising the rectovaginal septum (Figure 8.2). An enterocele or rectocele results from a stretching or actual separation or tear of the rectovaginal fascia, leading to a bulging of the posterior vaginal wall noted on examination during a Valsalva maneuver. Trauma from vaginal childbirth commonly leads to transverse defects above the usual location of the connection to the perineal body (Figure 8.3) (8,13). In addition, patients may present with lateral, midline, or high transverse fascial defects. Separation of the rectovaginal septum fascia from the vaginal apex results in the development of an enterocele as a hernia sac without fascial lining and filled with intraperitoneal contents (Figure 8.4).

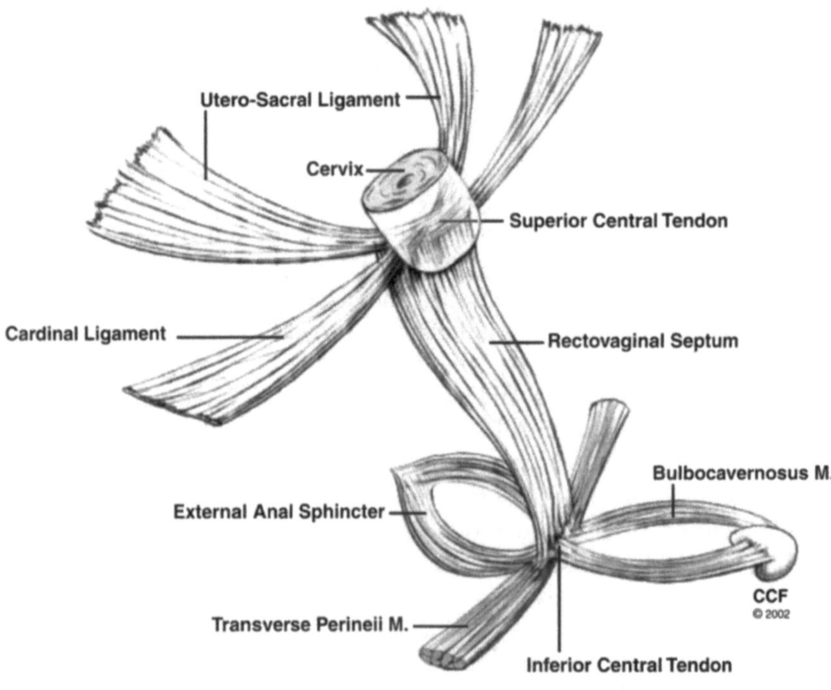

FIGURE 8.2. Diagrammatic representation of the rectovaginal septum including its attachment to a "superior tendon" and an "inferior tendon."

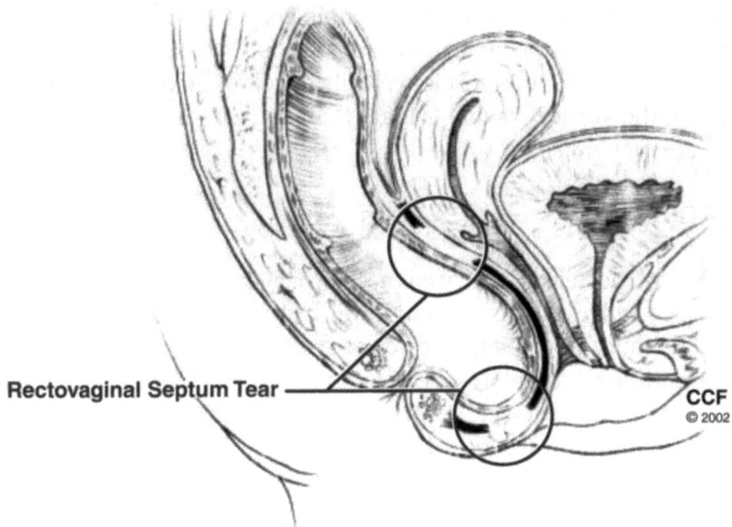

FIGURE 8.3. Fascial tears of the rectovaginal septum can occur superiorly or inferiorly at sites of attachment to a central tendon.

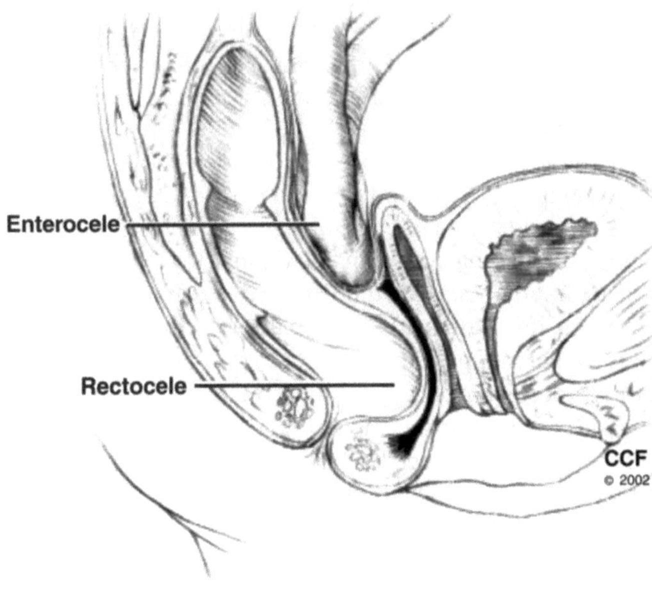

FIGURE 8.4. Enteroceles can develop from weakness of the rectovaginal septum along its cephalad portion, whereas rectoceles develop from weakness along its inferior portion.

The levator plate extends from the pubic bone to the sacrum/coccyx and provides support for the change in vaginal axis from vertical to horizontal along the mid vagina. A rectocele typically develops at, or below, the levator plate along the vertical vagina (Figure 8.1).

Symptoms

Symptoms of posterior wall weakness typically result in pelvic/perineal pressure or a bulge with associated lower back pain (enterocele) or a need to digitally reduce or splint the posterior vaginal bulge or perineum in order to either initiate or complete a bowel movement (rectocele). Accumulation of stool within the rectocele reservoir leads to increasing degrees of perineal pressure and obstructive defecation. In the absence of digital reduction, women will note incomplete emptying, which leads to a high degree of frustration and a vicious cycle of increasing pelvic pressure, the need for stronger Valsalva efforts, enlargement of the rectocele bulge, and increasing perineal pressure. Rectal digitation is not commonly self-reported by patients with a symptomatic rectocele unless asked by the physician.

The symptom of constipation is not clearly understood by the practicing gynecologist. Its vague nature, coupled with a poor understanding of the complexity of colonic function, results in a lack of interest on the gynecologists' part to further evaluate the symptom of constipation. Unfortunately, this may result in surgical treatment of abnormal bowel function via a posterior colporrhaphy when conservative therapy for constipation may have otherwise achieved a satisfactory outcome. The persistence of abnormal defecation may be responsible for the high rectocele recurrence rate in some series with this operation (14).

An enlarging enterocele or rectocele will widen the levator hiatus and increase vaginal caliber (15). In addition, women with increasing degrees of prolapse have progressively larger genital hiatuses (16). This may lead to sexual difficulties, including symptoms of vaginal looseness and decreased sensation during intercourse. Whether this is due primarily to the enlargement of the vaginal introitus and levator hiatus or coexistent damage to the pudendal nerve innervating the pelvic floor musculature is unclear. A large enterocele or rectocele may extend beyond the hymenal ring. Once exteriorized, the patient is at risk for vaginal mucosal erosion and ulceration. Hemorrhoids also can be associated with a rectocele (12). They typically occur secondary to increased Valsalva efforts by the patient in order to effectuate a bowel movement.

Surgery to Correct an Enterocele

The goals of surgery to repair an enterocele include correction of a superior posterior vaginal wall bulge and restoration of fascial integrity to the entire posterior vaginal wall. Surgery for enterocele often is approached vaginally, but also may be performed abdominally. The choice of approach depends on concomitant pathology or additional types of pelvic organ prolapse that require repair, as well as the surgeon's preference. No reports exist in the literature that compare the outcomes between the different types of repairs.

The traditional vaginal enterocele repair requires a midline incision in the posterior vaginal wall from the introitus to the level of the vaginal apex. The enterocele sac is then dissected off the posterior vaginal mucosa, underlying rectovaginal septum, and anterior rectal wall. The enterocele sac is sharply opened and explored to confirm the absence of intraperitoneal contents. If intraperitoneal contents are adherent to the sac, they are sharply dissected free. Nonabsorbable sutures are then placed in a purse-string fashion to close the enterocele sac. Several sutures may be required depending on the size of the sac. The excess peritoneum is then trimmed. Other concomitant repairs may then be performed as clinically indicated, and the posterior vaginal wall is closed as described for rectocele repair (13) (vide infra).

The McCall culdoplasty is another vaginal technique designed to repair enteroceles. This procedure allows for apical support of the vagina and closes the cul-de-sac. Following a vaginal hysterectomy, previously cut uterosacral ligaments are plicated together along with the intervening peritoneum overlying the sigmoid colon and the apical posterior vaginal mucosa. The first suture is placed as high as possible on the uterosacral ligaments, and successive sutures are placed until the cul-de-sac is closed. The number of sutures depends on the size of the enterocele and cul-de-sac. Permanent suture material is used. Reported complications have included ureteral injury, infection, and subsequent vault prolapse (17). If the patient had a previous hysterectomy, extra care must be taken in identifying the uterosacral ligaments and ureters prior to plicating the peritoneum.

Discrete fascial defect repair is growing in popularity as a means to correct enteroceles akin to the concept as practiced endorectally by coloproctologists. The concept of this surgical repair is to identify and correct discrete tears or breaks in the endopelvic fascia. Breaks in the fascial attachments at the apex of the vagina will cause an enterocele so that intraperitoneal contents will protrude though the fascial defects (Figure 8.3). Similar to hernia repairs performed by general surgeons, the technique involves identifying the discrete fascial tears, reducing the hernia, and then closing the defect. This may be accomplished vaginally, abdominally, or laparoscopically (13).

The Moschcowitz procedure, the Halban procedure, and uterosacral ligament plication are three types of enterocele repairs approached abdominally. The Moschcowitz procedure (18) involves placing a series of purse-string sutures to close the cul-de-sac. The sutures incorporate the posterior vaginal wall, the right and left pelvic sidewall peritoneum, and the anterior serosa of the sigmoid colon. Three or four sutures usually are required. One complication of this surgery is ureteral obstruction, as the ureter may be pulled medially in the suture. The Halban procedure also obliterates the cul-de-sac; however, the sutures are placed in a longitudinal fashion. Instead of incorporating peritoneum overlying the pelvic sidewalls, a series of sutures are placed along the anterior serosa of the sigmoid, down to the most inferior portion of the cul-de-sac, and then up along the posterior vaginal wall. This technique may decrease the chance of ureteral obstruction; however, there are no reported series comparing these techniques. Uterosacral ligament plication involves plicating the uterosacral ligaments together, along with the posterior vaginal wall, in a fashion analogous to the McCall technique. Three to five sutures usually are required to close the cul-de-sac.

Surgery to Correct a Rectocele

Gynecologic indications for rectocele repair extend beyond the presence of a symptomatic, non-emptying rectocele (Table 8-1). In recent surveys, 100% of gynecologists would repair a rectocele in the absence of gastrointestinal symptoms, whereas only 6% of colorectal surgeons would repair these asymptomatic cases (4–6). As such, the gynecologic goals of rectocele repair procedures also vary (Table 8-2). While less than half of colorectal surgeons approach a rectocele repair vaginally, 95% to 100% of gynecologists repair rectoceles vaginally (4–6). The vaginal approach to rectocele repair potentially allows for correction of vaginal, as well as rectal, symptomatic dysfunction.

Posterior Colporrhaphy Technique

Posterior colporrhaphy commonly is performed in conjunction with a perineoplasty to address a rectocele or relaxed perineum with a widened

TABLE 8-1. Indications for rectocele repair.

1. Obstructive defecation symptoms
2. Lower pelvic pressure and heaviness
3. Prolapse of posterior vaginal wall
4. Pelvic relaxation with enlarged vaginal hiatus

TABLE 8-2. Goals of surgery to repair a rectocele.

Re-establish:
1. Endopelvic fascial integrity from apex to perineum
2. Levator plate integrity
3. Anterior rectal wall support
4. Normal vaginal caliber and length
5. Integrity of perineal body

genital hiatus. Preoperatively, the severity of the rectocele is assessed, as well as the desired final vaginal caliber. Allis clamps are placed on the inner labia minora/hymen remnants bilaterally and then approximated in the midline. The resultant vagina should loosely admit two to three fingers. A triangular incision over the perineal body is made between the Allis clamps and sharp dissection is then performed to separate the posterior vagina from the underlying rectovaginal fascia. A midline incision is made along the length of the vagina to a site above the superior edge of the rectocele.

The dissection is carried laterally to the lateral vaginal sulcus and the medial margins of the puborectalis muscles (Figure 8.5). The rectovaginal fascia with or without the underlying levator ani muscles is then plicated with interrupted sutures while depressing the anterior rectal wall (Figure 8.6). Typically, absorbable sutures are placed along the length of the

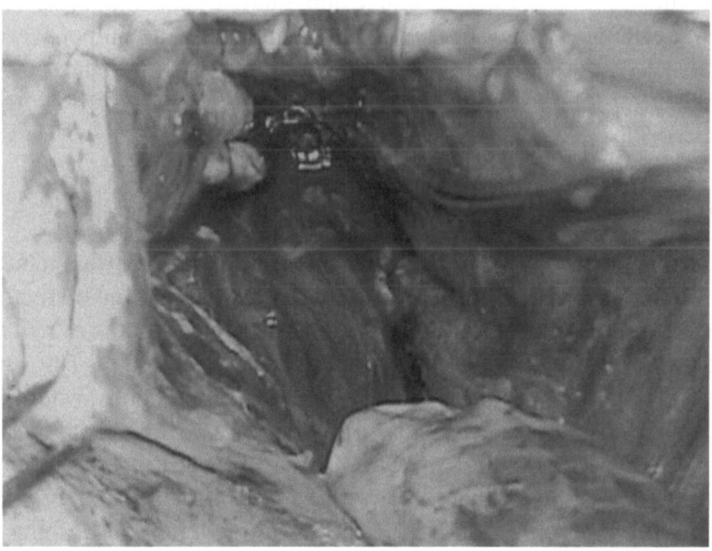

FIGURE 8.5. Surgical dissection is carried to the lateral vaginal sulcus in order to identify the fascia, which will be plicated for correction of posterior vaginal wall weakness.

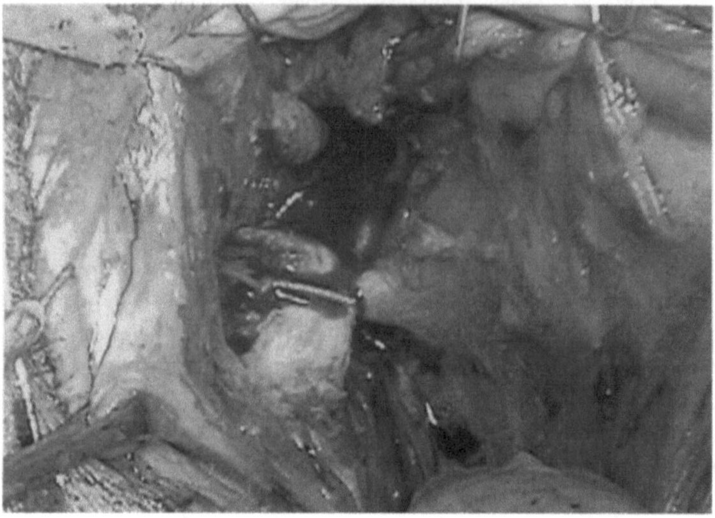

FIGURE 8.6. Multiple interrupted sutures are used to approximate the endopelvic fascia overlying the levator muscles in the midline.

rectocele until plication to the level of the perineal body is complete. Excess vaginal mucosa is carefully trimmed and then re-approximated. A concomitant perineoplasty may be performed by plicating the bulbocavernosus and transverse perineal muscles. This reinforces the perineal body—or inferior central tendon—and provides enhanced support to the corrected rectocele.

Discrete Fascial Defect Repair Technique

Discrete tears or breaks in the rectovaginal fascia or rectovaginal septum have been described and may contribute to the formation of rectoceles (Figure 8.3) (8). The intent of the discrete facial defect repair of rectoceles is to identify the fascial tears and re-approximate the edges. The surgical dissection is similar to the traditional posterior colporrhaphy, whereby the vaginal mucosa is dissected off the underlying rectovaginal fascia to the lateral border of the levator muscles. Instead of plicating the fascia and levator muscles in the midline, however, the fascial tears are identified and repaired with interrupted sutures. Richardson (8) described pushing anteriorly with a finger in the rectum in order to identify areas of rectal muscularis that are not covered by the rectovaginal septum, thereby locating fascial defects and identifying fascial margins with re-approximation. A perineoplasty may be necessary if a widened vaginal hiatus is present.

TABLE 8-3. Outcomes for posterior colporrhaphy.

Author	Number of patients	Mean follow-up (months)	Improvement in pelvic pressure symptoms	Anatomic correction rates	Improvement in evacuation difficulty	Postoperative dyspareunia rates
Paraiso (20)	102	10	89%	61%	82%	Increased from 2% to 12%
Mellgren (21)	25	12	N/A	96%	88%	Increased from 6% to 19%
Kahn (22)	171	42.5	51%	76%	62%	Increased from 18% to 27%
Lopez (23)	25	61.2	75%	92%	91%	Increased from 6% to 33%

Results of Surgical Repair

The posterior colporrhaphy has been the traditional approach to rectocele repair by gynecologists. Although commonly performed, it has been described as "among the most misunderstood and poorly performed" gynecologic surgeries (19). Although many authors have reported satisfactory anatomic results, conflicting effects on bowel and sexual function postoperatively have been noted (Table 8-3). Several authors have reported high sexual dysfunction rates—up to 50%—with women reporting dyspareunia or apareunia after posterior colporrhaphy (24). Many authors have suggested that the significant rate of postoperative dyspareunia may be due to the plication of the levator ani muscles; this has led several authors to advocate (and popularize) the discrete fascial defect repair. Several groups have reported a similar anatomic cure rate with this surgery, along with significant improvement in quality of life measures. Unlike the traditional posterior colporrhaphy, all these series have reported less postoperative dyspareunia (Table 8-4) with significant improvement in splint-

TABLE 8-4. Outcomes for the discrete fascial defect repair.

Author	Number of patients	Mean follow-up (months)	Improvement in pelvic pressure symptoms	Anatomic correction rates	Improvement in evacuation difficulty	Postoperative dyspareunia rates
Cundiff (25)	69	24	87%	82%	63%	Decreased from 29% to 19%
Glavind (26)	67	3	N/A	100%	85%	Decreased from 12% to 6%
Kenton (27)	46	12	90%	77%	54%	Decreased from 26% to 2%
Porter (28)	125	18	73%	82%	55%	Decreased from 67% to 46%

ing, vaginal pressure, and stooling difficulties. However, rates of fecal incontinence and constipation may be unchanged postoperatively.

These studies show promising anatomical and functional results; however, long-term prospective studies are required. Thus far, the incidence of postoperative dyspareunia with the discrete fascial defect repair is less than the traditional posterior colporrhaphy in nonrandomized comparisons (12), with some reported skepticism about the ability to adequately demonstrate and repair discrete fascial tears (29).

Other Techniques and Results

The use of synthetic mesh interposition to correct a rectocele at the time of abdominal sacrocolpopexy for vaginal vault prolapse has been reported (29). This simplifies the surgical approach for patients with both vaginal vault prolapse and rectocele, as it eliminates the need for a concomitant vaginal procedure. A continuous piece of mesh is placed abdominally from the perineal body to the vaginal vault. The mesh is then attached to the anterior longitudinal ligament overlying the sacral promontory in a tension-free fashion. Fox and Stanton, using this technique, treated 29 patients and noted continued bowel symptoms, including constipation and incomplete defecation (29). Others have noted a similar persistence of—or even an increase in—bowel symptoms in 39% of patients who underwent this type of surgery (30).

Adopting the principles of hernia repair by the general surgeons, reconstructive pelvic surgeons have reported reinforcement of pelvic organ prolapse repairs with synthetic and biologic prostheses. Synthetic mesh is used widely for anti-incontinence surgery and abdominal sacrocolpopexy to repair vaginal vault prolapse. Although high success rates have been reported, erosion of the mesh and infection has been associated with these repairs (31,32). Autologous grafts and allograft prostheses, including fascia lata, rectus sheath, and dermal grafts, have been employed for these surgeries, as well as reinforcement of cystocele repairs to reduce these complications (33). Few complications have been associated with these grafts, and they have a comparable success rate to synthetic materials. Xenograft materials—including bovine pericardium, porcine skin and small intestinal mucosa—also have been used to reinforce these repairs; however, no extended reports on complications and success rates exist in the literature.

Few studies have reported on the use of graft materials to reinforce posterior compartment defects. Sand et al. reported on 132 women undergoing either standard rectocele repairs or rectocele repairs reinforced with Polyglactin 910 mesh (an absorbable mesh) and found no difference in recurrence rates between the two groups (34). Two small observational studies on the use of Marlex mesh for rectocele repair did not report erosion or recurrence (35,36), whereas Sullivan and colleagues (37) reported on 236 women undergoing total pelvic mesh repair with Marlex for all types of pelvic support defects, including enteroceles and rectoceles. Through an abdominal approach, a strip of Marlex was used to reinforce the rectovaginal septum. Defecation difficulty improved in 76% of patients, but 28% of patients required postoperative surgical correction of rectoceles. There were no recurrences of enteroceles and only 3% complained of postoperative dyspareunia.

Laparoscopic rectocele repair involves opening the rectovaginal space and dissecting inferiorly to the perineal body. The perineal body is sutured to the rectovaginal septum and rectovaginal fascial defects are identified and closed. The advantages reported include improved visualization and more rapid recovery with both decreased pain and hospitalization. Disadvantages include difficulty with laparoscopic suturing, increased operating time and expense, and an extended "learning curve" time necessary to master the laparoscopic surgical techniques (38).

Few reports describing outcomes of laparoscopic surgery for pelvic organ prolapse exist in the literature. Lyons and Winer (39) described the use of polyglactin mesh in laparoscopic rectocele repair in 20 patients, with 80% reporting relief of both prolapse symptoms and the need for manual assistance to defecate. Further studies are needed to assess this surgical approach for rectocele repair.

Transrectal Repairs

Colorectal surgeons typically prefer a transrectal or transperineal approach to rectocele correction. Initial reports described the procedure in the lithotomy position (40). The rectal mucosa is mobilized and pulled outward until taut. A two-layer suture closure is performed of the defect underlying the rectal mucosa. The redundant anterior rectal mucosa is then removed to diminish a postoperative "mass effect" resulting in occasional persisting evacuatory difficulty. The formation of scars at the suture line adds to the support.

A transrectal repair of the rectocele with multilayer closure, but with resection of the lateral quadrants of the mucosal prolapse rather than the anterior quadrant, has been described (41). In addition, the rectovaginal septum can be repaired through a transanal approach, particularly if there is other associated anal pathology. The levator ani muscle and rectovaginal fascia are plicated separately. Ninety-eight percent of 355 patients reported improvement in this study by Sehapayak. In terms of bowel function, 14% continued to use laxatives, 35% had occasional straining, and 49.5% were asymptomatic. This study, however, did not report on postoperative sexual function. Complications included infection and a rectovaginal fistula. This author warns against performing this procedure for enteroceles or high rectoceles, or combining it with transvaginal surgery because of the risk of infection and rectovaginal fistula—complications that are not seen with vaginal rectocele repairs where the rectal mucosa is neither incised nor excised. Maintaining rectal mucosal integrity appears to significantly reduce infectious morbidity.

Rectocele operations performed transanally versus transvaginally have been compared in only one study (42), where complications occurred equally in the two groups of patients. In all, 54% had postoperative constipation and 34% overall had incontinence to gas, liquid, or stool. Sexual dysfunction was reported in 22% of patients. The only significant difference between the transvaginal and endorectal groups was that the patients undergoing transvaginal repair had more persistent pain.

Conclusions

The gynecologic indications for enterocele and rectocele repair are more numerous compared with the traditional colorectal indications because gynecologists primarily address vaginal symptoms when repairing a rectocele. Here, obstructive defecation symptoms are only some of a list of accepted indications. Preoperative evaluation typically only includes clinical assessment gained from the history and physical examination, and gynecologists rarely depend on defecography to plan a reconstructive procedure for rectoceles. Overall, surgical correction success rates are quite high when using a vaginal approach for rectocele correction. Vaginal dissection results in better visualization and access to the endopelvic fascia and levator musculature, which allows for a "firmer" anatomic correction. In addition, maintaining rectal mucosal integrity appears to reduce the risk of postoperative infection and fistula formation. More comprehensive data collection is necessary to better understand the effect of various surgical techniques on vaginal, sexual, and defecatory symptoms in these patients who may present with complex symptomatology where the rectocele and/or enterocele represent the dominant clinical finding.

References

1. Gonzalez-Argente FX, Jain A, Nogueras JJ, Davila GW, Weiss EG, and Wexner SD. Prevalence and severity of urinary incontinence and pelvic genital prolapse in females with anal incontinence or rectal prolapse. Dis Colon Rectum. 2001;44:920–6.
2. Jackson SL, Weber AM, Hull TL, Mitchinson AR, and Walters MD. Fecal incontinence in women with urinary incontinence and pelvic organ prolapse. Obstet Gynecol. 1997;89:423–7.
3. Meschia M, Buonaguidi A, Pifarotti P, Somigliana E, Spennacchio M, and Amicerelli F. Prevalence of anal incontinence in women with symptoms of urinary incontinence and genital prolapse. Obstet Gynecol. 2002;4:719–23.
4. Kapoor, Davila GW, Wexner SD, and Ghoniem G. Int Urogynecol J. 2001;12:S53.
5. Mizrahi, Kapoor, Nogueras JJ, Weiss E, Wexner SD, and Davila GW. ASCRS. 2002.

6. Davila GW, Ghoniem GM, Kapoor DS, and Contreras-Ortiz O. Pelvic floor dysfunction management practice patterns: a survey of members of the international urogynecological association. Int Urogynecol J. 2002;13:319–25.
7. Hall AF, Theofrastous JP, Cundiff GW, Harris RL, Hamilton LF, Swift SE, and Bump RC. Interobserver and intraobserver reliability of the proposed International Continence Society, Society of Gynecologic Surgeons and American Urogynecologic Society pelvic organ prolapse classification system. Am J Obstet Gynecol. 1996;175:1467–71.
8. Richardson AC. The rectovaginal septum revisited: Its relationship to rectocele and its importance in rectocele repair. Clin Obstet Gynecol. 1993;36:976–83.
9. Uhlenhuth E, Wolfe WM, Smith EM, and Middleton EB. The rectogenital septum. Surg Gynecol Obstet. 1948;86:148–63.
10. Milley PS and Nichols DH. A correlative investigation of the human rectovaginal septum. Anat Rec. 1969;163:443–52.
11. Delancey JOL. Anatomic aspects of vaginal eversion after hysterectomy. Am J Obstet Gynecol. 1992;166:1717–24.
12. Zbar AP, Lienemann A, Fritsch H, BeerGabel M, and Pescatori M. Rectocele: pathogenesis and surgical management. Int J Colorectal Dis. 2003;18:369–84.
13. Shull BL and Bachofen CG. Enterocele and rectocele. In: Walters MD and Karram MM, editors. Urogynecology and reconstructive pelvic surgery. 2nd ed. St. Louis: Mosby; 1999. p. 221–34.
14. Brubaker L. Rectocele. Curr Opin Obstet Gynecol. 1996;8:376–9.
15. Kahn MA and Stanton SL. Techniques of rectocele repair and their effects of bowel function. Int Urogynecol J. 1998;9:37–47.
16. Delancey JOL and Hurd WW. Size of the urogential hiatus in the levator ani muscles in normal women and women with pelvic organ prolapse. Obstet Gynecol. 1998;91:364–8.
17. Given FT Jr. "Posterior culdeplasty": revisited. Am J Obstet Gynecol. 1985; 153:135–9.
18. Moschcowitz AV. The pathogenesis, anatomy and cure of prolapse of the rectum. Surg Gynecol Obstet. 1912;15:7–12.
19. Nichols DH. Posterior colporrhaphy and perineorrhaphy: separate and distinct operations. Am J Obstet Gynecol. 1991;164:714–21.
20. Paraiso MF, Weber AM, Walters MD, Ballard LA, Piedmonte MR, and Skibinshi C. Anatomic and functional outcome after posterior colporrhaphy. J Pelvic Surg. 2001;7:335–9.
21. Mellgren A, Anzen B, Nilsson BY, et al. Results of rectocele repair; a prospective study. Dis Colon Rectum. 1995;38:7–13.
22. Kahn MA and Stanton SL. Posterior colporrhaphy: its effects on bowel and sexual function. Br J Obstet Gynaecol. 1997;104:82–6.
23. Lopez A, Anzen B, Bremmer S, et al. Durability of success after rectocele repair. Int Urogynecol J. 2001;12:97–103.
24. Francis WJ and Jeffcoate TN. Dyspareunia following vaginal operations. J Obstet Gynaecol Br Emp. 1961;68:1–10.
25. Cundiff GW, Weidner AC, Visco AG, Addison WA, and Bump RC. An anatomic and functional assessment of the discrete defect rectocele repair. Am J Obstet Gynecol. 1998;179:1451–7.
26. Glavind K and Madsen H. A prospective study of the discrete fascial defect rectocele repair. Acta Obstet Gynecol Scand. 2000;79:145–7.

27. Kenton K, Shott S, and Brubaker L. Outcome after rectovaginal reattachment for rectocele repair. Am J Obstet Gynecol. 1999;181:1360–3.
28. Porter WE, Steele A, Walsh P, Kohli N, and Karram MM. The anatomic and functional outcomes of defect-specific rectocele repairs. Am J Obstet Gynecol. 1999;181:1353–8.
29. Fox SD and Stanton SL. Vault prolapse and rectocele: assessment of repair using sacrocolpopexy with mesh interposition. Br J Obstet Gynaecol. 2000;107: 1371–5.
30. Taylor GM, Ballard P, and Jarvis GJ. Vault prolapse and rectocele: assessment of repair using sacrocolpopexy with mesh interposition. Br J Obstet Gynaecol. 2001;8:775–6.
31. Birch C and Fynes MM. The role of synthetic and biological prostheses in reconstructive pelvic floor surgery. Curr Opin Obstet Gynecol. 2001;14:527–35.
32. Iglesia CB, Fenner DE, and Brubaker L. The use of mesh in gynecologic surgery. Int Urogynecol J. 1997;8:105–15.
33. Øster S and Astrup A. A new vaginal operation for recurrent and large rectocele using dermis transplant. Acta Obstet Gynecol Scand. 1981;60:493–5.
34. Sand PK, Koduri S, and Lobel RW. Prospective randomized trial of Polyglactin 910 mesh to prevent recurrences of cystoceles and rectoceles. Am J Obstet Gynecol. 2001;184:1357–64.
35. Parker MC and Phillips RKS. Repair of rectocoele using Marlex mesh. Ann R Coll Surg Eng. 1993;75:193–4.
36. Watson SJ, Loder PB, and Halligan S. Transperineal repair of symptomatic rectocele with marlex mesh: a clinical, physiological and radiological assessment of treatment. J Am Coll Surg. 1996;183:257–61.
37. Sullivan ES, Longaker CJ, and Lee PYH. Total pelvic mesh repair: a ten-year experience. Dis Colon Rectum. 2001;44:857–63.
38. Paraiso MFR, Falcone T, and Walters MD. Laparoscopic surgery for enterocele, vaginal apex prolapse and rectocele. Int Urogynecol J. 1999;10:223–9.
39. Lyons TL and Winer WK. Laparoscopic rectocele repair using polyglactin mesh. J Am Assoc Gynecol Laparosc. 1997;4:381–4.
40. Marks MM. The rectal side of the rectocele. Dis Colon Rectum. 1967;10:387–8.
41. Sehapayak S. Transrectal repair of rectocele: An extended armamentarium of colorectal surgeons. Dis Colon Rectum. 1985;6:422–33.
42. Arnold MW, Stewart WRC, and Aguilar PS. Rectocele: four years' experience. Dis Colon Rectum. 1990;33:684–7.

Editorial Commentary

The physical examination of these patients is geared towards the detection of rectocele, enterocele, and graded uterovaginal prolapse. The surgical treatment is tailored and needs to be multidisciplinary in the absence of randomized controlled trials. Gynecologists have accepted that defect-specific repair is a feature of rectocele treatment but long-term data are as yet unavailable and it is also unclear whether transvaginal approaches provide equivalent results to endorectal surgery. Here, although postoperative sexual dysfunction appears more common following transvaginal surgery, the transvaginal technique is probably indicated if there is a concomitant cystocele or attendant vaginal prolapse. The somewhat traditional addition by gynecological surgeons of a levatorplasty to narrow the genital hiatus and provide a vaginal buttress is now recognized in many cases to worsen evacuatory dysfunction in these patients.

AZ

Chapter 9
Assessing the Postoperative Patient with Evacuatory Dystunction

Chapter 9.1
Assessing the Postoperative Patient with Evacuatory Dysfunction: Disordered Defecation of the Neorectum and Neorectal Reservoir

Tracy L. Hull

Introduction

The technical ability to avoid a permanent stoma has evolved over the past 20 years. In the majority of cases when the rectum—and even the entire colon—require surgical excision for various conditions, such as rectal cancer, ulcerative colitis, or familial polyposis, it is possible to join bowel to the anal area. This in turn allows the patient to defecate per anus. However, even though the patient avoids a stoma, nearly all will have some element of defecation dysfunction. This chapter will be divided into two sections:

1. defecation dysfunction after rectal resection with a low colorectal or coloanal anastomosis, and
2. defecation dysfunction after a proctocolectomy and pelvic ileal pouch.

Defecation Dysfunction after Rectal Resection with Low Anastomosis

Traditionally, surgical treatment requiring resection of the distal half to two-thirds of the rectum required a permanent colostomy. Changing attitudes regarding the limited distal spread of rectal cancer and technical advances doing anastomosis led surgeons to attempt to restore continuity with tumors, even in the distal rectum. During the early era of anterior rectal resection with a low anastomosis, surgeons were concerned mainly with effectiveness of cancer clearance and the safety of the anastomotic technique. Bowel function was not a primary focus. However, as surgeons learned that they could safely save the anal sphincters and avoid a permanent stoma, they also came to realize that there was a price. Most patients had preservation of fecal continence, but bowel dysfunction proved disabling for some, both socially and in the work place.

Bowel dysfunction in this group of people has been termed, anterior resection syndrome. It encompasses stool frequency, urgency, and soilage

(1). More specifically, after a low straight colorectal or coloanal anastomosis, patients may have frequent stooling, urgency, nocturnal bowel movements, and fragmentation of stooling (the sensation that the bowel is not fully evacuated and the person needs to defecate small amounts of stool repeatedly in a short space of time). It is known that frequency decreases with time for some patients, especially over the first year (2); however, some patients still had reduced quality of life due to their bowel dysfunction (see Chapter 7.2).

The main reason for the bowel dysfunction has been attributed to alterations in pelvic physiology and the loss of the rectal reservoir capacity. One of the physiologic alterations demonstrated by several authors is reduced mean anal resting pressure (3,4). The etiology of this is debatable, but may be due to injury to the internal sphincter muscle during passage of the circular stapling device or during the mucosectomy (5). Pelvic nerve damage also is speculated as a possible cause (6). Another contributing factor may be a problem with sensitivity in the upper anal canal. These issues are covered in other parts of this book. In one study by Miller et al. (7), the upper anal canal was found to be less sensitive in those with poor function postoperatively after an anterior resection compared with those with acceptable bowel function. Others feel the observed loss of the rectoanal inhibitory reflex may be a significant contributing factor to poor function (8).

The loss of the rectal reservoir has been targeted as a major factor leading to bowel dysfunction. In a straight low anastomosis, the colon, which replaces the rectal reservoir, is denervated and is of small caliber, compliance, and capacity when compared with the normal rectum. Addressing this, two separate units in 1986 described incorporating a colonic J pouch anastomosed to the anal area to improve neorectal function and capacity (9,10). It has been demonstrated in prospective randomized trials that the addition of a colonic J pouch significantly reduces stool frequency, at least in the early postoperative period (11,12). However, the long-term advantage of the colonic J pouch has been questioned. Advantages of the colonic J pouch at one year may not be apparent by two years, as has been shown by some investigators examining the number of daily bowel movements, tenesmus, urgency, and the incontinence score (2); however, others have shown improvement in the night-time number of bowel movements and continence favoring the colonic J pouch group, even after five years (13).

There are no ideal methods to assess outcome and function after a colonic pouch. The number of bowel movements is a target that can be counted; however, when looking at functional outcome parameters such as incontinence, there is lack of a standardized universally accepted tools. Therefore, comparison between studies is difficult. Manometry has been looked at, but probably offers little in guidance because the primary goal is the assessment of the patient's quality of life. Likewise, no universally accepted tool exists to measure quality of life in this group of patients.

Therefore, in patients without optimal outcome, as deemed by their own concerns, identifying the problem with an accurate history is the first step, and there really is no current literature to support many of these treatment schemes that are discussed in the following paragraphs; nonetheless, many are clinically extremely helpful.

Incontinence

Incontinence is dealt with in other chapters and its assessment and management applies equally well to these postoperative cases as it does in patients presenting with primary or postobstetric incontinence. Suffice to say that after low anterior resection, its etiology is multifactorial. I will not elaborate on this problem except to emphasize that patient education regarding perianal skin protection is highly important and often is neglected.

Frequency of Bowel Movements/Fragmentation/Urgency

One goal of the colonic J pouch is to decrease the frequency of stooling or the need to evacuate small amounts of stool repeatedly in a short period of time. Even with a colonic J pouch, this can still pose a problem. It usually does improve over the first year, but not always. Additionally, pelvic external irradiation—especially if given postoperatively—can make these symptoms worse, most notably the symptom of fecal urgency. The first step is to rule out a stricture, which may contribute to these symptoms. Medical therapy is tried next, where fiber, in the form of agents such as Metamucil, Citrucel, or Konsyl, may solidify stool and improve defecation. I start with a teaspoon at bedtime and increase up to a teaspoon three times daily if improvement continues to be seen. The next line of medication to use is Imodium or Lomotil. For some, using one pill each morning is sufficient; however, up to eight daily can be used. Even eight daily of both Imodium and Lomotil are needed by a small number of patients. All patients need to individualize their needs and there is no formula except that of trial and error. For instance, if a patient has problems with night-time defecation, two pills before bedtime are appropriate. Additionally, if night-time defecation is a significant problem, reducing the size of meals after 6:00 pm is helpful.

A cleansing enema, especially in the morning, may help those with fragmentation in an effort to fully cleanse the left colon. One option is to use a Fleet enema and keep the container after use. It can be reused four or five times and filled with tepid tap water until the plastic cracks and is no longer useable. When reusing it, a water-soluble lubricant will be needed to aid in inserting the tip. Using a commercial enema kit and filling it with tepid tap water to an amount of 200 to 250 cubic centimeters is another acceptable route of delivery. Air should be purged from the tubing and the tip well lubricated with water-soluble lubricant prior to anal insertion. The bag is hung at shoulder height to allow gravity to assist in the instillation of the water. Patients are encouraged to hold the enema for one to two minutes before evacuation. Occasionally, patients find small tap-water enemas twice daily to be more helpful. For patients who feel they incompletely empty, using an asepto syringe similar to that used to rinse out the lower bowel—if possible after each bowel movement—eliminates that sensation. We typically do not use evacuation suppositories, as we have not had good relief of symptoms with their use.

Patients with incapacitating urgency or frequency usually do well with B and O suppositories. Because they contain belladonna, it is important to avoid prescribing them to patients with glaucoma. It also is not recommended for those with severe hepatic or renal disease, bronchial asthma, narcotic idiosyncrasies, acute alcoholism, or convulsive disorders. I use the strength 15A, which contains 30 milligrams of opium. Sometimes even using half is sufficient. To cut them in half, they need to be refrigerated and cut with a serrated knife. I recommend half or one each morning. Another suppository can be repeated for twice-daily use if needed; however, the majority of patients do well with one each morning. Because it contains powdered opium, there is the theoretical concern of addiction; however, these suppositories are used in patients who are incapacitated due to their stool fragmentation. The dramatic improvement in quality of life, from reduced reliance of being in the bathroom, must be considered strongly to outweigh the concern of addiction.

Inability to Evacuate

Problems with evacuation were reported more frequently when the colonic J pouch was constructed with limbs of similar length to the pelvic ileal pouch. However, through randomized studies, the ideal length of the colonic J pouch has been found to be five to six centimeters (14,15). One speculation as to why the large colonic J pouch may have evacuation difficulty is a horizontal inclination that develops over the first year (16). Even with the smaller pouch, some patients will have problems with evacuation. It is important to verify that the anastomosis is open and rule out recurrence of cancer in the pelvis. Treatment usually consists of an enema routine as described above.

Additional Considerations

Anastomotic Complications

Anastomotic complications have been shown to be reduced with the colonic J pouch. In a randomized study, significantly fewer patients had an anastomotic leak when compared with straight anastomosis (2% vs. 15% $p = 0.03$) (12). In this study, symptomatic anastomotic strictures were similar in both groups. Other studies have found anastomotic leak rates similar between colonic J pouch patients and those with a straight anastomosis (17,18). Joo et al. (2) also found a fourfold decrease in anastomotic complications in the colonic J pouch group. This was not statistically significant in their small number of patients. Improved blood flow to the side of the colon versus an end-to-end anastomosis as shown by laser Doppler flowmetry during surgery is speculated as to why the leak rate is less (19).

Coloplasty

In approximately 25% of patients at our institution (unpublished Cleveland Clinic Cleveland, Ohio data), the colonic J pouch is not technically feasible (20). The reasons for this include:

1. A bulky colonic pouch from excessive fat in the mesentery, which would not fit through the pelvis (especially in a narrow male pelvis);
2. Limitations in the ability to reach the pelvic floor (usually due to a fatty mesocolon, which hinders the pouch mobility); and
3. Difficulty pulling a bulky colonic J pouch through long tight anal muscles.

In 1997, Z'graggen et al. (21) described a "novel" colonic reservoir; the coloplasty preliminary work from our institution showed no difference in complications using the coloplasty technique compared with a straight anastomosis or colonic J pouch (22). Evaluation of the first 69 coloplasty patients showed that they had significantly less stools in 24 hours (3.8 vs. 4.8 $p = 0.04$) and less clustering of stools compared with straight anastomosis ($p = 0.2$). Coloplasty patients used less anti-diarrheal medication compared with the J pouch ($p = 0.02$) or straight anastomosis ($p = 0.03$) patients (23). Further work is underway, but it appears that patients with a coloplasty have functional outcome similar to those with a colonic J pouch, and perhaps even superior in some respects. This issue has been addressed recently by Fürst and colleagues (24), who also found similar functional results between the two types of procedures and no basic differences in anorectal manometry or maximal neorectal volumes.

Defecation Dysfunction after Proctocolectomy and Pelvic Ileal Pouch

After more than two decades, the pelvic ileal pouch has become the gold standard for reconstruction after a total proctocolectomy for ulcerative colitis or familial polyposis. Extensive experience and reports about various technical aspects and functional outcome are found in the literature. Certain complications seen with pelvic pouches will be discussed.

Leak

Estimates of anastomotic leak vary. It ranges from 3% to 12% and higher (25–27). The amount of experience a surgeon has performing the pelvic pouch procedure may influence the leak rate (and even the overall complication rate), where it appears to be more frequent after a hand-sewn anastomosis (10.5% vs. 4.6%, $p < 0.001$) (25). Symptoms include ileus, fever, increased white blood cell count, malaise, anal pain, anal drainage, and incontinence. An anastomotic leak occurring after 30 days also may signal undiagnosed Crohn's disease.

Initial treatment consists of drainage of sepsis and usually a proximal ileostomy if none has been performed at the time of initial surgery. Placing a small mushroom catheter through the defect may allow for drainage and for the cavity to collapse and heal. The catheter then can be removed and healing confirmed by gastrograffin enema examination before stoma closure. Pouch advancement (28), oversewing the defect after placing antibiotic powder in the cavity, or use of fibrin glue all are potential treatments; however, no extensive studies exist to indicate their success. Persistent leaks may need to be addressed with a total redo pouch, as will be discussed later. Early drainage of peri-pouch sepsis is likely to limit the disturbance in neorectal compliance, which contributes to poor postoperative function. In this respect, there is merit in very early examination under anesthesia in patients who develop fever or anal discharge after ileal or colonic pouch–anal anastomosis, and it is advisable here to place the mesenteric axis of the ileum away from the midline posteriorly during the initial anastomosis in order to ensure that posterior transpouch or transanastomotic drainage can be performed safely (29).

A leak from the tip of the J pouch is a commonly overlooked problem (30). It may become symptomatic before or after ileostomy closure, typically presenting as an anterior upper-pelvic abscess. On pouch endoscopy, subtle findings such as granulation tissue or edema at the suture or staple line may be the only clue. Usually, the abscess is amenable to percutaneous drainage; however, definitive treatment usually requires re-resection of the tip of the J, as it almost never heals with simple drainage alone.

Pelvic Sepsis

Overall, pelvic sepsis occurs in 5% to 6% of pelvic pouch patients (31,32). It is important to address the problem early to avoid pelvic fibrosis, as this can lead to impaired pouch function (32). Drainage usually can be performed percutaneously; however, sometimes transabdominal drainage is required. It is important to aggressively rule out a fistula as the initiating source of the sepsis before closing a stoma. This is done with a gastrograffin enema and commitment to early pouch endoscopy.

Residual Anastomotic Sinus

Occasionally, when a gastrograffin enema is obtained prior to ileostomy closure, an anastomotic sinus is visualized. Many patients are asymptomatic and the majority of these sinuses will close with time, where even waiting six to nine months may be appropriate. In the event it does not close, an advancement pouch flap can be used to close the opening. Fibrin glue has been tried, but results are not definitive as yet in the literature. Simply unroofing the sinus tract into the pouch also has been used successfully as a definitive treatment (33).

Results after Successful Anastomotic Leak Treatment

Variable reports have been seen regarding function after successful treatment of a leak. MacRae et al. (26) found that a leak was the most common cause for pouch failure; they showed that leaks after stapled anastomosis did better than following hand-sewn techniques. Breen and colleagues (34) showed no difference in function in this circumstance, and our data has shown that 60% of cases had an ultimately successful outcome, although multiple surgical procedures may be needed to correct the leak (35). Aggressive treatment of the sepsis is needed at the outset to prevent fibrosis of the pouch, which may have the most detrimental effect on pelvic pouch function, even after the leak has been corrected.

Pelvic Pouch Hemorrhage

About 3% of patients will have severe bleeding from the inside of the pelvic pouch in the postoperative period (27). Prevention by inspection of the staple line after construction and before the anastomosis will avoid this problem in some patients. Treatment starts by verifying normal coagulation parameters. An adult rigid proctoscope is passed into the pouch to evacuate all clots. Lavage with iced saline is performed next. A 25–30 French urethral catheter is passed into the pouch and instilled with 50 to 75 cubic centimeters of 1:100 000 epinephrine solution. This concentration is obtained by taking one milliliter 1:1 000 epinephrine and placing it into a 100-cubic centimeter bag of normal saline. The catheter is clamped for 30 to 60 minutes and the pulse and blood pressure are monitored every 10 to 15 minutes. This is repeated several times if the bleeding persists. If there continues to be bleeding, an examination under anesthesia is performed in an attempt to isolate and oversew the bleeding point.

Stricture

Narrowing at the pouch anal anastomosis is common. It is reported 10% to 18% of the time, and not all cases are symptomatic (27,34,35). Nearly all patients will form a “web” at the anastomosis, which requires dilatation prior to stoma closure. This usually can be done with a digital examination in the office.

Refractory strictures, which are symptomatic, may be due to tension or ischemia at the anastomosis during pouch construction. It also may be associated with previous or ongoing occult sepsis, so careful examination in the operating room combined with a gastrograffin enema may help demonstrate the problem. Additionally, Crohn’s disease must be kept in the differential diagnosis. Initial treatment with repeat dilatation—in the operating room if needed—should be undertaken. Other treatments such as endoscopic endoballoon dilatation with intravenous (IV) sedation may be tried, and self-dilatation with a Hegar type 14 or 15 dilator daily for one to two months may prevent symptomatic recurrence. Other nonoperative treatments have included anal catheterization.

A common surgical procedure to correct a refractory stricture is the pouch advancement. Because full pouch advancement and correction may be attained by transanal dissection, the patient is placed in the Kraske position and trial dissection is conducted. It usually requires circumferential mucosectomy (if that had not been done when the pouch initially was constructed) and advancement of the full thickness pouch through the anal canal to the dentate line. The surgeon must be prepared to reposition the patient in order to open the abdomen and mobilize the pouch from the transabdominal route if needed. More operative tips regarding this condition are provided under the section on redo pelvic pouches below. Some patients require pouch excision, ileostomy, or conversion to a continent ileostomy for these refractory strictures.

Portal Vein Thrombosis

A surprising finding of portal vein thrombosis has been found in some patients who have a computed tomography (CT) scan for abdominal pain, fever, leukocytosis, and/or ileus. At our institution, of 702 patients where ileal pouch–anal anastomoses have been performed from 1997 through 2000, 94 had CT scans. Of these, 42 (45%) had portal vein thrombosis. In 45 of the 94 patients with CT scans, an area of sepsis was detected in the abdomen. Twenty of these 45 patients had portal vein thrombosis. However, 22 of these 94 had no septic focus, and only portal vein thrombosis was found. Of the 42 with portal vein thrombosis, only eight were treated, but the long-term effects are unknown. This diagnosis should be suspected in patients with symptoms of sepsis, but where no focus is found on CT. Perhaps this subset should be aggressively treated with anticoagulation (36).

Pouch Failure Requiring Redo Pelvic Pouch

Pouch failure requiring a complete redo transabdominally of the pouch occurs for various reasons. Successful results have been reported 50% to 100% of the time (ulcerative colitis 95% and Crohn's disease 60%) (37–40). Postoperative quality of life using the SF 36 has shown patients to have results within one standard deviation of the normal population.

This type of surgery is a huge undertaking. There should be an attempt to eradicate sepsis prior to the redo surgery. The patient and surgeon must be highly motivated. It is optimal to wait at least six months from any prior abdominal surgery to allow for the normal postoperative inflammation to subside fully. Preoperatively, the patient is marked for a stoma if one is not already in place. It is important to allow plenty of time for the surgery and secure the required help to perform the procedure. Due to anatomic wandering of the ureters from previous pelvic surgery, ureteric stents may be beneficial, and in anticipation of significant bleeding, blood should be available.

The conduct of the surgery is variable. It is sometimes easier to begin with transanal mobilization and disconnection of the pouch from the anus before starting the abdominal mobilization. As with other redo pelvic surgery, using a big incision and entering the abdomen above the umbilicus is beneficial. Positioning the patient in stirrups with their arms by their sides gives added mobility to the surgeon while dissecting. Lighted retractors help with illuminating the deep pelvis.

While mobilizing from the abdominal standpoint, it is important to be aware of the pouch mesentery. It is sometimes helpful to dissect behind the superior mesenteric vessels. In patients with chronic sepsis, the tissue encountered deep in the pelvis may be fibrotic and hard. Dissection with long sturdy scissors and the bovie diathermy will be needed. After the pouch is disconnected, the decision to repair the existing pouch and reconnect it—construction of a new pouch—is sometimes a difficult decision. Here, there are no easy guidelines. If fibrotic areas associated with the underlying problem of the pouch can be resected and a pouch of acceptable capacity can be refashioned, it is acceptable to preserve the existing pouch. It is usually the rule that a hand-sewn anastomosis will be needed for a redo pouch. Placing drains in the presacral space and omentum to cover any areas of phlegmon may improve results. A loop ileostomy should always be used at completion.

Results of complete redo pouches show variable success rates. Cohen et al. (38) found of 24 patients that 14 could have their pouches reused and ten needed completely new pouches constructed. Eighty-three percent were satisfied with their outcome. Ogunbiyi et al. (41) reported a 50% success rate. Reports agree that sepsis should be eradicated prior to redo surgery and a motivated surgeon and patient are essential for a successful outcome.

An accurate estimate of the number of pouch failures leading to pouch excision is difficult to obtain. In our database of over 2000 patients, it is about percent. In the literature, the most common etiologies are a leak at the ileal pouch–anal anastomosis, unrecognized Crohn's disease, poor functional results, and pelvic sepsis (26,42,43).

Crohn's disease in a pelvic pouch occurs from 3% to 10% of the time in various series (27,39), and any patient with "chronic pouchitis" should be suspected of having underlying undiagnosed Crohn's disease. Successful treatment with long-term antibiotics, immune modulators (6-MP), and Infliximab may help with pouch salvage. Functioning pouches (in those found to have unsuspected Crohn's disease) at five years have been reported in 50% to 70% of patients (39).

Pouchitis

Making the diagnosis of pouchitis is not simply done by examining the pelvic pouch. It is important to listen to the patient and their symptoms, as pouchitis can occur in a relatively noninflamed pouch. Similarly, on routine examination, an inflamed pouch may be totally asymptomatic and require no treatment. The most common clue is a relative sudden change in defecation pattern including increased frequency, urgency, loose or watery stool, or blood in the stool (44). Patients also may report symptoms resembling a viral syndrome or pelvic pressure and pain. Two scoring systems have been developed to aid in diagnosis of pouchitis: the Heidelberg Pouchitis Activity Index and the Mayo Clinic's Pouchitis Disease Activity Index (45). Both systems look at clinical information, endoscopy, and histologic features, but weigh each area differently to provide a score. The patient is then felt to have pouchitis if their score is above a certain level. Heuschen et al. (45) scored suspected pouchitis patients using both tools. The authors felt the sensitivity and specificity of the Heidelberg Pouchitis Activity Index were satisfactory; however, the cut-off point for diagnosis of pouchitis would need to be lowered to obtain an acceptable specificity and sensitivity for the Pouchitis Disease Activity Index. Interestingly, the authors suggested that the diagnosis of pouchitis alone should be based on endoscopic and histologic features without consideration of the clinical features.

Pouchitis occurs almost exclusively in patients who have had a pouch for ulcerative colitis as opposed to those with familial polyposis. At the Mayo Clinic, from their series of 1310 patients, 48% of patients had at least one episode of pouchitis (46). Other series have reported 20% to 50% (47) of pelvic pouch patients presenting with pouchitis. It is important to remember that all patients with a long-standing pelvic pouch develop various degrees of "colonization" of the pouch. The mucosa microscopically takes on characteristics of the colon with changes such as villous atrophy and mucin changes ("colonic metaplasia") (48). How this will affect long-term function or influence the development of pouchitis is unknown at present.

The etiology of pouchitis remains unknown. Multiple factors have been cited, including immune alterations, bacterial overgrowth, a deficiency of mucosal nutrients, and transient ischemia to name a few (47). It is conceivable that all factors play a role; however, until more definitive studies have been conducted, the exact etiology will remain unknown.

Treatment of pouchitis begins with exclusion of pelvic sepsis, anastomotic stricture, or inflammation of the transition zone (cuffitis). Crohn's disease also must be considered. When doing endoscopy of a pouch, all inflammatory changes should stop at the transition of the afferent limb of the bowel into the pouch. Inflammation proximal to this should raise the suspicion of Crohn's disease.

Irritable pouch syndrome also has been described and is defined as patients with symptoms of pouchitis without meeting the cut-off for the Pouchitis Disease Activity Index (49). Of 61 consecutive pouchitis patients, 42% were diagnosed with irritable pouches. This group of patients responded to treatment with anti-diarrheal agents, anti-cholinergics, and/or antidepressants.

Metronidazole is probably the most frequently prescribed first-line medication for pouchitis. The usual oral dose is 750 to 1500 milligrams daily for seven to ten days. Improvement usually is seen within 24 to 36 hours. Due to side-effects of peripheral neuropathy, nausea, and antabuse-like effects if alcohol is consumed, alternative antibiotics have been used. Ciprofloxacin has been the most common, but others have been effective, including amoxicillin–clavulanic acid, erythromycin, and tetracycline. Additionally, oral steroids, steroid enemas, 5 aminosalicylic acid (both topically and orally) have been effective. We have found that low-dosage antibiotics such as metronidazole or ciprofloxacin are effective in preventing chronic or recurrent pouchitis, and we also have successfully used medication such as 6-MP in this retractory group of pouchitis patients. This array of successful treatment options only points to the fact that the mechanism of pouchitis is not currently understood.

Conclusion

Miraculous advances in surgical techniques have prevented countless patients from living with a permanent stoma after rectal resection or total proctocolectomy. When counseling patients preoperatively, it is important to communicate realistic functional expectations because surgery is not perfect and nearly all surgeries have some element of defecation dysfunction afterwards. Postoperatively, it is essential to work with patients to individualize treatment régimes. In turn, this will optimize their function and quality of life. Not every patient will achieve satisfactory results, and some will require a permanent stoma to improve their quality of life.

When performing pelvic ileal pouches, awareness and counseling of the array of possible complications is necessary. Diligent evaluation when problems are suspected can frequently locate and treat the culprit. This is essential in order to prevent permanent problems in the pouch. Redo pouches are clearly feasible if the surgical expertise exists; therefore, this type of redo surgery should only be attempted by committed surgeons and motivated patients.

References

1. Ortiz H and Armendariz P. Anterior resection: do the patients perceive any clinical benefit? Int J Colorectal Dis. 1996;11:191–5.
2. Joo JS, Latulippe JF, Alabaz O, Weiss EG, Nogueras JJ, and Wexner SD. Long-term functional evaluation of straight coloanal anastomosis and colonic J-pouch. Dis Colon Rectum. 1998;41:740–6.
3. Williamson MER, Lewis WG, Finan PJ, Miller AS, Holdsworth PJ, and Johnston D. Recovery of physiologic and clinical function after low anterior resection of the rectum for carcinoma; myth or reality? Dis Colon Rectum. 1995;38:411–8.
4. Horgan PG, O'Connell PR, Shinkwin CA, and Kirwan WO. Effect of anterior resection on anal sphincter function. Br J Surg. 1989;76:783–6.
5. Molloy RG, Moran KT, Coulter J, Waldron R, and Kirwan WO. Mechanism of sphincter impairment following low anterior resection. Dis Colon Rectum. 1992;35:462–4.
6. Williams N and Seow-Choen F. Physiological and functional outcome following ultra-low anterior resection with colon pouch-anal anastomosis. Br J Surg. 1998;85:1029–35.
7. Miller AS, Lewis WG, Williamson MER, Holdsworth PJ, Johnston D, and Finan PJ. Factors that influence the outcome after coloanal anastomosis for carcinoma of the rectum. Br J Surg. 1995;82:1327–30.
8. O'Riordain MG, Molloy RG, Gillen P, Horgan A, and Kirwan WO. Rectoanal inhibitory reflex following low stapled anterior resection of the rectum. Dis Colon Rectum. 1992;35:874–8.
9. Lazorthes F, Fages P, Chiotasso P, Lemozy J, and Bloom E. Resection of the rectum with construction of a colonic reservoir and colo-anal anastomosis for carcinoma of the rectum. Br J Surg. 1986;73:136–8.
10. Parc R, Tiret E, Frileux P, Moszkowski E, and Loygue J. Resection and colo-anal anastomosis with colonic reservoir for rectal carcinoma. Br J Surg. 1986;73:139–41.
11. Ho YH, Tan M, and Seow-Choen F. Prospective randomized controlled study of clinical function and anorectal physiology after low anterior resection: comparison of straight and colonic J pouch anastomosis. Br J Surg. 1996;83:978–80.
12. Hallbook O, Påhlman L, Krog M, Wexner SD, and Sjodahl R. Randomized comparison of straight and colonic J pouch anastomosis after low anterior resection. Ann Surg. 1996;224:58–65.
13. Harris CJ, Lavery IC, and Fazio VW. Function of a colonic J pouch continues to improve with time. Br J Surg. 2001;88:1623–7.

14. Lazorthes, Gamagami R, Chiotasso P, Istvan G, and Muhammad S. Prospective, randomized study comparing clinical results between small and large colonic J-pouch following coloanal anastomosis. Dis Colon Rectum. 1997;40:1409–13.
15. Hida J, Yasutomi M, Fujimoto K, Okuno K, Leda S, Machidera N, Kubo R, Shindo K, and Koh K. Functional outcome after low anterior resection with low anastomosis for rectal cancer using the colonic J-pouch: prospective randomized study for determination of optimum pouch size. Dis Colon Rectum. 1996;39:986–91.
16. Hida J, Yasutomi M, Maruyama T, Tokoro T, Uchida T, Wakano T, and Kubo R. Horizontal inclination of the longitudinal axis of the colonic J-pouch: defining causes of evacuation difficulty. Dis Colon Rectum. 1999;42:1560–8.
17. Ortiz H, Miguel MD, and Armendariz P. Coloanal anastomosis: are functional results better with a pouch. Dis Colon Rectum. 1995;38:375–7.
18. Hallbook O, Nystrom P, and Sjodahl R. Physiologic characteristics of straight and colonic J-pouch anastomoses after rectal excision for cancer. Dis Colon Rectum. 1997;40:332–8.
19. Hallbook O, Johansson K, and Sjodahl R. Laser Doppler blood flow measurement in rectal resection for carcinoma—comparison between the straight and colonic J-pouch reconstruction. Br J Surg. 1996;83:389–92.
20. Harris GJ, Lavery IJ, and Fazio VW. Reasons for failure to construct the colonic J pouch. What can be done to improve the size of the neorectal reservoir should it occur? Dis Colon Rectum. 2002;45:1304–8.
21. Z'graggen K, Maurer CA, Mettler D, Stoupis C, Wildi S, and Buchler MW. A novel colonic reservoir for rectal construction: description of the technique. Gastroenterology. 1997;112:A1487.
22. Mantyh CR, Hull TL, and Fazio VW. Coloplasty in low colorectal anastomosis: manometric and functional comparison to straight and colonic J pouch anastomosis. Dis Colon Rectum. 2001;44:37–42.
23. Zutshi M, Remzi F, Lavery I, Hull T, Senagore A, Church J, Strong S, Delaney C, and Fazio V. Functional outcome and complications of coloplasty pouch for low coloanal and colorectal anastomosis. Podium presentation at American Society of Colon and Rectal Surgeons; 2002 Jun 6; Chicago, Illinois.
24. Fürst A, Suttner S, Agha A, Beham A, and Jauch K-W. Colonic J-pouch *vs.* coloplasty following resection of distal rectal cancer. Early results of a prospective, randomized, pilot study. Dis Colon Rectum. 2003;46:1161–6.
25. Ziv Y, Fazio VW, Church JM, Lavery IC, King T, and Ambrosetti P. Stapled ileal pouch anal anastomoses are safer than handsewn anastomoses in patients with ulcerative colitis. Am J Surg. 1996;171:320–3.
26. MacRae HM, McLeod RS, Cohen Z, O'Connor BI, and Ton ENC. Risk factors for pelvic pouch failure. Dis Colon Rectum. 1997;40:257–62.
27. Belliveau P, Trudel J, Vasilevsky C, Stein B, and Gordon PH. Ileoanal anastomosis with reservoirs: complications and long-term results. Can J Surg. 1999;42: 345–52.
28. Zinicola R, Wilkinson KH, and Nicholls RJ. Ileal pouch-vaginal fistula treated by abdominoanal advancement of the ileal pouch. Br J Surg. 2003;90:1434–5.
29. Nicholls RJ. Personal communication. 1998.
30. Dayton MT and Larsen KP. Outcome of pouch-related complications after ileal pouch-anal anastomosis. Am J Surg. 1997;174:728–32.

31. Johnson E, Carlsen E, Nazir M, and Nygaard K. Morbidity and functional outcome after restorative proctocolectomy for ulcerative colitis. Eur J Surg. 2001; 167:40–5.
32. Beart R. Ulcerative colitis: complications of pelvic pouch. In: Fazio VW, editor. Current therapy in colon and rectal surgery. Philadelphia: BC Decker; 1990. pp. 180–2.
33. Whitlow CB, Opelka FG, Gathright JB, and Beck DE. Treatment of colorectal and ileoanal anastomotic sinuses. Dis Colon Rectum. 1997;40:760–3.
34. Breen EM, Schoetz DJ, Marcello PW, Roberts PL, Coller JA, Murray JJ, and Rusin LC. Functional results after perineal complications of ileal pouch-anal anastomosis. Dis Colon Rectum. 1998;41:691–5.
35. Ozuner G, Hull T, Lee P, and Fazio VW. What happens to a pelvic pouch when a fistula develops? Dis Colon Rectum. 1997;40:543–7.
36. Remzi FH, Fazio VW, Oncel M, Baker ME, Church JM, Ooi BS, Connor JT, Preen M, and Einstein D. Portal vein thrombi after restorative proctocolectomy. Surgery. 2002;132;655–62.
37. Thompson-Fawcett MW, Jewell DP, and Mortensen NJ. Ileoanal reservoir dysfunction: a problem-solving approach. Br J Surg. 1997;84:1351–9.
38. Cohen Z, Smith D, and McLeod R. Reconstructive surgery for pelvic pouches. World J Surg. 1998;22:342–6.
39. Fazio VW, Wu JS, and Lavery IC. Repeat ileal pouch-anal anastomosis to salvage septic complications of pelvic pouches: clinical outcome and quality of life assessment. Ann Surg. 1998;228:588–97.
40. Dayton MT. Redo ileal pouch-anal anastomosis for malfunctioning pouches—acceptable alternative to permanent ileostomy? Am J Surg. 2000;180:561–565.
41. Ogunbiyi OA, Korsgen S, and Keighley MR. Pouch salvage. Long-term outcome. Dis Colon Rectum. 1997;40:548–52.
42. Gemlo BT, Wong DW, Rothenberger DA, and Goldberg SM. Ileal pouch-anal anastomosis: patterns of failure. Arch Surg. 1992;127:784–7.
43. Foley EF, Schoetz DJ, and Roberts PL. Rediversion after ileal pouch-anal anastomosis: causes of failures and predictors of subsequent pouch salvage. Dis Colon Rectum. 1995;38:793–8.
44. Simchuk EJ and Thirlby RC. Risk factors and true incidence of pouchitis in patients after ileal pouch-anal anastomoses. World J Surg. 2000;24:851–6.
45. Heuschen UA, Allemeyer EH, Hinz U, Autschback F, Uehlein T, Herfarth C, and Heuschen G. Diagnosing pouchitis: comparative validation of two scoring systems in routine follow-up. Dis Colon Rectum. 2002;45:776–88.
46. Meagher AP, Farouk R, and Dozois RR. J ileal pouch-anal anastomosis for chronic ulcerative colitis: complications and long-term outcome in 1310 patients. Br J Surg. 1998;85:800–3.
47. Stocchi L and Pemberton JH. Pouch and pouchitis. Gastroenterol Clin North Am. 2001;30:223–41.
48. Merrett MN, Soper N, Mortensen N, and Jewell DP. Intestinal permeability in the ileal pouch. Gut. 1996;39:226–30.
49. Shen B, Achkar JP, Lashner BA, Ormsby AH, Brzezinski A, Soffer EE, Remzi RH, Bevins CL, and Fazio VW. Irritable pouch syndrome: a new category of diagnosis for symptomatic patients with ileal pouch-anal anastomosis. Am J Gastroenterol. 2002;97:972–7.

Editorial Commentary

Dr. Hull is an alumnus of the Colorectal Residency Program at the Cleveland Clinic in Cleveland, Ohio, and is currently a staff member in that department. In her role in the Anorectal Physiology Laboratory, she is exposed to large numbers of patients referred to the laboratory with defaecation dysfunction after rectal resection with ileoanal anastomosis. Accordingly, in her chapter she brings a wealth of personal wisdom as a referral centre for this problem were she highlights that the amount of rectum resected is indeed in direct correlation with postoperative function or in fact dysfunction. She also has taken the opportunity in her chapter to highlight the fact that, when technically feasible, a colonic J-pouch is a far better reconstructive option than is a "straight coloanal" anastomosis. However, if a patient has been referred after straight anastomosis without a J-pouch, then a variety of therapeutic options exist. She also discusses the newer technique of coloplasty as well as ultimately some of the evacuatory problems noted after pelvic pouch surgery. Her chapter will certainly form a cornerstone for any surgeon who performs or manages patients who have had lower anastomoses for either the colon or the small bowel to the rectum or anus.

SW

Chapter 9.2
Evaluation and Management of Postoperative Fecal Incontinence

HOMAYOON AKBARI and MITCHELL BERNSTEIN

Introduction

Fecal incontinence—or the involuntary loss of gas, liquid, or solid stool—can result in a significantly reduced quality of life. The prevalence of fecal incontinence in the general population has been estimated to be 2.2%, with much higher rates in the elderly and nursing-home populations (1,2). The diagnosis and subsequent management of these patients is often difficult, requiring extensive physical, physiologic, and anatomic assessment prior to the initiation of therapy. An overview of the anatomy and physiology of continence and a detailed discussion of the etiology, diagnosis, and management of postoperative fecal incontinence follows. This chapter should be read in conjunction with the overview of fecal incontinence. (Chapter 7.1).

Anatomy and Physiology

Anal continence is dependent upon a complex interaction of many factors. Whereas the musculature of the pelvic floor and anal sphincters is critical to the maintenance of fecal continence, stool volume and consistency, the reservoir function of the rectum, sensory and motor innervation of the anorectum, along with reflex and ascending neural pathways, all have a role.

The integrity of the anal sphincters is essential to the maintenance of anal continence. The internal anal sphincter (IAS) is a thickening of the circular smooth muscle of the rectum within the anal canal. The IAS is responsible for approximately 80% of the resting tone of the anal canal and is tonically contracted. The IAS is under the control of the autonomic nervous system, with excitatory sympathetic innervation from the hypogastric plexus and inhibitory parasympathetic innervation from the sacral parasympathetic nerves (nervi erigentes). Under resting conditions, the basal tone of the IAS prevents the passage of gas and stool. When rectal distension occurs, the rectoanal inhibitory reflex (RAIR) is initiated via the sacral parasympathetic nerves. This allows for relaxation of the IAS and the passage of stool. If defecation does not occur, then the IAS will regain tone during rectal accommodation.

The external anal sphincter (EAS) is comprised of striated muscle that surrounds the anal canal. The EAS comprises three muscles: the subcutaneous, superficial, and deep portions. It has been proposed that the EAS can be considered to be continuous with the puborectalis superiorly (3). Innervation of the external sphincter is from the somatic nervous system via the inferior rectal branch of the internal pudendal nerve. In addition, motor innervation to the EAS may be supplied by the perineal branch of S4. While the EAS contributes only 20% of resting tone, it is responsible for maximal voluntary control. Rectal distension results in an involuntary contraction of the EAS, as does increased intra-abdominal pressure, such as during a Valsalva procedure (4). Voluntary contraction of the EAS can be maintained for 45 to 60 seconds before fatigue sets in, during which time rectal accommodation and increased compliance of the colon diminish afferent output to the spinal cord defecation reflex center, resulting in a decreased urge to defecate and return of basal IAS tone.

In addition to the sphincter apparatus, the integrity of the pelvic floor musculature plays a critical role in maintaining continence. The pelvic floor comprises the levator ani muscle, which in turn can be subdivided into its component muscles—the ischiococcygeus, iliococcygeus, pubococcygeus, and puborectalis. The levators extend from the pubic bone to the ischial spine, originating from the arcus tendineus of the obturator fascia. The levator hiatus, through which the vagina, urethra, and rectum pass, is found between the two limbs of the pubococcygeus. During defecation, contraction of the levator ani elevates the pelvic floor and widens the levator hiatus. The puborectalis—the inferior most portion of the levator complex—forms a sling around the rectum, which acts to pull the anorectal junction anteriorly, creating the anorectal angle. During defecation, the puborectalis relaxes, thereby widening and straightening the anorectal angle. Innervation to the levator complex is via the S2–4 sacral roots, as well as the perineal branch of the pudendal nerve. The puborectalis is innervated by the inferior rectal branch of the pudendal nerve. A recent study demonstrated the significance of levator ani contraction in incontinent patients. Poor levator ani contraction was found to have a strong relation to the severity of incontinence and to be predictive of response to treatment (5).

Etiology of Fecal Incontinence

Fecal incontinence may result from a disturbance in any of the aforementioned factors. Thus, incontinence may result from direct injury to the sphincter complex or pelvic floor musculature, autonomic or somatic neuropathy, or loss of an adequate rectal reservoir.

Post-surgical fecal incontinence is most often the result of injury to the anal sphincters during anorectal surgery. Endoanal sonography has demonstrated that approximately 50% of patients have sphincter defects following anorectal surgery; of these patients, 70% to 75% do not complain of anal incontinence. However, in those patients who do complain of postoperative incontinence, sphincter defects are identified in virtually all cases (6,7). The surgical management of anal fistulas, fissures, and hemorrhoids may all result in postoperative fecal incontinence (8).

The highest incidence of postoperative fecal incontinence follows surgery for anal fistulas (7). Inappropriate division of the external and internal sphincters, particularly in high trans-sphincteric fistulas, is the most frequent cause of incontinence following anal surgery. In one large retrospective study, 45% of patients experienced some degree of anal incontinence following fistula surgery (9). Fistulas that are at a particularly high risk for fecal incontinence following fistulotomy are those with posterior midline internal openings, high trans-sphincteric fistulas, and those with secondary tracts or extensions (10). In females, primary fistulotomy for anterior fistulas predisposes to incontinence due to the relatively shorter sphincter anteriorly. While primary fistulotomy is most often the cause of incontinence, "seton fistulotomy" can result in functional continence disturbance. Cutting setons in the management of high trans-sphincteric fistulas have long been shown to be associated with a relatively high rate (44%–63%) of anal incontinence (11,12).

Internal anal sphincterotomy in the management of fissure in ano also may result in some degree of anal incontinence (13). The IAS is not responsible for voluntary control; therefore, its division does not typically result in total anal incontinence. More commonly, with its role in maintaining 80% of the resting anal tone, excessive division of the IAS typically results in gas incontinence and fecal soiling or staining. Nyam and Pemberton reported a 33% incidence of such symptoms in men and a 53% incidence in women in the immediate post-sphincterotomy period. Long term, the same authors reported that 6% of patients suffered from gas incontinence, 8% fecal soiling, and 1% incontinence for solid stool (14). While a 6% to 10% rate of incontinence to flatus, stool, or both, generally is quoted following internal sphincterotomy, a wide range (1.5%–35%) has been noted by others (15,16). Posterior and anterior midline sphincterotomies yield a higher rate of incontinence than do lateral internal sphincterotomies, as they typically cause a keyhole deformity. Such a deformity permits the leakage of liquid stool and the involuntary passage of gas. For this reason, the use of the midline sphincterotomy should be condemned and has been largely abandoned.

To minimize the chance of creating postoperative incontinence, the amount of IAS divided should be limited. In our practice, the length of the fissure is used as a guide, dividing as much internal sphincter as the fissure is long. Although the lateral internal sphincterotomy remains the "gold standard" by which the efficacy of other therapies, including topical nitroglycerin and botulinum toxin injections, is measured, we try to avoid its use in young women of childbearing age. Such women are susceptible to sphincter injury—overt or occult—at the time of vaginal delivery; combined with a prior sphincterotomy, incontinence may result. The importance of the IAS in continence function has been highlighted recently (17,18). It has been shown previously that in patients with demonstrated EAS atrophy, recovery of IAS function (i.e., recovery of the rectoanal inhibitory wave) is more rapid than in controls or patients with chronic constipation, suggesting an inherent importance in intrinsic IAS function for the production of continence (19,20). Moreover, it has been shown that the constitutive coronal length of the subcutaneous EAS, which normally overlaps the termination of the IAS, may be deficient in some patients with chronic anal fissures, implying that internal anal sphincterotomy may render the distal anal canal relatively unsupported in these patients, resulting in soiling (21). Zbar et al. also have shown recently that deliberate IAS preservation in cutting seton use for high trans-sphincteric fistula-in-ano (by rerouting the seton through the intersphincteric space) may be associated with improved postoperative function (22). Each of these findings shows an important place for IAS preservation in the avoidance of incontinence—a finding confirmed if endoanal distraction is avoided during perineal surgery (23,24).

Hemorrhoidectomy likewise may have a deleterious effect on sphincter function and anal continence. Anal incontinence following hemorrhoidectomy has been shown to correlate with sonographic evidence of internal, external, or combined sphincter defects (25). More recently, endoanal sonography has been used to study the sphincter complex following "stapled" hemorrhoidectomy. Sonographic evidence of IAS fragmentation following stapled hemorrhoidectomy was seen in 15% of patients, all of whom were asymptomatic (26). Although no functional effects were seen six months following surgery in a separate study, long-term effects on continence remain to be seen (27). Patients who develop an ectropion following hemorrhoid surgery often will complain of incontinence. In fact, an ectropion results in the classic "wet" anus, in which patients have constant staining from the exposed anal mucosa without true fecal incontinence. This issue is complex. In some cases, there is clearly sphincter damage at the time of hemorrhoidectomy; in others, perirectal sepsis can cause destructive sphincter atrophy (25). In other studies, there may be no sphincter damage at all and the incontinence is a subtle distortion of IAS dysfunction, perhaps accentuating preexisting low anal pressures that are observed with substantial hemorrhoidal prolapse (8).

Among females, the leading cause of sphincter dysfunction is obstetrical trauma. Indeed, the rate of fecal incontinence is eight times greater in women, reflecting the incidence of incontinence following pregnancy and vaginal delivery (28). Sphincter lacerations are not always apparent at the time of delivery. Sphincter injury not clinically evident at the time of delivery, but sonographically evident, has been shown to be predictive of incontinence three months post partum (29). In addition, up to 44% of multiparous women who are asymptomatic have occult sphincter lacerations documented by endoanal sonography (30).

Postobstetric fecal incontinence is not solely related to damage to the sphincter complex sustained during delivery; instead, it is often multifactorial. Structural damage to the sphincter complex may be coupled with pudendal neuropathy and pelvic floor dysfunction. The latter of these two manifest more commonly in multiparous women and in older patients. In a large study in which 949 women were assessed after childbirth, 3.1% were found to be incontinent of stool and 25% of flatus three months after childbirth (31). Sphincter lacerations were highest in primiparous women, women who had median episiotomies, and those with forceps or vacuum delivery. Birth weight was not predictive of sphincter injury.

Pudendal neuropathy—a known complication of pregnancy and vaginal delivery—also contributes to post-partum fecal incontinence (32,33). Although transient in most women, persistent alterations in motor latencies have been noted (34). Risk factors for pudendal nerve damage include multiparity, forceps delivery, and increased duration of the second stage of labor (35). Sphincter lacerations combined with a pudendal neuropathy cause a decrease in resting and squeeze pressures (33–37), which manifest as fecal incontinence.

Diagnosis

History and Physical Examination

The evaluation of the incontinent patient should always start with a detailed history and physical examination. Although many patients have difficulty discussing incontinence issues due to the societal taboos surrounding it, a thorough history can be obtained with gentle and direct questioning. The onset of incontinence should be established and a history of antecedent anorectal or gynecological surgery obtained. A detailed obstetric history should be obtained from female patients, including the number of vaginal deliveries, associated sphincter injuries, duration of labor(s), and use of episiotomies and/or instrumentation during delivery. The degree of incontinence (i.e., gas, liquid stool, and/or solid stool) and any progression of symptoms should be addressed. Sensation of passing stool should be assessed, as it may indicate a neurogenic component to the incontinence, particularly in the older or diabetic patient. The Cleveland Clinic Florida has developed an incontinence scoring system that may be useful in objectifying the subjective history (38). The effects of incontinence on the patient's quality of life should be investigated, as this may guide the nature of future intervention.

Physical examination should start with a complete inspection of the anus and perineum. Scars from previous surgeries should be noted. Gentle spreading of the buttocks may demonstrate a patulous anus, perineal body disruption, or attenuation. Any mucosal ectropion or Whitehead and keyhole deformities should be noted. Any palpable defects in the sphincter are noted on digital rectal examination. Resting tone is noted and the patient should be asked to squeeze on the examining finger to assess motion of the sphincter complex and the squeeze pressure generated. In female patients, a bi-digital examination allows for a more accurate assessment of the perineal body.

Endoanal Ultrasound

Endoanal ultrasound provides excellent visualization of the internal and external anal sphincters and is an invaluable tool in the evaluation of patients suffering from fecal incontinence. Isolated or combined internal and/or external anal sphincter injuries can be assessed. Although the accuracy of endoluminal ultrasound is user dependent, excellent correlation with pathological findings has been reported with experienced users (39).

In addition to identifying defects, sonographically documented sphincter injuries have been shown to correlate with the severity of symptoms (40). Men with sphincter defects on ultrasound have been shown to have worse sphincter function and to be less likely to respond to nonoperative therapy compared with women with fecal incontinence and no sphincter defect on ultrasound (41).

In our laboratory, we use the 3535 ultrasound scanner from B & K Medical. The 1850 probe with a 360-degree rotating 10-megahertz (MHz) transducer attached offers the best resolution of the sphincter complex. The ultrasound probe is used to image the entire anal canal. The probe is inserted to the level of the upper anal canal, identified by the U-shaped puborectalis muscle, which is visualized as a mixed echogenicity structure lateral and posterior to the anal canal. Then the probe is withdrawn slowly while imaging the internal and external anal sphincters. The IAS is seen as a uniform hypoechoic inner ring at the level of the mid anal canal. The EAS appears as a broad ring of mixed echodensity surrounding the hypoechoic internal sphincter (Figure 9.2.1). The EAS is usually thinner anteriorly. In women, visualization of the anterior sphincter may be enhanced by digital pressure applied to the posterior vaginal wall (Figure 9.2.2). As the probe is withdrawn into the distal anal canal, the IAS is no longer visualized.

In patients with postoperative fecal incontinence, defects of either the IAS, EAS, or both may be seen on endoanal sonography. Following fistulotomy, defects in both the internal and external anal sphincters are usually visualized (Figure 9.2.3). Isolated IAS defects are seen following hemorrhoid surgery, anal dilation procedures, and sphincterotomies.

Magnetic Resonance Imaging

Magnetic resonance imaging (MRI) of the anal canal is possible with both surface phased-array coils and with an endocoil. More detailed studies are

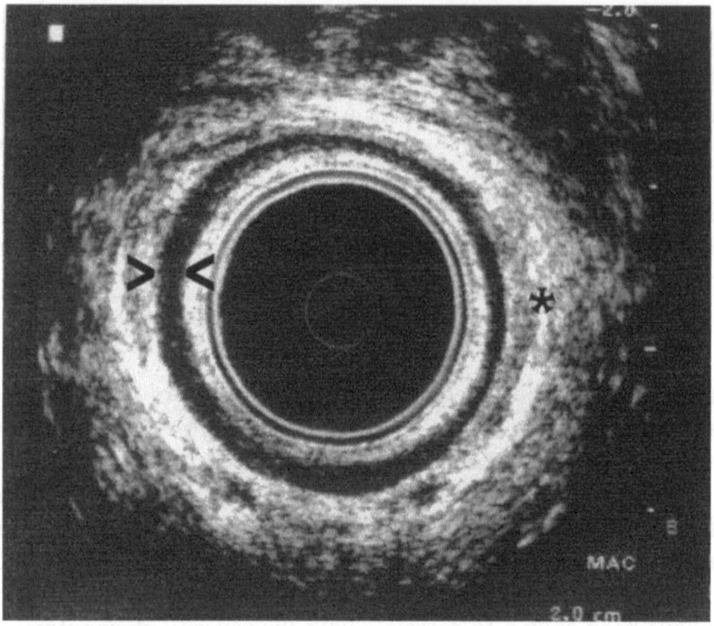

FIGURE 9.2.1. Endoanal ultrasound of the mid anal canal. The IAS is visualized as a continuous hypoechoic ring (marked by two arrow heads). The mixed echogenic thicker external sphincter is marked by the asterisk.

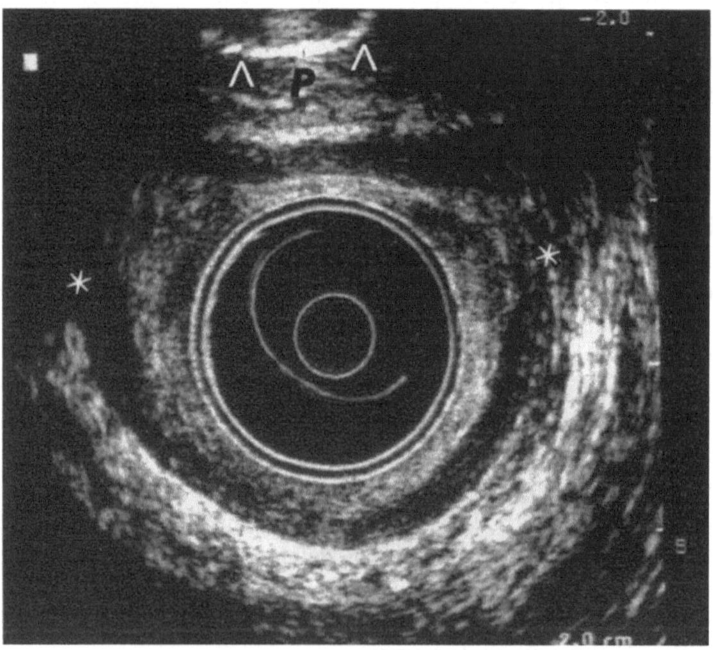

FIGURE 9.2.2. Endoanal ultrasound image of a large postobstetric injury. The ends of the sphincter are marked by asterisks. The perineal body (P) and anterior scar are better visualized with the examiners digit (marked by arrowheads) in the distal vagina.

possible with endoanal coils (42). Whereas more anatomically detailed studies may be possible with MRI, there are conflicting reports comparing endoanal ultrasound with MRI (43–45). Generally, the IAS is less-well visualized on MRI, whereas the EAS is better visualized. Magnetic resonance of the anal canal to image the sphincter complex is used in our practice on the rare occasion when adequate sphincter imaging is not possible with endoanal sonography.

Anal Manometry

Anorectal manometry is used to quantify objectively the pressures generated the length of the anal canal, as well as to assess the integrity of the anorectal sensory response. In our laboratory, we use an eight-channel water-perfused catheter, with each channel connected to a pressure transducer. The channels are staggered at 0.5-centimeter intervals and arranged in a radial array. The catheter is manually withdrawn in 0.5-centimeter intervals and resting and squeeze pressures along the entire length of the anal canal are recorded. Resting pressures are reflective of IAS function,

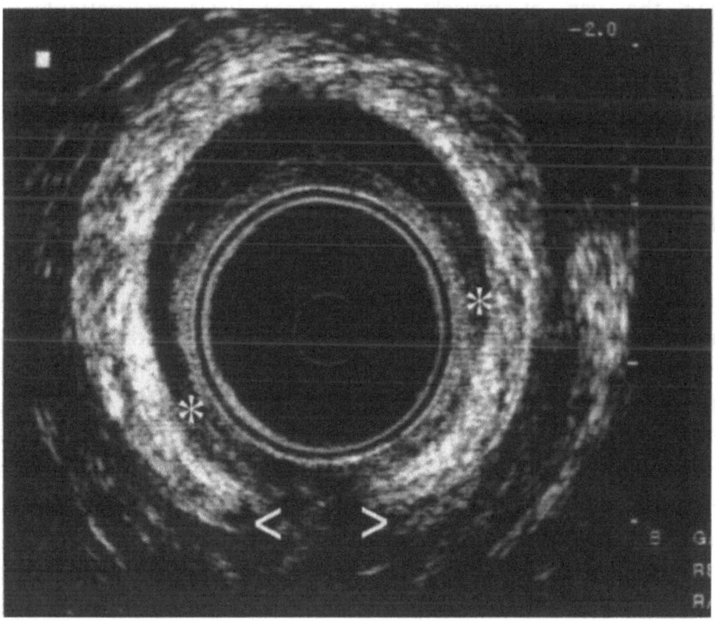

FIGURE 9.2.3. Endoanal ultrasound image of the mid anal canal in a male with fecal incontinence following a posterior fistulotomy. Defect in external sphincter is marked by arrowheads. The internal sphincter has retracted (ends marked with asterisks) and bunched anteriorly.

whereas active squeeze pressures measure EAS function. Thus, isolated EAS injury is characterized by low squeeze pressures and near-normal resting pressures, whereas the opposite is seen in isolated IAS injury (46). The effective length of the anal canal—often referred to as the high-pressure zone (HPZ)—is also measured. The anorectal sensory response [rectoanal inhibitory reflex (RAIR)] is documented by insufflating a balloon within the rectum and monitoring for a drop in the resting pressure. Other catheter/probe systems include solid-state probes with micro-transducers, which directly measure pressure without the hydrostatic interface, or balloon catheters, where the resting and squeeze pressures are measured with an inner and outer balloon.

Anal manometry has been shown to correlate well with ultrasound studies. In one large study examining postobstetric incontinence, reduced squeeze pressures were seen in patients with isolated external and combined internal and external anal sphincter defects. Reduced resting pressures also were recorded in patients with combined defects, but no pressure changes were noted in isolated IAS defects (47). Reduced resting—but not squeeze pressures—is more likely to reflect post-surgical incontinence following fistula surgery (48). While the prospective function of physiology testing remains debatable, the use of preoperative anal manometry has been shown to improve the functional outcome in fistula surgery by decreasing the use of muscle-cutting procedures in patients with sphincter dysfunction (49). While low pressures may be associated with functional incontinence, it should be noted that both resting and squeeze pressures decrease with age, particularly in women with no functional deficit (50,51).

Pudendal Nerve Terminal Motor Latency

The pudendal nerve supplies motor innervation to the EAS and puborectalis. Pudendal nerve terminal motor latency (PNTML) measures conduction time from the ischial spine to the anal verge. The study is performed using a stimulating and recording electrode on the index finger. The index finger is inserted in the anal canal and the pudendal nerve is stimulated at the level of the ischial spine. The recording electrode is located at the base of the finger and records external sphincter contraction. The time between stimulation and contraction is then calculated. Normal PNTML is 2.0 ± 0.2 milliseconds. In the postoperative incontinent patient, increased PNTML is seen following obstetrical injury and in older individuals with perineal descent or rectal prolapse. Prolonged latencies are seen in 70% of patients with fecal incontinence (52), and a pudendal neuropathy combined with abnormal manometry is associated more often with solid stool incontinence compared to leakage in patients with no neuropathy (53). A normal PNTML study has been shown to be a predictor of a good functional result following sphincteroplasty (54).

Treatment

The treatment of fecal incontinence should be directed by the etiology, severity of incontinence, and degree to which the patient's quality of life is diminished. Patients with multiple co-morbidities, those who wish to avoid surgery, and patients with mild incontinence (i.e., leakage of liquid stool) may be managed medically with dietary modifications. In addition, patients awaiting operative intervention and undergoing testing may benefit from medical intervention prior to their definitive procedure. Medical treatments include dietary modifications to produce firmer, bulkier stool, decreasing gastrointestinal (GI) motility with pharmacological agents, the use of enemas and bowel regimen management, and biofeedback. Many of these issues are discussed in other chapters in this book. Surgical treatment consists of either operations aimed at repair of the sphincter or operations aimed at replacement of the sphincter with endogenous or exogenous tissues. Finally, at the extreme of operative management is diversion with colostomy.

Medical Management

Dietary Modifications and Anti Diarrheals

Dietary modification should start with limiting or eliminating foods that encourage loose or frequent bowel movements. Many patients at the time of presentation have already learned to avoid these foods, which include caffeine, fruit juices, and certain vegetables. Diarrhea or loose stools may increase the severity of incontinence, particularly in the elderly patient. This may be caused by medications, including cholesterol-lowering drugs and certain cardiac medications such as digitalis. Food intolerance such as gluten sensitivity and lactose intolerance also may be contributing factors. A careful review of medication history and testing for food intolerance may benefit these patients.

The use of fiber supplements designed to make the stool firmer and bulkier, and therefore easier to control, may be helpful, particularly in patients with leakage of liquid stool. Although there are no studies directly examining the use of bulking agents in fecal incontinence, there is much anecdotal evidence. We use commercially available polycarbophil tablets (FiberCon; Wyeth Pharmaceuticals, Collegeville, Pennsylvania). Patients are instructed to titrate the number of pills to achieve an acceptable balance between relief of symptoms and constipation. Powder and pill preparations of methylcellulose and psyllium also are available and may be used.

Bowel regimen management can be employed along with dietary modifications to permit bowel evacuation at a socially acceptable time. Suppositories and enemas may be used to stimulate rectal evacuation at an acceptable time, allowing the patient more freedom. Typically, patients will empty themselves prior to leaving the house, thereby decreasing the chances of an accident. Oral laxatives are not beneficial because of the unpredictability as to when the laxative effect will be achieved.

Anti-diarrheals may be useful in dehydrating the stool and in slowing colonic transit. Dehydrating agents such as kaolin/pectin act by absorbing excess fluid. Colonic transit is decreased with opiate derivatives such as loperamide (Imodium; McNeil Consumer Healthcare, Fort Washington, PA) and diphenoxylate-atropine (Lomotil; Searle, Chicago, IL), codeine, and tincture of opium. Loperamide has been shown to decrease the frequency of incontinence and increase basal sphincter tone by a direct agonist action (55,56). Similar effects on sphincter tone have not been noted with diphenoxylate atropine. Given its dual action on sphincter tone and colonic transit, the over-the-counter loperamide is our first-line drug in patients with fecal incontinence, especially with liquid seepage. Patients may be started on a prophylactic dose of loperamide, or its use may be intermittent, with use prior to social events or leaving the house.

Biofeedback

Biofeedback therapy, first introduced by Kegel over a half century ago to strengthen the perineal musculature (57), is an attractive option for the management of fecal incontinence in the motivated patient. Patients with some intact anorectal sensation and contractility of the EAS are most ideally suited to biofeedback therapy. Biofeedback consists of a six- to eight-week course of intensive training with a biofeedback therapist utilizing either manometry with rectal distension or manometry and electromyography (EMG) without rectal distension to strengthen the anal sphincter and its response to rectal distension. Repetitive exercise of the EAS with visual and/or audio feedback results in increased muscle strength and control. Therapy using rectal distention permits for a learned increase in sphincter tone in response to rectal filling. Response rates of 65% to 75% have been reported in a meta-analysis examining both coordination training and strength training (58). Success with biofeedback has been shown to be independent of patient age, initial severity of symptoms, etiology of incontinence, and the results of physiology testing (59). The use of newer home biofeedback units may improve long-term effects.

Surgical Management

Sphincter Repair

Sphincter repair is possible in patients with a localized sphincter defect in which either direct apposition or an overlapping sphincteroplasty permits re-approximation of the functional sphincter. Sphincter repair is best done at the time of injury if recognized, such as after obstetrical injury. However, sphincter repair may be performed months or years after injury, although functional outcomes after apposition or overlapping repair of an atrophied muscle may be disappointing.

Primary repair of a defect recognized at the time of injury may be performed with either direct apposition or an overlapping sphincteroplasty. Most obstetric injuries recognized at the time of delivery are repaired with an end-to-end apposition of the muscle. Up to 50% of women experience some degree of anal incontinence and have sonographic evidence of a sphincter defect following these repairs (60). Primary overlapping repairs have been reported to have more favorable outcomes (61); however, this has recently been challenged in a large randomized study in which no functional difference between the two repairs was noted (62).

Delayed primary and secondary repair of sphincter injuries are most commonly repaired by overlapping sphincteroplasty. Preoperatively, the patient is given a mechanical bowel preparation and an enema the morning of surgery. The patient is positioned in the prone jack-knife position, with the buttocks taped apart, and a curvilinear incision is made, usually anteriorly for obstetric injuries, although it may be made posteriorly for defects secondary to anorectal surgery. Then the anoderm is elevated off of the underlying sphincter and scar. The sphincter is then mobilized, proximally to the anorectal ring and laterally to the mid lateral line. For posterior repairs, lateral mobilization is limited due to the posterolateral location of the pudendal nerves as they enter the sphincter complex. Once the sphincter has been mobilized, the scar is divided with preservation of scar tissue for future suture placement. The two ends are then overlapped and secured with 2-0 absorbable horizontal mattress sutures. The buttock tapes are released prior to suturing to permit a more accurate assessment of the repair, which should accommodate a fingertip comfortably. The muscle ends should be under minimal tension when overlapped and excessive tension indicates inadequate mobilization of the sphincter muscle. We include an anterior levatorplasty to our sphincter repair procedures, although this is controversial. The mobilized sphincter is retracted posteriorly by gentle traction on the sutures—which are left uncut and tagged—and the levators are approximated with 2-0 absorbable sutures. All suture ends are then cut. The incision in the anoderm is left open unless a perineal reconstruction is necessary. In our experience, the closed space is prone to infection, which can jeopardize the sphincter repair.

Functional improvement can be expected in 65% to 90% of patients following an overlapping sphincteroplasty (63,64). Subjectively, excellent to good results may be expected in 50% to 75% of patients (65,66). The long-term outcomes of sphincteroplasty recently have been called into question. Halverson and Hull have reported that 54% of patients were incontinent to liquid or solid stool at a mean follow-up of 69 months following sphincteroplasty (67). Poor outcomes are associated with EAS atrophy [(68) predictable by preoperative endoanal MRI or by three-dimensional (3D) reconstructed endoanal sonography] and by previous repairs. Pudendal neuropathy has been reported to be predictive of poor functional outcome following anterior overlapping sphincteroplasty (69), although this has been debated in more recent studies (70).

Isolated IAS injuries that result in disabling fecal soiling and leakage are notoriously difficult to repair owing to the thin nature of the IAS muscle. Dissection and manipulation often result in more damage to the muscle. Once mobilized, overlapping of the muscle has not traditionally yielded improvements in symptoms, as the repair rarely holds up (71).

We have recently developed an operative procedure for patients with incapacitating fecal soilage and an isolated IAS injury. Our operative approach to such injuries begins with a full mechanical bowel preparation. The patient is brought to the operating room and placed in the prone jack-knife position with the buttocks taped apart. With a large Hill–Ferguson retractor placed into the anal canal, the defect in the IAS is readily palpable. A curvilinear incision is made just distal to the intersphincteric groove. The incision extends laterally to beyond the defect and to where the IAS is felt to be present. This often requires an incision involving close to half the circumference of the anal canal. A flap of mucosa and submucosa is raised for four to five centimeters. The two ends of the retracted IAS are clearly identified. The buttock tapes are released and a layered closure of the defect is employed. Two and sometimes three layers are generally needed to bring the IAS together in a tension-free repair (Figures 9.2.4 and 9.2.5). The patients are maintained on a bowel regimen that includes stool softeners for up to one month postoperatively.

To date, we have performed this "internal anal sphincteroplasty" on 16 patients with favorable results (results unpublished). The most common etiology of isolated IAS injury in our patients was an internal sphinctero-tomy, with fistulotomy the next most common cause. Ten patients had significant improvement in their incontinence score and symptoms, two had modest improvement in both incontinence score and symptoms, and four had no improvement.

Muscle Transposition

In patients with large defects that are not amenable to sphincteroplasty, a muscle encirclement procedure may be used. Thiersch first proposed the use of an encirclement device in the nineteenth century for the treatment of rectal prolapse. Several decades later, the use of muscle-encircling procedures was introduced with the gluteus muscle transposition procedure.

Gluteus Muscle Transposition

The gluteus muscle is a broad muscle that originates from the ilium, sacrum, and coccyx, and inserts into the iliotibial band of the femur. Its primary function is in extension and lateral rotation of the hip; however, it is also acts as an accessory muscle for voluntary control of evacuation. The inferior portion of the gluteus muscle on each side is mobilized through

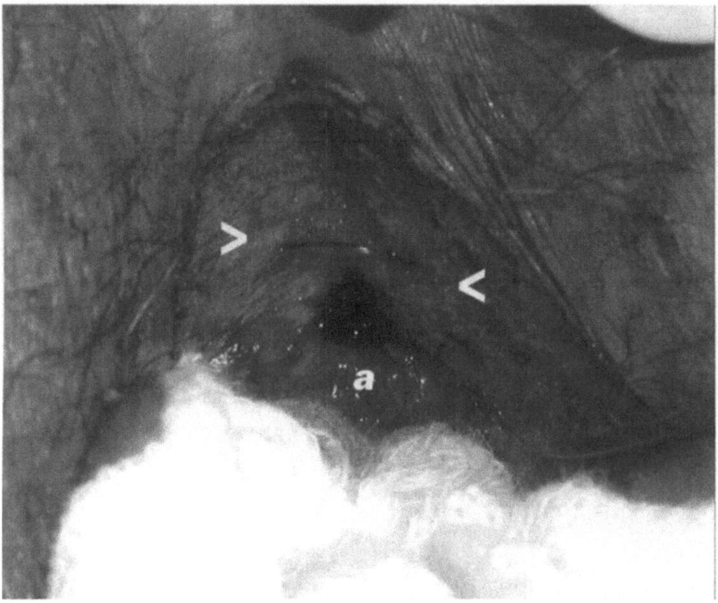

FIGURE 9.2.4. Intraoperative photograph demonstrating defect in internal sphincter between arrowheads. Initial suture of first layer of internal sphincteroplasty can be seen. Anal mucosal flap (a) is being retracted by an assistant.

bilateral oblique incisions and detached from its sacrococcygeal origin. The inferior gluteal artery and nerve are carefully preserved as the muscle is mobilized laterally. The resultant mobilized muscle will have a superior and inferior limb with the attached fascia. Two lateral perianal curvilinear incisions are made and subcutaneous tunnels are created around the anus. The two limbs of the gluteus muscle are then passed through these tunnels on each side, overlapped, and sutured together. All wounds are primarily closed. The gluteus muscle transposition procedure has resulted in good outcomes in 60% of patients (72,73). Following gluteus muscle transposition, Pearl et al. reported manometric increases in squeeze but not resting pressures (74). In spite of an increase in squeeze pressures, only two of seven patients were continent to liquid stool.

Gracilis Muscle Transposition

The use of the gracilis muscle to encircle the anal canal and treat fecal incontinence was first described by Pickrell and coworkers in 1952 (75). The gracilis muscle—part of the adductor group of thigh muscles—is a superficial muscle on the medial aspect of the thigh that arises from the inferior ramus of the pubis and ischium and inserts into the upper tibia below the tibial tuberosity. The procedure involves mobilization of the muscle in the thigh through three incisions (76). More recently, this mobilization has been

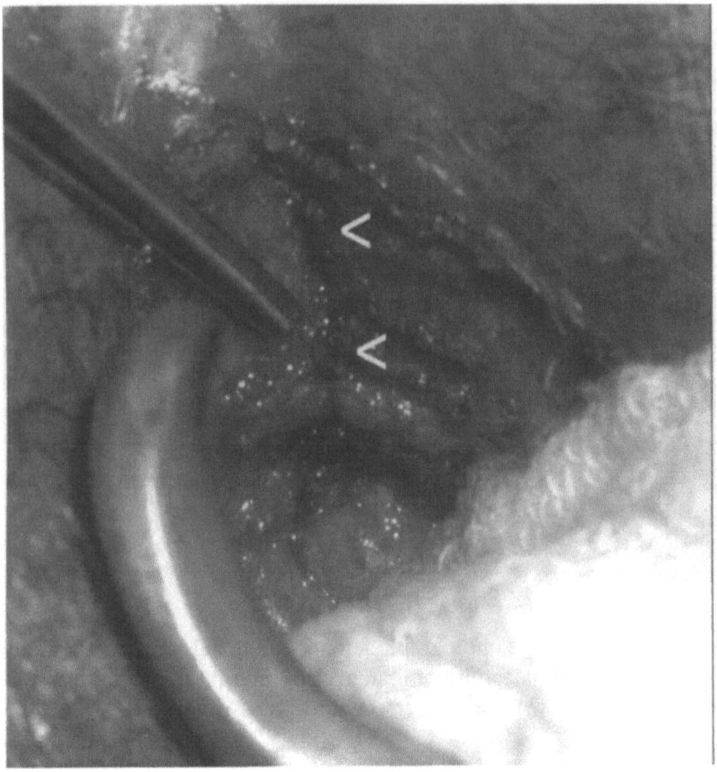

FIGURE 9.2.5. Intraoperative photograph demonstrating approximated internal sphincter following internal anal sphincteroplasty. The suture line is marked by arrowhead.

performed with the aid of an endoscope providing limited skin incisions (77). The mobilization is continued distally and the tendinous insertion is divided. The divided muscle is then delivered through the upper thigh incision with its proximal neurovascular bundle intact. Two curvilinear incisions are made anterior and posterior to the anus and an extrasphincteric tunnel encircling the anal canal is created. The muscle is tunneled from the upper thigh incision and is wrapped around the anal canal and sutured with non-absorbable sutures to the contralateral ischial tuberosity. To avoid a "loose wrap," the thigh from which the muscle was harvested is placed in the adducted position prior to suturing the tendon to the ischial tuberosity. All incisions are closed primarily.

Good functional results with continence to liquid and solid stool have been reported in 50% of patients immediately following gracilis muscle transposition. These results appear to hold up over time, where Corman reported excellent results in seven of 14 patients at five years of follow-up (78).

Dynamic Graciloplasty (See Chapter 10.2)

The gracilis muscle is a fast-twitch skeletal muscle with predominately type II fibers compared with the EAS, which has a predominance of type I fatigue-resistant muscle fibers. Active contraction of the EAS to control the passage of stool is possible with "adduction"; however, sustained contractions are not possible. As such, the EAS is not able to compensate fully for the loss of sustained contractions with muscle loss or injury. Animal studies have demonstrated that chronic low-frequency stimulation of fast-twitch muscles can convert them into fatigue-resistant slow-twitch muscles. Baeten first reported the use of chronic stimulation to improve functional outcome following graciloplasty (79). The ability to use the gracilis muscle to create a dynamic neosphincter has renewed interest in its use in patients with fecal incontinence. An electrical stimulator is implanted subcutaneously in the anterior abdominal wall and connected to an implanted electrode attached either to the main nerve of the muscle or the muscle itself in proximity to the nerve. The stimulator continually stimulates the muscle with low frequency to convert it into a slow-twitch muscle. Once transformation of the muscle has occurred, the stimulator can be reprogrammed to a high-frequency stimulator to permit tonic contraction of the gracilis neosphincter. The stimulator can be turned off with a hand-held remote to permit evacuation. Following dynamic graciloplasty, Baeten et al. reported a 73% success rate in restoring continence in 52 patients (80). A recent large multicenter trial with 115 patients recently reported success—defined as a greater than 50% decrease in frequency of incontinent episodes—in 62% of patients (81).

Dynamic graciloplasty results in a functionally more physiologic neosphincter than either the non-dynamic gracilis or gluteus muscle transposition procedures. However, like its predecessors, the procedure has a high morbidity. Postoperative complications include wound seromas, muscle tendon rupture, perineal sepsis, stimulator malfunction, electrode displacement, and fecal impaction. Given the high morbidity and disfigurement, we have abandoned dynamic graciloplasty as an operative option in fecal incontinence. Patients who have large defects or a combined neuropathy and sphincter injury and are not suitable candidates for a sphincter repair procedure are offered the artificial bowel sphincter.

Artificial Bowel Sphincter (See Chapter 10.3)

For more than 25 years, artificial urinary sphincters have been used with good success for the treatment of urinary incontinence. In 1987, Christiansen and Lorentzen (82) implanted a urinary sphincter around the anus in a patient with severe fecal incontinence with the intention of restoring continence through an active and controllable device. Since then, two types of artificial sphincters have been used to treat patients with severe fecal incontinence. A modification of the AMS 800 urinary sphincter (AMS,

Minneapolis, MN) was used until 1996, at which time the artificial bowel sphincter (ABS) (AMS, Minneapolis, MN) became available and has since been the device of choice for implantation. Results have been largely favorable, with an overall initial success rate of around 75%. The most common complications encountered in the initial experiences included device erosion, infection, and mechanical failures in one of the three components of the device. The Acticon Neosphincter has a fluid-filled silicone cuff that is placed around the anal canal, a reservoir balloon that is placed in the space of Retzius, and a control pump that is placed in the scrotum or labia. The control pump is squeezed nine to twelve times to deflate the cuff, permitting evacuation. The cuff passively refills from the balloon reservoir, once again establishing continence.

Initial reports on the safety and efficacy of the ABS reported success rates of 70% to 75% with complication rates of 30% to 45% (83,84). In a recent large North American trial, 112 patients had the Acticon Neosphincter implanted. Patients were evaluated at six and twelve months following implantation, where 46% of the patients required revisional surgery, 37% required removal of the device, but where 85% of patients with the device in place at twelve months had a successful outcome (85). The artificial anal sphincter may significantly enhance quality of life in patients with anal incontinence. Complications include evacuation difficulties, infection, and cuff erosion. Because of the high morbidity and complication rates, patient selection is critical to a successful outcome. The Food and Drug Administration approved the Acticon Neosphincter in 2001 for use in adults with intractable fecal incontinence.

Conclusion

Fecal incontinence severely affects patients' quality of life. The management of patients with postoperative incontinence is a difficult challenge, but also a rewarding one. Postoperative fecal incontinence is seen most frequently following inappropriate division of the sphincter muscles during fistulotomy or following obstetrical trauma. A thorough history and examination, along with physiological and radiographic studies, allows for accurate diagnosis and targeted therapy. A detailed discussion with the patient on the expected outcomes and complications is essential in avoiding unrealistic expectations and disappointments. Therapies range from minor dietary modifications to the implantation of artificial sphincters. Patients with co-morbidities or patients who do not wish to undergo surgery are managed medically, with dietary modification, and, where appropriate, biofeedback therapy. Many patients are able to achieve adequate control over their incontinence and resume active lifestyles.

Patients who are considered for surgery should undergo appropriate testing in an anorectal physiology laboratory. The selective use of endoanal ultrasonography, anorectal manometry, and PNTML testing are invaluable in the evaluation of these patients. Sonography helps to localize the site of injury, which may not always be palpable as a defect on examination. Manometry permits quantification of remaining sphincter function and the effective length of the sphincter. Pudendal nerve testing helps predict functional outcome following surgery.

Sphincter injuries are best managed by overlapping sphincteroplasty. Patients with intact pudendal nerves fare better than those with a neuropathy. While most often discussed in the context of anterior sphincter injuries, it can be employed successfully with posterior injuries. Isolated internal sphincter injuries can result in significant seepage of liquid stool. They are difficult to manage given the anatomy of the muscle. We have recently developed a layered internal sphincteroplasty at our institution, which has had good preliminary results. Here, it is potentially possible that isolated IAS injury may increase in incidence with the introduction of newer less-extensive operative day-case procedures for hemorrhoids where no attempt is made to separate the sphincter muscle from the submucosal venous plexus. In these procedures, including Ligasure hemorrhoidectomy and endoanal stapled mucosectomy, the histological examination of some resected specimens has shown smooth muscle in the sample, although this has not correlated with clinical incontinence.

The development of the ABS has heralded a new era in incontinence surgery. Previously, patients not amenable to sphincteroplasty would have medical management or muscle-encirclement procedures as their only options. The permanent disfigurement of these surgical procedures combined with a 50% to 60% success rate made these an unattractive option to many surgeons and patients. Although the ABS has a complication rate of 30% to 40% and a success rate of 50% to 75%, it permits the construction of a neosphincter without the disfigurement of a muscle transposition procedure. It is hoped that with further research and refinement it will continue to improve as an option.

References

1. Nelson R, Norton N, Cautley E, Furner S. Community based prevalence of anal incontinence. JAMA. 1995;274:559–61.
2. Nelson R, Furner S, and Jesudason V. Fecal incontinence in Wisconsin nursing homes: Prevalence and associations. Dis Colon Rectum. 1998;41:1226–9.
3. Goligher JC. Surgery of the anus, rectum and colon. 4th ed. London: Bailliere Tindall; 1980.
4. Duthie HL. Dynamics of the rectum and anus. Clin Gastroenterol. 1975; 4:467–77.
5. Fernandez-Fraga X, Azpiroz F, and Malagelada JR. Significance of pelvic floor muscles in anal incontinence. Gastroenterology. 2002;123:1441–50.
6. Felt-Bersma RJ, van Baren R, Koorevaar M, Strijers RL, and Cuesta MA. Unsuspected sphincter defects shown by anal endosonography after anorectal surgery. A prospective study. Dis Colon Rectum. 1995;38:249–53.
7. Stamatiadis A, Konstantinou E, Theodosopoulou E, and Mamoura K. Frequency of operative trauma to anal sphincters: evaluation with endoanal ultrasound. Gastroenterol Nurs. 2002;25:55–9.

8. Zbar AP, BeerGabel M, Ciappa AC, and Aslam M. Fecal incontinence after minor anorectal surgery. Dis Colon Rectum. 2001;44:1610–23.
9. Garcia-Aguilar J, Belmonte C, Wong WD, Goldberg SM, and Madoff RD. Anal fistula surgery. Factors associated with recurrence and incontinence. Dis Colon Rectum. 1996;39:723–9.
10. van Tets WF and Kuijpers HC. Continence disorders after anal fistulotomy. Dis Colon Rectum. 1994;37:1194–7.
11. Hamalainen KP and Sainio AP. Cutting seton for anal fistulas: high risk of minor control defects. Dis Colon Rectum. 1997;40:1443–6.
12. Graf W, Pahlman L, and Ejerblad S. Functional results after seton treatment of high transsphincteric anal fistulas. Eur J Surg. 1995;161:289–91.
13. Zbar AP, Aslam M, and Allgar V. Faecal incontinence after internal sphincterotomy for anal fissure. Tech Coloproctol. 2000;4:25–8.
14. Nyam DC and Pemberton JH. Long-term results of lateral internal sphincterotomy for chronic anal fissure with particular reference to incidence of fecal incontinence. Dis Colon Rectum. 1999;42:1306–20.
15. Oh C, Divino CM, and Steinhagen RM. Anal fissure: 20-year experience. Dis Colon Rectum. 1995;38:378–82.
16. Khubchandani IT and Reed JF. Sequelae of internal sphincterotomy for chronic fissure in ano. Br J Surg. 1989;76:431–4.
17. Sangwan YP and Solla JA. Internal anal sphincter: advances and insights. Dis Colon Rectum. 1998;41:1297–311.
18. Zbar AP, Jayne DG, Mathur D, Ambrose NS, and Guillou PJ. The importance of the internal anal sphincter (IAS) in maintaining continence: anatomical, physiological and pharmacological considerations. Colorectal Dis. 2000;2:193–202.
19. Zbar AP, Aslam M, Gold DM, Gatzen C, Gosling A, and Kmiot WA. Parameters of the rectoanal inhibitory reflex in patients with idiopathic fecal incontinence and chronic constipation. Dis Colon Rectum. 1998;41:200–8.
20. Kaur G, Gardiner A, and Duthie GS. Rectoanal reflex parameters in incontinence and constipation. Dis Colon Rectum. 2002;45:928–33.
21. Zbar AP, Kmiot WA, Aslam M, Williams A, Hider A, Audisio RA, Chiappa AC, and deSouza NM. Use of vector volume manometry and endoanal magnetic resonance imaging in the adult female for assessment of anal sphincter dysfunction. Dis Colon Rectum. 1999;42:1411–8.
22. Zbar AP, Ramesh J, Salazar R, and Pescatori M. Conventional cutting versus internal anal sphincter-preserving seton for high trans-sphincteric fistula: a prospective, randomized manometric and clinical trial. Tech Coloproctol. 2003;7:89–94.
23. van Tets WF, Kuijpers JF, Tran K, Mollen R, and van Goor H. Influence of Parks' anal retractor on anal sphincter pressures. Dis Colon Rectum. 1997;40:1042–5.
24. Zimmerman DD, Gosselink MP, Hop WC, Darby M, Briel JW, and Schouten WR. Impact of two different types of anal retractor on fecal continence after fistula repair: a prospective, randomized, clinical trial. Dis Colon Rectum. 2003;46:1674–9.
25. Abbasakoor F, Nelson M, Beynon J, Patel B, and Carr ND. Anal endosonography in patients with anorectal symptoms after haemorrhoidectomy. Br J Surg. 1998;85:1522–4.

26. Ho YH, Seow-Choen F, Tsang C, and Eu KW. Randomized trial assessing anal sphincter injuries after stapled haemorrhoidectomy. Br J Surg. 2001;88:1449–55.
27. Altomare DF, Rinaldi M, Sallustio PL, Martino P, De Fazio M, Memeo V. Long-term effects of stapled haemorrhoidectomy on internal anal function and sensitivity. Br J Surg. 2001;88:1487–91.
28. Kamm MA. Obstetric damage and faecal incontinence. Lancet. 1994;344:730–3.
29. Faltin DL, Boulvain M, Trion O, Bretones S, Stan C, and Weil A. Diagnosis of anal sphincter tears by postpartum endosonography to predict fecal incontinence. Obstet Gynecol. 2000;95:643–7.
30. Sultan AH, Kamm MA, Hudson CH, Tomas JM, and Bartram CI. Anal-sphincter disruption during vaginal delivery. N Engl J Med. 1993;329:1905–11.
31. Eason E, Labrecque M, Marcoux S, and Mondor M. Anal incontinence after childbirth. CMAJ. 2002;166:326–30.
32. Allen RE, Hosker GL, Smith AR, and Warrell DW. Pelvic floor damage and childbirth: A neurophysiological study. Br J Obstet Gynecol. 1990;97:770–9.
33. Snooks SJ, Swash M, Setchell M, and Henry MM. Injury to the innervation of pelvic floor sphincter musculature in childbirth. Lancet. 1984;2:546–50.
34. Sato T, Konishi F, Minakami H, et al. Pelvic floor disturbance after childbirth: vaginal delivery damages the upper levels of sphincter innervation. Dis Colon Rectum. 2001;44:1155–61.
35. Snooks SJ, Swash M, Henry MM, and Setchell M. Risk factors in childbirth causing damage to the pelvic floor innervation. Int J Colorectal Dis. 1986;1:20–4.
36. Snooks SJ, Henry MM, and Swash M, Anorectal incontinence and rectal prolapse: Differential assessment of the innervation to puborectalis and external anal sphincter muscles. Gut. 1985;26:470–6.
37. Tetzschner T, Sorensen M, Rasmussen OO, Lose G, and Christiansen J. Pudendal nerve damage increases the risk of fecal incontinence in women with anal sphincter rupture after childbirth. Acta Obstet Gynecol Scand. 1995;74:434–40.
38. Jorge JMN and Wexner SD. Etiology and management of fecal incontinence. Dis Colon Rectum. 1993;36:77–97.
39. Sultan AH, Nicholls RJ, and Kamm MA Anal endosonography and correlation with in vitro and in vivo anatomy. Br J Surg. 1993;80:508–11.
40. Damon H, Henry L, Barth X, and Mion F. Fecal incontinence in females with a past history of vaginal delivery: significance of anal sphincter defects detected by ultrasound. Dis Colon Rectum. 2002;45:1445–50.
41. Chen H, Humphreys MS, Kettlewell MG, Bulkley GB, Mortensen N, and George BD. Anal ultrasound predicts the response to nonoperative treatment of fecal incontinence in men. Ann Surg. 1999;229:739–43.
42. Stoker J, Bartram CI, and Halligan S. Imaging of the posterior pelvic floor. Eur J Radiol. 2002;12:779–88.
43. Malouf A, Halligan S, and Bartram CI. Prospective assessment of the accuracy of endoanal MRI endosonography in patients with fecal incontinence. AJR Am J Roentgenol. 2000;175:741–5.
44. Rociu E, Stoker J, Eijkemans MJ, Schouten WR, and Lameris JS. Fecal incontinence: Endoanal US versus endoanal MR imaging. Radiology. 1999;212:453–8.
45. Schafer A, Enck P, Furst G, Kahn T, Frieling T, and Lubke HJ. Anatomy of the anal sphincters: Comparison of the anal endosonography to magnetic resonance imaging. Dis Colon Rectum. 1994;37:777–81.

46. Lestar B, Penninckx F, and Kerremans R. The composition of anal basal pressure: an in vivo and in vitro study in man. Int J Colorectal Dis. 1989;4;118–22.
47. Chaliha C, Sultan AH, Bland JM, Monga AK, and Stanton SL. Anal function: Effect of pregnancy and delivery. Am J Obstet Gynecol. 2001;185:427–32.
48. Lunniss PJ, Kamm MA, and Phillips RK Factors affecting continence after surgery for anal fistula. Br J Surg. 1994;81:1382–5.
49. Pescatori M, Maria G, Anastasio G, and Rinallo L. Anal manometry improves the outcome of surgery for fistula-in-ano. Dis Colon Rectum. 1989;32:588–92.
50. Loening-Baucke V and Anuras S. Effects of age and sex on anorectal manometry. Am J Gastroenterol. 1985;80:50–3.
51. Enck P, Kuhlbusch R, Lubke H, Frieling T, and Erckenbrecht JF. Age and sex and anorectal manometry in incontinence. Dis Colon Rectum. 1989;32:1026–30.
52. Roig JV, Villoslada C, Lledo S, et al. Prevalence of pudendal neuropathy in fecal incontinence. Results of a prospective study. Dis Colon Rectum. 1995;38:952–8.
53. Kafka NJ, Coller JA, Barrett RC, et al. Pudendal neuropathy is the only parameter differentiating leakage from solid stool incontinence. Dis Colon Rectum. 1997;40:1220–7.
54. Gilliland R, Altomare DF, Moreira H, Oliveira L, Gilliland JE, and Wexner SD. Pudendal neuropathy is predictive of failure following anterior overlapping sphincteroplasty. Dis Colon Rectum. 1998;41:1516–22.
55. Read M, Read NW, and Barber DC. Effects of loperamide on anal sphincter function in patients complaining of chronic diarrhea with fecal incontinence and urgency. Dig Dis Sci. 1982;27:807–14.
56. Sun WM, Read NW, and Verlinden W. Effects of loperamide oxide on gastrointestinal transit time and anorectal function in patients with chronic diarrhoea and faecal incontinence. Scand J Gastroenterol. 1997;32:34–8.
57. Kegel A. Progressive resistance exercise in the functional restoration of the perineal muscles. Am J Obstet Gynecol. 1948;56:242–5.
58. Heyman S, Jones KR, Ringel Y, Scarlett Y, and Whitehead WE. Biofeedback treatment of fecal incontinence: a critical review. Dis Colon Rectum. 2001;44:728–36.
59. Rieger NA, Wattchow DA, Sarre RG, et al. Prospective trial of pelvic floor retraining in patients with fecal incontinence. Dis Colon Rectum. 1997;40:821–6.
60. Sultan AH, Kamm MA, Hudson CN, and Bartram CI. Third degree obstetric anal sphincter tears: risk factors and outcome of primary repair. BMJ. 1994;308:887–91.
61. Sultan AH, Monga AK, Kumar D, and Stanton SL. Primary repair of obstetric anal sphincter rupture using the overlap technique. Br J Obstet Gynaecol. 1999;106:318–23.
62. Fitzpatrick M, Behan M, O'Connell PR, and O'Herlihy C. A randomized clinical trial comparing primary overlap with approximation repair of third degree obstetric tears. Am J Obstet Gynecol. 2000;183:1220–4.
63. Engel AF, van Baal SJ, and Brummelkamp WH. Late results of anterior sphincter plication for traumatic faecal incontinence. Eur J Surg. 1994;160:633–6.
64. Fleshman JW, Peters WR, Shemesh EI, Fry RD, and Kodner, IJ. Anal sphincter reconstruction: anterior overlapping muscle repair. Dis Colon Rectum. 1991;34:739–43.
65. Wexner SD, Marchetti F, and Jagelman DG. The role of sphincteroplasty for fecal incontinence reevaluated: a prospective physiologic and functional review. Dis Colon Rectum. 1991;34:22–30.

66. Karoui S, Leroi AM, Koning E, Menard JF, Michot JF, and Denis P. Results of sphincteroplasty in 86 patients with anal incontinence. Dis Colon Rectum. 2000;43:813–20.
67. Halverson AL and Hull TL. Long-term outcome of overlapping anal sphincter repair. Dis Colon Rectum. 2002;45:345–8.
68. Briel JW, Stoker J, Rociu E, Lameris JS, Hop WC, and Schowten WR. External anal sphincter atrophy on endoanal magnetic resonance imaging adversely affects continence after sphincteroplasty. Br J Surg. 1999;86:1322–7.
69. Gilliland R, Altomare DF, Moreira H Jr., Oliveira L, Gilliland JE, and Wexner SD. Pudendal neuropathy is predictive of failure following anterior overlapping sphincteroplasty. Dis Colon Rectum. 1998;41:1516–22.
70. Buie WD, Loery AC, Rothenberger DA, and Madoff RD. Clinical rather than laboratory assessment predicts continence after anterior sphincteroplasty. Dis Colon Rectum. 2001;44:1255–60.
71. Leroi AM, Kamm MA, Weber J, Denis P, and Hawley PR. Internal anal sphincter repair. Int J Colorectal Dis. 1997;12:243–5.
72. Prochiantz A and Gross P. Gluteal myoplasty for sphincter replacement: principles, results and prospects. J Pediatr Surg. 1982;17:25–30.
73. Devesa JM, Vicente E, Enriquez JM, et al. Total fecal incontinence: a new method of glutcus maximus transposition. Preliminary results and report of previous experience with similar procedures. Dis Colon Rectum. 1992;35:339–49.
74. Pearl RK, Prasad ML, Nelson RL, Orsay CP, and Abcarion H. Bilateral gluteus maximus transposition for anal incontinence. Dis Colon Rectum. 1991;34:478–81.
75. Pickrell KL, Broadbent TR, Masters FW, et al. Construction of a rectal sphincter and restoration of anal continence by transplanting the gracilis muscle. Ann Surg. 1952;135:853–62.
76. Christiansen J, Sorensen M, and Rasmussen OO. Gracilis muscle transposition for fecal incontinence. Int J Colorectal Dis. 1996;11:15–8.
77. Khan M, Southern S, and Ramakrishnan V. Endoscopic harvest of the gracilis muscle. Plast Reconstr Surg. 2001;107:294.
78. Corman ML. Gracilis muscle transposition for anal incontinence. Br J Surg. 1985;72(Suppl):S21–2.
79. Baeten C, Spaans F, and Fluks A. An implanted neuromuscular stimulator for fecal continence following previously implanted gracilis muscle: Report of a case. Dis Colon Rectum. 1988;31:134–7.
80. Baeten CGMI, Geerdes BP, Adang EMM, et al. Anal dynamic graciloplasty in the treatment of intractable fecal incontinence. N Engl J Med. 1995;332:1600–5.
81. Wexner SD, Baeten C, Bailey R, et al. Long-term efficacy of dynamic graciloplasty for fecal incontinence. Dis Colon Rectum. 2002;45:809–18.
82. Christiansen J and Lorentzen M. Implantation of artificial sphincter for anal incontinence. Lancet. 1987;2;244–5.
83. Lehur PA, Michot F, Denis P, et al. Results of artificial sphincter in severe fecal incontinence. Report of fourteen consecutive implantations. Dis Colon Rectum. 1996;39:1352–5.
84. Wong WD, Jensen LL, Bartolo DC, and Rothenberger DA. Artificial anal sphincter. Dis Colon Rectum. 1996;39:1345–51.
85. Wong WD, Congliosi SM, Spencer MP, et al. The safety and efficacy of the artificial bowel sphincter for fecal incontinence: results from a multicenter cohort study. Dis Colon Rectum. 2002;45:1139–53.

Editorial Commentary

Drs. Akbari and Bernstein succinctly describe the investigative and management approach towards postoperative fecal incontinence. The vast majority of this problem occurs secondary to injudicious sphincter injury (or division) after comparatively minor anorectal surgery; mostly for complex (or recurrent) anorectal fistulas or following standard or newer forms of haemorrhoidectomy and haemorrhoidopexy. Although sphincter injury (both to the IAS and EAS) is the commonest problem here, the factors contributing to postoperative fecal incontinence can be complex and multifactorial. In some cases, postoperative destructive perirectal sepsis is the culprit but in others, subtle derangements in anorectal manometry are important as are pre-existent constitutive differences in the orientation of the distal EAS. In this latter circumstance, unwise IAS division (sphincterotomy) will leave the distal anal canal unsupported resulting in troublesome seepage.

Some anorectal surgery alters the dynamics of anal closure occasionally leading to guttering defects which are difficult to treat effectively and there is much in the operative decision making and conduct of fistulectomies and deliberate sphincterotomies that would prevent postoperative incontinence and that has serious medicolegal significance for the coloproctologist, even when the surgery contemplated is considered minor in nature. The profusion of new haemorrhoidectomy techniques aimed at minimizing the anal trauma, postoperative pain and hospital stay, is the potential for IAS damage and the relatively poor results with IAS repair (including sphincteroplasty as described in this chapter) and IAS bolstering techniques (such as autologous lipofilling or silcone injection), demand that IAS injury should be avoided at all costs during the conduct of such surgeries.

In the case of poor functional outcome following coloanal anastomosis, the etiology of postoperative incontinence is even more complicated where there may be secondary anastomotic strictures (with overflow), capacitance problems with the neorectal reservoir, inadvertent sphincter injury following excessive endoanal manipulation or distraction and an unrecognized ano- and rectovaginal fistula. The treatment of patients involves a sophisticated assessment of sphincter and perineal body integrity and the exclusion of low fistulas and complex perirectal sepsis as well as the expertise necessary to repair all of these problems, sometimes as staged procedures. The latest physiological and imaging data highlights the clinical importance of the IAS in the maintenance of continence (particularly where there is attendant EAS atrophy) and here like many things in anorectal surgery prevention of damage is far better than the current remedies available for salvage.

AZ

Chapter 10
Postoperative Assessment of the Neosphincter

Chapter 10.1
An Overview

Donato F. Altomare, Marcella Rinaldi, and
Altomarino Guglielmi

Introduction

The restoration of continence using an anal neosphincter has been a major goal for colorectal surgeons in the last century. Several techniques have been described ranging from Thiersch's anal ring to the more recent electrostimulated gracilis neosphincter and to the artificial anal sphincter. The assessment of some of these new surgical technologies—particularly when there are postoperative problems—is covered elsewhere in this book; this chapter is designed to provide an overview of the highlights of the neosphincter approach.

The surgery for fecal incontinence traditionally bears a significant percentage of failure, probably because it has focused almost exclusively on the correction of what has been considered to be the main mechanism for the control of defecation—namely, the anal sphincter. Continence is the result of a highly complex physiological mechanism involving motor and sensory nerve pathways along with primary sphincter mechanisms. For this reason, restoration of a damaged sphincter in the presence of other possible causes of incontinence rarely results in completely normal continence, particularly over the long-term. In fact, continence should not be regarded simply as a retention mechanism, but it should also include the ability to defecate normally—in other words, to expel feces at the chosen time and in the proper place and manner (1). A significant proportion of patients suffering from fecal incontinence develop some form of obstructed defecation, complicating analysis and final evaluation of the results of surgery for incontinence.

The indications for anal neosphincter surgery, which originally was devised to treat patients with fecal incontinence, have been extended to include the more complex total anorectal reconstruction after removal of the anorectum due to cancer or trauma. In fact, although the number of Miles'-type operations has dramatically fallen in the last 20 years, about 10% of rectal cancer patients still require this operation for curative intent (2). Another category of patients who potentially can benefit from an anal neosphincter reconstruction is those with anorectal malformations.

The strong regard for quality of life issues (covered elsewhere in this book as it pertains to the principal symptom of fecal incontinence) has prompted colorectal surgeons to experiment with the implementation of biotechnology and electrostimulation devices, with the detailing of new and expensive operations aimed at assisting these patients to overcome the socially and psychologically disabling condition of fecal incontinence.

Surgical Options Overview

Although several attempts have been made in the past to use different muscles converted to act as a neoanal sphincter, the most widely accepted techniques at the moment are the graciloplasty, the gluteoplasty, and the artificial anal sphincter.

Graciloplasty (See Chapter 10.2)

The most reliable skeletal muscle for use as a neoanal sphincter is the gracilis because of its anatomical position in the medial part of the thigh, its length, and the presence of a single proximal vascular and nerve supply. Pickrell first described this operation in 1952 (3) to treat children with neurological fecal incontinence. After a long period of neglect of the technique, in 1972, Simonsen (4) published his excellent 77% success rate with total anorectal reconstruction using the gracilis neoanal sphincter in 24 patients operated for rectal cancer, and Corman (5) independently reported a 70% success rate in adult incontinent patients where this muscle was used to augment sphincter function.

In the three decades following its original description, this kind of operation again declined, and there were only sporadic case reports of its use. The technique was then resumed and improved upon by Cavina and colleagues (6), using temporary external electrostimulation to sustain muscle trophism and function and using both muscles (one to reconstruct the pelvic floor and one as a true anal neosphincter) in patients undergoing the Miles' operation for rectal cancer. The operation, however, did not become popular with colorectal surgeons, probably because this muscle is unreliable when required to function as a sphincter and because it rapidly becomes fatigued, becoming atrophic with the passage of time like any unstimulated muscle. Interest in the operation revived when, at the end of the 1980s, Williams et al. (7) and Baeten et al. (8) independently developed a dynamic fatigue-resistant anal neosphincter. This involved using permanent, chronic low-frequency electrostimulation by means of a totally implantable pulse generator in order to convert fatigue-prone type II muscle fibers into fatigue-resistant type I fibers. Although Williams' suggestion to stimulate the gracilis nerve in order to spare the battery and deliver the electrical impulses simultaneously to all the motor units was very attractive, Baeten's option of directly stimulating the muscle became more widely accepted thanks to the lower risk of lead displacement.

The main indications for this kind of surgery include anal sphincter damage, which is not suitable for direct repair, idiopathic anal incontinence, anorectal malformations, total anorectal reconstruction following Miles' operation, and failure of previous attempts at sphincter repair. It is contraindicated in the presence of inflammatory bowel diseases or psychological/cognitive inability to manage the device. The presence of a heart pacemaker should not be considered a contraindication for this procedure, as successful experiences without side effects have already been described.

Gluteoplasty

Because of its synergistic function in the continence mechanism, the gluteus maximus muscle could be the most suitable muscle for use as a surrogate for a damaged or nonfunctioning anal sphincter. However, owing to the high percentage of failure and postural damage, this operation is very rarely performed nowadays, where, since 1902, only 13 series of patients operated on using the gluteoplasty procedure have been reported. Recently, Devesa reported a 59% success rate in a pooled analysis of 71 patients operated on with nine different adynamic gluteoplasty techniques (9). An attempt to stimulate the muscle electrically was made at the end of the past century, but the high variability of the vascular and nerve supply makes the gluteus maximus less reliable than the gracilis muscle. It appears from early work by Guelinckx et al. (10) that the neurovascular pedicle of a gluteoplasty is somewhat more reliable following muscle transposition around the anal sphincter in the cadaver. More recently, this approach has been supplemented with a fascia lata graft (11).

Artificial Bowel Sphincter (See Chapter 10.3)

This hydraulic device is derived from the more commonly used AMS (American Medical System) urinary artificial sphincter. It consists of three components: an inflatable pump located around the anus, a control pump located in the scrotum or the labium majus, and a pressure balloon that enables maintenance of the pressure in the anal cuff. The cuff is filled with radiopaque liquid and closes the anal canal, thus restoring continence. When patients feel the desire to defecate, they can empty the cuff by pressing the pump and moving the liquid into the balloon, which will slowly and spontaneously channel the liquid back into the anal cuff within some minutes.

As with graciloplasty, the technique can be applied in patients with a nonfunctioning but intact anal sphincter, as well as with sphincter lesions not amenable to direct repair; this procedure has recently been adopted for total anorectal reconstruction following the Miles' operation (12).

Smooth Muscle Neoanal Sphincter

For selected patients undergoing total anorectal reconstruction, a number of passive anal sphincters have been created using smooth muscle obtained from the colon itself. At least three techniques have been described, each of which causes passive closure of the neoanus. In the technique described by Schmidt (13) in 1982 for the creation of a continent abdominal colostomy, the mucosa of the last 10 centimeters of the terminal colon is removed and the seromuscular layer is divided longitudinally and sutured circumferentially around the terminal colon. This technique has been applied by other authors to the perineal colostomy after some modifications, with "good results" being reported (14). Holschneider and Hecker proposed an original technique for recreation of an internal anal sphincter (IAS) by plicating and suturing a four- to eight-centimeter segment of distal colon denuded of its mucosa (15), and Gamagami et al. (16) proposed a neointernal anal sphincter using an isolated cylinder of smooth muscle obtained from a resected part of the colon applied to the terminal colon before its suture to the perineum—a procedure recently reported to recreate a high-pressure zone (HPZ) within the anal canal in a porcine model (17). These approaches have used reversed smooth muscle plications with or without incisions in the demucosated colonic wall (18) or incontinuity plications that rely on a similar mechanism to the wraps around the gastroesophageal junction as provided by Nissen-style fundoplications. It has been suggested that such attempts at IAS replacement may find a place in low rectal cancers, where deliberate IAS resection is part of the oncologic procedure. It is likely that the reversed (so-called type I) IAS plication procedure using a demucosated segment folded back on itself may prove more suitable in humans considering the length and thickness of plication required after IAS resection; however, these matters will be the subjects of further research.

Direct Perineal Colostomy

Other authors have proposed a direct perineal colostomy without any sphincter mechanism, with the first such report being made by the French group headed by Chiotasso (19), whereas, in 1995, Lazaro da Silva (20) described an original technique featuring a circular interruption and suture of the colonic muscle layer with the intention of creating mucosal valves and inhibiting the peristaltic motility resultant from the discontinuation of the intermuscular enteric nervous system during rectoanal resection.

Antegrade Colonic Enema with Perineal Colostomy

Hughes and Williams were the first to see the potential need for a colonic washout system and a colonic conduit with the neoanal sphincter procedure in order to prevent obstructed defecation after electrostimulated graciloplasty for fecal incontinence (21). However, this operation is quite complex and is not free from major complications. Instead, the association of the Malone antegrade colonic enema using the terminal ileum according to the Marsh and Kiff technique (22) has been proposed in association with a simple perineal colostomy without any sphincter mechanism (Altomare, unpublished data). Periodical complete emptying of the bowel enables the patient to be free of episodes of either constipation or incontinence.

Assessment of Functional Results

The objective evaluation of the functional results after anal neosphincter operation, both for incontinent patients and perineal colostomy patients, is very controversial and is being actively debated among experts. In fact, it is necessary to evaluate the degree of continence obtained without ignoring the difficulty in the evacuation process that can be experienced by many of these patients. Assessment of the functional results must address the two faces of the same coin—namely, control of the passage of feces per anum (in other words, the ability to postpone defecation until desired—continence) and the ability to evacuate completely and without trouble when desired (defecation). One of the major confounding factors in assessment of the outcome from anal neosphincter surgery is the lack of common standardized criteria for the evaluation of continence and the ability to defecate. Here, the performance of anal manometry does not provide a complete idea of the clinical situation; therefore, the results are unsuitable as clinical criteria. Perfectly continent patients have been observed with relatively low postoperative anal pressures, and others remain incontinent despite an apparently well-functioning anal sphincter.

Assessment of Functional Results by Scoring Systems

Various scoring systems have recently been introduced in order to express qualitative data into a semiquantitative environment, both for continence and constipation, combining the frequency of symptoms with the severity of the disturbance. Several scoring systems to evaluate the degree of continence have, in fact, been proposed in the past few years, and this makes comparison of the results between the various case series difficult (see Chapter 7.2). The most widely used scores of incontinence in clinical practice are the Cleveland Clinic Florida Continence grading Scale (score 0 to

20) (23) and the American Medical System score proposed by Wong et al. (24). The latter score is believed to be more precise and detailed, as only one clinical situation corresponds to each possible score. For example, a score of 91 identifies incontinent patients who have experienced bowel leakage of solid stool with a greater frequency than once per week, but less than once per day in the previous four weeks.

Unfortunately, only the most recent articles on neoanal sphincter surgery have adopted one of these systems, so the results from different centers are not really comparable. Other scores also have failed to take into account fecal urgency in some cases, which may be modified by proximity to a toilet and the ability of anti-diarrheal use to ameliorate reported symptoms (25). In a systematic review reported by Chapman in 2002 (26) on the 37 articles published in English on the electrostimulated graciloplasty for fecal incontinence, the complication rate was seen to be generally very high, with a total of 387 complications being reported in 347 patients with a mean of 1.12 events per patient. These complications particularly featured infections (28%) and hardware-related (15%) problems. With regard to the functional results, all the articles were considered of low evidence quality (grade IV of the hierarchy of evidence) and the percentage of patients achieving "satisfactory continence" ranged from 42% to 85%. Moreover, the definition of satisfactory continence was not applied consistently across these articles, ranging from full continence to continence only to solid feces. Furthermore, approximately 7% of patients suffered from severely obstructed defecation after surgery.

After short-term follow-up, the clinical results of the artificial anal sphincter implant in terms of the control of continence are encouraging, ranging between 55% and 83% (24,27–31). However, in the long term, a reduction of the success rate is expected because of the risk of late infections, failure of the device, or rectal perforation/extrusion. In a long-term review of a group of 28 patients implanted in Italy, the success rate dropped from 75% to about 50%, with a significant proportion of patients being those whose neosphincter had to be deactivated because of obstructed defecation (unpublished personal data). In fact, another major concern with the artificial bowel sphincter (ABS) is the common complaint of difficult evacuation. This inconvenience is also common after graciloplasty. It is difficult to understand why the problem arises; however, it can affect between 17% and 50% of patients (24,30,31), although the use of laxatives and/or enemas and a proper diet can help in the management of difficult evacuation after this procedure. Sometimes the problem is due to an undetected rectocele or rectal intussusception—disorders that previously were clinically irrelevant in the presence of fecal incontinence. Therefore, a full preoperative proctologic investigation, including defecography, should be recommended, with simultaneous correction of any potential defecatory problems at the time of ABS implantation.

Very recently, the Acticon ABS implant has been applied to the perineal colostomy after Miles' operation, with even better short-term results being reported than for fecal incontinence. Romano and colleagues (12) have recently described a two-stage operation with a perineal colostomy using a silastic anal sling immediately following the Miles' operation and a covering ileostomy, then followed by the ABS implant and closure of the ileostomy during the second stage. They have reported a good grade of continence in four of the five patients treated after a follow-up period ranging from six to twenty-two months.

The problem of impaired evacuation is particularly relevant for patients with total anorectal reconstruction after Miles' operation, in whom several kinds of anatomic and neurological disruption to the physiology of defecation have been surgically introduced. These include:

1. Changes in anorectal angle width: Minor or even absent changes in the anorectal angle width can be documented in these patients using dynamic defecography during pushing maneuvers. This result is due to the absence of the puborectalis muscle and the fibrotic tissue in the pelvic floor area. The persistence of an acute anorectal angle during straining to defecate can contribute to evacuation difficulties experienced by these patients. Such an acute angle needs a propulsive pressure three times greater than the resting anal pressure for stool to be forced.
2. Changes in the propulsive effect of the Valsalva maneuver: This maneuver is essential for starting and maintaining defecation because the increased intra-abdominal pressure is transmitted to the rectal ampulla. In patients with a perineal colostomy, this maneuver is less effective due to the lack of a functioning pelvic floor muscle.
3. Variations in the ano-colic reflex: This is an intramural reflex that is particularly active in children and animals and consists of a strong sigmoidorectalis contraction in response to anal stimulation (the passage of the first fecal bolus). Removal of the anus interrupts this reflex mechanism.
4. Alteration in contraction of the neorectum: The strength of contraction of the colon is less than that of the rectum because of the width and architectural organization of the muscle layer. Moreover, the loss of the compliance mechanism, which is mediated by the sacral parasympathetic nerves, contributes heavily to postoperative defecatory disturbances.
5. Altered sensitivity of the neorectum: Normal sensitivity of the rectal ampulla is essential for "correct" defecation, as demonstrated by the severe defecatory problems, including fecaloma formation and obstructed defecation experienced by diabetic or neurological patients. This sensitivity is usually lost or severely damaged after total anorectal reconstruction.

In the case of patients submitted to total anorectal reconstruction, the information on the degree of continence is even less reliable because less-detailed descriptions of the results tend to be obtained from both surgeons and patients. Patients are generally more prone to accept an imperfect degree of (neo) anal continence rather than a permanent abdominal colostomy. However, it is obvious that some criteria used in older reports to define the results of this kind of surgery as "good"—such as the patients' degree of satisfaction, the ability to control solid feces only, or a generic classification—can no longer be accepted. Using these standards, it would appear superficially at least that the functional results following direct perineal colostomy without an anorectal sphincter implant are better than for the electrostimulated gracilis neosphincter.

In these cases, the functional results frequently have been described in terms of manometric data and the number of defecations per day, and it is only recently that more objective scoring systems of the severity of the disease have started to be more routinely used. Two scoring systems for chronic constipation have been proposed recently in the medical literature—namely, the Cleveland Clinic Score by Agachan et al. (32) and the K.E.S.S. (Knowles-Eccersley-Scott-Symptom) score (33). The latter has been prospectively validated and was developed by discriminant function analysis of a series of complaints that coincide in chronically constipated patients. Currently, these scoring systems have not been applied to patients presenting with evacuatory difficulty following neosphincter surgery. Most of these patients spend a lot of time at the toilet and need daily enemas, digitations, and laxatives. It is evident that a functional evaluation based simply on the continence parameter is insufficient, as it does not consider the other face of the same coin—the ability to defecate properly. These points were discussed in a recently published article that proposed a new scoring system specific for neosphincter patients (34). As shown in Tables 10.1-1 and 10.1-2, the score consists of two variables, I (incontinence) and E (evacuation). Two degrees of incontinence are considered and combined with the frequency of episodes of incontinence, but the score is weighted in such a way that, for example, daily incontinence to gas is comparable to a major incontinence occurring less than once per week. For the variable E, three degrees are considered—namely, incomplete or failed evacuation, prolonged straining, and the need for enemas or digital evacuation. In this case, too, the severity of the symptoms is combined with their frequency.

This score has not been clinically applied so far, but other authors have proposed a modification of this scoring system, combining the two scores

TABLE 10.1-1. Incontinence scoring system for sphincter replacement patients.

Frequency	Incontinence for gas or minor straining	Incontinence for liquid or solid stool
Never	I	I
<1/week	II	II
≥1/week to <1/day	II	III
≥1/day	II	IV

See Madoff and Baeten (34).

TABLE 10.1-2. Evacuation scoring system for sphincter replacement patients.

Frequency	Incomplete or failed evacuation	Strain >30 minutes	Enemas, irrigation, or digital evacuation
Never	I	I	I
<1/week	II	II	II
≥1/week to <1/day	III	III	III
≥1/day	IV	IV	IV

See Madoff and Baeten (34).

into one and proposing a method that might enable the physician to correct the subjective evaluation and bias provided by the postoperative patient (35).

Assessment of Functional Results by Quality of Life (QoL) Index

Quality of life (QoL) questionnaires are considered an important tool in medicine, and particularly in functional surgery. Apart from a scoring system to evaluate the degree of continence obtained after anal neosphincter surgery, the true success of the operation is best expressed by the patient's degree of satisfaction, and hence their improvement in quality of life. Several socioeconomic and health-related factors can contribute to the quality of life. For example, gas leakage could be well tolerated by a farmworker who is used to working outside with little social contact, but not by a teacher, whereas a housewife could better tolerate the need for prolonged straining at the toilet to empty the bowel as opposed to a business man. It is clear, therefore, that the same functional result may be considered good or poor according to its impact on the patient's quality of life.

On the other hand, changes in the quality of life of incontinent patients are not necessarily related to a significant improvement of the continence score, as it may depend on other social factors. Here, an improvement in the continence grading scale from 18 to 14, for example, although potentially significant, would not change the patient's lifestyle, and therefore would not impact quality of life. Furthermore, the experience of obstructed defecation after neoanal sphincter surgery for fecal incontinence can severely affect the QoL, sometimes even more than the fecal incontinence for which the procedure was performed.

A Fecal Incontinence Quality of Life (FIQL) questionnaire that includes four domains—coping behavior, embarrassment, lifestyle, and depression, each of which is evaluated using some questions scored from 0 to 4 according to the agreement expressed by the patient—has been described and prospectively validated by Rockwood et al. (36). This useful tool should now be applied routinely to evaluate the functional results in incontinent patients. Only a few recent articles (24,30) have considered the impact of this operation on the patients' quality of life using the FIQL instrument. An attempt to better evaluate the QoL in incontinent patients has been made by Byrne and colleagues (37), where QoL indexes eight categories of daily activities (i.e., job and work, home duties, travel, etc.) and where patients are asked to rate each activity important to them on a scale from 0 to 10. They are then asked to score their ability to perform each of these activities on a 0 to 10 scale. The QoL score is then calculated by summing the product of each important activity and the performance ability divided by 10 and subsequently divided again by the sum of the score obtained for the chosen activities. This yields the weighted QoL mean score, ranging from 0 to 1.

Conclusions

The main problem in assessing anal function in patients with a neoanal sphincter, particularly those after total anorectal reconstruction following Miles' operation, is the onset of defecatory disturbance, which can sometimes be even more troublesome than anal incontinence. No QoL questionnaires have yet been drawn up for patients with obstructed defecation or combined functional disorders. There is a strong need for such a tool, which would make it possible to perform a better evaluation of the results of these newer operations and to compare different groups of patients undergoing different anal neosphincter procedures.

References

1. Baeten CGM. Surgical treatment of anal incontinence. Br J Surg. 1998;85:723–24.
2. Tolmos J, Vargas HI, Lim S, and Stamos M. A forty-year experience with anal carcinoma: changing trends and impact of multimodality therapy. Am Surg. 1997;63:918–22.
3. Pickrell K, Broadbent R, Masters F, and Metzger JT. Construction of a rectal sphincter and restoration of anal continence by transplanting the gracilis muscle. Ann Surg. 1952;135:853–62.
4. Simonsen OS, Stolf NAG, Aun F, Raia A, and Habr-Gama A. Rectal sphincter reconstruction in perineal colostomies after abdominoperineal resection for cancer. Br J Surg. 1976;63:389–91.
5. Corman ML. Follow-up evaluation of gracilis muscle transposition for fecal incontinence. Dis Colon Rectum. 1980;23:552–5.
6. Cavina E, Seccia M, Evangelista G, Chiazugi M, Buceianti P. Construction of continent perineal colostomy by using electrostimulated gracilis muscles after abdominoperineal resection: personal technique and experience with 32 cases. Ital J Surg Sci. 1987;17:305–14.

7. Williams NS, Patel J, George BD, Hallan RI, Watkins S. Development of an electrically stimulated neoanal sphincter. Lancet. 1991;338:1166–9.
8. Baeten CG, Konsten J, Spaans F, et al. Dynamic graciloplasty for treatment of faecal incontinence. Lancet. 1991;338:1163–5.
9. Devesa JM and Fernandez JM. Bilateral Gluteoplasty for anal incontinence. Sem Colon Rectal Surg. 1997;8:103–9.
10. Guelinckx PJ, Sinsel NK, and Gruwez JA. Anal sphincter reconstruction with the gluteus maximus muscle: anatomic and physiologic considerations concerning conventional and dynamic gluteoplasty. Plast Reconstr Surg. 1996;98: 293–304.
11. Farid M, Moneim HA, Mahdy T, and Omar W. Augmented unilateral gluteoplasty with fascia lata graft in fecal incontinence. Tech Coloproctol. 2003;7:23–8.
12. Romano G, LaTorre F, Cutini G, Bianco F, Esposito P, and Montori A. Total anorectal reconstruction with the artificial bowel sphincter: report of eight cases. A quality of life assessment. Dis Colon Rectum. 2003;46:730–4.
13. Schmidt E. The continent colostomy. World J Surg. 1982;6:805–9.
14. Fedorov VD, Odaryuk TS, Shelygin YA, Tsazkov PV, Fzolov SA. Method of creation of a smooth-muscle cuff at the site of the perineal colostomy after extirpation of the rectum. Dis Colon Rectum. 1989;32:562–6.
15. Holschneider AM and Hecker WCh. Reverse smooth muscle plasty: a new method of treating anorectal incontinence in infant with high anal and rectal atresia. J Pediatr Surg. 1981;16:917–20.
16. Gamagami RA, Chiotasso P, and Lazorthes F. Continent perineal colostomy after abdominoperineal resection: outcome after 63 cases. Dis Colon Rectum. 1999;42:626–31.
17. Lorenzi M, Vernillo R, Garzi A, Vindigni C, D'Onofrio P, Angeloni GM, Stefanoni M, Picchianti D, Genovese A, Lorenzi B, and Iroatulam AJN. Experimental internal anal sphincter replacement with demucosated colonic plication. Tech Coloproctol. 2003;7:9–16.
18. Holschneider AM, Amano S, Urban A, et al. Free and reverse smooth muscle plasty in rats and goats. Dis Colon Rectum. 1985;28:786–94.
19. Chiotasso P, Schmitt L, Juricic M. Acceptation des stomies perinéales [meeting abstract]. Gastroenterol Clin Biol. 1992;16:A200.
20. Lazaro da Silva A. Abdominoperineal excision of the rectum and anal canal with perineal colostomy. Eur J Surg. 1995;161:761–4.
21. Hughes SF and Williams NS. Continent colonic conduit for the treatment of faecal incontinence associated with disordered evacuation. Br J Surg. 1995;82: 1318–20.
22. Marsh PJ and Kiff ES. Ileocaecostomy: an alternative surgical procedure for antegrade colonic enema. Br J Surg. 1996;83:507–8.
23. Jorge JMN and Wexner SD. Etiology and management of fecal incontinence. Dis Colon Rectum. 1993;36:77–97.
24. Wong WD, Congliosi SM, Spencer MP, et al. The safety and efficacy of the artificial anal sphincter. Results from a multicenter cohort study. Dis Colon Rectum. 2002;45:1139–53.
25. Vaizey CJ, Carapeti E, Cahill JA, and Kamm MA. Prospective comparison of faecal incontinence grading systems. Gut. 1999;44:77–80.
26. Chapman AE, Geerdes B, Hewett P, et al. Systematic review of dynamic graciloplasty in the treatment of faecal incontinence. Br J Surg. 2002;89:138–53.

27. Vaizey CJ, Kamm MA, Gold DM, Bartram CI, Halligan S, and Nicholls RJ. Clinical, physiological, and radiological study of the new purpose-designed artificial bowel sphincter. Lancet. 1998;352:105–9.
28. Lehur PA, Roig JV, and Duinslaeger M. Artificial anal sphincter: A prospective clinical and manometric evaluation. Dis Colon Rectum. 2000;43:1100–6.
29. O'Brien P and Skinner S. Restoring control: the artificial bowel sphincter (ABS) in the treatment of anal incontinence. Dis Colon Rectum. 2000;43:1213–6.
30. Altomare DF, Dodi G, La Torre F, Romano G, and Rinaldi M. Artificial anal sphincter for severe fecal incontinence. A multicentre retrospective analysis of 28 cases. Br J Surg. 2001;88:1841–6.
31. Devesa JM, Rey A, Hervas PL, et al. Artificial anal sphincter. Complications and functional results of a large personal series. Dis Colon Rectum. 2002; 45:1154–63.
32. Agachan F, Chen T, Pfeifer J, Reissman P, and Wexner SD. A constipation scoring system to simplify evaluation and management of constipated patients. Dis Colon Rectum. 1996;39:681–5.
33. Knowles CH, Scott SM, Legg PE, Allison ME, and Lunnis PJ. Level of classification performance of KESS (symptom scoring system for constipation) validated in a prospective series of 105 patients. Dis Colon Rectum. 2002;45:842–3.
34. Madoff RD, Baeten CGMI, Christiansen J, et al. Standards for anal sphincter replacement. Dis Colon Rectum. 2000;43:135–41.
35. Violi V, Boselli AS, De Bernardinis M, Costi R, Tzivelli M, and Roncoroni L. A patient-rated, surgeon-corrected scale for functional assessment after total anorectal reconstruction. An adaptation of the working party on anal sphincter replacement scoring system. Int J Colorectal Dis. 2002;17:327–37.
36. Rockwood TH, Church JM, Fleshman JW, et al. Fecal incontinence quality of life scale: quality of life instrument for patients with fecal incontinence. Dis Colon Rectum. 2000;43:9–16.
37. Byrne CM, Pager CK, Rex J, Roberts R, and Solomon MJ. Assessment of quality of life in the treatment of patients with neuropathic fecal incontinence. Dis Colon Rectum. 2002;45:1431–6.

Editorial Commentary

Dr. Altomare (an alumnus of the Department of Colorectal Surgery at Cleveland Clinic Florida) describes his extensive experience with neosphincters for faecal incontinence. The most commonly used options include the stimulated and nonstimulated graciloplasty, the nonstimulated gluteoplasty, the artificial bowel sphincter, the smooth muscle neoanal sphincter, the direct perineal colostomy and the antegrade enema with perineal colostomy. Dr. Altomare and colleagues describe the scoring system and the method of evaluation of each of these operations and discuss in detail the physiologic alterations and aberrations which are part of the postoperative findings in these patients. In addition, he addresses the quality of life considerations that are a result of these changes.

SW

Chapter 10.2
Managing Functional Problems Following Dynamic Graciloplasty

Cornelius G.M.I. Baeten and Mart J. Rongen

Dynamic graciloplasty is a technique for patients with severe fecal incontinence who cannot be treated with other methods. The technique is based upon a much older operation described by Pickrell (1). In this operation, a gracilis muscle is wrapped around the anus. The main artery, vein, and nerve of this muscle are preserved. This muscle can only contract by will and closes the anal canal, and active voluntary contraction is only possible for a few minutes. The gracilis contains a majority of type II fibers that are very fatigable. Type II fibers can be changed into type I fibers by electrical stimulation (2). Every muscle is composed of a certain proportion of type I and II fibers dictated by the nerve leading to this muscle. The electrical stimulation "tricks the nerve" and the muscle changes towards the properties of the stimulated nerve. The same will happen when the nerves of two muscles are transected and are crosswise anastomosed. The muscles will both change to the characteristics of each other.

The problem that patients with fecal incontinence treated with a conventional graciloplasty have to overcome are twofold:

1. They have to concentrate on contracting the muscle. Psychologically, this is only possible for a very short time.
2. The muscle fatigues and the patients have to find a toilet in a few minutes, otherwise the muscle will relax and stool is lost.

Combining Pickrell's technique (3) with the idea that a muscle can be changed by low-frequency electrical stimulation made it possible to change the gracilis muscle into a nonfatigable muscle (4) that contracts, because it is forced to do so on demand of the stimulator. Cerebral attention is no longer necessary. The combination of conventional graciloplasty with electrical stimulation is called *dynamic graciloplasty*. The only cerebral activity is to register a call to stool and to take the remote control to switch "off" the stimulator. No stimuli will go to the muscle, the muscle will then relax, the anus opens, and the patient can defecate. After defecation, the stimulator can be switched "on" again with the same remote control so that the anus will close again.

In the literature, the successful outcome of dynamic graciloplasty varies from 56% to 80% (5–8). This success rate is acceptable because this technique is used as a last resort for patients who have already been treated unsuccessfully in various other ways. Dynamic graciloplasty is used in patients with severe fecal incontinence in whom diets, constipating drugs, biofeedback therapy, anal repair, and other operations have failed. The success can be obtained at the cost of many complications, most of which are treatable (9,10). Some of the problems seen in dynamic graciloplasty can be considered functional and form the subject of this chapter. The most important functional problems are: (A) non-contractility of the gracilis muscle, (B) persisting incontinence, and (C) constipation.

Non Contractility of the Gracilis

When after dynamic graciloplasty the muscle does not contract sufficiently, or not at all, it is important to find the cause and to ascertain whether it is a primary muscle problem or a stimulation problem. The difference can be found in a very simple way. The gracilis still has its own intact nerve and the patient is able to contract the muscle voluntarily.

When a voluntary contraction of the gracilis wrap is possible, the problem is not a muscle problem, but probably represents a stimulation failure. In a voluntary contraction, all the motor units in the gracilis are recruited and the muscle will give its maximal force. A contraction based upon electrical stimulation can, at its best, generate the same force as in a voluntary contraction, but it is more likely that the generated force will be suboptimal. The force is dependent on the number of motor units that can be activated by electrical stimulation. Every motor unit consists of a nerve fiber connected to one or more muscle fibers. The number of nerve fibers located in the electrical field between the electrodes determines the number of muscle fibers that will contract. This force is dependent on the localization of the electrode next to the nerve, on the amplitude, on the pulse width and frequency of the stimulation (Figure 10.2.1).

With higher amplitude, more motor units will be activated up to a maximum. When all fibers in the nerve are stimulated, a further increase in amplitude will not generate more force. Initially, poor contraction is most likely based upon a bad positioning of the electrode; the solution is reinsertion of the lead. A secondary poor contraction can be based upon dislocation of the electrode or on two physiological phenomena.

1. Fibrosis will be formed around the electrode and higher amplitude is necessary to generate the same contraction force (11).
2. The muscle fibers will be changed from type II to type I. Type 1 fibers are less forceful.

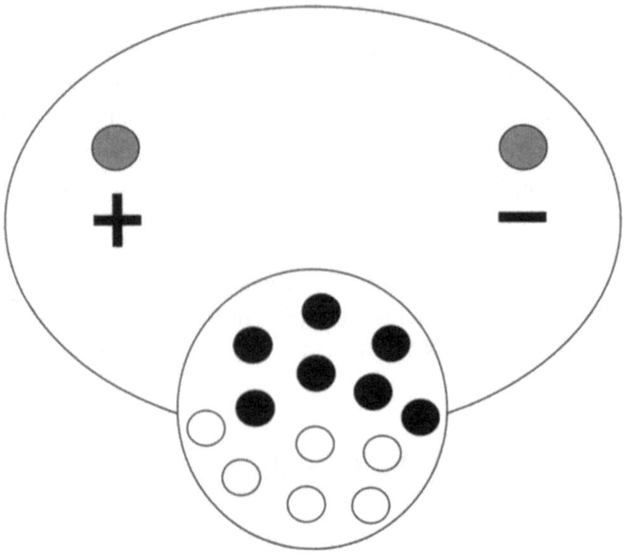

FIGURE 10.2.1. Electrically stimulated graciloplasty design. The circles represent motor units (shaded circles are conversion to Type I fibers for continuous contraction).

Another reason for loss of contraction could be a possible breakage of the electrode. In our experience with 300 patients and 600 electrodes, this has never happened; the solution in such a case is electrode replacement. On one occasion, our unit experienced damage to the isolation sheath and a leakage of current leading to weak contraction of the muscle. The solution here was replacement of the electrode. Loss of contraction also can occur when the electrode is distracted from the muscle. Dislocation means that the electrode generates an electrical field, but the nerve to the gracilis is no longer in the vicinity of this field. We have observed this once in a patient who played with the stimulator located in a subcutaneous pocket, where she turned the stimulator around and the electrodes twisted around and were torn out of the gracilis. The therapy there was reinsertion of the electrode.

Weak contraction can be seen when the amplitude is too low, meaning that the amplitude is close to the threshold. The threshold is the lowest amplitude with which a reaction of the muscle can be seen; the therapy was to reprogram the stimulator to a higher amplitude. Non-contraction of course is seen when the battery is empty. In that case, the programming of the stimulator is no longer possible. For the most part, the nearing end of the battery can be detected a few months earlier during programming. The solution here is simple: the implantable pulse generator (IPG) has to be replaced. The longevity of the stimulator is dependant upon the programmed amplitude and frequency, and in our experience, this lasts for a median of about eight years (8). The programming of the stimulator itself is not very difficult. Changes can be made in amplitude, frequency, pulse width, the polarity of the electrodes, and in the IPG. The impedance can be measured, providing an indication whether or not the electrodes are intact or dislocated. Almost all stimulation problems are potentially solvable.

When the problem of poor or non-contractility is not a stimulation problem, the cause is most likely a malfunction of the muscle itself. The test to determine this has already been discussed. When no voluntary contraction is possible, something is primarily wrong with the muscle. The gracilis muscle is the most superficial adductor in the upper leg and is innervated by a branch of the obturator nerve. This nerve is always accompanied by the branches of the obturator artery and vein. These three structures reach the gracilis muscle invariably eight centimeters from the origin of the gracilis. In freeing the gracilis muscle for the transposition around the anus, the nerve, artery, and/or vein can be damaged. These structures can also be damaged by traction in the transposition position. Damage of the nerve leads to atrophy, occlusion of the artery and necrosis, whereas damage to the vein leads to significant muscle congestion. This damage can lead to the disappearance of the entire muscle or to its deterioration into a fibrotic string around the anus so that the contractile function is lost. This problem has never been seen in our experience of over 300 dynamic graciloplasties. The gracilis also has peripheral arteries and veins. The number of peripheral arteries varies between patients, and in one patient even between the left and the right sides.

These peripheral structures have to be divided in order to make an adequate functioning gracilis wrap. In most cases, this division creates no problem for the survival of the muscle because the vessels of the gracilis form one vascular network that can sufficiently vascularize the whole muscle from the main proximal artery and vein (12). Nevertheless, in some muscles, the division leads to hypoperfusion of the distal part and to its distal fibrosis. When the distal part cannot contract, this leads to malfunction of the dynamic graciloplasty. This problem is seen in a small percentage of patients. The solution is a new graciloplasty from the other side or the application of another technique such as the artificial bowel sphincter (ABS) (13) (see Chapter 10.3).

Non-contractility of the gracilis seems to be present when the wrap is too loose. The muscle is not able to constrict the anal canal sufficiently. The same phenomenon occurs when the attachment of the distal tendon of the muscle to the periosteum of the pubic bone loosens. In these cases, re-attachment or shortening of the tendon can be a solution. During graciloplasty, it is always difficult to judge how tight the wrap must be, and as a general rule, we place one finger between the anus and the gracilis wrap and then suture the distal tendon tightly to fit against the pubic bone.

Non-contractility is also seen when the patient is under general anesthesia and muscle relaxants are used. This, of course, will disappear when the patient is awakened. General neurological diseases seldom afflict the gracilis muscle, and even in cases of paresis of the whole leg, the gracilis stays functional.

Persisting Incontinence

One of the most frustrating findings after graciloplasty is when the patient is not able to control stool despite a well-contracting muscle. One has to realize that continence is much more than only the function of the sphincters. When a patient with fecal incontinence is analyzed and a deficient sphincter is found, it is logical that this is an indication to restore that function with an anal repair, a dynamic graciloplasty or an ABS. Other reasons for incontinence can be under-detected at that stage. When we assess patients with incontinence after a successful restoration of sphincter function, problems of hyposensibility, deficient rectal capacity, or rectal compliance with loose consistency of the stool become more prominent. Therapies to improve rectal sensibility are not always successful, and the only thing that can be done is to try physiotherapy with rectal balloons. A balloon can be placed into the rectum and inflated with several different volumes of air. The patient can try to concentrate on feeling low filling volumes. The stool consistency can be influenced by diets or constipating drugs, and the capacity of the rectum can be enlarged by gradual rectal filling with balloon distension or by operations to augment the rectum. A good technique is to bring down a vascular-intact bowel loop and to suture this onto the opened frontal side of the rectum in the same way as urologists create a bladder augmentation (e.g., cecocystoplasty) (14). However, even with these extra therapies in quite a number of cases, patients often stay incontinent and operations to restore the sphincter function are blamed for this poor outcome. However, they often are successful in improving sphincter function, although they cannot make up for the other deficient factors. Combinations of sphincter restoration and conservative therapy often ultimately result in success.

Constipation

One of the most frequent functional problems after dynamic graciloplasty is constipation. The first thought, of course, is that the wrap is too tight, forming an obstruction. This indeed can happen once in a while, but is actually quite rare. We have seen such a stenosis in only five cases in 300 patients (1.6%). Therapy for this condition includes detachment of the gracilis tendon, resulting in a good outcome in two of these five patients so that the cut tendon allowed the gracilis to retract over a small distance. The gracilis probably was connected to the surrounding tissue in such a way that a complete retraction did not occur. Two patients stayed continent after this procedure.

In most cases, the constipation is seen in patients who have a normal accessible anus and anal manometry shows normal values. We found constipation without stenosis in 16% of our cases. It is very frustrating for the patients when incontinence for feces is replaced by severe constipation. Here, transit studies in these patients often give an indication for slow-transit constipation without outlet obstruction. One can speculate how this is possible, where many patients have a history of constipation first developing in their youth. Severe constipation may lead to expulsion difficulties and destruction of the anal sphincters. These patients then become incontinent despite their firm stool and hidden constipation. When patients are seen in the phase of incontinence, therapies like dynamic graciloplasty are provided in specialist units. This restores the sphincter function; however, the original problem resurfaces. There is no absolute proof of this, but it provides an acceptable explanation of this problem.

The treatment for this constipation is initially dietary therapy and laxative drugs. In most cases, this is sufficient, but some patients require enemas. Here, water enemas can be used in small volumes with a syringe or in large volumes with the aid of a pump. This retrograde lavage (15) of the colon is almost always successful. The median time to clean the bowel is usually about 20 minutes. Two patients in our series had no success with this retrograde lavage and complained that only the distal part of the colon was effectively emptied. In these patients, we used a Malone appendicostomy for antegrade lavage (16). This resulted in one good and one poor outcome. Of course, one can argue that patients who need to lavage the colon after dynamic graciloplasty probably have "pseudoincontinence" and do not need their graciloplasty in the first place. Nevertheless, these patients benefit from the tighter anus that makes it possible to instill the fluid into the colon without leakage. During the time between two separate lavages, these patients remained continent. Another form of antegrade lavage is described by the group headed by Professor Norman Williams (17). They divided the sigmoid colon and constructed an end-to-side anastomosis of the proximal part to the distal part. Here, the transected distal portion was then invaginated and anastomosed to the skin of the abdomen as a continent stoma for antegrade tap-water irrigation. Although good results have been described with this procedure, the extra intervention is complex when compared with the Malone procedure.

Conclusions

Graciloplasty has been used in one form or another for fecal incontinence since 1946, although electrically stimulated graciloplasty designed to convert fatigable fibers into fatigue-resistant fibers has only been introduced and studied in the last 15 years. In well-selected patients, there is a durable success in over 70% of cases (18). Disturbances of evacuation are a problem in up to one-fifth of cases, although this is usually a temporary problem. We still require parameters that are more likely to accurately predict successful outcome following this procedure. It may well be that dynamic graciloplasty might be successful in those patients where initial sacral neuromodulation has provided only limited response, and in this regard, dynamic graciloplasty has paved the way for improved understanding of the effects of electrical stimulation on the anal sphincter (19).

References

1. Pickrell KL, Broadbent TR, Masters FW, and Metzger JT. Construction of a rectal sphincter and restoration of continence by transplanting the gracilis muscle. Ann Surg. 1952;135(6):853–62.
2. Pette D. Fiber transformation and fiber replacement in chronically stimulated muscle. J Heart Lung Transplant. 1992;11:S299–S305.
3. Baeten C, Spaans F, and Fluks A. An implanted neuromuscular stimulator for fecal continence following previously implanted gracilis muscle. Report of a case. Dis Colon Rectum. 1988;31(2):134–7.
4. Konsten J, Baeten CG, Havenith MG, and Soeters PB. Morphology of dynamic graciloplasty compared with the anal sphincter. Dis Colon Rectum. 1993;36(6): 559–63.
5. Mander BJ, Wexner SD, Williams NS, Bartolo DC, Lubowski DZ, Oresland T, et al. Preliminary results of a multicentre trial of the electrically stimulated gracilis neoanal sphincter. Br J Surg. 1999;86(12):1543–8.
6. Seccia M, Menconi C, Balestri R, and Cavina E. Study protocols and functional results in 86 electrostimulated graciloplasties. Dis Colon Rectum. 1994;37(9): 897–904.
7. Mavrantonis C, Billotti VL, and Wexner SD. Stimulated graciloplasty for treatment of intractable fecal incontinence: critical influence of the method of stimulation. Dis Colon Rectum. 1999;42(4):497–504.
8. Rongen MJGMU, O; El Naggar K, Geerdes BP, Konsten J, and Baeten CGMI. Long term results of dynamic graciloplasty for fecal incontinence. Dis Colon Rectum. In press 2003.
9. Matzel KE, Madoff RD, LaFontaine LJ, Baeten CG, Buie WD, Christiansen J, et al. Complications of dynamic graciloplasty: incidence, management, and impact on outcome. Dis Colon Rectum. 2001;44(10):1427–35.
10. Geerdes BP, Heineman E, Konsten J, Soeters PB, and Baeten CG. Dynamic graciloplasty. Complications and management. Dis Colon Rectum. 1996;39(8): 912–17.
11. Rongen MJGM, Adang EM, Gerritsen van der Hoop A, and Baeten CI. One step versus two step procedure in dynamic graciloplasty. Submitted 1999.
12. Geerdes BP, Kurvers HA, Konsten J, Heineman E, and Baeten CG. Assessment of ischaemia of the distal part of the gracilis muscle during transposition for anal dynamic graciloplasty. Br J Surg. 1997;84(8):1127–9.

13. Wong WD, Congliosi SM, Spencer MP, et al. The safety and efficacy of the artificial bowel sphincter for fecal incontinence: results from a multicenter cohort study. Dis Colon Rectum. 2002;45(9):1139–53.
14. Williams NS, Ogunbiyi OA, Scott SM, Fajobi O, and Lunniss PJ. Rectal augmentation and stimulated gracilis anal neosphincter: a new approach in the management of fecal urgency and incontinence. Dis Colon Rectum. 2001;44: 192–8.
15. Briel JW, Schouten WR, Vlot EA, Smits S, and van Kessel I. Clinical value of colonic irrigation in patients with continence disturbances. Dis Colon Rectum. 1997;40(7):802–5.
16. Rongen MJ, van der Hoop AG, and Baeten CG. Cecal access for antegrade colon enemas in medically refractory slow-transit constipation: a prospective study. Dis Colon Rectum. 2001;44(11):1644–9.
17. Abercrombie JE and Williams NS. Total anorectal reconstruction. Br J Surg. 1995;82(4):438–42.
18. Rongen MJ, Uludag O, El Naggar K, Gerdes BP, Konsten J, and Baeten CG. Long-term follow-up of dynamic graciloplasty for fecal incontinence. Dis Colon Rectum. 2003;46:716–21.
19. Baeten CG, Bailey HR, Bakka A, et al. Safety and efficacy of dynamic graciloplasty for fecal incontinence: report of a prospective, multicenter trial. Dynamic Graciloplasty Therapy Study Group. Dis Colon Rectum. 2000;43:743–51.

Editorial Commentary

Dynamic graciloplasty has become a widely accepted option for the treatment of severe fecal incontinence in patients otherwise refractory for treatment and potentially destined for a stoma. The technique was largely championed and developed by Dr. Cornelius Baeten and therefore it is appropriate that along with his coworkers he has provided the information. He notes that the successful outcome of this operation varies from 56% to 80% and describes many of the reasons for failure of the operation to achieve its optimal goal, showing the significance of noncontractility in constipation which may occur following this operation. Although the dynamic graciloplasty is no longer available in the United States it is available throughout the rest of the world and many patients in the United States have already undergone this operation necessitating some familiarity with its complications and aftermath which directly affect outcome and case presentation to the coloproctologist working in a tertiary referral center.

SW

Chapter 10.3
Assessing the Functional Results of the Artificial Bowel Sphincter

T. CRISTINA SARDINHA and JUAN J. NOGUERAS

Introduction

Anal incontinence is defined as the uncontrolled passage of flatus or stool. This social, physical, and psychological disability affects one to two percernt of the American population (see Chapter 7). However, the true incidence of anal incontinence is clearly underestimated. Anal incontinence is the most frequent reason for nursing home admissions, leading to a major economic burden to the patient, their family, and society overall. The most common cause of anal incontinence is obstetric injury, followed by iatrogenic procedures and traumatic injuries to the perineum and anorectum (1). Anal incontinence may vary from mild to severe, and there are a diversity of classifications that have been reported to quantify its severity. We have adopted the Cleveland Clinic Florida incontinence score system (2), which assesses the degree of anal incontinence based on the frequency of uncontrolled loss of flatus, liquid, or solid stool. Moreover, it determines the social impact of anal incontinence.

The overall management of anal incontinence is based on the extent of neurologic and/or anatomic involvement of the anorectum. Options may vary from dietary modifications to fecal diversion. However, for patients with severe, irreparable anal incontinence, the surgical options are limited. In recent years, a new approach for the management of these difficult patients has emerged. Increasing numbers of reports have been published detailing outcomes after implantation of the artificial bowel sphincter (ABS) for fecal incontinence (3–8). A multicenter prospective study was carried out among 19 sites—13 in the United States, three in Canada, and three in Europe. Based on safety data from this clinical trial, the Food and Drug Administration (FDA) awarded the artificial anal sphincter approval as a Humanitarian Use Device in 1999. The device is currently available and designated as the Acticon™ Neosphincter (American Medical Systems).

Device Description

The American Medical System artificial bowel sphincter (ABS) is an implantable, fluid-filled, solid silicone elastomer device. The ABS consists of three components; namely, a cuff, a control pump (with septum), and a pressure-regulating balloon—each of which is attached to the other with kink-resistant tubing (Figure 10.3.1). The ABS simulates normal sphincter function by opening and closing the anal canal at the control of the patient.

The occlusive cuff is implanted around a segment of the anal canal, and when inflated, it occludes the canal by applying circumferential peranal pressure (Figure 10.3.2). The cuff is available in a variety of widths and lengths and the surgeon determines the appropriate size to be used in the

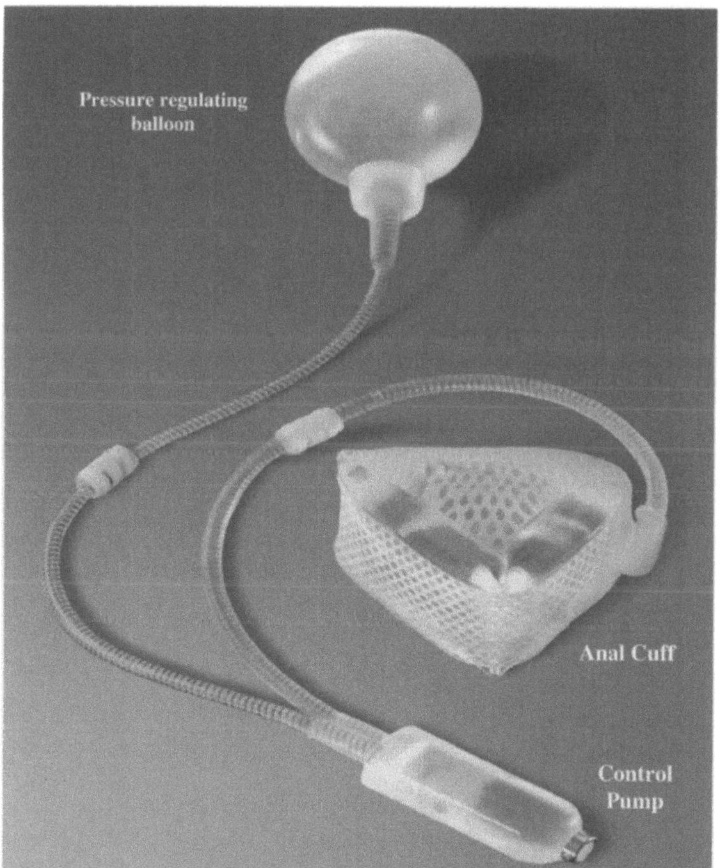

FIGURE 10.3.1. The ABS consists of three components: a cuff, a control pump (with septum), and a pressure-regulating balloon, each of which is attached to the other by kink-resistant tubing. (Courtesy of American Medical Systems.)

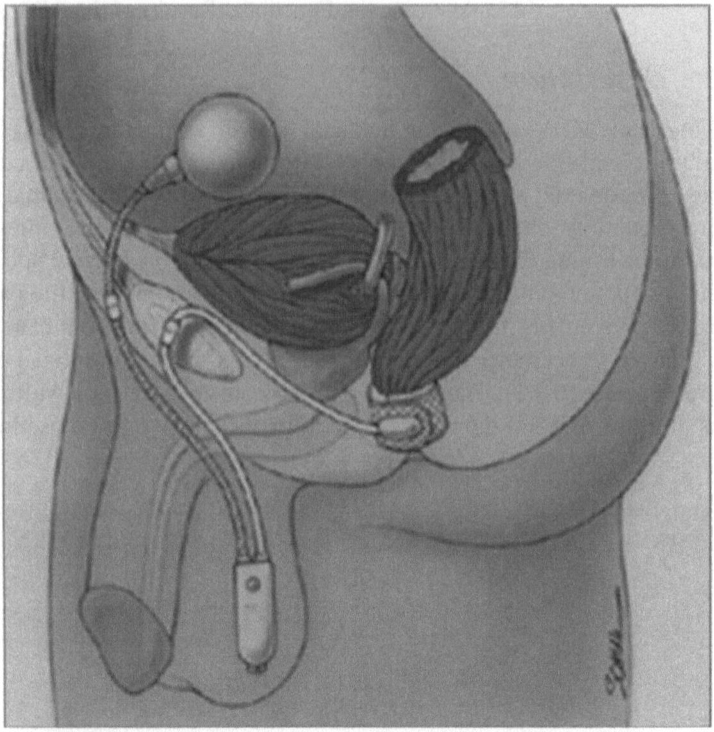

a

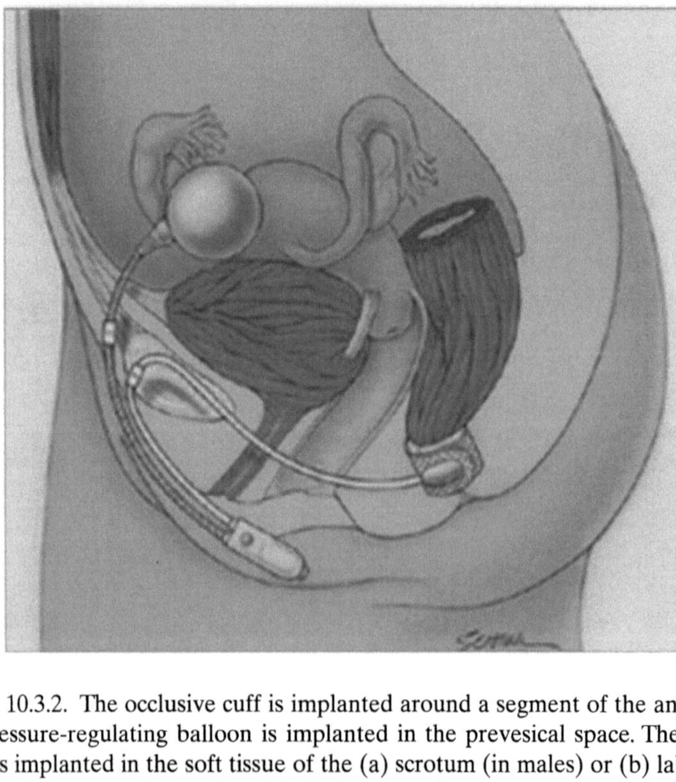

b

FIGURE 10.3.2. The occlusive cuff is implanted around a segment of the anal canal. The pressure-regulating balloon is implanted in the prevesical space. The control pump is implanted in the soft tissue of the (a) scrotum (in males) or (b) labium (in females). (Courtesy of American Medical Systems.)

patient by intraoperatively measuring the circumference and length of the anal canal. The pressure-regulating balloon is implanted in the prevesical space controlling the amount of pressure exerted by the occlusive cuff (Figure 10.3.2). This balloon is made of silicone elastomer and is available in a range of different pressure settings. The most commonly implanted balloons are in the ranges 91 to 100 and 101 to 110 centimeters H_2O. The control pump is implanted in the soft tissue of the scrotum (Figure 10.3.2a) or labium (Figure 10.3.2b) and is approximately 1.2 centimeters wide and 3.6 centimeters long. The upper part of the control pump contains the resistor and valves needed to transfer fluid to and from the cuff; it also contains the deactivation button. The patient squeezes and releases the bulb at the bottom half of the control pump to transfer fluid within the device (Figures 10.3.3–10.3.5). A septum at the bottom of the control pump is designed to allow the insertion of a small amount of fluid, if needed, in the postoperative period. The ABS prosthesis has color-coded tubing to help the surgeon create the correct tubing connections.

Preoperative Preparation

On the evening prior to surgery, the patient undergoes a standard mechanical and antibiotic bowel preparation. Once in the operating room, the patient is placed in the lithotomy position and the anal and genital area is shaved. A proctoscopic examination is performed to ensure adequate rectal

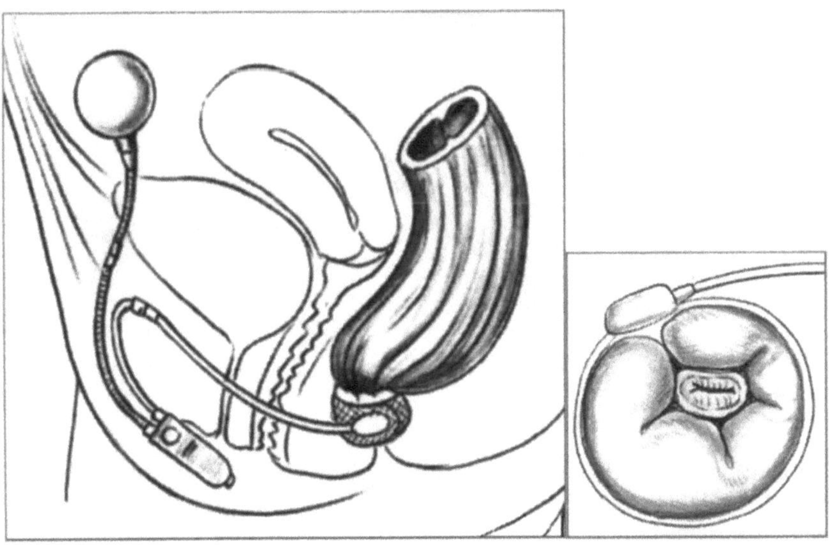

FIGURE 10.3.3. The ABS (Acticon™) at rest: the cuff is full and the sphincter is closed. (Courtesy of American Medical Systems.)

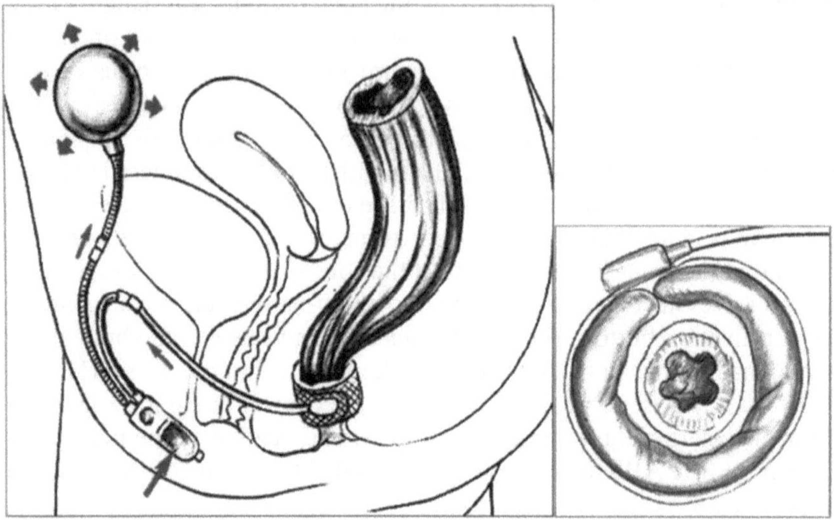

FIGURE 10.3.4. The ABS (Acticon™) at work: the pump empties the cuff and the sphincter opens, allowing a bowel movement. (Courtesy of American Medical Systems.)

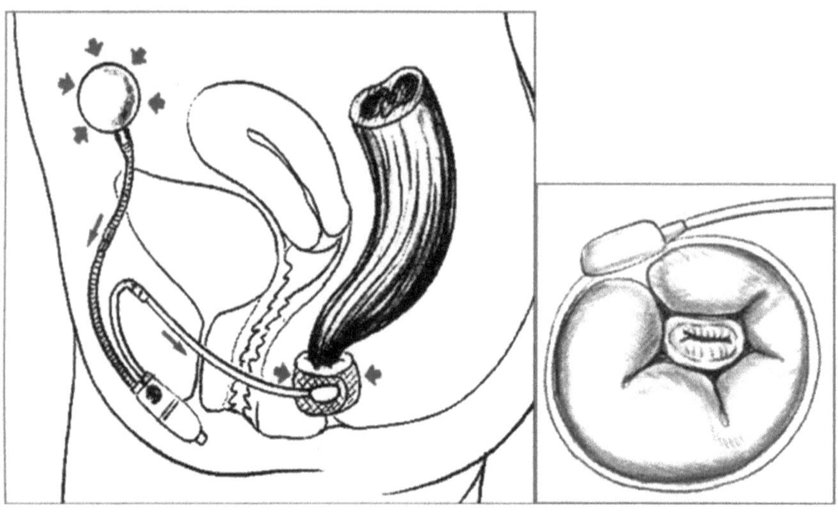

FIGURE 10.3.5. The ABS (Acticon™) with continence restored: the cuff refills automatically and the sphincter recloses to maintain continence. (Courtesy of American Medical Systems.)

cleansing and the rectum is irrigated with Betadine and saline. A Betadine-soaked gauze pad is placed in the rectum to minimize leakage. The authors prefer to tag the gauze pad with a large looped suture in order to facilitate its removal at the completion of the procedure.

Equipment Preparation

Silicone components actively attract dust and lint; therefore, one should avoid cloth drapes, which attract lint, and ensure that all surgical gloves are rinsed free of powder. In a separate stand, the components are filled with the appropriate filling solution. We prefer Cysto-Conray II, diluted 60 cubic centimeters of dye with 15 cubic centimeters of sterile water. The preparation of the components requires care and precision. For example, over-distension of the occlusive cuff will result in permanent cuff damage.

Intraoperative Steps

There are several important intraoperative steps involved in the implantation of the ABS; namely,

- making the skin incisions,
- encircling the anal canal,
- sizing the occlusive cuff,
- creating the pocket for the pressure-regulating balloon,
- creating the pocket for the control pump, and
- making all connections.

The surgeon must decide on the location of the perineal incisions. The two most popular options are a single anterior transverse incision or bilateral vertical para-anal incisions. Until very recently, European surgeons have favored the single anterior transverse perineal incision, claiming that this minimizes the risk of rectal perforation in a heavily scarred perineal body. Conversely, North American surgeons have preferred the bilateral vertical incisions. Over time, the bilateral incisions have been placed further laterally, allowing for adequate dissection in the ischiorectal fossa and sufficient distance between the incisions and the anus. The downside of the bilateral perianal incisions is the blind, blunt anterior dissection of the perineal body. Recently, the trend towards an anterior perineal incision among the various high-volume centers has been apparent. In our center, this incision is being used with greater frequency.

Using blunt dissection, a circumferential tunnel is created around the anal canal several centimeters deep into the ischiorectal fossa. The most difficult part of this maneuver is the anterior dissection, where extra care is taken to avoid a rectal perforation. Once a circumferential tunnel is created, the surgeon then must size the length and thickness of the anal canal so as to select the appropriately sized occlusive cuff using a cuff sizer. Several points are worth mentioning at this juncture. First, the tendency is to select a cuff that is too occlusive in the deactivated position. This is dangerous, as it may lead to pressure necrosis of the rectal wall and subsequent cuff erosion into the rectum. The authors always ensure that the cuff sizer places no pressure on the rectal wall.

The occlusive cuff is now implanted around the anal canal. The location of the cuff tubing should be on the same side as the control pump, so this must be preoperatively determined by asking the patient his/her preference. Most right-handed patients will prefer to have the control pump on their right side. A suprapubic incision is then made and the rectus fascia is divided. The linea alba is separated bluntly and a pocket is created in the prevesical space of sufficient size to accommodate the pressure-regulating balloon, where it is easier to insert the deflated balloon prior to its filling with the filling solution. Once properly situated, making a direct connection with the balloon pressurizes the occlusive cuff. To implant the control pump in the scrotum or labium majus, blunt dissection is then used to create a dependent pouch in a position above Scarpa's fascia. The tunnel is dilated with Hegar dilators up to a #14 size. The control pump is then placed in the pocket, ensuring that the deactivation button faces anteriorly and is palpable.

Once the components are in place, the tubings are connected. The device is now activated and must be deactivated prior to leaving the operating room. It will remain deactivated for the first six weeks postoperatively.

Clinical Experience

Christiansen and Lorentzen reported their initial experience with five patients with neurogenic incontinence treated with implantation of an 800 AMS® urinary sphincter around the anus (3). Continence was achieved for solid and semi-solid stool, but not for diarrhea. In a subsequent report by Christiansen and Sparso, the experience with 12 patients was described (4). Of the 10 patients available for follow-up evaluation with greater than six months follow-up, five had excellent results, three had good results, and two had acceptable results. Two patients required explantation of the device due to infection and four patients had a total of eight revisional procedures. Wong et al. reported their experience in 12 patients who underwent implantation of an artificial anal sphincter (5). Three infections and three mechanical complications occurred in four patients (33%). A successful outcome was achieved in eight patients (75%). Lehur et al. described their experience with 13 patients who underwent implantation of the artificial anal sphincter (6). After a median follow-up of 20 months, nine of ten patients with a functioning sphincter were continent for stool and five were also continent for gas. Sepsis occurred in two patients and three patients required device explantation.

Lehur et al. then published the experience of three European centers in 24 consecutive patients who underwent implantation with a minimum follow-up of six months (7). Of the 24 patients, seven had the device explanted, of which three were successfully reimplanted. Therefore, 20 patients (83%) had an implanted, activated device overall. Incontinence scores improved significantly postoperatively, both in the short term and in the long term. Overall, a high degree of satisfaction was achieved in 18 (75%) of these patients. O'Brien and Skinner reported an improvement in the Cleveland Clinic Florida (CCF) incontinence score from 18.7 ± 1.6 preoperatively to 2.1 ± 2.6 after activation of the ABS ($p < 0.0001$) (9).

Wong et al. published the results of a multicenter, prospective, nonrandomized trial under common protocol in which 112 of 115 patients were implanted (8). A total of 384 device-related or potentially device-related adverse events were reported in 99 enrolled patients. In 51 of the 112 implanted patients (46%), 73 revision operations were required. The infection rate necessitating surgical revision was 25%. Despite the high morbidity rate, a successful outcome was achieved in 85% of patients with a functioning device. The intention to treat success rate was overall 53%. Devesa et al. analyzed their data in 53 patients who underwent implantation of the Acticon™ neosphincter (10).

Perioperative events occurred in 26% of patients, including abnormal bleeding, vaginal perforation, rectal perforation, and even unobserved urethral perforation. Early complications included infection (15%) and wound complications (15%), whereas late complications included cuff and/or pump erosion (18%), infection (6%), impaction (22%), pain (8%), and mechanical failures (4%). The definitive explantation rate in this series was 19%, and of the remaining 43 patients with a device, only 60% continued to use the device. Ortiz et al. published their experience in 24 consecutive patients who underwent implantation of the Acticon™ neosphincter. The cumulative probability of device explantation was 44% at 48 months (11). Of the 15 patients with a functioning implant, there was significant improvement in the incontinence score and functional outcome. Lehur et al. also have demonstrated a significant improvement in quality of life after successful implantation in 16 consecutive patients (12).

A recent publication from the University of Minnesota reported the long-term results of 45 patients who underwent implantation of an ABS device. The study population was divided into two groups based on the time of implantation of the device. Group I (operated from 1989 to 1992) consisted of 10 patients. Of those, six had a functioning ABS (mean follow-up 91, range 29–143 months). Of the 35 patients in Group II (operated from 1997 to 2001), 17 had a functioning ABS (mean follow-up 39, range 12–60 months). The overall infection rate was 34%. Thirty-seven per cent of the study population required revisional surgery. The overall success for patients with severe fecal incontinence treated with the ABS was 49% (13). Despite a growing number of publications assuring the feasibility and safety of the ABS device for the surgical treatment of disabling anal incontinence, long-term results of this innovative approach are awaited and are currently anecdotal (14–17). Furthermore, problems such as device infection, impaired evacuation, and skin erosion still need to be minimized. Nonetheless, careful patient selection and an experienced surgical team are keystones for the successful outcome of the ABS device in the treatment of anal incontinence (18).

Moreover, further efforts are required to optimize the surgical therapy of anal incontinence, including improved technology and prospective randomized trials developed by specialized colorectal surgery centers, along with improvements in topical therapies for passive incontinence secondary to internal anal sphincter damage. Advances and outcomes in radiofrequency treatments (the SECCA procedure), (19) the PROCON intra-anal photosensor (20), and the ACYST™ (Carbon Medical Technology, Minnesota), which is a submucosal injection of pyrolytic carbon beads (212–500 μm) akin to the periurethral bead insertion used to assist urinary stress incontinence (21,22) are awaited. The role of the ABS device and its indications in total anorectal reconstruction is at present unclear (23).

References

1. Oliveira L and Wexner SD. Anal incontinence. In: Beck DE and Wexner SD, editors. Fundamentals of anorectal surgery. 2nd ed. London: WB Saunders: London; 1998. p. 115–52.
2. Jorge JMN and Wexner SD. Etiology and management of fecal incontinence. Dis Colon Rectum. 1993;36:77–97.
3. Christiansen J and Lorentzen M. Implantation of artificial sphincter for anal incontinence: Report of five cases. Dis Colon Rectum. 1989;32:432–6.
4. Christiansen J and Sparso B. Treatment of anal incontinence by an implantable prosthetic anal sphincter. Ann Surg. 1992;215:383–6.
5. Wong WD, Jensen LL, Bartolo DC, and Rothenberger DA. Artificial anal sphincter. Dis Colon Rectum. 1996;39:1345–51.
6. Lehur PA, Michot F, Denis P, et al. Results of artificial sphincter in severe anal incontinence: Report of 14 consecutive implantations. Dis Colon Rectum. 1996;39:1352–5.
7. Lehur PA, Roig JV, and Duinslaeger M. Artificial anal sphincter: Prospective clinical and manometric evaluation. Dis Colon Rectum. 2000;43:1100–6.
8. Wong, WD, Congilosi SM, Spencer MP, Corman ML, Tan P, Opelka F, Burnstein M, Nogueras JJ, Bailey HR, et al. The safety and efficacy of the artificial bowel sphincter for fecal incontinence: results from a multicenter cohort study. Dis Colon Rectum. 2002;45:1139–53.
9. O'Brien PE and Skinner S. Restoring control. The Acticon Neosphincter ® artificial bowel sphincter in the treatment of anal incontinence. Dis Colon Rectum. 2000;43:1213–16.
10. Devesa JM, Rey A, Hervas PL, et al. Artificial anal sphincter: complications and functional results: a large personal series. Dis Colon Rectum. 2002;45:1154–63.

11. Ortiz H, Armendariz P, DeMiguel M, Ruiz MD, Alos R, and Roig JV. Complications and functional outcome following artificial anal sphincter implantation. Br J Surg. 2002;89:877–81.
12. Lehur PA, Zerbib F, Neunlist M, Glemain P, and Bruley des Varannes S. Comparison and anorectal function after artificial anal sphincter implantation. Dis Colon Rectum. 2002;45:508–13.
13. Parker SC, Spencer MP, Madoff RD, Jensen LL, Wong WD, and Rothenberger DA. Artificial bowel sphincter. Long-term Experience at a single institution. Dis Colon Rectum. 2003;46:722–9.
14. Michot F, Costaglioli B, Leroi AM, and Denis P. Artificial bowel sphincter in severe fecal incontinence. Outcome of prospective experience with 37 patients in one institution. Ann Surg. 2003;237:52–6.
15. Altomare DF, Dodi G, LaTorre F, Romano G, Melega E, and Rinaldi M. Multicentric retrospective analysis of the outcome or artificial anal sphincter implantation for severe fecal incontinence. Br J Surg. 2001;88:1487–91.
16. DiBsise JK. In charge of incontinence: Not quite there yet. Am J Gastrenterol. 1999;94:2008.
17. Christiansen J. The artificial anal sphincter. Can J Gastroenterol. 2000;14(suppl D):152–4.
18. Madoff RD, Baeten CGMI, Christiansen J, Rosen HR, Williams NS, Heine JA, Lehur PA, Lowry AC, Lubowski DZ, Matzel KE, Nicholls RJ, Seccia M, Thorson AG, Wexner SD, and Wong WD. Standards for anal sphincter replacement. Dis Colon Rectum. 2000;43:135–41.
19. Efron JE, Corman ML, Fleshman J, Barnett J, Nagle D, Birnbaum E, Weiss EG, Nogueras JJ, Sligh S, Rabine J, and Wexner SD. Safety and effectiveness of temperature-controlled radio-frequency energy delivery to the anal canal (Secca procedure) for the treatment of fecal incontinence. Dis Colon Rectum. 2003;46:1606–18.
20. Giamundo P, Welber A, Weiss EG, Vernava AM 3rd, Nogueras JJ, and Wexner SD. The procon incontinence device: a new nonsurgical approach to preventing fecal incontinence. Am J Gastroenterol. 2002,97.2328–32.
21. Weiss EG, Efron J, Nogueras JJ, and Wexner SD. Submucosal injection of carbon coated beads is a successful and safe office based treatment of fecal incontinence. Dis Colon Rectum. 2002;45:A46–7.
22. Madjar S, Covington-Nichols C, and Secrest CL. New periurethral bulking agents for stress urinary incontinence: modified technique and early results. J Urol. 2003;170(6 Pt 1):2327–9.
23. Romano G, La Torre F, Cutini G, Bianco F, Esposito P, and Montori A. Total anorectal reconstruction with the artificial bowel sphincter: report of eight cases. A quality of life assessment. Dis Colon Rectum. 2003;46:730–4.

Editorial Commentary

Dr. Sardinha, (an alumnus of the Cleveland Clinic Florida at the Department of Colorectal Surgery) and Dr. Juan Nogueras (one of the faculty members since 1991) have described in a very detailed manner the technique of artificial bowel sphincter implantation. Certainly the outline of intraoperative steps in this procedure as well as the general preoperative and intraoperative considerations are very helpful to anyone contemplating performing or already performing this procedure. Drs. Sardinha and Nogueras have also evaluated the world literature to provide an authoritatively written and comprehensively referenced current and complete compendium on the subject of the artificial bowel sphincter and in particular have offered very useful illustrations and drawings to facilitate performance of this technique.

SW

Chapter 11
Functional Problems in the Patient with a Neurological Disorder

JEANETTE GAW and WALTER E. LONGO

Introduction

Bowel function and continence are regulated by a number of factors. These include the intrinsic enteric nervous system, autonomic and voluntary nervous system, hormones, and luminal contents. Patients with neurologic diseases are beleaguered by abnormal colorectal function. The most common complaints are constipation and fecal incontinence. These can have a devastating effect on their social lives and significantly impact upon their quality of life. Bowel dysfunction was rated as a moderate to severe life-limiting problem by close to half of the patients with a spinal cord injury (1). In order to manage these patients properly, a thorough understanding of normal physiology that controls bowel function is essential. Knowledge of the different alterations that occur with each neurologic disorder also is important in managing neurogenic bowel dysfunction.

Normal Physiology of Colonic Motility

Colorectal Motility

One of the main functions of the colon is to transport contents from the ileum to the anus. Contractions of the smooth muscles in the circular and longitudinal layers of the bowel are responsible for luminal transport. There are two types of contractions: phasic and tonic (2). Phasic contractions increase intraluminal pressures whereas tonic contractions are less well defined. Haustral contractions are an important type of phasic contraction. These are localized, segmental contractions that cause mixing of colonic contents and allow absorption of water and electrolytes. Another type of phasic contraction is the mass contraction. Mass contractions affect large segments of the colon and cause propulsion of contents towards the rectum. A gastrocolic response is a mass contraction that is stimulated by a meal.

Colonic motility is coordinated by three factors; namely, myogenic, chemical, and neurogenic (3). The enteric smooth muscles are interconnected by gap junctions, producing a syncytium of smooth muscle. The myogenic transmission occurs through these connections. Most intestinal smooth muscle displays autorhythmicity, which causes colonic wall contractions. Chemical control of colonic contractile activity is achieved through neurotransmitters and hormones. These substances may act through a paracrine or endocrine fashion and include peptides, amines, acetylcholine, prostaglandins, and sex steroids. These promote or inhibit colonic contractions through the action on the central nervous system, autonomic nervous system, enteric nervous system, or by direct action on muscle cells. The neurogenic control of colonic motility is through both the intrinsic nervous system and the autonomic nervous system.

Intrinsic Colonic Nervous System

Colonic contractions and function are coordinated by the intrinsic colonic nervous system. The intrinsic colonic nervous system consists of approximately 100 million neurons within the myenteric plexus (Auerbach's plexus) and submucosal plexus (Meissner's plexus) (4). The myenteric plexus is located between the circular and longitudinal muscles. It consists of unmyelinated fibers and postganglionic parasympathetic cell bodies. Part of its function is to regulate peristalsis and the secretory function of the mucosa. The submucosal plexus, on the other hand, innervates the muscularis mucosa, intestinal endocrine cells, and submucosal blood vessels. Additionally, it relays local sensorimotor responses to the myenteric plexus, prevertebral ganglia, and the spinal cord.

The enteric ganglia are not merely relay stations for signals from the central nervous system. They are interconnected and are capable of processing information much like the central nervous system. The intrinsic nervous system of the colon may be thought of as containing several preprogrammed modules of behavior. In turn, these are affected by the sympathetic and parasympathetic nervous systems, hormones, and luminal contents (5). With this system, a few parasympathetic efferent fibers can activate blocks of integrated circuits within the intrinsic colonic nervous system, thereby affecting motility throughout the colon (5).

Extrinsic Colonic Nervous System

The extrinsic nervous control of the colon is provided by the autonomic nervous system (6). The autonomic nervous system is subdivided into the sympathetic and parasympathetic nervous system.

Sympathetic Nervous System

The sympathetic innervation of the colon parallels the blood supply. The lateral columns of T5 to T12 provide sympathetic innervation to the right colon, whereas the lateral columns of T12 to L3 innervate the left colon and upper rectum. The preganglionic fibers pass through the white rami communicantes to the sympathetic chain. For the right colon, following the sympathetic chain, the fibers travel via the thoracic splanchnic nerves to synapse at the celiac and superior mesenteric plexi. The postganglionic fibers then travel along the superior mesenteric artery and its branches to the right colon. In contrast, for the left colon and the upper rectum, the fibers after the sympathetic chain travel via the lumbar splanchnic nerves to join the preaortic plexus and synapse at the inferior mesenteric plexus. Just as the innervation of the right colon follows its vasculature, the postganglionic fibers then travel via the inferior mesenteric artery to the left colon and upper rectum.

The sympathetic innervation of the lower rectum and the anal canal is supplied by the aortic plexus and the two lateral lumbar splanchnic nerves. The nerves combine to form the superior hypogastric plexus—the presacral nerve—and descends into the pelvis. It then divides into two hypogastric nerves that can be found at the sacral promontory. It continues on caudally to supply the lower rectum and anal canal.

In general, colonic and rectal motility and contractility are inhibited by sympathetic stimulation. Sympathetic stimulation of the internal anal sphincter (IAS) was classically thought to cause a constriction (7), although there is some evidence that under some circumstances it may cause a relaxation (8).

Parasympathetic Nervous System

The parasympathetic nervous supply of the colon comes from the vagus nerve and the sacral parasympathetic nerves. The right colon is supplied by the posterior vagus nerve, which passes through the celiac plexus to the preaortic and superior mesenteric plexus. Again, the nerve fibers follow the blood supply to innervate the right colon to the mid transverse colon (6). The left colon and the anorectum are innervated by the sacral parasympathetic centers in S2 to S4. The nervi ergentes originate from the sacral parasympathetic centers and join the pelvic plexi of the sympathetic system on the pelvic side wall. From there, it travels along the presacral nerve to the inferior mesenteric plexus and is distributed along the inferior mesenteric artery (6). Stimulation of the parasympathetic system results in an increase in colonic tone, motility, and relaxation of the IAS.

Somatic Innervation

The somatic pudendal nerve (S2–S4) innervates the pelvic floor. The external anal sphincter (EAS) is controlled by the inferior rectal branch of the internal pudendal nerve and the perineal branch of S4. In about one-third of the population, there is a direct branch from the fourth sacral nerve to the EAS as well (9). The puborectalis muscle is innervated by a direct branch from S3 and S4. The levator ani is supplied on its pelvic side by the fourth sacral nerves whereas its perineal surface is innervated by the interior rectal branches of the pudendal nerves.

Sensation of the anal canal is supplied by the inferior rectal branch of the pudendal nerve. Pain can be felt from the anal verge to within 1.5 centimeters proximal to the dentate line (9).

Hormonal Regulation

Hormonal control of colonic function is very complex and is still poorly understood (10). There is an extensive endocrine system with at least 15 gastrointestinal hormones already identified. These are synthesized in both endocrine and paracrine cells and also are found in enteric neurons, where they are also potential neurotransmitters.

The regulatory effects on the colon of only a handful of hormones are known (6). Gastrin has trophic effects on colonic mucosa in addition to a stimulatory effect on colonic motility. Cholecystokinin is also well studied and has been shown to increase colonic motility. Motilin can increase colonic contractions as well. Other hormones have an inhibitory effect on colonic motility. These include peptide YY (PYY), glucagon, somatostatin, and possibly secretin (10). The exact roles of these hormones still need to be elucidated. Additionally, it is unclear whether a neurologic disorder or denervation of the colon from a spinal cord injury alters the local colonic effects of these hormones.

Luminal Contents

The contents of stool can affect the secretion and absorption of the colonic epithelium. This is demonstrated by the diarrhea caused by the malabsorption of bile salts in patients with terminal ileitis or ileal resections (11). Several other compounds, in addition to bile acids, have direct regulatory effects on colonic function (6). These include oleic acid and volatile fatty acids, which are products of the bacterial breakdown of carbohydrates.

Mechanisms of Continence

Fecal continence is maintained by several factors, both mechanical and neurologic. Stool volume and consistency play an important role in maintaining anal continence. Some patients are variably continent to solid, liquid, or gas. By changing the stool consistency and volume, some patients may be rendered continent.

Another mechanical factor is the reservoir function of the rectum. The valves of Houston slow down the progression of stool and provide a barrier effect. Rectal capacity and adaptive compliance are also important for an effective reservoir function.

An important component for maintaining continence is the angulation of the anorectal angle. This is normally maintained at 80 to 90 degrees by the continuous tonic activity of the puborectalis muscle (10). In order to defecate, this angle needs to be straightened. In addition, this angle may help to maintain continence during sudden increases in intra-abdominal pressure (coughing, laughing, or straining) because this tends to increase the angulation. This flap valve theory has now been challenged as an important factor during increases in intra-abdominal pressure in a normal subject. Instead, a reflex contraction of the EAS may be what maintains continence during sudden increases in intra-abdominal pressures (12). The flap valve mechanism may play a more important role in subjects compromised with a decreased anal pressure.

Anal resting pressure is maintained by the IAS, EAS, and the hemorrhoidal complex. The resting pressure is between 40 and 80 millimeters Hg and is higher than the basic intrarectal pressure. This differential in pressure assists in the maintenance of continence. The IAS is the major contributor to this resting high-pressure zone (HPZ). In addition, the EAS maintains a tonic activity that contributes to the resting pressure. Increases in intra-abdominal pressure, rectal distension, and perianal stimulation tend to augment its activity. Of note, voluntary contraction of the EAS can only be maintained between 40 and 60 seconds; that is, it is fatigable (10).

The hemorrhoidal complex is a vascular cushion located in the left lateral, right anterolateral, and right posterolateral areas of the anal canal. These have the ability to expand and contract, thereby contributing to anal continence (13).

Anorectal Sensibility and Rectoanal Inhibitory Reflex (RAIR) (See Chapters 2.2 and 2.8)

Anorectal sensibility is necessary to discriminate between gas, liquid, or solid. It allows awareness to contract the EAS in order to postpone defecation. When feces reach the rectum with colonic mass movements, the rectal wall stretches; this causes reflexive relaxation of the IAS. This is called the rectoanal inhibitory reflex (RAIR). Gowers first described this phenomenon in 1877 when he also observed that this reflex seemed to be intact in two patients with flaccid paralysis caused by spinal cord injuries. This and subsequent studies suggest that the RAIR is mediated through the intrinsic nervous system with intramural nerve fibers from the rectum to the IAS. It probably also is influenced by the autonomic nervous system. With the reflexive relaxation of the IAS, the rectal contents can then descend into the anal canal, where sampling can occur to determine whether the contents are solid, liquid, or gas. The EAS is then contracted to maintain continence.

Defecation Reflex

Distension of the rectum stimulates contractions of the colon and rectum. This is known as the defecation reflex and involves the sacral segments of the spinal cord. A voluntary increase in abdominal pressure assists the defecation reflex to evacuate the rectum. In addition, a squatting position tends to straighten the puborectalis angle. However, if it is not a socially acceptable time or place to defecate, the EAS is constricted to maintain continence and the rectum accommodates, allowing the urge to defecate to pass.

Alterations in the Spinal Cord Patient

Bowel dysfunction is one of the most devastating sequelae of spinal cord injury. The most frequent symptoms reported are nausea, diarrhea, constipation, and fecal incontinence (14,15). These have severe ramifications socially and psychologically (1,14). In one survey, about half of the patients became dependent on others for toileting and their bowel dysfunction was a significant source of emotional distress (14).

Neurogenic bowel dysfunction in spinal cord injury patients can be classified into two groups based upon the level of injury: lower motor neuron and upper motor neuron lesions (16). Lower motor neuron bowel syndrome results from an injury to the spinal cord at the level of the conus medullaris and cauda equina. These patients have an areflexic bowel because the spinal reflex is interrupted. Only the intrinsic bowel nervous system remains intact and the bowel tends to be flaccid. On the other hand, patients with an upper motor neuron bowel dysfunction have a lesion above the level of the conus medullaris. These patients tend to have a hyperreflexic bowel. Here, the reflex arch between the colon and the spinal cord remains intact; however, the voluntary control of the EAS muscle is interrupted and the sphincter tends to remain tightly closed.

Spinal Shock

When a transection of the spinal cord occurs, all sensory and motor functions below that level are lost. In addition, for the first few weeks, there is also a temporary loss of spinal reflexes. This phenomenon is called spinal shock and may last a variable period of time. Close to 10% of patients will develop a prolonged ileus as a manifestation of spinal shock (6). During the period of spinal shock and adynamic ileus, the patient should not take anything by mouth. Manual disimpaction and enemas are required to empty the rectum. Eventually, a return of reflex activity is seen followed by an exaggerated reflex activity.

Gastrocolic Reflex

The gastrocolic reflex is an increase in both small bowel and colonic propulsion initiated by feeding. The response is increased by a fatty or proteinaceous meal and is mediated by cholinergic motor neurons. The term "gastrocolic reflex" is a misnomer in that the stomach is probably not the source of the cholinergic stimulus. Even when the stomach and esophagus are excluded, the response is still present (16). The stimulus may be central, intrinsic (within the colon itself), or hormonally mediated (16). The gastrocolic response after spinal cord injury may be blunted or absent (17). This may be secondary to an absent central vagal stimulation or an impaired release of motilin (16); however, there is some evidence that the gastrocolic response still may be present in some patients with complete transection of their spinal cord (18). The discrepancy in results may be due to the variability of the techniques used to measure rectosigmoid motility (6).

Colorectal Compliance

Colonic compliance is decreased in patients with supraconal spinal cord injuries (17,19). Colonic pressures in these patients were observed to exceed 40 millimeters Hg with rapid infusion of only 300 cubic centimeters of water whereas normal subjects required only 2200 cubic centimeters instillation. This reflects the hyperreflexic nature of an upper motor neuron lesion; however, a slow infusion or intermittent rectal infusion produces colonic compliance that is close to normal (20). Rectal compliance is also lower than normal in spinal cord-injured patients (21).

Colonic Motility

Colonic transit times are significantly prolonged in patients with spinal cord injury (22). The colonic segment affected depends in part on the level of spinal injury. Supraconal lesions affect the transit time of the proximal colon significantly while affecting the rectosigmoid area to a lesser degree. On the other hand, conal or cauda equinal lesions cause a more significant prolongation of the rectosigmoid transit time while affecting the proximal colon somewhat less (23); however, an increase in colonic transit time may not necessarily correlate with the degree of intestinal symptoms in spinal cord-injured patients (22).

Anorectal Function

The studies of anorectal physiologic alterations in patients with spinal cord lesions have had mixed results. In general, patients with supraconal lesions may have stronger rectal contractions and their RAIR may be more robust

(2). These effects, combined with the fact that these patients may have little to no anorectal sensation and no voluntary control of the EAS, creates an increased risk of fecal incontinence.

Patients with cauda equinal and conal lesions may have symptoms of obstructed defecation (16). This results from an interruption of the reflex arc between the rectal wall and the spinal cord. The RAIR may be absent (24), resulting in a lack of reflexive relaxation of the IAS when the rectal wall is stretched. Patients do not have spinal cord-mediated peristalsis, which results in a flaccid colon and rectum. Because of the decreased reflex, it is also harder to stimulate defecation; however, patients with lower motor neuron lesions also may experience fecal incontinence. The pelvic musculature, including the levator ani, lacks tone and results in a descended perineum. The rectal angle becomes more obtuse, thereby opening the rectal lumen (16). These factors, combined with the lack of anorectal sensation and voluntary control of the EAS, may all result in fecal incontinence.

Alterations in Spina Bifida

Spina bifida also results in both constipation and fecal incontinence. The lesion is usually either conal or cauda equinal because most of the myelomeningoceles are either sacral or lumbosacral. As with patients with traumatic cord injuries of the same level, this results in obstructed defecation. In addition, reduced resting anal pressure, anal squeeze pressure, and anorectal sensation can result in secondary fecal incontinence.

Patients with spina bifida also may have hydrocephalus, which results in intellectual deficits, potentially contributing to fecal incontinence. In addition, these patients may develop a tethered cord, which seems to be associated with a worse bowel function. However, it is difficult to ascertain whether the tethering itself results in a worse bowel function or whether this is a result of complex associated anorectal malformations. Surgery to untether the cord does not seem to improve overall rectal function (25). Bowel function may be affected permanently in myelodysplasia, whereas that after surgery for Hirschsprung's disease (HD) and anorectal malformations is more self-limiting and less severe (26). Objective assessment of these patients has recently advocated the use of saline enema testing and fecoflowmetry as a measure of rectal irritability, compliance, and evacuatory efficiency (27).

Alterations in Multiple Sclerosis

Multiple sclerosis is a progressive neurologic disease that results from multiple demyelinating lesions within the central nervous system. This causes a variety of symptoms, which include bowel dysfunction. Constipation is reported in 40% to 50% of the patients, whereas 50% have reported an episode of fecal incontinence in the previous three months, with 20% to 30% having at least one episode of incontinence every week (28–30).

The abnormalities noted are similar to patients with spinal cord injuries. However, the lesions are usually numerous and result in a combination of supraconal and conal disease. Constipation may result from a prolonged colonic transit time (31) and a frequently absent gastrocolic response (32). There is also an element of paradoxical puborectalis contraction (anismus) in some of the patients, resulting in anal outlet obstruction (33). Fecal incontinence may result in some cases from reduced anal resting pressure, anal squeeze pressure, and anorectal sensibility (34–37). This is compounded by a reduced rectal compliance and increased rectal wall irritability (31,38,39).

Alterations in Patients with Central Nervous System Disorder

Parkinson's Disease

Parkinson's disease is characterized by a loss of pigmented neurons in the central nervous system (CNS), which results in a loss of their dopamine neurotransmitters. The patients develop dystonia of their striated muscles. As a result of these abnormalities, they develop a resting tremor, rigidity, and bradykinesia and have difficulty initiating automatic and voluntary movements such as swallowing. The loss of dopaminergic neurons is not limited to the CNS, where there is also a loss of dopamine neurotransmitters in the enteric nervous system (40), resulting in a prolonged colonic transit time and constipation (41). In addition, because the EAS is a striated muscle, these patients also develop dystonia, resulting in paradoxical contraction of the sphincter during defecation, which appears to be reversible with dopaminergic medication (42). Patients with Parkinson's disease also may develop fecal incontinence as a result of decreased anal resting pressure and squeeze pressure.

Stroke

Fecal incontinence is associated with the severity of the stroke (43). Between 31% and 40% of patients develop fecal incontinence within two weeks of their stroke; however, this number goes down to about 3% to 9% after six months follow-up (44). Patients who develop fecal incontinence have a higher risk of death within six months compared with those who remain continent, although the reasons for this finding are complex and multifactorial (43). Constipation is also a major problem in patients with stroke where, in one stroke rehabilitation center, 60% of the patients experienced constipation (44).

Cerebral Palsy

The entire gastrointestinal tract is affected by cerebral palsy. Patients develop swallowing disorders, abnormal esophageal motility, and reflux esophagitis. Constipation and fecal incontinence are also frequent problems (45). The colonic transit time also has been demonstrated to be prolonged (45).

Therapeutic Measures

The derangements of colorectal function that are seen in patients with neurologic diseases are usually multifactorial. The lesions in the nervous system, which affect colorectal motility and anorectal function, are compounded by dietary changes, immobility, and medications. All of these factors need to be taken into account when evaluating and managing a patient with a neurologic disorder and associated bowel dysfunction.

A comprehensive and individualized treatment plan should include a regimen that takes into consideration the patient's diet, activity level, medications, and personal schedule. The program also should include dietary modification, medications, and procedures to stimulate scheduled evacuation of stool. This type of bowel care is important so that patients can empty their colons at appropriate times, and therefore avoid constipation, as well as fecal leakage. A regularly scheduled stool evacuation also avoids inspissation of stool, dilatation of the colon, and reduced peristalsis.

Diet

A diet that includes a high amount of fiber (20–30 grams) is generally encouraged. Fiber is found in foods such as whole grains, fruits, and vegetables. It allows the stool to form bulk and to retain water. This in turn facilitates the passage of stool through the colon.

However, the recommendation of increasing the intake of fiber is based on an assumption that patients with neurologic bowel dysfunction will react the same way to fiber as those with normal bowel. This may not be uniformly true and fiber may indeed have an opposite effect. In a study of bran supplements in patients with spinal cord injury, the overall colonic transit time was prolonged and there was no change in either evacuation time or stool weight (46). In patients with Parkinson's disease, fiber supplements increased stool frequency and weight, but did not affect colonic transit or anorectal function (47). However, there were both subjective and objective improvements in the symptoms of constipation (47). Additionally, adding fiber to the diet should modify the consistency of stool, thereby preventing either really hard stools or diarrhea. Theoretically, this should improve continence. It has been recommended that patients with spinal cord injuries should have at least 15 grams of fiber daily (48). Given the lack of evidence and the possible adverse effects, the increase in fiber should be monitored carefully with regard to its effect on each individual patient's bowel response.

Medications

A variety of medications can be used in the management of bowel dysfunction. However, medications should not be used automatically as part of a bowel regimen because some patients respond to dietary modifications and increased fluid intake alone (49). The major classes of medications include synthetic fiber supplements, stool softeners, laxatives, and prokinetic agents.

Fiber Supplements

As mentioned above, fiber is an important component in a bowel regimen, as it tends to modify stool consistency by absorbing water. A dietary fiber of at least 30 grams a day is recommended. Fiber supplements are useful when patients are unable to take this amount in their diet. Supplements include psyllium (Fiberall, Konsyl, Metamucil, Naturacil), ispaghula husk, methylcellulose (Citrucel), and calcium polycarbophil (Fibercon). Different fiber supplements may have different efficacies. These are usually fairly well tolerated, with little adverse effects except for bloating and flatulence; however, an adequate amount of fluid intake also is required to prevent stool inspissation, intestinal obstruction, esophageal obstruction, and fecal impaction.

Stool Softeners

Docusate (Colace, Surfak) is a commonly used stool softener. It lowers the surface tension of the stool, thereby allowing water and lipids to enter the stool substance. It also may irritate the mucosa and stimulate secretion of mucus and water; however, it does not have any discrete laxative activity. It is recommended for patients who cannot form soft stools despite dietary and fluid-intake modifications. Soft stools are especially important for patients who should avoid straining, such as those with hemorrhoids or with autonomic dysreflexia.

Laxatives

Laxatives are stimulants that enhance colonic motility. There are several classes of laxatives. These include stimulants, saline derivatives, and hyperosmolar laxatives.

Stimulant laxatives exert a direct affect on the colon to increase motility by stimulating the myenteric complex. In addition, they also alter electrolyte transport and increase intraluminal fluid, thereby increasing propulsion. Stimulants include anthraquinones (senna, cascara), and polyphenolic derivatives include bisacodyl (Dulcolax) and phenolphthalein (Ex-Lax). They cause a bowel movement between six and twelve hours. Side-effects include abdominal cramping and electrolyte disturbances. Long-term adverse effects include melanosis coli and cathartic colon. Melanosis coli is a colonoscopic and histologic finding of unknown significance. It is a staining of the colonic mucosa from macrophage ingestion of the pigments from the stimulant. Cathartic colon, on the other hand, is a condition in which the colon becomes less responsive to the laxatives over time. It may be secondary to damage to the myenteric plexus. Bisacodyl also comes in suppository form and may be better tolerated. Used as a suppository, bisacodyl acts as a rectal stimulant.

Another class of laxatives is saline laxatives, which are derived from salts such as magnesium, potassium, or sodium. These include magnesium hydroxide (Milk of Magnesia), magnesium citrate solution, and sodium phosphate (Fleet's phosphosoda). The mechanism of action of these agents involves the drawing of fluid into the small intestine, increasing colonic motility. These agents typically cause evacuation within two to six hours; however, these are fairly potent agents and may result in severe abdominal cramping and watery bowel movements. Side effects may include hypermagnesemia, hyperkalemia, dehydration, and congestive heart failure. Sodium phosphate may cause hyperphosphatemia, hypocalcemia, and hypokalemia, especially in the elderly and in those with a decreased creatinine clearance (50). A gentler stimulant should be used initially as part of a routine bowel program.

Another class of laxatives is the hyperosmolar laxatives, which include lactulose (Chronulac), sorbitol, and polyethylene glycol (PEG) electrolyte solutions (Golytely, Miralax). These are metabolized in the colon into short-chain amino acids, which then draw fluid intraluminally through osmosis. Lactulose and sorbitol may cause abdominal cramping and flatulence; however, these agents do not generally cause mucosal irritation or electrolyte imbalances.

Prokinetic Drugs

The most commonly studied prokinetic drug is cisapride. It is a serotonin agonist that stimulates gastrointestinal motility. The use of cisapride in patients with neurological diseases has been studied and has been shown to reduce the colonic transit times in patients with spinal cord lesions (51–53). These properties have led some authors to recommend the use of cisapride to prevent constipation. Most of these reports are small in patient numbers and do not provide conclusive evidence to support this claim at this time (54). Additionally, cisapride has been shown to cause a rare but life-threatening arrhythmia (torsades de pointes) and has been withdrawn from the market in some countries (55). The drug, therefore, should be reserved only for those with severe slow-transit constipation and who have failed other modalities.

Another prokinetic agent is metoclopramide (Reglan). It increases gastric motility and has been used to resolve the ileus that results from an acute spinal cord injury (56); however, it does not seem to affect colonic motility. Adverse reactions to metoclopramide include extrapyramidal symptoms, which are related to dose and duration.

Rectal Stimulation

Patients with hyperirritability of the rectal wall—such as those with supraconal lesions (traumatic cord injury, multiple sclerosis, or spina bifida)—may utilize this property to induce rectal contractions. This may be achieved using digital stimulation, suppositories, or enemas. An appropriate time and place may then be chosen to defecate, thereby emptying the colon to avoid social embarrassment.

Digital stimulation involves inserting either a lubricated, gloved finger or an adapted plastic device into the rectum. The finger or device is then rotated against the rectal wall. In addition, direct gentle pressure can be placed on the sacrum to relax the puborectalis muscle.

Rectal stimulants such as suppositories may be used if digital stimulation fails. Glycerine suppositories generally cause evacuation in 15 to 30 minutes by irritating the mucosa and causing rectal contractions through hyperosmotic stimulation. Bisacodyl (Dulcolax) also comes as a suppository and is available in two formulations: hydrogenated vegetable base and PEG base. There is some evidence that the PEG-based bisacodyl can shorten the time required for bowel care (57). Another suppository is a CO_2 suppository (Ceo-Two), which acts by causing rectal distension with the production of carbon dioxide. The rectal distention then causes reflex colonic peristalsis. There is also a mechanical effect in that the carbon dioxide can cause expulsion of stool. This suppository may not be effective in some patients with a patulous anal sphincter because the gas may escape without causing the necessary rectal distention; however, it might be useful in patients with a lower motor neuron defect who lack the rectal reflex, but who need mechanical mechanisms to eliminate stool.

If digital stimulation and suppositories become ineffective, then an enema may be used. Enemas include preparations such as sodium phosphate (Fleet), which is a mucosal irritant as well. There are also enemas that are made specifically for patients with neurologic bowel dysfunction. These include Theravac mini-enemas, which only contain four milliliters of fluid containing docusate sodium and benzocaine as an additive. Benzocaine can anesthetized the rectal mucosa and hopefully prevent autonomic dysreflexia. For any of these mucosal irritants to be effective, the agents should be placed in contact with the rectal wall. However, long-term use of enemas may result in an enema-dependent colon. Additionally, enemas may result in rectoanal trauma, bacteremia, and autonomic dysreflexia.

Patients with lower motor neuron defects—such as from trauma or spina bifida—have areflexic bowel and a patulous EAS. Their bowel routine may involve digital removal of stool from the rectum. The digital stimulation also may stimulate local peristalsis. Theoretically, because these patients lack a spinal reflex, enemas and suppositories would not be effective. With an intermittent Valsalva maneuver and use of abdominal wall contractions, the stool in the colon also may empty into the rectum, where digital evacuation completes the process.

On the other hand, patients who have upper motor neuron deficits have an intact rectocolic reflex following the initial four to six weeks of spinal shock. However, they are limited by the lack of conscious control of the EAS and a lack of rectal sensation. The EAS may be spastic, and those with high cord transections cannot generate an adequate abdominal contraction to aid defecation. A bowel regimen involves scheduled evacuations because they may not feel the urge to defecate. Rectal stimulation may be performed digitally or by suppository or enema. Digital stimulation also is used to relax the puborectalis muscle and the spastic EAS.

Enema Continence Catheter

The enema continence catheter was first described by Shandling and used in children with constipation or fecal incontinence secondary to spina bifida (58). It is a catheter with an inflatable balloon that is inserted into the rectum. The enema is then administered and the inflated balloon allows retention of the enema fluid despite the patulous anal sphincter. It has been shown to improve the symptoms of bowel dysfunction in children with spina bifida by 50% to 100% (59,60). Satisfaction rates by the parents and children are very high. This has led some investigators to evaluate this method in adults with fecal incontinence or constipation. The enema continence catheter improved the symptoms of 73% of patients with fecal incontinence and 40% of those with constipation (61).

Most adult patients were able to administer the enema by themselves; it generally took 30 to 45 minutes. The method requires careful instruction, and therefore requires a motivated patient. Some patients with high thoracic lesions may experience autonomous hyperreflexia, and perforation of an insensate rectum is also a risk.

Antegrade Colonic Enema

Malone first described a procedure that creates a continent, catheterizable appendicostomy for antegrade colonic wash outs (62,63). The original description of the procedure involved implanting the tip of the appendix into the cecum in a non-refluxing manner and then bringing the base out to the abdominal wall. Since then, the procedure has been revised by merely bringing the distal tip of the appendix out through the abdominal wall (58). Alternatively, in patients without an appendix, a tubularized cecal flap may be created (64). An antegrade enema then can be administered by inserting a catheter through the appendicostomy. By emptying the colon and rectum, symptoms of constipation and fecal incontinence may be improved.

This procedure was originally developed by Malone for children. Since then, there have been several studies among children with spina bifida and anorectal malformations. The success rate has been reported between 50% and 90% (62,63,65). Small studies have been performed on adults with fecal incontinence and constipation, including those with spinal cord injuries (66). Overall, the procedure resulted in high satisfaction rates. The mean time to perform the antegrade enema was 30 minutes in one study, and the amount of water used was between 500 cubic centimeters and 2000 cubic centimeters. Although the patient population studied was small and diverse, over 80% of patients with fecal incontinence and constipation reported improvements of their symptoms (63,67).

The complications of the procedure are minor and include stomal stenosis, appendiceal necrosis, and leakage of stool from the stoma. These are managed with local care and are not associated with a high morbidity. In addition, patients may have some abdominal discomfort during the washout; however, if the patient cannot tolerate the washouts, they may simply stop using the stoma and it will obliterate after a few months. Although the immediate complications associated with the procedure are minor, long-term results are still lacking.

The success of the antegrade colonic enema has led some investigators to develop less-invasive procedures. A percutaneous cecostomy inserted with radiologic guidance has been described (68). In addition, percutaneous endoscopic cecostomy (PEC) also has been described (69). Although both studies were pilot studies involving a very small number of cases, the results have been encouraging.

Biofeedback

Biofeedback training may be used to improve EAS function, as well as anorectal sensibility. This technique may only be used on patients who have some residual voluntary control of the EAS and some anorectal sensation. A small anal probe is inserted into the anal canal. The patient is then instructed to squeeze or relax. The pressure is transduced and displayed so that the patient may learn how to squeeze or relax.

Biofeedback also may be used to improve anorectal sensibility. This is done by inserting a balloon into the rectum and slowly distending the balloon. The patients then indicate when they first feel something. Over a period of weeks, the patients can gradually sense rectal distension at smaller volumes.

Biofeedback therapy seems to improve symptoms of constipation and fecal incontinence in children with spina bifida, although the same results can be achieved by behavior modification (70,71). Because patients who have multiple sclerosis may have bowel dysfunction secondary to pelvic floor incoordination and decreased anal squeeze and anorectal sensibility, biofeedback seems to be an ideal treatment. This was studied recently in a small group of patients (72) where it appears to help some patients with mild to moderate disability or with quiescent disease.

Electric Nervous Stimulation

Brindley originally described the method of sacral anterior root stimulation for bladder dysfunction using an intrathecally implanted device (73). Because stimulation of the sacral roots (S2–S4) also results in stimulation of the hindgut, it also has been used to improve bowel dysfunction. Stimulation increases left colon motility and induces emptying of the left colon. Rectal contractions are stimulated and result in defecation in some patients with spinal cord injuries (74). In another study of patients with supraconal lesions, the patients reported improvement in constipation, a decrease in time of bowel care, and half achieved unassisted defecation (75). Implantation of electrodes extradurally has been approved by the Food and Drug Administration (FDA) in the United States. It also seems to be efficacious in reducing the time spent on bowel care (76). The implantation of these devices also is combined with posterior rhizotomy, which reduces autonomic dysreflexia, reflex urinary incontinence, and ureteric reflux. It should be noted that these are studies with a very small number of accrued patients. In addition, the EAS is also innervated by the somatic contribution of these sacral roots and may be stimulated to contract simultaneously, resulting in obstruction. Chia and his colleagues have observed that although most of their patients had an improvement in bowel function with sacral stimulation, all patients were unable to defecate during the stimulation because of a higher anal pressure compared with the rectal pressure (77). Defecation occurred immediately after the stimulation. Further studies are necessary and development of selective stimulation protocols is needed.

More recently, a less-invasive method involving magnetic stimulation of the sacral nerves has been described for patients with spinal cord injury (78). The method is an application of Faraday's law in that a change in the magnetic field induces an electrical field. A magnetic stimulator is placed either in the suprapubic area or in the lumbosacral area at specified amounts of time. Colonic transit time was shown to decrease and rectal pressure to increase. Although the number of patients in this study was small, there were anecdotal reports of significantly improved bowel symptoms.

Colostomy

Patients who fail all measures may require a colostomy. A colostomy usually is seen as an intervention that is performed when everything else has failed. This mostly stems from extrapolations on how permanent stomas appear to decrease the quality of life of patients who have cancer or inflammatory bowel disease. A permanent stoma, especially in cancer patients, seems to have a negative impact on their social lives and on their body image. However, this may not be the case with patients who have significant bowel dysfunction and whose lives are severely limited by this benign but distressing symptom. A colostomy can simplify bowel care and improve the patient's quality of life (79). In a study involving spinal cord patients, 100%

were satisfied with their colostomy and 70% wished that they had it done earlier (80). All patients reported that the stomas had improved their quality of life by shortening bowel care and increasing their independence. However, prior to recommending a colostomy, careful studies need to be conducted in order to identify the site of bowel dysfunction (colonic motility vs. rectal evacuation) and the level of the colostomy.

A recent study (81) examined the long-term outcome between left-sided and right-sided colostomies and ileostomies in spinal cord-injured patients with colonic dysmotility. A record of 41 patients with intestinal stomas—sigmoid colostomy, transverse colostomy, or ileostomy—were reviewed with focus on how colonic transit times (CTT) affected quality of life (QoL), health status (HS), and time to bowel care (TBC) pre- and post-stoma formation. Regardless of the stoma type, all patients had significant improvement in QoL and HS. Time to bowel care was shortened significantly by over 100 minutes. The study concluded that more abdominal symptoms (bloating, obstipation, and chronic abdominal pain), along with prolonged CTT, favored a more proximal site of fecal diversion.

Conclusions

Bowel dysfunction in patients with neurologic disorders is common. The symptoms of constipation and fecal incontinence have a tremendous impact on the quality of life of these patients. In order to successfully manage patients with neurogenic bowel dysfunction, one should take into account the unique needs and condition of each patient, along with the patient's lifestyle, level of activity, and social goals. Dietary modification and increased activity may be supplemented by pharmacologic agents. A scheduled and individualized bowel regimen is also important, and there are new treatment modalities that can improve the bowel function of these patients, as have been outlined in this chapter. Because of the complexity of the problems and the variability of symptoms, there is no hard data in terms of recommendations for managing these patients. The ideal bowel program for each individual often is achieved by trial and error. It is clear that meticulous attention to diet, hydration, use of bulk forming agents, exercise, and the selective use of stimulants remains a crucial part of bowel management in these cases. In refractory cases, the coloproctologist may give strong consideration to an intestinal stoma after appropriate patient and family counseling—a procedure that can be met with very satisfactory results and a normal quality of life in many cases.

References

1. Levi R, Hulting C, Nash M, and Seger A. The Stockholm spinal cord injury study. I. Medical problems in a regional SCI population. Paraplegia. 1995; 33:308–15.

2. Krogh K, Christensen P, and Lauberg S. Colorectal symptoms in patients with neurologic diseases. Acta Neurol Scand. 2001;103:335–43.
3. Bassotti G, Germani U, and Morelli A. Human colonic motility: physiological aspects. Int J Colorectal Dis. 1995;10:173–80.
4. Goyal RK and Hirano I. The enteric nervous system. New Engl J Med. 1996;334:1106–15.
5. Wood JD, Alpers DH, and Andrews PLR. Fundamentals of neurogastroenterology. Gut. 1999;45(Suppl II):II6–16.
6. Longo WE, Ballantyne GH, and Modlin IM. The colon, anorectum, and spinal cord patient: A review of the functional alterations of the denervated hindgut. Dis Colon Rectum. 1989;32:261–7.
7. Carlstedt A, Nordgren S, Fasth S, Appelgren L, and Hulten L. Sympathetic nervous influence on the internal anal sphincter and rectum in man. Int J Colorectal Dis. 1988;3:90–5.
8. Lubowski DZ, Nicholls RJ, Swash M, and Jordan MJ. Neural control of internal anal sphincter function. Br J Surg. 1987;74:668–70.
9. Nivatgongs S and Gordon PH. Surgical anatomy. In: Gordon PH and Nivatgongs S, editors. Principles and practice of surgery for the colon, rectum, and anus. 2nd ed. St. Louis: Quality Medical Publishing; 1999. p. 3–39.
10. Schouten WR and Gordon PH. Physiology. In: Gordon PH and Nivatgongs S, editors. Principles and practice of surgery for the colon, rectum, and anus. 2nd ed. St. Louis: Quality Medical Publishing; 1999. p. 41–86.
11. Hoffmann AF and Poley JR. Role of bile acid malabsorption in pathogenesis of diarrhea and steatorrhea in patients with ileal resection. I. Response to cholestyramine or replacement of dietary long chain triglyceride by medium chain triglyceride. Gastroenterology. 1972;62:918–34.
12. Bannister JJ, Gibbons C, and Read NW. Preservation of faecal continence during rises in intra-abdominal pressure: is there a role for the flap valve? Gut. 1987;28:1242–5.
13. Gibbons CP, Read NW, and Trowbridge EA. Anal cushions. Lancet. 1986; 2(8497):42.
14. Glickman S and Kamm MA. Bowel dysfunction in spinal-cord-injury patients. Lancet. 1996;347:1651–3.
15. Lynch AC, Wong C, Anthony A, Dobbs BR, and Frizelle FA. Bowel dysfunction following spinal cord injury: a description of bowel function in a spinal cord-injured population and comparison with age and gender matched controls. Spinal Cord. 2000;38:717–23.
16. Glick ME, Meshkinpour H, Haldeman S, Hoehler F, Downey N, and Bradley WE. Colonic dysfunction in patients with thoracic spinal cord injury. Gastroenterology. 1984;86:287–94.
17. Connell AM, Frankel H, and Guttman L. The motility of the pelvic colon following complete lesions of the spinal cord. Paraplegia. 1963;1:98–115.
18. Meshkinpour H, Nowroozi F, and Glick ME. Colonic compliance in patients with spinal cord injury. Arch Phys Med Rehabil. 1983;64:111–2.
19. MacDonagh R, Sun WM, Thomas DG, Smallwood R, and Read NW. Anorectal function in patients with complete supraconal spinal cord lesions. Gut. 1992;33:1532–8.
20. Lynch AC, Anthony A, Dobbs BR, and Frizelle FA. Anorectal physiology following spinal cord injury. Spinal Cord. 2000;38:573–80.

21. Leduc BE, Spacek E, and Lepage Y. Colonic transit time after spinal cord injury: any clinical significance? J Spinal Cord Med. 2002;25:161–6.
22. Krogh K, Mosdal C, and Laurberg S. Gastrointestinal and segmental colonic transit times in patients with acute and chronic spinal cord lesions. Spinal Cord. 2000;38:615–21.
23. Tjandra JJ, Ooi BS, and Han WR. Anorectal physiologic testing for bowel dysfunction in patients with spinal cord injuries. Dis Colon Rectum. 2000; 43:927–31.
24. Beuret-Blanquart F, Weber J, Gouverneur JP, Demangeon S, and Denis P. Colonic transit time and anorectal manometric anomalies in 19 patients with complete transection of the spinal cord. J Auton Nerv Syst. 1990;30:199–207.
25. Levitt MA, Patel M, Rodriguez G, Gaylin DS, and Pena A. The tethered spinal cord in patients with anorectal malformations. J Pediatr Surg. 1997;32: 462–8.
26. Rintala RJ. Fecal incontinence in anorectal malformations, neuropathy and miscellaneous conditions. Semin Pediatr Surg. 2002;11:75–82.
27. Kayaba H, Hebiguchi T, Itoh Y, Yoshino H, Mizuno N, Morii M, Adachi T, Chihara J, and Kato T. Evaluation of anorectal function in patients with tethered cord syndrome: saline enema test and fecoflowmetry. J Neurosurg. 2003;98(3 Suppl):251–7.
28. Hinds JP, Eidelmann BH, and Wald A. Prevalence of bowel dysfunction in multiple sclerosis. A population study. Gastroenterology. 1990;98:1538–42.
29. Sullivan SN and Eber GC. Gastrointestinal dysfunction in multiple sclerosis. Gastroenterology. 1983;84:1640–6.
30. Chia YM, Fowler CJ, Kamm MA, Henry MM, Lemieux MC, and Swash M. Prevalence of bowel dysfunction in patients with multiple sclerosis and bladder dysfunction. J Neurol. 1995;242:105–8.
31. Weber J, Grise P, Roquebert M, Hellot MF, Mihout B, Samson M, Beuret-Blanquart F, Pasquis P, and Denis P. Radiopaque markers transit and anorectal manometry in 16 patients with multiple sclerosis and urinary bladder dysfuntion. Dis Colon Rectum. 1987;30:95–100.
32. Glick ME, Meshkinpour H, Haldeman S, Bhatia NN, and Bradley WE. Colonic dysfunction in multiple sclerosis. Gastroenterology. 1982;83:1002–7.
33. Chia YW, Gill KP, Jameson JS, Forti AD, Henry MM, and Shorvon PJ. Paradoxical puborectalis contraction is a feature of constipation in patients with multiple sclerosis. J Neurol Neurosurg Psychiatry. 1996;60:31–5.
34. Sørensen M, Lorentzen M, Petersen J, and Christiansen J. Anorectal dysfunction in patients with urologic disturbance due to multiple sclerosis. Dis Colon Rectum. 1991;34:136–9.
35. Jameson JS, Rogers J, Chia YW, Misiewicz JJ, Henry MM, and Swash M. Pelvic floor function in multiple sclerosis. Gut. 1994;35:388–90.
36. Nordenbo AM, Andersen JR, and Andersen JT. Disturbances of ano-rectal function in multiple sclerosis. J Neurol. 1996;243:445–51.
37. Waldron DJ, Horgan PG, Patel FR, Maguirre R, and Given HF. Multiple sclerosis: assessment of colonic and anorectal function in the presence of faecal incontinence. Int J Colorectal Dis. 1993;8:220–4.
38. Haldeman S, Glick M, Bhatia NN, Bradley WE, and Johnson B. Colometry, cystometry, and evoked potentials in multiple sclerosis. Arch Neurol. 1982;39:698–701.

39. Singaram C, Ashraf W, Gaumintz EA, Torbey C, Sengupta A, Pfeiffer R, and Quigley EM. Dopaminergic defect of enteric nervous system in Parkinson's disease patients with chronic constipation. Lancet. 1995;346:861–4.
40. Edwards LL, Pfeiffer RF, Quigley EM, Hofman R, and Balluf M. Gastrointestinal symptoms in Parkinson's disease. Mov Disord. 1991;6:51–6.
41. Mathers SE, Kempster PA, Law PJ, Frankel JP, Bartram CI, Lees AJ, Stern GM, and Swash M. Anal sphincter dysfunction in Parkinson's disease. Arch Neurol. 1989;46:1061–4.
42. Ashraf W, Pfeiffer RF, and Quigley EM. Anorectal manometry in the assessment of anorectal function in Parkinson's disease: a comparison with chronic idiopathic constipation. Mov Disord. 1994;9:655–63.
43. Nakayama H, Jorgensen HS, Pedersen PM, Raaschou HO, and Olsen TS. Prevalence and risk factors of incontinence after stroke: The Copenhagen stroke study. Stroke. 1997;28:58–62.
44. Robain G, Chennevelle JM, Petit F, and Piera JB. Incidence of constipation after recent vascular hemiplegia: a prospective cohort of 152 patients. Rev Neurol. 2002;158:589–92.
45. Del Guidice E, Staiano A, Capano G, Romano A, Florimonte L, Miele E, Ciarla C, Campanozzi A, and Crisanti AF. Gastrointestinal manifestations in children with cerebral palsy. Brain Dev. 1999;21:307–11.
46. Cameron KJ, Nyulasi IB, Collier GR, and Brown DJ. Assessment of the effect of increased dietary fibre intake on bowel function in patients with spinal cord injury. Spinal Cord. 1996;34:277–83.
47. Ashraf W, Pfeiffer RF, Park F, Lof J, and Quigley EM. Constipation in Parkinson's disease: objective assessment and response to psyllium. Mov Disord. 1997;12:946–51.
48. Consortium for Spinal Cord Medicine. Neurogenic bowel management in adults with spinal cord injury. Washington, DC: Paralyzed Veterans of America; 1998.
49. Chen D and Nussbaum SB. The gastrointestinal system and bowel management following spinal cord injury. Phys Med Rehabil Clin North Am. 2000;11:45–56.
50. Beloosesky Y, Grinblat J, Weiss A, Grosman B, Gafter U, and Chagnac A. Electrolyte disorders following oral sodium phosphate administration for bowel cleansing in elderly patients. Arch Intern Med. 2003;163:803–8.
51. Geders JM, Ganig A, Baumann WA, and Korsten MA. The effect of cisapride on segmental colonic transit time in patients with spinal cord injury. Am J Gastroenterol. 1995;90:285–9.
52. Longo WE, Woolsey RM, Vernava AM, Virgo KS, McKirgan L, and Johnson FE. Cisapride for constipation in spinal cord injured patients: a preliminary report. J Spinal Cord Med. 1995;18:240–4.
53. de Groot GH and de Pagter GF. Effects of cisapride on constipation due to a neurologic lesion. Paraplegia. 1988;26:159–61.
54. Weisel PH, Norton C, and Brazzelli M. Management of faecal incontinence and constipation in adults with central neurologic diseases (Cochrane Review). In: The Cochrane Library, Issue 3, 2002. Oxford: Update software.
55. Wysowski DK and Bacsanyi J. Cisapride and fatal arrhythmias. N Engl J Med. 1996;335:290–1.
56. Miller F and Fenzli TC. Prolonged ileus with spinal cord injury responding to metoclopramide. Paraplegia. 1981;19:34–5.

57. Steins SA. Reduction in bowel program duration with polyethylene glycol-based bisacodyl suppositories. Arch Phys Med Rehabil. 1995;76:674–7.
58. Shandling B and Gilmour RF. The enema continence catheter in spina bifida: successful bowel management. J Pediatr Surg. 1987;22:271–3.
59. Liptak GS and Revell GM. Management of bowel dysfunction in children with spinal cord disease or injury by means of the enema continence catheter. J Pediatr. 1992;120:190–4.
60. Scholler-Gyure M, Nesselaar C, van Wieringen H, and van Gool JD. Treatment of defecation disorders by colonic enemas in children with spina bifida. Eur J Pediatr Surg. 1996;6:32–4.
61. Christensen P, Kvitzau B, Krogh K, Buntzen S, and Laurberg S. Neurogenic colorectal dysfunction—use of new antegrade and retrograde colonic wash-out methods. Spinal Cord. 2000;38:255–61.
62. Malone PS, Ransley PG, and Kiely EM. Preliminary report: the antegrade continence enema. Lancet. 1990;336:1217–8.
63. Griffiths DM and Malone PS. The Malone antegrade continence enema. J Pediatr Surg. 1995;30:68–71.
64. Kiely EM, Ade-Ajayi N, and Wheeler RA. Caecal flap conduit for antegrade continence enemas. Br J Surg. 1994;81:1215.
65. Roberts JP, Moon S, and Malone PS. Treatment of neuropathic urinary and faecal incontinence with synchronous bladder reconstruction and the antegrade continence enema procedure. Br J Urol. 1995;75:386–9.
66. Yang CC and Steins SA. Antegrade continence enema for the treatment of neurogenic constipation and fecal incontinence after spinal cord injury. Arch Phys Med Rehabil. 2000;81:683–5.
67. Krogh K and Laurberg S. Malone antegrade continence enema for faecal incontinence and constipation in adults. Br J Surg. 1998;85:974–7.
68. Shandling B, Chait PG, and Richards HF. Percutaneous caecostomy: a new technique in the management of faecal incontinence. J Pediatr Surg. 1996;31:534–7.
69. De Peppo F, Iacobelli BD, De Gennaro M, Colajacomo M, and Rivosecchi M. Percutaneous endoscopic cecostomy for antegrade colonic irrigation in fecally incontinent children. Endoscopy. 1999;31:501–3.
70. Whitehead WE, Parker L, Bosmajian L, Morrill-Corbin ED, Middaugh S, Garwood M, Cataldo MF, and Freeman J. Treatment of fecal incontinence in children with spina bifida: comparison of biofeedback and behavior modification. Arch Phys Med Rehabil. 1986;67:218–24.
71. Ponticelli A, Iacobelli BD, Silveri M, Broggi G, Rivosecchi M, and De Gennaro M. Colorectal dysfunction and faecal incontinence in children with spina bifida. Br J Surg. 1998;81:117–9.
72. Wiesel PH, Norton C, Roy AJ, Storrie JB, Bowers J, and Kamm MA. Gut focused behavioural treatment (biofeedback) for constipation and faecal incontinence in multiple sclerosis. J Neurol Neurosurg Psychiatry. 2000;69:240–3.
73. Brindley GS, Polkey CE, Rushton DN, and Cardozo L. Sacral anterior root stimulators for bladder control in paraplegia: the first 50 cases. J Neurol Neurosurg Psychiatry. 1986;49:1104–14.
74. Binnie NR, Smith AN, Creasey GH, and Edmond P. Constipation associated with chronic spinal cord injury: The effect of pelvic parasympathetic stimulation by the Brindley stimulator. Paraplegia. 1991;29:463–9.

75. MacDonagh RP, Sun WM, Smallwood R, Forster D, and Read NW. Control of defecation in patients with spinal injuries by stimulation of sacral anterior nerve roots. BMJ. 1990;300:1494–7.
76. Creasey GH, Grill JH, Korsten M, U HS, Betz R, Anderson R, and Walter J. Implanted Neuroprosthesis Research Group. An implantable neuroprosthesis for restoring bladder and bowel control to patients with spinal cord injuries: a multicenter trial. Arch Phys Med Rehabil. 2001;82:1512–9.
77. Chia YW, Lee TK, Kour NW, Tung KH, and Tan ES. Microchip implants on the anterior sacral roots in patients with spinal trauma: does it improve bowel function? Dis Colon Rectum. 1996;39:690–4.
78. Lin VW, Hsiao IN, Zhu E, and Perkash I. Functional magnetic stimulation of the colon in persons with spinal cord injury. Arch Phys Med Rehabil. 2001; 82:167–73.
79. Stone JM, Wolfe VA, Nino-Murcia M, and Perkash I. Colostomy as treatment for complications of spinal cord injury. Arch Phys Med Rehabil. 1990;71:514–8.
80. Rosito O, Nino-Murcia M, Wolfe VA, Kiratli BJ, and Perkash I. The effects of colostomy on the quality of life in patients with spinal cord injury: a retrospective analysis. J Spinal Cord Med. 2002;25:174–83.
81. Safadi BY, Rosito O, Nino-Murcia, et al. Managing colonic dysmotility in the spinal cord patient population: which stoma works better? Association of VA Surgeons; 3 May 200. Abstract #13.

Editorial Commentary

There is reasonably little current data concerning the anorectal and colonic function of patients with diabetic autonomic neuropathy or in those suffering from Parkinsonism, except for sporadic reports concerning EAS fatigue which may contribute to evacuatory difficulty. Drs. Gaw and Longo succinctly outline in their chapter an epidemiologic assessment of bowel dysfunction in patients with a range of neurological disorders, although here too there is a paucity of data pertaining to long-term functional outcome in patients undergoing meningocele and myelomeningocele repair or in the extended follow-up following the reconstruction of congenital anorectal anomalies.

For the coloproctologist, referrals of patients with evacuatory problems after spinal surgery or following spinal injury represent difficult cases, since there is not that much in the literature to guide assessment or treatment. In some of these patients who do not respond to intermittent enemas or who have been treated with defunctioning stomas elsewhere for ease of management, the assessment may require sphincter electromyography and simulated distal limb stomal challenge to determine the integrity of the outlet musculature on the one hand and rectal sensitivity and capacitance on the other so as to guide either delayed stomal closure or in those with sufficient manual dexterity and motivation, selected use of an antegrade colonic conduit.

AZ

Chapter 12
Psychological Assessment of Patients with Proctological Disorders

ANNALISA RUSSO and MARIO PESCATORI

Introduction

Many patients with evacuatory disorders have underlying psychological problems and troubled psychological histories. It is often hard to know whether the colorectal symptomatology predates the psychological or psychiatric disorder or whether the converse is true. Studies on the bowel function of patients with defined psychological problems such as clinical depression, however, have been somewhat disappointing in that they have failed to categorize specific problems (1,2). What is evident is that colorectal symptomatology has a profound effect on the quality of life of the patient and their perceived symptoms, providing an equilibrating channel for the presentation of organic problems to the coloproctologist. In our opinion, it is an inherent value for the dedicated colorectal unit to have as part of their management team a psychologist with specific interest in these disorders and in their objective assessment (3).

During the past few years, the improvements in the field of colorectal surgery have proceeded more rapidly than they have in the past, mainly due to the development of new technologies such as laparoscopic colectomy, which carries less trauma and shorter hospitalization than open colorectal resection, and endoanal ultrasound, which permits a better evaluation of anorectal sepsis and rectal cancer staging. The recovery of proctological patients following surgical treatments is shortening, and given that the sensitive site of proctological disorders causes obvious relational and social discomfort, the length of convalescence has an important impact on the patient's quality of life. Although surgery may be carried out successfully from a technical standpoint, the patient's perception of outcome may be not as good as was expected by the clinician. This discrepancy is frequently not due to the surgical treatment itself, but more to ancillary problems often related to the psychological and functional aspects surrounding recovery.

In effect, the surgical considerations alone may not be sufficient to completely solve the most complicated of problems, and other factors must be evaluated with alternative approaches in a multidisciplinary context for optimal results. Psychological factors such as anxiety, stress, and emotional disorders can affect the surgical outcome to such a profound extent that the mental health of some patients has to be considered the principal priority. This psychological paradigm is of prime importance in the assessment of some poor postoperative functional outcomes, in health-related quality of life in patients with fecal incontinence, patients presenting with the principal symptom of proctalgia (frequently in the absence of significant clinical signs), and in the psychological overlay of many patients who have presented to pelvic floor clinics with inflammatory bowel diseases, irritable bowel syndrome (IBS), and evacuatory difficulty. Some of these issues are discussed in this chapter.

Postoperative Complications

We quote the example of two females over 50 years of age on whom we operated by using a Block obliterative suture procedure for rectocele who required re-operation for postoperative complications (4). Their persistent proctalgia was likely to be psychogenic and they were the only two out of 45 cases operated on using the simple and safe Block procedure who needed an early re-intervention in our series. One of them developed a sense of guilt caused by an extra-conjugal relationship with anal intercourse and the other one experienced significant psychological distress consequent upon her mother's death.

The transitory absence of anal contraction is very uncommon as a primary cause of significant fecal incontinence, which we have observed in two abused women. Both were referred to our gastroenterology department with fecal incontinence; one patient had been sexually abused by her father and the other physically abused by her husband. In both cases, anal contraction was absent on digital examination and during manometry, but anal endosonography and electrophysiological studies were normal. Anal contraction was restored following biofeedback, with both patients recovering from fecal incontinence (5).

Fecal Incontinence and Quality of Life

Fecal incontinence (FI) is a relatively common and profoundly disabling condition that increases significantly in the elderly (6). Surgeons place more emphasis on physiological aspects, but patients are more affected by leakage, hygiene, and social embarrassment. Byrne et al. (7) showed the importance of evaluation of the quality of life in patients with neuropathic FI. Their results on patients' perception of their own quality of life were compared with St. Mark's and Pescatori quantitative scores of incontinence. In patients with neuropathic fecal incontinence, the most frequent quality of life concern was the ability to go shopping and to socialize outside the home without concern about the location of the nearest toilets.

Because these results demonstrate the important impact of fecal incontinence on social interactions, qualitative assessment of incontinence may permit improvement in postoperative sphincter function after surgery or during biofeedback training, particularly in functional FI where there is recurrent uncontrolled passage of fecal material in the absence of neurologic or structural etiologies (8). This differs from FI due to neurological injury, where impaired perception of rectal distension has been noted in both children and adults.

Family History

Assessment of the family history can be as important as the clinical assessment. The following case report can help to better understand how psychological assessment can help the patient after surgery and where it also can avoid inappropriate operations. A 32-year-old female was the only daughter in a protective family. She had an unexpected proposal of marriage and she wanted to recover from an illness prior to marriage (she had had "congenital" fecal incontinence requiring a sphincteroplasty). After surgery, her anus was tight and she was perfectly continent on discharge. Bulk laxatives and pelvic floor exercises were strongly suggested. Two months later, she presented with a patulous anus and recurrent incontinence as a result of self-digitations and straining at stool. Despite our recommendations, she did not perform any pelvic floor rehabilitation and she did not take any laxatives. The psychological consultation revealed that when she came back home, she broke her engagement and then her relatives did not want to take care of her anymore. Consequently, she thought that the only way to still be considered the target of attention by her family again was to restore the "illness." She did not really want to be cured, and for this reason, she intentionally damaged the sphincteroplasty.

Magni et al. (9) reported another interesting contribution that demonstrates how the family history is crucial. He studied the psychological and clinical pattern of 29 women who underwent laparoscopy for chronic pelvic pain (CPP). Eleven patients with CPP without evident organic pathology had a higher mean score on the Zung self-rating depression scale and more somatic symptoms, which usually accompany depression, than 18 patients in whom organic disease was present. They also showed a higher number of depressive disorders in personal anamnesis and in the family history. On the basis of those results and comparing a group of women affected by another type of idiopathic chronic pain, the authors reported that CPP without organic pathology might be an expression of a depressive disorder. Therefore, it is mandatory to explore the patient's psychological pattern prior to and not after surgery if psychological problems are suspected.

Proctalgia

When psychologically assessed, our patients with chronic proctalgia revealed a higher level of anxiety than age-matched controls. This has allowed us to identify both state anxiety and trait anxiety, where it is important to understand which personality characteristics are typical in patients who present with some proctological disorders, highlighting which psychological disorders follow the treatment of certain forms of colorectal disease (10). These patients tended to have more primitive defensive strategies and lack of personality formation in standard testing when compared with age-matched control patients without proctologic problems. Historically, people with proctalgia and attendant genital pain tend to experience ancillary psychosomatic illnesses. Persistent chronic symptoms with lack of demonstrable pathological findings and frequent consultations and treatment failure may support such a psychosomatic diagnosis (11).

Cancer

Cancer can be considered an archetype of this category of disorders in its interaction with psychological overlay. The self-efficacy theory can explain how quality of life is very important after a surgical treatment through the Cancer Behavior Inventory (12), which is a valid approach for the measurement of self-efficacy behavior related to coping with cancer. Cancer patients tend to feel more efficacious about their coping capacity, although this is impaired when they become depressed or anxious (12). This level of depression is higher in cancer patients and in cancer survivors, and both the Structured Clinical Interview for DSM III-R (SCID) and the Hamilton Depression Rating Scale (HAMD) show that patients who are depressed are more likely to have metastatic disease and pain than non-depressed patients. These assessment scales also are able to identify suicidal ideation, where those with non-efficacious coping strategies have related major depressive symptoms (13). Suicidal ideation (at least) is potentially predictable, where demographic and medical variables such as social support appear to be the most important predictors for good quality of life in cancer survivors. Once these predictors are defined, selected psychotherapy can be efficacious in improving the quality of life of cancer sufferers (14).

According to a study on posttraumatic stress disorder (PTSD) in cancer survivors, the psychological symptoms of children and adolescent cancer survivors change in the decades following successful treatment (15). Posttraumatic symptomatology during young adulthood, when people mature and make important transitions, can affect quality of life. When posttraumatic symptoms occur in cancer survivors, care providers and family members should be prepared to strengthen support mechanisms when these symptoms develop. Using protocol-based family systems frameworks, psychologists offer system-oriented consultation to these patients, along with their family and health care team (15).

The environment and the family of the patient also have an important and crucial role in remission. In pediatric oncology, for example, behavioral and cognitive–behavioral interventions for pain and distress during invasive procedures can be applied to the whole family to help them cope with the negative aspects of the treatment (16), where increased symptoms of PTSD in survivors of childhood cancer and their parents have been reported (17,18).

Inflammatory Bowel Disease (IBD)

"Neuroticism," depression, anxiety, and hypochondriasis are common symptoms that have been assessed in IBD patient groups. Although is known that the family can influence the individual experience of illness, the impact of the family on the course of IBD has not been widely investigated (19); however, there is evidence that the patient's adjustment is more difficult if family relationships are unstable (20). Conversely, there is easier adjustment when a strong social support is present. Moreover, family life itself is affected by the course of the patient's IBD. Research has demonstrated how Expressed Emotions (EE) of the family members can play a key role in helping the patient adjust within the community, whereas patients whose relatives are critical and hostile tend to have more relapses than those whose relatives do not show these "high EE" components (21,22).

An extreme example of how psychological trauma can trigger and worsen an organic illness is represented by the sad clinical history of an introverted young colleague born in a small quiet village in southern Italy, whose mother died when he was 12 years old. A few months later, he started complaining of abdominal pain, diarrhea, and rectal bleeding, and the diagnosis of ulcerative colitis was made. After an effective course of medical treatment, he was relatively well for 10 years. At the age of 22, he was left by his girlfriend when he suddenly experienced an exacerbation of his symptoms. At sigmoidoscopy, his rectum was severely inflamed. He was admitted to the hospital and underwent a course of intensive medical treatment that included steroids. He subsequently did well and started working as a postgraduate surgeon in the University hospital of a big Italian city; however, due to his stressful life and the lack of an adequate financial income, he left the hospital and its appealing clinical and research work and went back to his home village. There, he was dissatisfied due to a frustrating—and for him—boring job and started complaining of colitic symptoms, developing episodes of frank cholangitis. A consultant gastroenterologist found associated liver disease with a foreshortened colon; colectomy was strongly advised but refused at that time by the patient. After five years, at the age of 37, he developed severe jaundice and died of cholangiocarcinoma. Research has demonstrated the relationship between IBD and psychological distress. Patients with active IBD have reported higher scores for psychological distress, somatization, obsessive–compulsive symptoms, depression, phobic anxiety, and psychotic behavior (23).

Irritable Bowel Syndrome (IBS)

Kolosky et al. (24) have shown important psychological factors associated with irritable bowel syndrome (IBS), where they noted a significant link between stress and gastrointestinal symptoms compatible with IBS. No less important are other factors related to IBS; namely, specific personality traits, psychological abuse, abnormal illness behavior, disrupted social supports, and coping skills along with particular sociodemographic characteristics. Indeed, the Truelove IBD classification includes postinflammatory, alimentary, and psychological factors (25–27).

Psychosocial factors such as personality, psychiatric diagnoses illness behavior, life stress, and psychological distress can all help distinguish patients with IBS from patients without this disorder (28). Furthermore, specific psychosocial difficulties (e.g., a history of physical abuse, maladaptive coping, etc.) can predict poor health outcome in this group with persistent pain, worse daily function, higher psychological distress, more days in bed, and more frequent visits to surgeons or physicians (29).

The observation that patients with IBS and patients with anxiety disorders—generalized anxiety disorder, panic disorder, posttraumatic stress disorder, and other psychiatric disorders such as major depression—have many autonomic symptoms supports the concept that psychiatric disorders and gastrointestinal disorders may have a common pathophysiology (30). This might assist in the subcategorization of IBS patients.

Here, controlled studies also have demonstrated that psychotherapy, stress management, and hypnosis can be effective in some patients with IBS, where some behavioral treatments are more effective than medical therapies, particularly if there is associated fecal incontinence and/or vomiting (31).

Chronic Constipation

Chronic constipation may severely affect quality of life and often is ultimately and complexly related to psychological problems. Close questioning during examination may reveal interesting and useful information for the physician and also may reveal beliefs and myths by the patient concerning bowel function, whereas many patients with chronic constipation describe a fear of not defecating every day or even a view that fecal matter is toxic (32).

The family environment may be dramatically related to the onset of "psychogenic" constipation, as shown by the case of a 23-year-old female who presented to our unit with severe slow-transit constipation and occasional mucous soiling. She had had unsuccessful operations between the ages of 12 and 17, including a Soave pull-through procedure and a right hemicolectomy. Surprisingly, none of her doctors had suggested a psychological consultation, which would have revealed that the patient had experienced sexual anal abuse by her mother's companion for five years when she was a child. Eventually, her constipation was managed by restorative proctocolectomy with an ileal pouch, followed by biofeedback training and psychotherapy.

Constipation may uncommonly require surgical intervention, but the surgeon should be aware of the importance of a psychological consultation (see Chapter 6.2). Many factors can predict the success or the failure of surgery and can help to understand persistent organic and psychosomatic symptoms. The existence of violence—both sexual and nonsexual—is a very important factor in the history where significant numbers of women who have been victims of sexual abuse can later present with gastrointestinal disorders. In this respect, 20% of sexually abused children will present with abdominal pain or constipation (33), and abdominal pain, constipation, and appetite disorders appear to be typical reactions to sexual abuse (34,35).

Psychological consultation is also crucial in the investigation of other important aspects of the patient's life, in particular, his/her quality of sleep. Patients with psychosomatic illnesses report fewer dreams during psychotherapy (36), and depressed people sleep much more than manic patients. These findings may be important in the etiology of constipation and IBS in these patients where patients with IBS tend to have abnormal rapid eye movement (REM) sleep (37). Moreover, higher levels of hysteria are more common in severely constipated subjects (38), where constipation and irritable bowel syndrome correlate with anxiety and personality profiles (39), as well as higher degrees of hypochondriasis (40).

In this respect, a direct link between mean transit time in the ascending colon and levels of anxiety measured by Minnesota Multiphasic Personality Inventory (MMPI) has previously been demonstrated (41,42), where, on multiple regression analysis, constipated patients with delayed colonic transit tend to show higher levels of anxiety, whereas those with colonic inertia, in which there is a lack of colonic motility, are correlated more frequently with higher levels of paranoia.

The "Iceberg Syndrome"

Many patients presenting with chronic constipation but without colonic transit disorders have an evacuatory dysfunction dominated by rectocele. Rectocele rarely requires an operation and patients frequently need rehabilitation to manage their pelvic floor dysfunction (chronic constipation and/or fecal incontinence), as well as psychological support to treat any associated anxiety and depression. Sometimes the common complaints attributed to rectoceles themselves are more often related to occult associated diseases including pudendal neuropathy, rectal mucosal intussusception, and/or concomitant peritoneocele.

These diseases are more difficult to diagnose; therefore, rectocele should be considered the "tip of the iceberg" whereas related disorders—including significant psychological/psychiatric problems—are the "underwater rocks" that may result in failure of rectocele surgery.

Here, descending perineum syndrome (DPS), pudendal neuropathy (PN), FI, and rectoanal intussusception may represent some of these "underwater rocks"; each condition may be complicated by enterocele, uterovaginal prolapse, or post-hysterectomy vault prolapse. This view highlights the need for a total pelvic workup of patients where rectocele itself is considered the dominant clinical finding, but where a multidisciplinary assessment is needed (43).

When the perineum descends more than 2.5 centimeters on straining, the patient can be labeled as having DPS (44). Chronic obstructed defecation and vaginal deliveries are most commonly associated with DPS and PN, consequent upon stretching of the pudendal nerves. As pudendal nerves carry both motor and sensory fibers, sphincter dysfunction (FI) and proctalgia are the commonest concomitant complaints. Pudendal neuropathy-related proctalgia can be treated by transanal electrostimulation, biofeedback, antidepressant therapy, acupuncture, or hypnosis, but due to its associated psychological component, it is unlikely to be effectively cured in many cases.

In this regard, our group has found a larger number of cases with altered preoperative psychological patterns who present either with surgical failures or with symptom recidivism where a preoperative "psychodiagnosis" had been made. Here, formal psychotherapy or psychological support, yoga, hypnosis, relaxation techniques, or pharmacological support—anxiolytics, hypnotics, and/or antidepressants—can improve results (10,45). Equally, the successful functioning of a dedicated pelvic floor unit—given the types of tertiary referrals—has been shown to benefit from a specialist psychologist—or psychiatrist—with a definitive interest in psychosomatic disorders and their impact on bowel habit. This has carried over into childhood practice, where dedicated proctological management of children with chronic constipation and encopresis has proved beneficial (46).

In conclusion, rectocele is just the "tip of the iceberg." A careful recognition of the "underwater rocks" as complex associated conditions requires analysis, which is fundamental in saving the "surgical ship" (patient) when dealing with the "Iceberg Syndrome." A multidisciplinary "crew" involving a gastroenterologist, a radiologist, a neurologist, a psychologist, and a trained biofeedback physiotherapist, combined with selected conservative surgery, can achieve the best clinical and functional results (43).

The following includes some of the testing and techniques used in our unit.

The Draw a Person Test

The draw-a-person test is one of the many tests we have used in patients affected by chronic constipation who present with typical emotional disorders such as anxiety, depression, and relational problems. After proctological intervention, patients often experience anal pain. The literature and our clinical experience have demonstrated that postoperative pain is strongly related to preoperative anxiety and stress levels. Pain is a relevant psychological component affecting the postoperative course, increasing the risk of complications such as urinary retention. The patients' quality of life evaluation is also important after surgical treatment, where investigation of personality changes may be of value if pain persists and is resistant to other surgical or medical treatments. Both the draw-a-person and the draw-the-family test originally described by Karen Machover (47) have been used by us in constipated patients to define how patients see themselves and their surroundings and to broadly judge the outgoing nature of their personality, helping us select some potentially recalcitrant patients who may benefit from psychological therapy (47–49). Although very subjective, this test (Figure 12.1) can provide insight into the intellectual nature of some patients, providing indirect evidence of verbalization skills, and in children, some information regarding parent bonding and identification (33).

Guided Imagery

When serious personality disorders occur, patients may not readily respond to psychopharmacologic and psychotherapeutic interventions. To reduce pain in patients undergoing surgical treatment, we, along with others, have used Guided Imagery, where it has been reported that Guided Imagery improves pain-related outcomes and reduces analgesic requirements and in-hospital stay following colorectal (50) and anal (45) surgery. Here, patients listen to a tape with music and a relaxing text before, during, and after surgery (51). In our recent trial, three parameters were investigated: a) postoperative pain, b) the quality of sleep, and c) the first micturition (45). This cheap and noninvasive intervention showed a significant reduction in postoperative pain, improved quality of sleep, and perceived ease of first micturition in a group of patients undergoing a range of proctological procedures (45).

Pelvic Floor Rehabilitation

In our unit since October 1992, patients with fecal incontinence or severe chronic constipation have been primarily selected for an intensive phase of biofeedback treatment protocol modified in our unit as the first rung of the treatment algorithm (52). This program includes Combined Rehabilitation

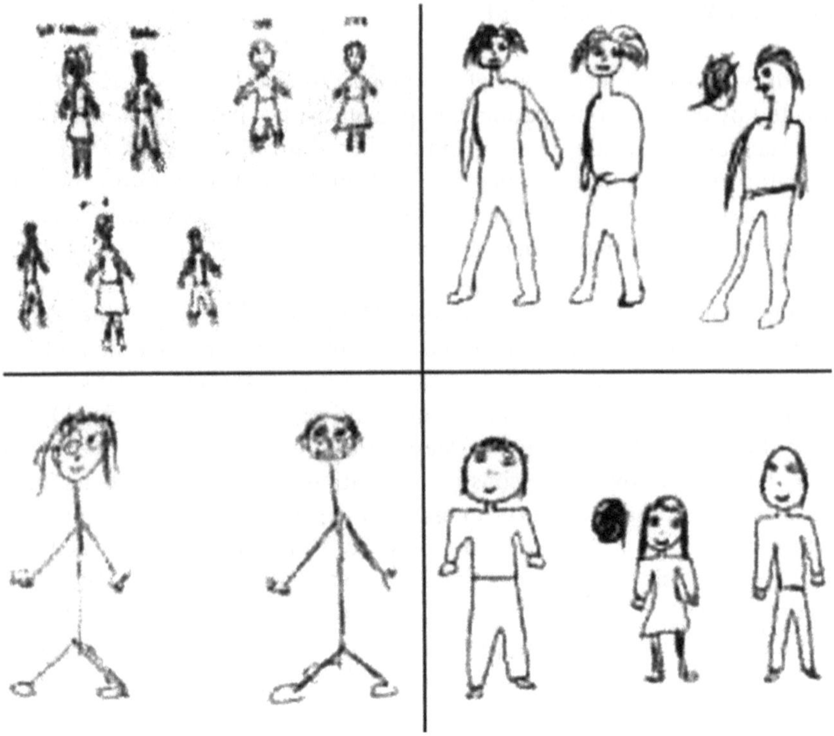

FIGURE 12.1. Upper left: chronic constipation; little figures; absence of corrections; upper right: controls: normal dimensions, presence of corrections; lower left: chronic constipation, figure excessively schematic; lower right: controls: figures graphically complete.

(CR) using a combination of three procedures: 1) biofeedback, 2) physiotherapy, and 3) electrostimulation (53).

Biofeedback improves cortical control of the pelvic floor muscles, physiotherapy improves muscle strength and coordination, and electrostimulation improves muscle resistance. Here, a synergistic effect that reinforces the continence mechanisms is expected, using the combination of these three techniques where follow-up has shown a significant improvement in the mean continence score after CR rehabilitation in an unselected group of the first 65 patients treated in this manner between October 1992 and October 1994 with a substantial improvement in post-treatment manometry (53). This approach has been reproduced with similar clinical improvements in selected patients with FI as treated by other units (54) using a multimodal combination of volumetric rehabilitation, electrostimulation, and pelviperineal kinesitherapy.

In our coloproctology unit, we also take into consideration other aspects of the well-being of our patients, such as their nutrition. Well-being indeed depends upon correct nutrition, especially after surgical treatment or other less-invasive treatments. As patients learn to correctly use their internal or external musculature during biofeedback, they also can help themselves in learning to feed their body correctly with a balanced nutritional program, highlighting potentially unrecognized food intolerances.

Conclusions

A multidisciplinary team, which includes either a psychologist or a psychiatrist, should follow these specialized patients from their first visit to the final steps of their treatment and the definitive resolution of their problem using a "holistic approach." The great advantage of a team psychologist—and a psychological perspective—in a dedicated coloproctology unit is in "flagging" patients who are likely, by virtue of their preexisting psychological and biosocial problems, not to benefit from surgery or to have symptom recidivism after surgery. Moreover, it is crucial that patients be afforded a range of non-surgical therapies for pelvic floor dysfunction as part of this holistic approach. The factors that are predictive for non-surgical success are still being evaluated in many units.

References

1. Garvey M, Noyes R, and Yates W. Frequency of constipation in major depression: relationship to other clinical variables. Psychosomatics. 1990;31: 204–6.
2. Nehra V, Bruce BK, Rath-Harvey DM, Pemberton JH, and Camilleri M. Psychological disorders in patients with evacuation disorders and constipation in a tertiary practice. Am J Gastroenterol. 2000;95:1755–8.
3. Devroede G. Psychophysiological considerations in subjects with chronic idiopathic constipation. In: Wexner SD and Bartolo DCC, editors. Constipation: etiology, evaluation and management. London: Butterworth Heinemann; 1995. p. 103–34.
4. Ayabaca SM, Zbar AP, and Pecatori M. Anal continence after rectocele repair. Dis Colon Rectum. 2002;45:63–9.
5. Berkelmans I, Leroi AM, Weber J, and Denis P. Fecal incontinence with transitory absence of anal contraction in two sexually or physically abused women. Eur J Gastroenterol. 1996;8:235–8.
6. Mavrantonis C and Wexner SD. A clinical approach to fecal incontinence. J Clin Gastroenterol. 1988;27:108–21.
7. Byrne CM, Pager CK, Rex J, Roberts R, and Solomon MJ. Assessment of quality of life in the treatment of patients with neuropathic fecal incontinence. Dis Colon Rectum. 2002;45:1431–6.
8. Whitehead WE, Wald A, Diamant NE, Enck P, Pemberton JH, and Rao SSC. Functional disorders of the anus and rectum. Gut. 1999;Suppl II:1155–9.
9. Magni G, Salmi A, De Leo D, and Ceola A. Chronic pelvic pain and depression. Psychopathology. 1984;17:132–6.

10. Renzi C and Pescatori M. Psychological aspects in proctalgia. Dis Colon Rectum. 2000;43:535–9.
11. Wesselman U, Burnett AL, and Heinberg LJ. The urogenital and rectal pain syndrome. Pain. 1997;73:269–94.
12. Merluzzi TV, Nairn RC, Hegde K, Martinez Sanchez MA, and Dunn L. Self-efficacy for coping with cancer: revision of the cancer behaviour inventory (version 2.0). Psycho-oncology. 2001;10:206–17.
13. Ciaramella A and Poli P. Assessment of depression among cancer patients: the role of pain, cancer and treatment. Psycho-oncology. 2001;10:156–65.
14. Parker PA, Baile WF, De Moor C, and Cohen L. Psychosocial and demographic predictors of quality of life in a large sample of cancer patients. Psycho-oncology. 2003;12:183–93.
15. Rourke MT, Stuber ML, Hobbie WL, and Kazak AE. Posttraumatic stress disorder: understanding the psychosocial impact of surviving childhood cancer into young adulthood. J Pediatric Nurs. 1999;16:115–6.
16. Kazak AE, Simms S, and Rourke MT. Family system practice in pediatric psychology. J Pediatric Psychol. 2002;27(2):133–43.
17. Kazak AE, Barakat L, Meeske K, et al. Posttraumatic stress, family functioning and social support in survivors of childhood cancer and their mothers and fathers. J Consult Clin Psychol. 1997;65:120–9.
18. Kazak AE. Effective psychosocial intervention for children with cancer [editorial]. Med Pediatr Oncol. 1999;32:292–3.
19. Vaughn CE, Leff J, and Sarner M. Relatives' expressed emotion and the course of inflammatory bowel disease. J Psychosom Res. 1999;47:461–9.
20. McMahon AW, Schmitt P, Patterson JF, and Rothman E. Personality differences between inflammatory bowel disease patients and their healthy siblings. Psychosom Med. 1973;35:35–91.
21. Brown GW, Birley JLT, and Wing JK. Influence of family life on the course of schizophrenic disorders: a replication. Br J Psychiatry. 1976;121:241–58.
22. Vaughn CE and Leff J. The influence of family and social factors on the course of psychiatric illness: a comparison of schizophrenic and depressed neurotic patients. Br J Psychiatry. 1976;129:125–37.
23. Sewitch MJ, Abrahamowicz M, Bitton A, Daly D, Wild GE, Cohen A, Katz S, Szego PL, and Dobkin PL. Psychological support and disease activity in patients with inflammatory bowel disease. Am J Gastroenterol. 2001;96:1470–9.
24. Koloski NA, Talley NJ, and Boyce PM. Predictors of health care seeking for irritable bowel syndrome and nonulcer dyspepsia: a critical review of the literature on symptom and psychological factors. Am J Gastroenterol. 2001;96:1340–9.
25. Sullivan ES, Jenkins PL, and Blewett AE. Irritable bowel syndrome and family history of psychiatry disorder: a preliminary study. Gen Hosp Psychiatry. 1995;17:43–6.
26. Kaplan DS, Masand PS, and Gupta S. The relationship of irritable bowel syndrome (IBS) and panic disorder. Ann Clin Psychiatry. 1996;8:81–8.
27. DelvauxM, Denis P, and Allemand H. Sexual abuse is more frequently reported by IBS patients than by patients with organic digestive diseases or controls. Results of a multicentre inquiry. Eur J Gastroenterol. 1997;9:345–52.
28. Sandler DS, Drossman DA, Nathan HP, and McKee DC. Symptom complaints and health care seeking behaviour in subjects with bowel dysfunction. Gastroenterology. 1984;87:314–8.

29. Drossman DA. Do psychological factors define symptom severity and patient status in Irritable Bowel Syndrome? Am J Med. 1999;107:41–50.
30. Lydiard RB and Falsetti SA. Experience with anxiety and depression treatment studies: implications for designing irritable bowel syndrome clinical trials. Am J Med. 1999;107:65–73.
31. Whitehead WE. Behavioral medicine approaches to gastrointestinal disorders. J Consult Clin Psychol. 1992;60:605–12.
32. Strickland MC and Heymen S. Psychiatric treatment of constipation. In: Wexner SD and Bartolo DCC, editors. Constipation: etiology, evaluation & management. London: Butterworth Heinemann; 1994.
33. Devroede G. Psychological considerations in subjects with chronic idiopathic constipation. In: Wexner SD and Bartolo DCC, editors. Constipation: etiology, evaluation & management. London: Butterworth Heinemann; 1994.
34. Rimsza ME, Berg RA, and Locke C. Sexual abuse: somatic and emotional reactions Child Ab Negl. 1988;12:201–8.
35. Leroi AM, Bernier C, Watier A, et al. Prevalence of sexual abuse among patients with functional disorders of the lower gastrointestinal tract. Int J Colorectal Dis. 1995;10:200–6.
36. Kristal H. Alexithymia and psychotherapy. Am J Psychother. 1979;33:17–31.
37. Kumar D, Thompson PD, Wingate DL, Vesselinova-Jenkins CK, and Libby G. Abnormal REM sleep in the irritable bowel syndrome. Gastroenterology. 1992;103:12–7.
38. Devroede G, Bouchoucha M, and Girard G. Constipation, anxiety and personality. What carries first? In: Bueno L, Collins S, and Junior JL, editors. Stress and digestive motility. London: JohnLibbey; 1989. p. 55–60.
39. Devroede G, Roy T, Bouchoucha M, et al. Idiopathic constipation by colonic dysfunction: relationship with personality and anxiety. Dig Dis Sci. 1989; 34:1428–33.
40. Drossman DA, McKee DC, Sandler RS, et al. Psychological factors in the irritable bowel syndrome. A multivariate study of patients and non patients with irritable bowel syndrome. Gastroenterology 1988;95:701–8.
41. Devroede G. Constipation and sexuality. Med Asp Human Sex. 1990 Feb:40–6.
42. Ripetti V, Caputo D, Ausania F, Esposito E, Bruni R, and Arullani A. Sacral nerve neuromodulation improves physical, psychological and social quality of life in patients with fecal incontinence. Tech Coloproctol. 2002; 6:147–52.
43. Pescatori M. Anal rectoceles and the Iceberg Syndrome. Urodynamica. Forthcoming 2004.
44. Parks AG, Porter NH, and Hardcastle J. The syndrome of the descending perineum. Proc R Soc Med. 1966;59:477–82.
45. Renzi C, Peticca L, and Pescatori M. The use of relaxation techniques in the perioperative management of proctological patients: preliminary results. Int J Colorectal Dis. 2000;15:313–6.
46. Loening-Baucke V, Cruikshank B, and Savage C. Defecation dynamics and behavior profiles in encopretic children. Pediatrics. 1987;80:672–9.
47. Machover K. Personality projection in the drawing of the human figure: a method of personality investigation. Springfield: Charles Thomas; 1949.
48. Castellazzi VL and Nannini MF. Il disegno della figura umana come tecnica proiettiva. Rome: Libreria Ateneo Salesiano; 1992.

49. Renzi C and Pescatori M. Family drawing with clinical approach to patients with chronic constipation: preliminary data. Neurogastroenterology. 2002;56–8.
50. Tusek DL, Church JM, Strong SA, Grass JA, and Fazio VW. Guided imagery: a significant advance in the care of patients undergoing elective colorectal surgery. Dis Colon Rectum. 1997;40:172–8.
51. Mathias JM. Guided imagery tapes help surgical patients. OR Manager. 1998;14:18–9.
52. Perozo SE, Ferrara A, Patankar SK, Larach SW, and Williamson PR. Biofeedback with home trainer programme is effective for both incontinence and pelvic floor dysfunction. Tech Coloproctol. 1997;5:6–9.
53. Peticca L, Pietroletti R, Ayabaca SM, and Pescatori M. Combined biofeedback physiotherapy and electrostimulation for fecal incontinence. Tech Coloproctol. 2000;4:157–61.
54. Pucciani F, Iozzi L, Masi A, Cianchi F, and Cortesini C. Multimodal rehabilitation for faecal incontinence: experience of an Italian center devoted to faecal disorder rehabilitation. Tech Coloproctol. 2003;7:139–47.

Editorial Commentary

Drs. Russo and Pescatori nicely discuss the importance of specialized psychological input in a working colorectal unit where it is recognized that the flagging of major pretreatment depression and anxiety in patients with pelvic floor dysfunction and evacuatory difficulty who undergo rectocele repair prevents suboptimal functional results. The exact interaction between biofeedback therapies, multimodal pelvic floor rehabilitation and definitive psychotherapy is at present unknown as is the relationship between sexual dysfunction and abuse in patients presenting with evacuatory difficulty or significant proctalgia.

The specialist coloproctologist will frequently have a "gut feeling" about some patients likely to fare badly from surgery or who necessitate psychologic or psychiatric input even though they present with functional anorectal disorders which clearly have demonstrable pelvic/perineal pathology which would normally in their own right be suitable for operative repair or reconstruction. This clinical inkling is a hard thing to quantify or evaluate by an evidence base but it is clear at the present time that there is very little available hard data which can actually guide the colorectal surgeon. Other cases sometimes seen in adult clinics include young patients presenting with encopresis where the principal problem along with inadequate evacuation is a strong psychological overlay secondary to sexual abuse and compounded by significant attendant family psychopathology. These young patients often present with a complex range of symptoms attributable to evacuation difficulty and manifesting as repetitive obsessive behavioural habits or extended forms of gastrointestinal somatization.

AZ

Chapter 13
A Practical Guide to Running an Anorectal Laboratory

Joseph T. Gallagher, Sergio W. Larach, and Andrea Ferrara

Introduction

The anorectal laboratory is an invaluable addition to the practice of any coloproctologist, enabling the specialist to provide unique services for patients in a competitive market. The Colon and Rectal Clinic of Orlando is a private practice performing solely colon and rectal surgeries and treatments with an anorectal laboratory first established in 1990. Based on the management of this anorectal laboratory, it was our intention to provide a workable model for a community-based private practice physiology center offering such specialist diagnostic and therapeutic services. There are many excellent institutionally based anorectal laboratories around the world; however, many are not practicable for translation into private colorectal practice.

Goals of an Anorectal Laboratory

The goals in development of an anorectal laboratory are as follows:

1. Provision of a comprehensive assessment of patients referred to the clinic with functional disorders;
2. To provide guidance with both surgical and non-surgical management of such functional disorders, as well as broad and specific management principles that may include changes in lifestyle, diet, toileting details, etc.,
3. To provide actual treatment (and audit), including biofeedback therapies,
4. To coordinate evaluation and treatment as part of a team approach incorporating gastroenterologists, urologists, or urogynecologists as indicated. In this respect, even though the coloproctologist directs the evaluation of all the patients presenting to the anorectal laboratory, most patients will not undergo surgery.

Staffing Issues

A successful anorectal laboratory requires a team approach, with personnel having different areas of expertise. However, there are two key positions required to establish an anorectal laboratory. All patients undergo an initial consultation by a colon and rectal surgeon before they are evaluated by the anorectal laboratory or before starting biofeedback treatment. The coloproctologist will then manage and direct future tests, as well as direct overall care of the patient. It is important in this respect to establish an initial clinical diagnosis of a functional disorder and to ensure that the patient does not have any additional diagnoses that are likely to significantly impact on the overall success of treatment. Another required participant for a successful anorectal laboratory is a trained and certified biofeedback therapist who can provide treatment as directed by the surgeon (1,2). Ideally, all of the procedures and staff of the anorectal laboratory would be conducted at one site in order to facilitate evaluation and treatment of patients with these disparate functional disorders.

The coloproctologist associated with the lab needs to be knowledgeable about and have an interest in functional disorders; his/her evaluation needs to be comprehensive (American system HCFA level 4 or 5). In addition to a complete physical examination (as extensively discussed in other parts of this book), the patient also should undergo an anoscopy and flexible sigmoidoscopy. Depending on the results of these evaluations, the patients with a functional disorder(s) can effectively be placed into diagnostic and therapeutic algorithms constructed for the unit as described by John Pemberton MD in his book, *The Pelvic Floor: Its Function and Disorders* (3). We feel it is important to supplement and reinforce this clinical evaluation with objective information obtained through the anorectal laboratory, where a similar approach has been offered by Smith (4). The guidelines for the running of an anorectal laboratory such as this may be assisted by data available concerning the management of an ambulatory anorectal service in terms of design, patient referral practice, patient selection, licensure, billing practice, and physician ownership (5).

Here, the surgeon's role is also one of interpretation of all anorectal physiology testing where the allied team performs anal manometry, endorectal ultrasound (ERUS), invasive electromyography (EMG), and pudendal nerve evaluation under direction of the coloproctologist and where the surgeon reviews all imaging studies. Initiation of conservative therapy and additional recommendations including diet, water intake, physical activity, toileting habits, and the like also are made during the initial consultation.

The certified biofeedback therapist will need specific training for pelvic floor dysfunction in order to be able to provide audited biofeedback therapy. This subject is considered in detail in Chapter 6.5. In our lab, the therapist is actually an employee of the clinic. The therapist collects and reviews the patient's diet diary and will administer the psychological profile (where necessary) and collate functional scoring tests (including sexual function, constipation, and an incontinence index). The therapist performs the manometry and biofeedback and counsels (and notates) the patient on dietary recommendations and toileting habits.

A radiologist is required for the smooth functioning of the lab—preferably one with a special interest in colorectal functional disorders. In our unit, we have a specialized radiologist from our major institutions who performs and interprets the radiologic tests performed for these functional disorders. Having such a dedicated radiologist has increased the efficiency and consistency of our radiographic evaluations in complex cases and has standardized algorithms of management where the coordination of findings is completed by the surgeon.

A urogynecologist, urologist, or gynecologist are also becoming important parts of the anorectal laboratory because about 30% of patients with anorectal functional disorders also have urinary dysfunction and because the vast majority of patients seen are female. Here, sexual function/dysfunction is a vital part of the evaluation. These physicians perform their own comprehensive evaluation and also will perform and interpret urodynamic studies where indicated. They also may perform any surgical corrective procedures as indicated for urinary dysfunction and assist in consultation of surgeries where transvaginal surgery may be used.

Ideally, a dietician should be available to counsel and evaluate each patient as part of the team approach, where dietary diaries are a very important part of the work-up of functional disorders. We currently use the local hospital dieticians as indicated and rely heavily on our biofeedback therapist to review these diaries, to reinforce good colonic dietary practices, and to counsel for dietary recommendations. In the best of all worlds, a psychologist should be available to evaluate and possibly counsel patients with functional disorders, as these complaints can sometimes be hallmark signs or symptoms of an underlying psychological disorder that should be addressed. Certain patients may be able to make significant improvements with changes in their toileting or dietary habits and with counseling; we are fortunate in our lab because our biofeedback therapist is also a certified mental health counselor, administering a SCL-90-R test for the prediction success with biofeedback therapies (2).

Testing and Equipment

The anorectal laboratory will need to establish it own controls for normal values. Reports generated from the lab will need to be standardized in order to facilitate communication between the team and increase the ability to review the collected information. The equipment used for anal physiology testing is constantly improving and the information collected that each unit has the most experience with tends to be used in clinical practice. Surveys have shown a shift in the demographics of both manometric and endosonographic use throughout both the United Kingdom and the United States (6).

Computerized anorectal manometry uses an eight-channel perfusion catheter with automated catheter withdrawal. This uses a computer program that is windows based (see Chapter 2.3). The standardized information retrieved from this test includes sphincter pressures at rest and squeeze, mean resting and squeeze sphincter asymmetry, high-pressure zone (HPZ) length, rectal sensation, paradoxical firing during strain, and the balloon rectoanal inhibitory reflex (RAIR). These tests are performed in the office by the therapist under the supervision of a surgeon and show high correlation with conventional manometry in both health and disease (7).

Computerized noninvasive EMG uses an intra-anal or surface sensor. This test determines the short peaks evaluation, ten-second contraction test, endurance and constipation profile, and is performed during the same visit as the computerized manometry by the biofeedback therapist. Pudendal nerve latency and invasive EMG are performed by the physician in a surgery center or a hospital outpatient neurological center. Invasive EMG is conducted using a single concentric needle electrode placed in the left lateral sphincter complex with the patient in the lithotomy position. The report includes motor unit potential (MUP) evaluation and a graphic evaluation of pelvic floor dysfunction. Pudendal nerve latency motor latency is determined using a standardized St. Mark's pudendal electrode glove (see Chapter 2.9).

Anal ultrasound is performed by the physician in the office. The cost of this machine for the office is approximately 22 000 US dollars. It has proven highly sensitive in the detection of internal anal sphincter (IAS) and external anal sphincter (EAS) defects in patients presenting with fecal incontinence and provides a thorough evaluation of all sphincter components in a standardized fashion.

As an allied service, the radiology department should be able, where necessary, to perform defecography, colonic transit studies, small bowel series, solid and liquid scintigraphic gastric emptying analyses, and hydrogen breath tests. Guidelines have been internationally established with radiology departments to ensure a standardization of imaging analysis for functional disorders (8). Most of the imaging is performed at a single center dedicated to conducting the imaging in a standard fashion with concise written reports. Having an imaging center familiar with specialized imaging for functional disorders improves the consistency of the results, as well as minimizes patient discomfort.

Biofeedback therapy is performed by the therapist, as has already been discussed. Before each session, the therapist reviews the dietary diary and the patient's toileting activities since the last visit. The biofeedback sessions will be given in four treatments over a course of up to two months. Patients may need additional treatments with secondary decay of benefit over time (see Chapter 6.5). Most biofeedback patients use an anal surface electrode and abdominal surface sensors; however, some patients will require an internal anal sensor for optimal results (2). The patient is allowed to sit in their street clothes in front of the monitor and is expected to do therapeutic Kegels and advanced Kegels at home. Depending on the patient, they may also receive an anal sensor to be used at home. Clinical improvement is monitored and recorded at each visit.

Additional tests may include comprehensive stool evaluation, where alternative therapies such as probiotics may be prescribed. Further tests and treatments potentially offered by the anorectal laboratory in the future may include radiofrequency anal canal treatments and percutaneous sacral nerve stimulation for fecal incontinence, 24-hour ambulatory anorectal motility studies, and selected pelvic magnetic resonance imaging (MRI). All of these tests and treatments are currently under evaluation and cost analysis. As these tests become universally accepted and standardized, they can be added to the armamentarium of the surgeon for the sophisticated treatment of patients presenting with functional pelvic disorders (9,10).

A successful anorectal laboratory will require a sound financial business plan. Cost analysis will have to be performed, taking into account state laws, local laws, and regulations. Financial success will have to be determined on an individual basis considering the size of the practice and local reimbursements for performing the test, interpretation of the test, and the stratified compensation for team members. There are many potential benefits that need to be assessed, including predicted increases in the practice patient base and the projected ability to offer services unique to a colon and rectal surgery practice in accordance with agreed surgical and gastroenterological society standards (11). The bare minimum to start an anorectal laboratory requires a dedicated physician interested in functional disorders and the ability to offer biofeedback therapy. Equipment costs can be prohibitive; the cost can be partially deferred and offset through increasing the volume of patients undergoing evaluation by the anorectal laboratory or possibly through local hospital equipment purchasing strategies.

References

1. Pantankar SK, Ferrara A, Levy JR, Larach SW, Williamson PR, and Perozo S. Biofeedback in colorectal practice: A multicenter, statewide, three-year experience. Dis Colon Rectum. 1997;40:827–31.
2. Patankar SK, Ferrara A, Larach SW, Williamson PR, Perozo SE, Levy JR, and Mills JA. Electromyographic assessment of biofeedback for fecal incontinence and chronic constipation. Dis Colon Rectum. 1997;40:907–11.
3. Pemberton JH, Swash M, Henry MH, and Lightner DJ. Algorithms. In: Pemberton JH, Swash M, and Henry MH, editors. The pelvic floor, its function and disorders. Philadelphia: Saunders; 2002. p. 4–10.

4. Smith LE. Practical guide to anorectal testing. 2nd ed. New York: Igaku-Shoin; 1995.
5. Bailey HR and Snyder MJ, editors. Ambulatory anorectal surgery. New York: Springer Verlag; 2000.
6. Karulf RE, Coller JA, Bartolo DC, Bowden DO, Roberts PL, Murray J, Schoetz DJ Jr, and Veidenheimer MC. Anorectal physiology testing. A survey of availability and use. Dis Colon Rectum. 1991;34:464–8.
7. Zbar AP, Aslam M, Hider A, Toomey P, and Kmiot WA. Comparison of vector volume manometry with conventional manometry in anorectal dysfunction. Tech Coloproctol. 1998;2:84–90.
8. Diamant NE, Kamm MA, Wald A, and Whitehead WE. A GA technical review on anorectal testing techniques. Gastroenterology. 1999;116:735–60.
9. Speakman CT and Henry MM. The work of an anorectal physiology laboratory. Baillieres Clin Gastroenterol. 1992;6:59–73.
10. Felt-Bersma RJ, Poen AC, Cuesta MA, and Meuwissen SG. Referral for anorectal function evaluation: therapeutic implications and reassurance. Eur J Gastroenterol Hepatol. 1999;11:289–94.
11. Rao SS, Azpiroz F, Diamant N, Enck P, Tougas G, and Wald A. Minimum standards of anorectal manometry. Neurogastroenterol Motil. 2002;14:553–9.

Editorial Commentary

I had the privilege of visiting the Colorectal Unit of Orlando some years ago and found an impressive combination of both specialized equipment and dedicated personnel. There are some guidelines provided in this chapter for the development and running of a successful anorectal laboratory which follow the recommendations in other units for the construction of an ambulatory proctologic service. I would emphasize some relatively neglected points. Regarding the socioeconomic aspects of the service, the office should be able to effectively deal with insurance companies. Specific request and reporting forms are valuable in the reporting of specialized findings, in the notation for clinical coloproctological conferences concerning medical and surgical patient management (and for medicolegal purposes) and for the academic collation and presentation of data. I believe that dynamic transperineal ultrasonography should be also available as it is quick and reproducible and is very helpful in the diagnosis of perineal descent, non relaxing puborectalis syndrome, recto-(peritoneo-entero)cele and sigmoidocele. Photographic equipment and video technology is essential for the recording of a database and for teaching purposes and images are necessary to support clinical and research presentations at congresses, workshops, and institutional meetings.

MP

Chapter 14
Medicolegal Aspects of Coloproctologic Practice

David E. Beck

Introduction

Our society has become increasingly litigious. Many people look to the American justice system to resolve problems, and if a bad outcome occurs, someone must be a fault. Some Americans view a poor outcome as a potential to "hit the lottery," and until tort reform is widely adopted, the number of malpractice suits will continue to expand and the cost of insurance will escalate. To minimize the risk of malpractice claims, the practicing physician must, in addition to practicing good medicine, exercise effective communication skills, establish rapport with the patient and their family, and accurately document their care (1). Despite doing all of this, a bad outcome still may result in the patient filing a malpractice claim (2). Research supports that patients who perceive their physician as having good communication and interpersonal skills are less likely to sue (3).

This chapter will provide a general overview of the legal process pertaining to medical malpractice and summarize risk-prevention techniques that prevent or help defend malpractice claims, with special emphasis on issues of interest to colorectal surgeons.

Physician–Patient Relationship

Technological advances and socioeconomic changes have dramatically changed medicine in the last few decades and encouraged specialization such as colon and rectal surgery. This fragmentation potentially decreases the opportunity to communicate effectively with patients, who also have become more demanding consumers (1). The media and lawyer advertising have made patients increasingly aware of their "rights" and fostered a sense of entitlement. Health systems and insurers contribute to the problem by creating incentives that discourage referrals to specialists and placing restrictions on the specialists that impede opportunities to establish rapport once referrals are made. Under such circumstances, it is important to make the most of each opportunity to listen to the patient, remember and use the patient's name, explain procedures in lay terms (avoid medical terminology), and take the time necessary to answer any and all questions. Mechanisms should be in place for the patient to contact the physician as needed. Office and hospital support staff must be trained and encouraged to assist the patient, support the physician–patient relationship, and communicate the physician's interest in the patient's well-being and concerns. This is especially important as colorectal surgeons perform outpatient procedures such as colonoscopy and anorectal procedures. It also may have implications where patients may be discharged earlier through deliberate "fast-track" policies applicable to colorectal resection (4). Making the effort to listen to a patient's questions and complaints is much less time consuming than defending a malpractice claim.

Additional resources for improving communication and relationships can be found in such texts as Dale Carnegie's *How to Win Friends and Influence People* and *Malpractice Prevention and Liability Control for Hospitals* by Orlikoff and Vanagunas (5,6).

The frequency of medical malpractice claims has been on the rise since the early 1970s (7). Recently, the increase in claims along with a slowdown of the economy, which reduced insurance company's income from investments, have forced several malpractice carriers to leave the market. The loss of reasonably priced coverage and, in some areas, the absence of coverage altogether have forced many providers to limit or close their practices. This situation will only worsen as long as we continue the contingency fee system in the absence of a loser pay provision. Until medicolegal tort reform becomes widespread, the well-trained and well-educated specialist must be aware of areas of treatment in colorectal disease that present an increased risk of malpractice claims (1,8).

High Risk Areas

Review of malpractice claims has identified certain aspects of colorectal disease that are at increased risk. The majority of claims are filed in the following categories (8):

1. Delay in diagnosis of colon and rectal cancer and appendicitis
2. Iatrogenic colon injury (e.g., colon perforation)
3. Iatrogenic medical complication during diagnosis or treatment
4. Sphincter injury with fecal incontinence resulting from anorectal surgery
5. Lack of informed consent.

The colorectal provider who is aware of these potential high-risk conditions can use risk-prevention strategies to avoid litigation (1). In particular, patient symptoms or lack of symptoms, as well as potential risk factors for colorectal cancer (i.e., rectal bleeding, change in bowel habit, positive family history), should be documented, along with recommendations for evaluation and screening (9). A patient's refusal to comply with recommendations also should be documented. Diagnostic evaluations are indicated in patients with significant symptoms. As no diagnostic study is perfect, additional or repeat diagnostic studies should be considered for patients with persistent symptoms or where re-referral occurs and there is limited or no access to prior investigations or reports.

As stated above, continence remains another high-risk medicolegal concern. Objective documentation of pre-therapy sphincter function (e.g., manometry, pudendal nerve terminal motor latency, or intra-anal ultrasound) can assist in the determination of when or if sphincter dysfunction has occurred. Finally, potential risks specific to colorectal procedures such as anastomotic leaks, bladder or sexual dysfunction, and interference with continence merit additional discussion with the patient and appropriate documentation in the medical records.

Informed Consent

Consent and informed consent are quite different concepts. Consent implies permission. Informed consent is assent given by the patient based on information or knowledge of the procedure and its inherent risks, benefits, and alternatives (1).

Courts have long recognized that every human being of adult years and sound mind has a right to determine what shall be done with his/her own body (10). The laws on informed consent vary somewhat from state to state; however, each patient should be allowed an exchange of information with the physician before a procedure is accomplished. Having the patient sign a form is not enough. Informed consent is only satisfied when consent was obtained after full disclosure of the risks, benefits, and alternatives of the procedure.

Many states use the "reasonable practitioner standard" to judge whether informed consent was obtained. This standard focuses on what a reasonable physician would disclose. The physician's duty is not to disclose all risks, but primarily those that are significant or material (1). A risk is material depending on the likelihood of occurrence or the degree of harm it presents. The focus is on whether a reasonable person in the patient's position probably would attach significance to the specific risk. This is the "reasonable patient standard."

In addition, most states require that a patient also prove causation (i.e., that he/she would not have consented to the procedure if informed of the risk) to prevail on a claim for lack of informed consent (1). In practice, it is difficult for a patient to convince a judge or jury that even though the surgery was needed to relieve pain or disease, he/she would not have consented if told of the risk (e.g., colon perforation). This is especially true if the patient has been informed of more serious risks such as death or paraplegia and agrees to the surgery. The question that must be answered by the judge or jury is whether a reasonable patient in the plaintiff's position would have consented to the treatment or procedure even if the material information and risks were discussed (1). The following points should always be discussed with the patient:

- The nature of the ailment, condition, or diagnosis being treated
- The general nature of the proposed treatment or procedure
- The likely prospects for success of the treatment (but no guarantee)
- The risks of failing to undergo the treatment
- The alternative methods of treatment (if any) and their inherent risks.

Obviously, good patient rapport coupled with accurate and complete charting are the best tools to deter suits based on informed consent and provide a heavy shield in defending them.

Documentation

While good communication and rapport with patients (i.e., treating a patient as you would like to be treated) is critical in deterring a lawsuit, complete and accurate documentation of patient care is invaluable in defending claims. In addition, good documentation may avert a potential claim when the plaintiff's attorney considering filing a suit reviews the record and notes that the care has been fully documented. Plaintiff attorneys are more likely to bring a suit when the case is poorly documented because they can more easily argue that what happened in the care of the patient was sinister and/or improper. When the documentation is clear and accurate, the plaintiff attorney may be deterred because what happened is easily proven from the record. Thus, judgment becomes the issue when documentation is accurate; physician judgment is usually easier to defend than a vague, evasive, and poorly documented chart (1).

The following charting guidelines help defend against malpractice claims:

A. Thorough and accurate charting—your primary shield to liability.
B. If an event results in litigation, your testimony is often not taken for up to two years after the event. The information in the chart provides the content and guidelines for your testimony.
C. Importantly, from a legal standpoint, if it is not charted, it was not done, observed, administered, or reported (1). In *Smith v State through Department of HHR* (11), the court stated:

"The experts concluded that decedent's condition required continued monitoring and that charting should have been done on a regular basis. The experts also agreed that the lack of documentation indicated that no one was properly observing the decedent, based on the standard maxim *not charted, not done.*

. . . The evidence indicates that the decedent was not adequately monitored in this case. The nurses did not specifically recall the patient, and thus the *best evidence of their actions would have been the documentation of the chart* (emphasis added)."

D. General charting guidelines (1)

1. If you are the treating or primary physician, make a daily entry on the chart.
2. Always sign, date, and time each entry.
3. Chart at the earliest time.
4. If a situation prevents you from charting until later, state why and that the record times are best estimates.
5. Chart all consultations.
6. Write legibly and spell correctly. Use accepted medical abbreviations.
7. Never alter the medical records.
8. Never black out or white out any entry on a chart. Should you make a mistake in charting, place a single line through the erroneous entry and label the entry "error in charting." Follow the hospital policy on charting. An addendum is acceptable if placed in sequence with the date and time made.
9. Chart professionally. Do not impugn or insult the patient. Do not impugn, insult, or criticize colleagues, co-workers, or support staff.
10. Always designate the dose, site, route, and time of medication administration.
11. Do not chart incident reports in your notes
12. Chart objectively rather than subjectively and avoid ambiguous terms (Table 14.1).
13. Document use of all restraints, safeguards, and patient positioning.
14. Document all patient noncompliance.
15. Document all patient education, discharge instructions, and patient responses.
16. Document the patient's status on transfer or discharge.
17. Ensure the patient's name is on each page of the medical chart.
18. Do not chart in advance.

TABLE 14.1 Subjective versus objective charting.

Subjective	Objective
Patient doing well	Patient denies any complaints. Awake, alert, and oriented. Vital signs stable; BP 100/70, P 72, R 18
Breath sounds normal	Respirations regular and unlabored. Breath sounds clear and equal bilaterally on auscultation. No rales or rhonchi noted.
Abdomen benign	Abdomen is flat, soft, and non-tender. Bowel sounds are of normal frequency and character. No masses or peritoneal signs are present.

E. In the ambulatory setting:

1. Chart the return visit date and that the date was provided to the patient.
2. Chart all cancelled and missed appointments.
3. Document all telephone conversations and their content.
4. Chart all prescriptions and refills, as well as patient teaching regarding prescriptions.
5. Chart follow-up and discharge instructions. If possible, have the patient or their representative cosign these instructions. This is especially true for outpatients who have been sedated (i.e., colonoscopy patients).

Malpractice Suit

Initial Phase

Once a patient initiates a claim for medical malpractice, the physician should immediately place a call to their risk manager or malpractice insurance carrier. An attorney usually will be selected and the physician should insist that the appointed counsel be experienced and have a well-established reputation in the handling of malpractice cases.

The physician should work closely with the defense attorney to review and analyze the allegations of the suit, with particular focus on the strengths and weaknesses of the case. This team effort often can substantially enhance the strength of the defense by educating the attorney on the medical aspects of the case (1).

The physician must remember that a malpractice case is a lengthy and potentially stressful process. The American system is adversarial and the rules have often been determined by legislators and lawyers. The physician defendant must understand that the process is lengthy, that the truth may not always be the goal, and that the physician's care rather than the physician is on trial. Although it may be impossible not to take the proceedings personally, the physician should try to keep the situation in a reasonable perspective.

Pretrial Discovery

During this phase, each side will discover the facts and opinions in the case. Written questions—or interrogatories—are generated and answered with written responses. Depositions—or sworn testimony—usually follow and are important to the outcome of the case. Prior to any testimony, the physician should be familiar with the facts of the case, previous medical care of the patient, and the allegations against the physician. This requires careful review of the medical records, medical data related to the case, and other depositions. The physician and the defense attorney should hold a conference prior to the deposition. This meeting should be long enough to discuss the case, as well as the medical and legal issues involved. The physician must remember that in our adversarial judicial system the purpose of the deposition is not to convince the plaintiff's attorney that the case should be dropped. The physician is present to answer questions and defend the care administered, not to educate the plaintiff's attorney.

The deposition is the physician's testimony, given under oath before a court reporter. The court reporter will make a written or video recording of the testimony. If video is used, the physician's appearance and demeanor are more important than if a written record in an informal setting is used. Attorneys for both defendant and plaintiff are present. Any party to the lawsuit may be present, but often the physician is the only party present (1). The testimony is recorded in question-and-answer form. Under the laws of discovery, the plaintiff attorney has the right to ask the defendant physician proper questions. The physician is present to discharge a legal obligation to answer proper questions.

As stated previously, the physician's deposition is very important. An effective presentation requires effort and close cooperation with the defense attorney. The physician must be his/her own person, but preparation is essential.

The following suggestions can be helpful:

1. Tell the truth; you must testify accurately.
2. Do not guess or speculate. If you do not know the answer, say so.
3. If you are not certain of what the attorney is asking, ask that the question be clarified or repeated. Do not attempt to rephrase the question for the interrogator (e.g., "If you mean such and such . . .").
4. Keep the answers short and concise. Do not volunteer information. Answer the question posed.
5. Be courteous. Avoid jokes and sarcasm.
6. Think about each question that is asked. Listen to each word. Formulate an answer, and then give the answer. Do not permit yourself to become hurried.
7. Do not argue with opposing counsel. If an argument is necessary, your attorney will do it for you.
8. If you realize that you have given an incorrect answer to a previous question, stop at that moment and say so; then correct your answer.
9. Be aware of questions that involve distances or time. If you make an estimate, make sure everyone knows it is an estimate.
10. Do not lose your temper, no matter how hard pressed. This may be a deliberate ploy. Do not fall for it.
11. Do not anticipate questions. Be sure to let the attorney completely finish the question and give your attorney time to object before you begin to respond.
12. Do not exaggerate or brag.

Aspects of Testimony

Memory

You have the right to refer to the chart or hospital records whenever you wish. Your memory is usually a composite of events you recall as jogged by your records. Be aware of attorney tactics such as generalities, ploys, and tricky questions.

Generalities

Often the plaintiff's attorney will begin with general questions such as, "Doctor, how do you treat X disease?" Usually, the lawsuit in which you are a party involves X disease or the plaintiff's attorney is trying to make it X disease. You really cannot answer this question and you should say just that such an answer is not possible (1). X disease probably occurs in various forms and you have not been provided with important information such as the patient complaints, history, physical examination, laboratory results, and the clinical impression. All these factors are needed to diagnose and treat intelligently and the question is too general to answer accurately.

Another common question is, "Doctor, what are the standards for making a diagnosis of X disease?" Again, you should advise that the question is too broad, as no details have been given. A physician does not immediately diagnose X or any other disease. You evaluate all the data in light of your formal training and clinical experience in considering or making a diagnosis. Patient signs and symptoms are innumerable. You must have specifics. One clinical presentation may require certain diagnostic studies to make the diagnosis, whereas others may be more certain from the history and physical examination.

A proper question is, "Doctor, what are the characteristics of X disease?" If your case involves X disease, you should know its characteristics, but you should point out that they are general characteristics and certainly will vary in specific instances. The point is, you must avoid generalities and demand specifics. Try to make the questioner stick to the specific case.

Ploys

Question: "Doctor, you have no memory of events independent of your records, do you?"

Appropriate response: "I have an excellent recall of the events when I refer to the records."

Question: "Doctor, if an event is not recorded in your records or in the hospital records, is it fair to say that event did not occur?"

Appropriate response: "That is incorrect. It is impossible for a physician to note everything that occurs. My records are for my own use to jog my memory. Thus I note pertinent highlights, which when later reviewed give me the complete picture at the time in question."

Remember that physicians treat patients, not charts (1). You may properly testify to the following:

1. What you actually recall
2. What you recall with the assistance of your records
3. What is recorded
4. What your routine or standard procedure is, even when such is not recalled or recorded.

Tricky Questions

Many plaintiff attorneys will use questions cleverly phrased to evoke a response that can later be used against the physician.

Possibilities. Questions phrased in terms of possibility invite speculation and are improper. The criterion is reasonable medical probability.

Question: "Doctor, isn't such and such possible?" Or "Couldn't such and such have happened?"
Appropriate response: "Most improbable."

Doing Things Differently. Almost all malpractice cases involve the "retrospectoscope" or Monday morning quarterbacking to suggest the physician knew things beforehand, that were only learned later, or that the physician has 100% control of the healing process.

Question: "Doctor, is there anything you would do differently now if you had Mrs. Y's case to treat again?"
Appropriate response: "My recommendations to Mrs. Y were based on her complaints, her history and findings at the time and on my clinical impression at the time. The course was appropriate on the basis of those factors."
Question: "Doctor you did not intend for Mrs. Y to have this complication did you?"
Appropriate response: "Of course, no harm to Mrs. Y was intended. At the time of my recommendation, there were good prospects for a good result. The procedure (or regimen) does have known complications and that is why the risks were explained to her beforehand."

Many other factors are involved in preparing for and successfully testifying by deposition or at trial (12). Effective and sincere testimony is critical to a successful defense in malpractice cases. Ineffective testimony can render a defensible case indefensible. A prepared physician who understands how to answer questions can avoid the plaintiff's tricks and ploys and substantially enhance the defense.

Expert Witnesses

Medicolegal cases are decided by judges or juries who rarely understand the complexities and issues involved in medical care. Therefore, each side in a lawsuit uses "expert witnesses" to testify. Jurisdictions vary in who may qualify as an "expert." Many states allow licensed physicians to testify on any aspects of medical care. Others have more specific requirements. Selection of an "expert" is very important. Their testimony helps to explain medical aspects and they render opinions on what care is appropriate or where it falls below standards (13). A credible expert will assist the defense attorney in identifying the strong and weak aspects of a case and help refute the plaintiff's expert. The defense expert should be knowledgeable of the case and well respected. An expert can help identify cases that would be difficult to defend and recommend settlement and avoidance of the risks of trial. Expert witnesses are appropriately compensated for their time, but "hired guns" or "experts" who testify for the money should be avoided.

Trial

After pretrial discovery, the physician should have a clear understanding of the evidence and witnesses—especially experts—who will be used against him/her at trial. Working with the defense attorney to rebut this evidence and to assist with selection of defense expert witnesses is strongly advised and helps the physician to prepare the defense.

At trial, the physician is observed carefully at all times by the judge and jury. The physician's trial testimony, mannerisms, and behavior are critical to a favorable verdict. A well-trained (15) and educated physician who portrays a sincere, conscientious, and caring attitude about the patient's well-being greatly increases the chances of a favorable verdict, even when severe complications have occurred and there may be questions of the appropriateness of the course of treatment chosen (1).

Conclusion

The defense of medical malpractice claims is similar to the defense of criminal cases. The physician stands accused and his/her reputation is usually an issue of great importance. The emotional costs to the physician are sometimes staggering. Until meaningful tort reform is widely enacted, physicians must understand that medical claims will increase and must be dealt with as an unfortunate aspect of the practice (14). In this environment, it is best to accept the reality of the medicolegal arena and use the best means available to aggressively defend and win the malpractice case.

References

1. Gay CF Jr. Medicolegal issues. In: Hicks TC, Beck DE, Opelka FG, and Timmcke AE, editors. Complications of colorectal surgery. Baltimore: Williams & Wilkins; 1996. p. 468–77.

2. Entmann SS, Glass CA, Hickson GB, Githens PB, Whetten-Goldstein K, and Sloan FA. The relationship between malpractice claims history and subsequent obstetric care. JAMA. 1994;272:1588–91.
3. Hickson GB, Clayton EW, Githens PB, and Sloan FA. Factors that prompted families to file medical legal malpractice claims following perinatal injuries. JAMA. 1992;267:1359–63.
4. Delaney CP, Fazio VW, Senagore AJ, Robinson B, Halverson AL, and Renzi FH. "Fast-track" postoperative management protocol for patients with high comorbidity undergoing complex abdominal and pelvic colorectal surgery. Br J Surg. 2001;88:1533–8.
5. Carnegie D. How to win friends and influence people. New York: Simon & Schuster; 1936.
6. Orlikoff J and Vanagunas A. Malpractice prevention and liability control for hospitals. Chicago: American Hospital Association; 1988.
7. Danzon PM. The frequency and severity of medical malpractice claims: New evidence. Law Contemp Probl. 1986:49:57–84.
8. Kern K. Medical malpractice involving colon and rectal disease; A 20-year review of United States civil court litigation. Dis Colon Rectum. 1993;36:531–9.
9. Feld AD. Medicolegal implications of colorectal cancer screening. Gastrointest Endosc Clin N Am. 2002;12:171–9.
10. Schloendorff v Society of New York Hospital, 2112NY125, 105 NE 92,93 (1914)
11. Smith v State through Department of HHR, 517 So2d 1072 (La App 3d Cir 1987)
12. Taraska JM. The physician as witness. In: Taraska JM, editor. Legal guide for physicians. New York: Matthew Bender; 1994. p. 1–56.
13. Gorski TF, Rosen L, Lawrence F, Helfrich D, and Reed JF 3rd. Usefulness of a state-legislated, comparative database to evaluate quality in colorectal surgery. Dis Colon Rectum. 1999;42:1381–7.
14. Taraska JM. Tort reform. In: Taraska JM, editor. Legal Guide for Physicians. New York: Matthew Bender; 1994. p. 57–64.
15. Prystowsky JB, Bordage G, and Feinglass JM. Patient outcomes for segmental colon resection according to surgeon's training, certification and experience. Surgery. 2002;132:663–72.

Editorial Commentary

Prevention is better than cure. This chapter eloquently covers how to avoid problems and what strategies to adopt when "trouble" looms. There is little clear evidence for example, that delayed colonic cancer referral impacts on cancer-specific outcome and much of the delays occur beyond the control of the colorectal surgeon. The biggest problem here is the missed cancer diagnosis when benign associated anorectal pathology is found and definitively treated and studies would suggest that one-stop flexible endoscopic services as part of a rectal bleeding clinic may be unsafe if strictly applied without follow-up to patients presenting with benign outlet bleeding (i.e., bright red, postdefecatory, painless bleeding without an attendant family history of colorectal neoplasia). Demographic studies have suggested that asymptomatic males over 40 years of age are better candidates for screening colonoscopy more for the diagnosis of adenomatous polyps (and their subsequent polypectomy) than for cancer. The coloproctologist today must be familiar with the profusion of new anorectal resectional and reconstructive techniques; a phenomenon aided in part by workshop attendance and CME accumulation as well as by mentorship programmes. However, it must be recognized that some of these new techniques (in hemorrhoid surgery for example), have brought a 'rash' of new and sometimes serious complications not normally associated with the older procedure. What is also evident is that superspecialization in rectal cancer surgery for example impacts on cancer-specific survival and locoregional recurrence rates. This clear value of specialization ***within*** the field of coloproctology itself may necessitate an extension to other important areas where the consequences of nonexpert surgery may be considerable; most notably, in complex pelvic floor disorders, multiply recurrent complicated perirectal sepsis and redo pouch surgery. This trend to refer within the specialty particularly in complicated functional disorders will also be a measure of the availability of and expertise with newer imaging methodologies and best-practice biofeedback and neurostimulation techniques.

AZ

Index

K

MIX
Papier aus verantwortungsvollen Quellen
Paper from responsible sources
FSC® C105338

If you have any concerns about our products,
you can contact us on
ProductSafety@springernature.com

In case Publisher is established outside the EU,
the EU authorized representative is:
Springer Nature Customer Service Center GmbH
Europaplatz 3, 69115 Heidelberg, Germany

Printed by Libri Plureos GmbH
in Hamburg, Germany